Gastrointestinal Surgery

Gastrointestinal Surgery

Editor: Benson Scott

AMERICAN
MEDICAL PUBLISHERS
www.americanmedicalpublishers.com

AMERICAN
MEDICAL PUBLISHERS
www.americanmedicalpublishers.com

Cataloging-in-Publication Data

Gastrointestinal surgery / edited by Benson Scott.
p. cm.
Includes bibliographical references and index.
ISBN 978-1-63927-491-8
1. Gastrointestinal system--Surgery. 2. Gastroenterology. 3. Surgery. I. Scott, Benson.
RD540 .G37 2022
61743--dc23

American Medical Publishers,
41 Flatbush Avenue,
1st Floor, New York,
NY 11217, USA

ISBN 978-1-63927-491-8 (Hardback)

Contents

Preface

Gastrointestinal (GI) diseases are the clinical conditions affecting the organs of the gastrointestinal tract. It consists of the esophagus, liver, pancreas, gallbladder, stomach and intestine. The management and treatment of many of these disorders require surgery. Gastrointestinal surgery can be of two types- upper GI surgery and lower GI surgery. Liver resection, pancreaticoduodenectomy and esophagectomy are upper GI surgeries. Colorectal surgery, colectomy and resections for rectal cancer are lower GI surgeries. Some of the other gastrointestinal surgical procedures are appendectomy, biliopancreatic diversion, enterostomy, gastroplasty, hepatectomy, liver transplantation, pancreatectomy, etc. Appendicitis is a potentially fatal condition if left unresolved, but is easily managed with surgery. A minor procedure called colonoscopy can detect colon cancer at an early stage. This book is a valuable compilation of topics, ranging from the basic to the most complex advancements in gastrointestinal surgery. It presents this complex subject in the most comprehensible and easy to understand language. This book will help new researchers by foregrounding their knowledge in this field.

Various studies have approached the subject by analyzing it with a single perspective, but the present book provides diverse methodologies and techniques to address this field. This book contains theories and applications needed for understanding the subject from different perspectives. The aim is to keep the readers informed about the progresses in the field; therefore, the contributions were carefully examined to compile novel researches by specialists from across the globe.

Indeed, the job of the editor is the most crucial and challenging in compiling all chapters into a single book. In the end, I would extend my sincere thanks to the chapter authors for their profound work. I am also thankful for the support provided by my family and colleagues during the compilation of this book.

Editor

1

WSES consensus conference: Guidelines for first-line management of intra-abdominal infections

Massimo Sartelli[1*], Pierluigi Viale[2], Kaoru Koike[3], Federico Pea[4], Fabio Tumietto[2], Harry van Goor[5], Gianluca Guercioni[6], Angelo Nespoli[7], Cristian Tranà[8], Fausto Catena[9], Luca Ansaloni[10], Ari Leppaniemi[11], Walter Biffl[12], Frederick A Moore[13], Renato Poggetti[14], Antonio Daniele Pinna[9], Ernest E Moore[12]

Abstract

Intra-abdominal infections are still associated with high rate of morbidity and mortality.

A multidisciplinary approach to the management of patients with intra-abdominal infections may be an important factor in the quality of care. The presence of a team of health professionals from various disciplines, working in concert, may improve efficiency, outcome, and the cost of care.

A World Society of Emergency Surgery (WSES) Consensus Conference was held in Bologna on July 2010, during the 1st congress of the WSES, involving surgeons, infectious disease specialists, pharmacologists, radiologists and intensivists with the goal of defining recommendations for the early management of intra-abdominal infections.

This document represents the executive summary of the final guidelines approved by the consensus conference.

Introduction

A World Society of Emergency Surgery (WSES) Consensus Conference was held in Bologna on July 2010, during the 1st congress of the WSES, involving surgeons, infectious disease specialists, pharmacologists, radiologists and intensivists with the goal of defining recommendations for the early management of intra-abdominal infections.

This document represents the executive summary of the final recommendations approved by the consensus conference.

The Surgical Infection Society and the Infectious Diseases Society of America have recently generated guidelines for the diagnosis and management of complicated intra-abdominal infections on 2010 [1]. IDSA guidelines represent an important reference for the management of intra-abdominal infections.

WSES guidelines represent a further contribution on this debated topic by specialists worldwide. The recommendations are formulated and graded according to the Grading of Recommendations Assessment, Development and Evaluation (GRADE) hierarchy of evidence [2,3] summarized in Table 1.

* Correspondence: m.sartelli@virgilio.it

[1]Department of Surgery, Macerata Hospital, Italy

Full list of author information is available at the end of the article

Principles of sepsis management

Severe sepsis and septic shock are the leading causes of multiple organ failure and mortality in noncoronary intensive care units (ICUs) [4,5].

Unfortunately, despite tremendous basic and clinical research efforts, mortality from septic shock remains unchanged at greater than 50%.

In an effort to improve sepsis-related mortality, several organizations have outlined evidence-based guidelines (EBGs) for the management of severe sepsis and septic shock [6].

Physicians have known about the existence of sepsis for centuries.

In 1992, the American College of Chest Physicians/Society of Critical Care Medicine (ACCP/SCCM) Consensus Committee developed definitions of patients with sepsis and its related disorders [7].

This Consensus represents the first attempt to create a universal language for diagnosing and treating sepsis.

Sepsis is defined as systemic inflammatory response syndrome (SIRS), resulting from infection.

Identifying patients with severe sepsis early and correcting the underlying microvascular dysfunction may improve patient outcomes. If not corrected, microvascular dysfunction can lead to global tissue hypoxia, direct tissue damage, and ultimately, organ failure.

Table 1 Grading of recommendations from Guyatt and colleagues [2]

Grade of recommendation	Clarity of risk/benefit	Quality of supporting evidence	Implications
1A			
Strong recommendation, high-quality evidence	Benefits clearly outweigh risk and burdens, or vice versa	RCTs without important limitations or overwhelming evidence from observational studies	Strong recommendation, can apply to most patients in most circumstances without reservation
1B			
Strong recommendation, moderate-quality evidence	Benefits clearly outweigh risk and burdens, or vice versa	RCTs with important limitations (inconsistent results, methodological flaws, indirect or imprecise) or exceptionally strong evidence from observational studies	Strong recommendation, can apply to most patients in most circumstances without reservation
1C			
Strong recommendation, low-quality or very low-quality evidence	Benefits clearly outweigh risk and burdens, or vice versa	Observational studies or case series	Strong recommendation but may change when higher quality evidence becomes available
2A			
Weak recommendation, high-quality evidence	Benefits closely balanced with risks and burden	RCTs without important limitations or overwhelming evidence from observational studies	Weak recommendation, best action may differ depending on circumstances or patient or societal values
2B			
Weak recommendation, moderate-quality evidence	Benefits closely balanced with risks and burden	RCTs with important limitations (inconsistent results, methodological flaws, indirect or imprecise) or exceptionally strong evidence from observational studies	Weak recommendation, best action may differ depending on circumstances or patient or societal values
2C			
Weak recommendation, Low-quality or very low-quality evidence	Uncertainty in the estimates of benefits, risks, and burden; benefits, risk and burden may be closely balanced	Observational studies or case series	Very weak recommendation; other alternatives may be equally reasonable

Systemic inflammatory response syndrome (SIRS)

SIRS is a reference for the complex findings that result from a systemic activation of the innate immune response, regardless of cause.

It includes the presence of more than one of the following manifestations:

- Temperature > 100.4°F or < 96.8°F (> 38°C or < 36°C)
- Heart rate > 90 beats/min
- Tachypnea, as manifested by a respiratory rate > 20 breaths/min or hyperventilation, as indicated by a $PaCO_2$ < 32 mm Hg
- Alteration of white blood cell count > 12,000 cells/mm^3, < 4,000 cells/mm^3, or the presence of > 10% immature neutrophils.

Sepsis

Sepsis is defined by the American College of Chest Physicians/Society of Critical Care Medicine (ACCP/SCCM) as SIRS resulting from infection.

Severe sepsis

Severe sepsis is sepsis associated with at least one acute organ dysfunction, hypoperfusion, or hypotension.

Septic shock

Septic shock occurs when sepsis-induced hypotension persists despite adequate fluid resuscitation.

Multiple organ dysfunction syndrome (MODS)

MODS includes altered functions of two or more organs in an acutely ill patient.

Pathophysiology

Abdominal sepsis occurs as result of intra-abdominal infection.

The pathophysiology of sepsis takes origin from the outer membrane components of both gram-negative organisms (lipopolysaccharide [LPS], lipid A, endotoxin) and gram-positive organisms (lipoteichoic acid, peptidoglycan). These outer membrane components are able to bind to the CD14 receptor on the surface of monocytes. By virtue of the recently described toll-like receptors, a signal is then transmitted to the cell, leading to the eventual production of the proinflammatory cytokines, including tumor necrosis factor (TNF), interleukin 1 (IL-1), IL-6, IL-8, and gamma interferon (IFN-), as well as other inflammatory mediators such as prostaglandins, leukotrienes, platelet activation factor, and nitrogen and oxygen intermediates. Most of these immunological mediators present multiple biologic effects, play a critical role in inflammation and immune responses, and have been recognized as key mediators in the pathogenesis of infectious diseases and, more particularly, the pathophysiologic alterations observed in endotoxic shock. As a result of the vicious cycle of inflammation, cardiovascular insufficiency and multiple organ failure occur and often lead to death [8-10].

Haemodynamic support

Septic shock is primarily maldistributive shock. Its pathogenesis involves a complex interaction among pathologic vasodilation, myocardial dysfunction, and altered blood flow distribution due to the inflammatory response to infection. It evolves into a progressive pathophysiological deterioration that culminates in hypotension poorly responsive to adequate fluid resuscitation accompanied by hypoperfusion and organ dysfunction.

It is associated with three major pathophysiological effects: vasodilatation, maldistribution of blood flow, and myocardial depression.

In septic shock, the absolute intravascular volume may be normal; however, because of acute vasodilatation, relative hypovolemia occurs. Differently from other types of shock that are primarily caused by decreasing intravascular volume (hypovolemic) or decreasing cardiac output (cardiogenic), a characteristic of septic shock is the maldistribution of blood flow in the microcirculation. In septic shock also myocardial depression may occur. The relative hypovolemia, myocardial depression, and maldistribution result in decreased oxygen delivery (DO_2) and subsequent tissue hypoxia.

Rivers and coll. [11] demonstrated that a strategy of early goal-directed therapy (EGDT) decreases the in-hospital mortality of patients who are taken to the emergency department in septic shock.

An organized approach to the haemodynamic support to sepsis includes use of fluid resuscitation, vasopressor therapy and inotropic therapy.

Patients with severe sepsis and septic shock may present ineffective perfusion. Poor tissues perfusion may cause a global tissue hypoxia, often associated to an elevated serum lactate level. A serum lactate value greater than 4 mmol/L (36 mg/dL) is correlated with poorer outcomes, even if hypotension is not yet present. Fluid resuscitation should be started as early as possible.

According to the Surviving Sepsis Campaign guidelines [6] during the first 6 hrs of resuscitation, the goals of initial resuscitation of sepsis-induced hypoperfusion should include all of the following as one part of a treatment protocol:

- Central venous pressure 8 to 12 mm Hg
- Mean arterial pressure (MAP) >65 mm Hg
- Urine output >0.5 mL/kg/hr
- Central venous (superior vena cava) or mixed venous oxygen saturation >70% or >65%, respectively

The early hypovolemic phase of sepsis must be always treated by providing appropriate high volume resuscitation.

The Surviving Sepsis Campaign guidelines [6] recommend that fluid challenge in patients with suspected hypovolemia be started with > = 1000 mL of crystalloids or 300-500 mL of colloids over 30 mins. More rapid administration and greater amounts of fluid may be needed in patients with sepsis-induced tissue hypoperfusion.

As the volume of distribution is less large for colloids than for crystalloids, resuscitation with colloids requires less fluid to achieve the same goals. A colloid equivalent is an acceptable alternative to crystalloid. Crystalloids are less expensive [6].

When an appropriate fluid challenge fails, to restore an adequate arterial pressure and organ perfusion, therapy with vasopressor agents should be started.

Vasopressor drugs maintain adequate blood pressure and preserve perfusion pressure for optimizing flow in various organs.

Both norepinephrine and dopamine are the first-line vasopressor agents to correct hypotension in septic shock. Both norepinephrine and dopamine can increase blood pressure in shock states, although norepinephrine seems to be more powerful. Dopamine may be useful in patients with compromised cardiac function and cardiac reserve [12], but norepinephrine is more effective than dopamine in reversing hypotension in patients with septic shock. Dopamine has also potentially detrimental effects on the release of pituitary hormones and especially prolactin, although the clinical relevance of these effects is still unclear and can have unintended effects such as tachyarrhythmias.

Dopamine has different effects based on the doses [13].

A dose of less than 5 μg/kg/min results in vasodilation of renal, mesenteric, and coronary districts. At a dose of 5-10 μg/kg/min, beta-1-adrenergic effects increase cardiac contractility and heart rate. At doses about 10 μg/kg/min, alpha-adrenergic effects lead to arterial vasoconstriction and increase blood pressure. Its major side effects are tachycardia and arrhythmogenesis.

The use of renal-dose dopamine in sepsis is a controversial issue. In the past, low-dose dopamine was routinely used because of the possible renal protective effects. Dopamine at a dose of 2-3 μg/kg/min was known to stimulate diuresis by increasing renal blood flow.

A multicentre, randomised, double-blind, placebo-controlled study about low-dose dopamine in patients with at least two criteria for the systemic inflammatory response syndrome and clinical evidence of early renal dysfunction (oliguria or increase in serum creatinine concentration), was published on 2000 [14]. Patients admitted were randomly assigned a continuous intravenous infusion of low-dose dopamine (2 µg/kg/min) or placebo administered through a central venous catheter. Administration of low-dose dopamine by continuous intravenous infusion to critically ill patients at risk of renal failure did not confer clinically significant protection from renal dysfunction.

A meta-analysis of literature from 1966 to 2000 for studies addressing the use of dopamine in the prevention and/or treatment of renal dysfunction was published on 2001 [15]. The Authors concluded that the use of low-dose dopamine for the treatment or prevention of acute renal failure was not justified on the basis of available evidence.

Norepinephrine is a potent alpha-adrenergic agonist with minimal beta-adrenergic agonist effects. Norepinephrine can successfully increase blood pressure in patients who are septic and remain hypotensive following fluid resuscitation. Norepinephrine is effective to treat hypotension in septic shock patients. In many studies norepinephrine administration at doses 0.01 to 0.3 µg/kg/min has been shown may be effective [16,17].

On 1993 Martin and coll. [18] published a randomized trial comparing norepinephrine vs dopamine. 32 volume-resuscitated septic patients were given either dopamine or norepinephrine to achieve and maintain normal hemodynamic and oxygen transport parameters for at least 6 h. Dopamine administration was successful in only 31% of patients, whereas norepinephrine administration was successful in 93%. Of the 11 patients who did not respond to dopamine, 10 responded when norepinephrine was added to therapy. Serum lactate levels were decreased as well, suggesting that norepinephrine therapy improved tissue oxygenation.

Recently a prospective trial by Patel and coll. compared dopamine to norepinephrine as the initial vasopressor in fluid resuscitated 252 adult patients with septic shock [19]. If the maximum dose of the initial vasopressor was unable to maintain the hemodynamic goal, then fixed dose vasopressin was added to each regimen. If additional vasopressor support was needed to achieve the hemodynamic goal, then phenylephrine was added. In this study dopamine and norepinephrine were equally effective as initial agents as judged by 28-day mortality rates. However, there were significantly more cardiac arrhythmias with dopamine treatment.

The Surviving Sepsis Campaign guidelines [6] state that there is no sufficient evidence to suggest which agent is better as initial vasopressor in the management of patients with septic shock.

Phenylephrine is a selective alpha-1 adrenergic receptor agonist primarily used in anesthesia to increase blood pressure. Although studies are limited [20], its rapid onset, short duration, and primary vascular effects make it an interesting agent in the management of hypotension associated with sepsis, but there are concerns about its potential to reduce cardiac output in these patients.

Epinephrine is a potent α-adrenergic and β-adrenergic agent that increases mean arterial pressure by increasing both cardiac index and peripheral vascular tone. The chief concern about the use of epinephrine in septic patients is the potential to decrease regional blood flow, particularly in the splanchnic circulation. On 2003 De Backer and coll. [21] published a trial to compare effects of dopamine, norepinephrine, and epinephrine on the splanchnic circulation in septic shock. In patients with severe septic shock, epinephrine administration increased global oxygen delivery and consumption. It caused lower absolute and fractional splanchnic blood flow and lower indocyanine green clearance, validating the adverse effects of therapy with epinephrine alone on the splanchnic circulation.

Epinephrine administration can increase blood pressure in patients who are unresponsive to first-line agents. It increases heart rate, and has the potential to induce tachyarrhythmias, ischemia, and hypoglycemia. Because of its effects on splanchnic circulation and its propensity to increase lactate concentrations, epinephrine has been considered a second-line agent [22].

A large (330 patients) randomized clinical trial published on 2007 by Annane and coll. [23] compared therapy with norepinephrine plus dobutamine (whenever needed) with epinephrine alone in septic shock. There was no evidence for a difference in efficacy and safety between epinephrine alone and norepinephrine plus dobutamine for the management of septic shock.

Vasopressin is a peptide hormone synthesized in the hypothalamus and is then transported and stored in the pituitary gland. Vasopressin mediates vasoconstriction via V1-receptor activation on vascular smooth muscle and mediates its antidiuretic effect via V2-receptor activation in the renal collecting duct system. In addition, vasopressin, at low plasma concentrations, mediates vasodilation in coronary, cerebral, and pulmonary arterial circulations.

Vasopressin infusion of 0.01 to 0.04 U/min in patients with septic shock increases plasma vasopressin levels to those observed in patients with hypotension from other causes, such as cardiogenic shock. Increased vasopressin levels are associated with a lesser need for other vasopressors. Urinary output may increase, and pulmonary vascular resistance may decrease. Infusions of > 0.04 U/min may lead to adverse, likely vasoconstriction-mediated events [24].

A large multicenter, randomized, double-blind trial comparing vasopressin versus norepinephrine infusion in patients with septic shock was published on 2008 [25]. A total of 778 patients underwent randomization (396 patients received vasopressin and 382 norepinephrine) and were included in the analysis. Low-dose vasopressin did not reduce mortality rates as compared with norepinephrine among patients with septic shock who were treated with catecholamine vasopressors.

According to the Surviving Sepsis Campaign guidelines [6] low doses of vasopressin (0.03 U/min) may be effective in raising blood pressure in patients refractory to other vasopressors and may have other potential physiologic benefits. Terlipressin has similar effects but is long lasting.

Dobutamine is frequently used in septic shock patients as an inotropic agent to increase cardiac output, stroke index, and oxygen delivery (Do_2). However, the lack of benefit, and even possible harm, of dobutamine administration to increase Do_2 to supranormal values in critically ill patients has raised questions regarding its use in the treatment of septic shock. Surviving Sepsis Campaign guidelines [6] recommend that a dobutamine infusion be administered in the presence of myocardial dysfunction as suggested by elevated cardiac filling pressures and low cardiac output.

Early intervention and implementation of evidence-based guidelines for the management of severe sepsis and septic shock improve outcomes in patients with sepsis. However, this is contingent on the early identification of sepsis. The early identification of sepsis is challenging because many of the signs and symptoms of sepsis are nonspecific. It is therefore necessary to identify those patients at highest risk for the development of sepsis and heighten our awareness for the development of sepsis in this population. In order to document the incidence of sepsis, assess its risk factors, and determine its impact on mortality in a general surgery population, the American College of Surgeons National Surgical Quality Improvement Project (NSQIP) dataset was analyzed [4]. The 2005-2006 NSQIP dataset contains prospectively collected clinical data and outcomes on 152.490 patients collected from 121 academic and community-based hospitals.

The analysis of the 2005-2006 NSQIP dataset identified 4 major risk factors for the development of sepsis or septic shock in general surgery patients: (1) age older than 60 years, (2) need for emergency surgery, (3) presence of any of the NSQIP comorbidities, and (4) male sex. These findings emphasized the need for early recognition through aggressive sepsis screening and rapid implementation of evidence-based interventions for sepsis and septic shock in general surgery patients with these risk factors.

Recently an analysis of 2005-2007 NSQIP dataset documented the incidence, mortality rate, and risk factors for sepsis and septic shock compared with pulmonary embolism and myocardial infarction in the general-surgery population [5]. Of 363.897 general-surgery patients, sepsis occurred in 8350 (2.3%), septic shock in 5977 (1.6%), pulmonary embolism in 1078 (0.3%), and myocardial infarction in 615 (0.2%). Thirty-day mortality rates for each of the groups were 5.4% for sepsis, 33.7% for septic shock, 9.1% for pulmonary embolism, and 32.0% for myocardial infarction. The septic-shock group had a greater percentage of patients older than 60 years. The need for emergency surgery resulted in more cases of sepsis and septic shock than did elective surgery. The presence of any comorbidity increased the risk of sepsis and septic shock 6-fold and increased the 30-day mortality rate 22-fold.

The incidences of sepsis and septic shock exceed those of pulmonary embolism and myocardial infarction. The risk factors for mortality included age older than 60 years, the need for emergency surgery, and the presence of any comorbidity. These findings confirmed the need for early recognition of patients at risk via aggressive screening and the rapid implementation of evidence-based guidelines.

Principles of surgical management

Source control encompasses all measures undertaken to eliminate the source of infection and to control ongoing contamination.

As a general principle, every established source of infection should be controlled as soon as possible. The urgency of intervention is determined by the rapidity of the evolution of clinical symptoms.

Control of the septic source can be achieved either by surgical or non surgical means.

Non-surgical interventional procedures imply percutaneous drainages of abscesses.

Ultrasound and CT guided percutaneous drainage of abdominal and extraperitoneal abscesses in selected patients are safe and effective [26-33].

However surgery is the most important therapeutic measure to control intra-abdominal infections.

Generally, the choice of the procedure depends on the anatomical source of infection, on the degree of peritoneal inflammation, on the generalized septic response and on the patient's general conditions.

Surgical source control entails resection or suture of a diseased or perforated viscus (e.g. diverticular perforation, gastroduodenal perforation), removal of the infected organ (e.g. appendix, gall bladder), debridement of necrotic tissue or resection of ischemic bowel.

In cases of IAI complicated by septic shock, a single operation may not be sufficient to achieve source control, necessitating re-exploration. Three methods of local mechanical management following initial laparotomy for source control are currently debated: open-abdomen, planned re-laparotomy and on-demand re-laparotomy.

Following removal of infected tissue, attention should always shift to the restoration of anatomy and functionality of the gastrointestinal tract.

Principles of antimicrobial management

Antimicrobial therapy plays an integral role in the management of intra-abdominal infections, especially in critical ill patients where empiric antibiotic therapy must be delivered as early as possible: in fact inadequate antimicrobial therapy is one of the variables most strongly associated to unfavorable outcome [6,34].

The initial antibiotic therapy for IAIs is always empiric because the patient is often critically ill and microbiological data (culture and susceptibility results) usually take at least 48 hours to become fully available.

The decision tree for the antimicrobial management of intra-abdominal infections depends mainly on three factors:

- Presumed pathogens involved and risk factors for major resistance patterns
- Clinical patient's severity
- Presumed/identified source of infection.

To predict the main pathogens involved and the related resistance patterns, infections are to be classed as community or hospital acquired.

During the past 2 decades the incidence of hospital-acquired infection caused by resistant microorganisms has significantly risen, probably in relationship with high level of antibiotic exposure and increasing rate of patients with one or more predisposing conditions such as recent exposure to antibiotics, high severity of illness, advanced age, co-morbidity, degree of organ dysfunction, low albumin level, poor nutritional status, immunodepression and presence of malignancy.

The major pathogens involved in community-acquired intra-abdominal infection are *Enterobacteriaceae, Streptococcus spp* and anaerobes (especially *B. fragilis*). Within the healthcare-associated infections, the spectrum of microorganism involved is broader, encompassing not only *Enterobacteriaceae, Streptococcus spp.* and anaerobes, but also *Enterococcus spp* and *Candida spp.*

The data regarding the role of *Candida spp* are actually conflicting: in a prospective multicenter epidemiological study conducted in 25 French centers, including more than 330 cases of peritonitis with positive microbiological cultures, two thirds of the health care-associated infections were associated to *Enterobacteriaceae* and one third to *Enterococcus spp*, while the isolation rate of *Candida spp* was less than 5% [35].

In contrast, in an observational study involving over 1182 patients with reliable microbiological data, the two genera of pathogens isolated from more than 25% of healthcare-associated infections and more commonly than from community-acquired infections were *Enterococcus spp* (29%) and *Candida spp* (33%) [36]. Apart from its epidemiological relevance, the clinical weight of *Candida spp* in peritonitis is high, since the isolation of the yeast from peritoneal fluid proved to be a variable independently associated to higher morbidity and mortality in a multiple-center, retrospective, case-control study conducted in critically ill patients admitted to 17 French ICUs [37].

More recently the same group confirmed the high mortality of candidal peritonitis (38%) in a prospective survey related on 93 patients admitted to ICU [38].

Enterococci are frequently responsible for hospital-acquired IAIs. During the past 2 decades the incidence of hospital-acquired enterococcal infection has significantly risen, probably in relationship with high level of antibiotic exposure and increasing number of patients with variable levels of immunosuppresion. In the aforementioned French survey, the prevalence of enterococcal isolation was significantly higher in the nosocomial cases of peritonitis and a significant increased incidence of fatal cases of peritonitis with positive cultures for enterococci was reported (20% versus 9% - $p < 0.003$) [35].

The threat of antimicrobial resistance has been identified as one of the major challenges in the management of intra-abdominal infections. The emergence of multidrug-resistant bacteria and the scanty pipeline of new antibiotics to fight them are, as of today, a concern especially for gram negative microorganisms, as highlighted in a recent report from the European Antimicrobial Resistance Surveillance System [39].

Hospital-acquired IAIs are commonly caused by more resistant bacteria, although the level of resistance is significant also in the community acquired infections.

The Study for Monitoring Antimicrobial Resistance Trends (SMART) program has been monitoring the activity of antibiotics against aerobic Gram-negative intra-abdominal infections. Hawser and coll. [40] reported susceptibility levels of key intra-abdominal pathogens in Europe for 2008, and showed that the options for effective empirical therapy of intra-abdominal infection have significantly reduced.

Coque and coll. highlighted the growing threat posed by increasing prevalence of extended-spectrum beta-lactamase (ESBL) producing Enterobacteriaceae all over Europe, even in countries traditionally showing low prevalence rates of resistance [41]. Increase of this resistance pattern has led to a progressive expansion of carbapenems use, because this class of antibiotics was traditionally considered the last resort for managing ESBL producers *Enterobacteriaceae.*

The inevitably increased carbapenem consumption has been associated to increasing carbapenemase production among *Enterobacteriaceae.* The recent rapid spread of serine carbapenemase in *Klebsiella pneumoniae* (KPC) is now an additional major threat for antimicrobial therapy in hospitals worldwide, and stresses the concept that the use of carbapenems must be mandatorily optimized in terms of indication and exposure [42].

Also *Acinetobacter spp* have worldwide shown similar alarming rates of increasing resistance to antibiotics. Today, Carbapenem-resistant A. baumannii-producing oxacillinases retaining susceptibility to only colistin and tigecycline is an ominous reality in hospitals worldwide and compounding this problem is the paucity of new antibiotics under development to address it [43].

In hospital acquired IAIs also *P. aeruginosa* plays an important - although less critical than in other settings - role. The high intrinsic antibiotic resistance of this pathogen, together with its extraordinary capacity for acquiring additional resistances through chromosomal mutations, should be always taken into consideration.

Among multidrug resistant Gram positive bacteria, Enterococci remain a challenge despite the availability of large number of antimicrobial agents theoretically active against this species. The clinical management of enterococcal infection remains challenging, mainly because no single agent could be anticipated to exert strong bactericidal activity against them.

Clinical patient's severity

This choice of the antimicrobial regimen poses serious problems for the management of critically ill patients. In patients with severe sepsis or septic shock an early correct empirical antimicrobial therapy has a significant impact on the outcome, independently by the site of infection [44].

This data confirm the results of Riché and coll. who demonstrated, in a prospective observational study involving 180 consecutive patients with secondary generalized peritonitis, a significantly higher mortality rate in septic shock (35 versus 8% for patients without shock) [45].

Recent international guidelines for the management of severe sepsis and septic shock (Surviving Sepsis Campaign) [6] recommend intravenous antibiotics within the first hour after severe sepsis and septic shock are recognized, use of broad-spectrum agents with good penetration into the presumed site of infection, and reassessment of the antimicrobial regimen daily to optimize efficacy, prevent resistance, avoid toxicity and minimize costs [6]. Full adherence to these recommendations requires that clinicians, in order to optimize antibiotic therapy in critically ill patients, be aware that it is not sufficient to make the correct choice on the basis of the anti-biogram or of a correct epidemiological evaluation of risk factor for microorganisms and resistance patterns, but it is also mandatory to implement timely administration of the right dose on the right schedule, according to the pathophysiological and immunological status of the patient and to the pharmacokinetics properties of the chosen drugs [46].

This concept is correct not only from a clinical point of view; in fact sub-optimal plasma levels of antimicrobials and/or suboptimal exposure to antimicrobials in the infection site represent the best condition to favor the emergence of resistant strains, with a consequent higher probability of therapeutic failure and increased human and social costs.

For example, in critically ill patients, higher-than-standard loading doses of b-lactams, aminoglycosides or glycopeptides should be administered to ensure optimal exposure at the infection site independently of the patient's renal function [47-49].

For lipophilic antibiotics such as fluoroquinolones and tetracyclines, the 'dilution effect' in the extracellular fluids during severe sepsis may be mitigated by the rapid redistribution of the drug from the intracellular compartment to the interstitium. In contrast to what happens with hydrophilic antimicrobials, standard dosages of lipophilic antimicrobials may frequently ensure adequate loading even in patients with severe sepsis or septic shock [47].

Once appropriate initial loading is achieved, daily reassessment of the antimicrobial regimen is warranted, because the pathophysiological changes that may occur could significantly affect drug disposition in the critically ill patients.

Conversely, it is less evident that higher than standard dosages of renally excreted drugs may be needed for optimal exposure in patients with glomerular hyperfiltration [47].

Therefore, selecting higher dosages and/or alternative dosing regimens focused on maximizing the pharmacodynamics of antimicrobials might be worthwhile, with the intent being to increase clinical cure rates among critically ill patients.

Indeed, different approaches should be pursued according to the mechanism of antimicrobial activity exhibited by each antimicrobial. Two patterns of bactericidal activity have been identified: time-dependent activity (where the time that the plasma concentration persists above the MIC of the etiological agent is considered the major determinant for efficacy) and concentration-dependent activity (where the efficacy is mainly related to the plasma peak concentration in relation to the MIC of the microorganism). In addition, these agents show an associated concentration-dependent post-antibiotic effect, and bactericidal action continues for a period of time after the antibiotic level falls below the MIC [50].

Beta-lactams, glycopeptides, oxazolidinones, and azoles exhibit time-dependent activity: the shorter the drug elimination half-life, the more frequent the daily dose fractioning must be. For these drugs the employ of intravenous continuous infusion, which ensures the highest steady-state concentration under the same total daily dosage, may be the most effective way of maximizing pharmacodynamic exposure [51-54].

On the other hand, quinolones, daptomycin, tigecycline, aminoglycosides, polienes and echionocandins exhibit concentration-dependent activity; therefore the entire daily dose should be administered in a once daily way (or with the lowest possible number of daily administrations) with the intent of achieving the highest peak plasma level. The use of extended-interval aminoglycoside dosing strategies for the treatment of moderate-to-severe infections encountered in critically ill surgical patients [55,56].

Classifications

Intra-abdominal infections (IAIs) include a lot of pathological conditions, ranging from uncomplicated appendicitis to faecal peritonitis.

From a clinical viewpoint IAIs are classified into uncomplicated and complicated [57].

In uncomplicated IAIs the infectious process only involves a single organ and does not proceed to the peritoneum.

In complicated IAIs, the infectious process proceeds beyond the organ, and causes either localized peritonitis (intra-abdominal abscess), or diffuse peritonitis.

Peritonitis is classified into primary, secondary or tertiary peritonitis [58].

Primary peritonitis is a diffused bacterial infection without loss of integrity of the gastrointestinal tract. It is rare. It mainly occurs in infancy and early childhood and in cirrhotic patients.

Secondary peritonitis, the most common form of peritonitis, is acute peritoneal infection resulting from loss of integrity of the gastrointestinal tract or from infected viscera. It is caused by perforation of the gastrointestinal tract (e.g. perforated duodenal ulcer), by direct invasion from infected intra-abdominal viscera (e.g. gangrenous appendicitis). Anastomotic dehiscences are common causes of peritonitis in the postoperative period.

Tertiary peritonitis is defined as peritonitis that persists after more than one failed source control procedure [59].

Intra-abdominal infections are also classified into community-acquired intra-abdominal infections (CA-IAIs) and healthcare-acquired intra-abdominal infections (HA-IAIs). CA-IAIs are acquired in community, whereas HA-IAIs develop in hospitalized patients or residents of long-term care facilities. They are characterized by increased mortality because of both underlying patient health status and increased likelihood of infection caused by multi drugs resistant organisms [59].

Moreover, in the classification of IAIs should be mandatory to introduce a grading of clinical severity, well represented by the sepsis definitions.

The updated sepsis definition is based on several clinical and bioumoral variables [60].

As is well demonstrated, there is an increased risk of death moving from the sepsis status to that of severe sepsis [61], and it appears reasonable to assume the latter as the breakpoint between a condition of clinical stability and a critically ill patient.

Diagnosis

Accurate physical examination and laboratory studies are able to identify most patients with intra-abdominal sepsis undergoing immediate laparotomy (1 C).

In the patient with abdominal sepsis early detection and treatment is essential to minimize complications [7].

Complicated intra-abdominal infections diagnosis is mainly a clinical diagnosis.

Abdominal pain may be acute or insidious.

Hypotension and hypoperfusion signs such as lactic acidosis, oliguria, and acute alteration of mental status are indicative of evolution to severe sepsis [7].

Abdominal rigidity suggests peritonitis and the need for urgent laparotomy.

Plain films of the abdomen are often the first imaging studies obtained in patients presenting with intra-abdominal infections.

Upright films are useful for identifying free air under the diaphragm (most often on the right) as an indication of a perforated viscus.

In adult stable patients not undergoing immediate laparotomy, computerized tomography (CT) is the imaging modality of choice for intra-abdominal infections in adults (recommendation 2 B).

Especially in children, the radiation associated with CT, should be always be considered.

In unstable patients not undergoing immediate laparotomy who may not undergo studies requiring them to leave the ICU or emergency room, then

ultrasound is the imaging modality of choice (recommendation 2 B).

When patients are stable, computerized tomography (CT) is the imaging modality of choice for most intra-abdominal processes [62,63].

Computed tomography (CT) of the abdomen and pelvis, when it is possible to perform, remains the diagnostic study of choice for intra-abdominal infections. CT should be performed with enteral and intravenous contrast [64].

Unstable Patients may not undergo studies that require trips away from the ICU or emergency department. In these patients intra-abdominal septic source may be detected by ultrasound (US) [65].

In experienced hands, the ultrasound can reliably diagnose most acute abdominal conditions in most patients.

Abdominal ultrasound has the advantage of being portable and may be helpful in the evaluation of right upper quadrant (eg, perihepatic abscess, cholecystitis, pancreatitis), right lower quadrant, and pelvic pathology (eg, appendicitis, tubo-ovarian abscess, Douglas abscess), but the examination is sometimes limited because of patient discomfort, abdominal distension, and bowel gas interference [66].

The value of both CT and US in the diagnostic work-up for intra-abdominal infections has been fully studied in relation to acute appendicitis. A meta-analysis by Doria and coll. evaluated the diagnostic performance of ultrasonography (US) and computed tomography (CT) for the diagnosis of appendicitis in pediatric and adult populations. This meta-analysis found that pooled sensitivity and specificity for diagnosis of appendicitis in children were 88% and 94%, respectively, for ultrasound studies and 94% and 95%, respectively, for CT studies. Pooled sensitivity and specificity for diagnosis in adults were 83% and 93%, respectively, for ultrasound studies and 94% and 94%, respectively, for CT studies.

From the diagnostic performance perspective, CT has a significantly higher sensitivity than US in studies of children and adults; from the safety perspective, however, the radiation associated with CT, especially in children, should be always considered [67].

Treatment

Schematically intra-abdominal infections have been divided into three groups.

- Community acquired extrabiliary intra-abdominal infections
- Community acquired biliary intra-abdominal infections
- Hospital acquired intra-abdominal infections

Extra-Biliary Community-Acquired Intra-Abdominal Infections

Source control

Gastro-duodenal perforation

In the case of a perforated peptic ulcer, surgery is the treatment of choice. In selected cases (pts younger than 70 ys old, no shock, no peritonitis, lack of spillage of the water-soluble contrast medium at gastroduodenogram) non-operative management may be attempted. After initial non operative management, no improvement of conditions within 24 hours is indication to surgery (Recommendation 1 A).

In case of perforated peptic ulcer, surgery is considered the standard method of source control [68,69], also because postoperative mortality and morbidity rates have improved significantly [70].

Studies about the natural history of gastroduodenal ulcer perforation between the second half of 19th and the first half of 20th century [71,72] reported that perforations of the stomach were sealed by adhesions to the surrounding viscera preventing leakage from the stomach into the peritoneum.

In 1946, Taylor presented the first series of successful outcome of patients with perforated peptic ulcer conservatively treated [73]. Nowadays conservative treatment, also known as "Taylor method", consists of naso-gastric aspiration, antibiotics, intravenous fluids and *H. pylori* eradication therapy [74-76].

Patients older than 70 years old are significantly less like to respond to conservative treatment than younger patients [77]; also major medical illness, shock on admission and longstanding perforation (>24 hrs) are significantly associated with higher mortality rate in case of perforated peptic ulcer [78-80].

During non operative management, rapid deterioration or no improvement of clinical conditions within 24 hours from starting treatment are absolute indications to surgical treatment [81,82].

Finally, delaying the time point of operation beyond 12 h after the onset of clinical symptoms will worsen the outcome in perforated peptic ulcer [83].

Simple closure with or without omental patch is an effective and safe operation in case of small perforated ulcers (<2 cm). *H. pylori* status should be determined when the patients recover from the acute episode and the bacterium should be eradicated in those who are infected. (Recommendation 1 A).

In case of large perforated ulcers, concomitant severe bleeding or stricture, resective gastro-duodenal surgery may be required. The need for resection is established by surgeon based on intraoperative findings (Recommendation 1 B).

In case of small perforated gastroduodenal peptic ulcer, no significant differences in immediate postoperative course were reported after simple closure or definitive surgery [84-87].

Different suture techniques for simple closure of the perforation were described: simple closure by interrupted sutures [88] simple closure by interrupted sutures covered with pedicled omentoplasty, closure with a pedicled omental plug drawn into the perforation [89] and finally closure with a free omental patch [90].

Many patients in the published studies received omental patch repair rather than simple suture, but there was nearly no comparative evidence available to decide which repair technique is superior. A trial by Lau and coll. compared patch repair with fibrin sealing without finding any differences [91].

After closure alone, long term recurrence rate of peptic ulcer was significantly higher than after definitive surgery [92-95].

Eradication of Helicobacter pylori after simple closure and omental patch for perforated duodenal and gastric ulcers prevents recurrence.

To determine whether eradication of Helicobacter pylori could reduce the risk of ulcer recurrence after simple closure of perforated duodenal ulcer, a randomized controlled trial was conducted by Ng and coll. [96]. After 1 year, ulcer relapse was significantly less common in patients treated with anti-Helicobacter therapy than in those who received omeprazole alone (4.8% vs. 38.1%).

The first two cases of primary gastric resection for ulcer perforation were described by von Haberer as early in 1919 [97].

The method was used extensively for several decades but it is now rarely used for treatment of ulcer perforation. The role of resectional surgery in case of perforated peptic gastroduodenal disease is not well established; many reports advocate gastrectomy only in selected patients, in case of large gastric perforations, with concomitant severe bleeding or stricture [98-101].

Laparoscopic repair of perforated peptic ulcer is safe and effective in centers with experience (Recommendation 1 A).

The p.o. outcome of laparoscopic approach does not significantly differ from that of open surgery, except for lower analgesic p.o. request.

In all studies the patients had small ulcers (mean diameter 1 cm) and all patients received simple suture, mostly with omental patch, or sutureless repair.

No experience was reported with emergency laparoscopic resection or laparoscopic repair of large ulcers.

One systematic review [102], one meta-analysis [103] and three randomized controlled trials [104-106] comparing open and laparoscopic approach to gastroduodenal perforations were published. The postoperative course after laparoscopic repair did not significantly differ from that of open repair, except for lower analgesic request.

Biopsy and frozen section should be performed in all gastric perforations when a pathologist is available (Recommendation 2 C)

If a patient has a curable tumor and acceptable general conditions (no shock, localized peritonitis, no comorbidities) the treatment of choice is gastrectomy (total or sub-total) with D2 lymph-node dissection; with poor general conditions and curable tumor is indicated a two-stage radical gastrectomy (first step simple repair and gastrectomy in a secondary elective intervention); with poor general conditions or non-curable tumor is indicated simple repair (Recommendation 2 C).

Treatment of choice of perforated gastric cancer is surgery. In most instances gastric carcinoma is not suspected as the cause of perforation prior to emergency laparotomy, and the diagnosis of malignancy is often made only by intraoperative or postoperative pathologic examination. The treatment should aim to manage both the emergency condition of peritonitis and the oncologic technical aspects of surgery.

Perforation alone does not significantly affect long term survival after gastrectomy [107], differed resection (i.e. two stage radical gastrectomy) does not affect long term outcome [108,109].

The presence of preoperative shock seems to be the most important negative prognostic factor for immediate postoperative survival after surgery for perforated gastric cancer [110].

Therefore, patients who have perforated gastric cancer should undergo appropriate gastric resection in spite of concurrent peritonitis unless the patient is hemodynamically unstable or has unresectable cancer [111-114].

Small bowel perforations

In patients with small bowel perforations, surgery is the treatment of choice. (Recommendation 1 A).

In case of small perforations, primary repair is preferable; when resection is required, the technique of anastomosis does not influence postoperative mortality or morbidity rates. (Recommendation 2 B).

Laparoscopic approach should be performed by a laparoscopically experienced surgeon in selected institutions (Recommendation 2 C).

Primary repair of perforated bowel is preferable to resection and anastomosis because it carries a lower complication rate [115,116] even if the better outcome may reflect the limited tissue injury in these patients. Primary repair should not be performed in patients who have malignant lesions, necrotic bowel, perforations associated with mesenteric vascular injuries, or multiple contiguous perforations [117].

When resection is required, the entire diseased segment is resected, leaving healthy, well perfused ends for anastomosis. The technique for the enteroenterostomy, whether stapled or hand-sewn, seems to have little impact on the anastomotic complication rate [118,119].

Primary bowel anastomosis must be considered cautiously in the setting of gross purulent or feculent peritonitis because of a high rate of serious complications [120,121]. Laparoscopic management of small bowel perforations was reported [122] but there was no comparative study with open surgery.

Acute Appendicitis

Acute appendicitis is the most common intra-abdominal condition requiring emergency surgery.

The Surgical Infection Society and the Infectious Diseases Society of America have generated guidelines for the management and treatment of complicated intra-abdominal infections on 2010 [1].

Operative intervention for acute, non-perforated appendicitis is the treatment of choice. Non-operative management of patients with acute, non-perforated appendicitis can be considered if there is a marked improvement in the patient's condition prior to operation (Recommendation 1 A).

Antibiotic treatment has been shown to be effective in treating selected patients with acute appendicitis. Three randomized controlled trials (RCTs) have compared the efficacy of antibiotic therapy alone with that of surgery for acute appendicitis [123-125]. A meta-analysis of these RCTs concluded that while antibiotics may be useful as primary treatment for selected patients, antibiotics are unlikely to replace appendectomy at present [126]. Selection bias and crossover to surgery in the RCTs suggest that appendectomy is still the gold standard therapy for acute appendicitis. A support for a less emergent approach comes from clinical trials analyzing time to perforation, which indicate this to be an unusual early event [127,128].

Both open and laparoscopic approaches to appendectomy are appropriate (Recommendation 1 A).

A systematic review that included 45 randomized trials compared the diagnostic and therapeutic effects of laparoscopic and conventional open appendectomy in the treatment of suspected acute appendicitis [129]. The most consistent findings were an approximately 50% reduction in wound infections but a threefold increase in intra-abdominal abscesses in the laparoscopic appendectomy group. However, subsequently, two large studies have shown that patients undergoing a laparoscopic technique were more likely to be readmitted within 28 days of surgery [130] and that the risk for a complication was higher in the laparoscopic appendectomy group with uncomplicated appendicitis [131]. Taken together, open appendectomy may be preferred, although laparoscopic appendectomy is useful in selected subgroups of patients. Use of either approach should be decided by the surgeon's expertise. The laparoscopic approach is useful for obese patients, elderly patients and patients whose diagnosis is uncertain, especially women of childbearing age.

Patients with perforated appendicitis should undergo urgent intervention (Recommendation 1 C).

Patients with a periappendiceal abscess can be managed with percutaneous image-guided drainage. Appendectomy is generally deferred in such patients (Recommendation 1 A).

If imaging studies demonstrate a periappendiceal abscess, CT- or ultrasound-guided percutaneous drainage can often be performed. Percutaneous drainage with or without interval appendectomy to treat periappendiceal abscess results in fewer complications and shorter overall length of stay [132-134].

The use of interval appendectomy after percutaneous abscess drainage or non-operative management of perforated appendicitis is controversial (Recommendation 2 C).

A survey using a postal questionnaire showed that 53% of surgeons performed routine interval appendectomy because they worried about recurrence [135]. However, the recurrence rate of appendicitis (10%-25%) and the complication rate of interval appendectomy (23%) are similar [135,136]. It was evident that the chances of missing malignancy are low and thorough investigation is better than interval appendectomy in detecting colonic cancer. These studies support the view that interval appendectomy is unnecessary in 75-90% cases.

Acute diverticulitis

Several major medical organizations, such as The American Society of Colon and Rectal Surgeons, The Society for Surgery of the Alimentary Tract, The American College of Gastroenterology, European Association of Endoscopic Surgeons, have proposed recommendations [137-141]. The practice parameters published by The American Society of Colon and Rectal Surgeons on 2006 are particularly useful [137]. The recommendations written here are generally consistent with them.

Complicated diverticulitis is defined as acute diverticulitis accompanied by abscess, fistula, obstruction, or free intra-abdominal perforation. Approximately 25% of patients diagnosed with diverticulitis for the first time present with complicated diverticulitis. Uncomplicated diverticulitis, accounting for 75% of cases, refers to diverticulitis without the complications noted above.

Hinchey Classification is used to describe perforations of the colon due to diverticulitis [142]. The classification is I-IV: Hinchey stage I - localized abscess (para-colonic),

Hinchey stage II - pelvic abscess, Hinchey stage III - purulent peritonitis (the presence of pus in the abdominal cavity), and Hinchey stage IV - fecal peritonitis.

Non-operative treatment, with bowel rest and antibiotics, is suggested in patients with uncomplicated diverticulitis (Recommendation 1 C).

Conservative treatment of acute uncomplicated diverticulitis is successful in 70 to 100 percent of patients [137]. Uncomplicated diverticulitis may be managed as an outpatient (dietary modification and oral antibiotics) for those without appreciable fever, excessive vomiting, or marked peritonitis, as long as there is the opportunity for follow-up. The patient should be able to take liquids and antibiotics by mouth. Hospitalization is indicated if the patient is unable to take liquids or has severe pain, or if symptoms fail to improve despite adequate outpatient therapy. Antibiotics should be selected to treat the most common bacteria found in the colon: gram-negative rods and anaerobic bacteria [143]. Non-operative treatment will resolve acute diverticulitis in 85 percent of patients, but approximately one-third will have a recurrent attack often within one year [144].

The decision to recommend elective sigmoid colectomy after recovery from acute diverticulitis should be made on a case-by-case basis (Recommendation 1 C).

The overall rate of recurrence appears to be approximately 10 to 30% within a decade after a first documented attack and that the majority of patients who have a single episode of diverticulitis will not have another [145]. In one report involving an average follow-up of 9 years with 2551 patients whose initial episode of diverticulitis was treated successfully without surgery, only 13% had recurrent attacks and only 7% required colectomy [146]. These observations imply that routine elective colectomy is probably unwarranted if the disease is successfully managed on initial presentation and that surgical treatment should be limited to patients whose symptoms persist despite conservative therapy [147]. Thus, continued observation may be appropriate for most patients who have repeated attacks of uncomplicated diverticulitis.

Systemic antibiotic treatment alone is usually the most appropriate treatment for patients with a small (<4 cm in diameter) diverticular abscess and image guided percutaneous drainage is for those with a large (>4 cm in diameter) one (Recommendation 2 B).

For patients in whom diverticulitis is complicated by peridiverticular abscess formation, the size of the abscess is an important determinant of the need for percutaneous drainage [145]. Many patients who have small pericolic abscesses (4 cm or less in diameter) without peritonitis (Hinchey stage 1) can be treated conservatively with bowel rest and broad-spectrum antibiotics [148]. For patients with peridiverticular abscesses that are larger than 4 cm in diameter (Hinchey stage 2), observational studies indicate that CT-guided percutaneous drainage can be beneficial [149-160]. This procedure typically eliminates or reduces the size of the abscess [148,151,152], with a reduction in pain, resolution of leukocytosis, and defervescence usually seen within several days [153]. Percutaneous drainage may allow for elective rather than emergency surgery, increasing the likelihood of a successful one-stage procedure. Patients whose abscess cavities contain gross feculent material tend to respond poorly, and early surgical intervention is usually required.

Elective colon resection should typically be advised if an episode of complicated diverticulitis is treated non-operatively (Recommendation 2 C).

After percutaneous drainage of a diverticular abscess, a later colectomy usually should be planned, because 41 percent of patients will otherwise develop severe recurrent sepsis [154]. Some, but not all, retrospective studies suggest that the number of recurrences is associated with the chance that emergency surgery will be required at some point in the future [155].

The resection should be carried proximally to the compliant bowel and extend distally to the upper rectum (Recommendation 1 C).

It is usually sufficient to remove only the most severely affected segment; however, the proximal margin of resection should be in an area of pliable colon without hypertrophy or inflammation [137]. Not all of the diverticula-bearing colon must be removed. Usually a sigmoid colectomy will suffice; however, occasionally the proximal resection margin must extend well into the descending colon or to the left transverse colon. Distally, the margin of resection should be where the taenia coli splay out onto the upper rectum. After sigmoid colectomy for diverticulitis, an important predictor of recurrent diverticulitis is a colosigmoid rather than a colorectal anastomosis [156,157].

When a colectomy for diverticular disease is performed, a laparoscopic approach is appropriate in selected patients (Recommendation 1 B).

Laparoscopic colectomy may have advantages over open laparotomy, including less pain, smaller scar, and shorter recovery [137]. There is no increase in early or late complications [158,159]. Cost and outcome are comparable to open resection [160]. Laparoscopic surgery is acceptable in the elderly [161] and seems to be safe in selected patients with complicated disease [162].

Urgent operation is required for patients with diffuse peritonitis or for those who fail non-operative management of acute diverticulitis (Recommendation 1 B).

If a patient presents with severe or diffuse peritonitis, emergency colon resection is necessary. Also, if sepsis does not improve with inpatient conservative treatment of acute diverticulitis or after percutaneous drainage, surgery is indicated [137]. Immunosuppressed or immunocompromised patients are more likely to present with perforation or fail medical management, so a lower threshold for urgent or elective surgery should apply to them [163]. The source control of diffuse peritonitis is discussed together in the next topic of large bowel perforations.

Large bowel perforations

No practice guideline has been proposed for the source control of large bowel perforation.

Causes of large bowel perforations include (1) penetrating foreign body perforation, (2) extrinsic bowel obstruction, (3) intrinsic bowel obstruction, (4) direct loss of bowel wall integrity without foreign body perforation, (5) intestinal ischemia, and (6) infection.

The principles of source control include: control of the site of perforation, evacuation of contamination, debridement of necrotic tissue, and re-establishment of functional anatomy. Many patients who have large bowel perforations develop sepsis with accompanying hemodynamic compromise, hypothermia, acidosis, and a coagulopathy [164]. These patients require rapid resuscitation and rapid surgery. The standard approach is known as damage control surgery. The goal is to rapidly obtain source control and peritoneal toilet without prolonging the surgery to restore functional anatomy or extensively mobilize tissues [165].

The decision whether to perform a proximal diverting procedure is based on the surgeon's assessment of the risks of anastomotic breakdown and other complications such as the patient's nutritional status, the quality of the tissues, the amount of bowel contamination, the extent of blood loss, and the intraoperative stability of the patient's condition [135,166].

Hartmann's procedure may be performed for the treatment of large bowel perforations (Recommendation 2 C).

Two-stage procedures are typically used in emergency situations with fecal peritonitis and in most cases with purulent peritonitis. A common approach is the Hartmann's procedure, which involves resection of the diseased colon, an end-colostomy, and creation of a rectal stump; this is followed by colostomy closure several months later [167,168]. Reversal of Hartmann's procedure is also associated with substantial morbidity and even mortality [169]. It is well known that patients with stomas may face both physical and psychological difficulties [170,171].

Primary anastomosis with or without proximal diverting stoma may be performed in selected patients (Recommendation 2 C).

It appears that resection and primary anastomosis, with or without proximal diverting stoma (colostomy or ileostomy), can be safely undertaken in selected patients who have phlegmons, abscess formation with localized peritonitis, diffuse purulent peritonitis, obstruction, or fistula formation [145,166,172,173]. Although data are not available from randomized trials, observational studies that include matched patients suggest similar overall mortality rates and lower risks of wound infection and postoperative abscess formation with a one-stage approach [168]. On-table colonic lavage may also be considered [174].

Antimicrobial therapy for extra-biliary community-acquired IAIs

Once the diagnosis of intra-abdominal infection is suspected, it is necessary to begin empiric antimicrobial therapy.

However routine use of antimicrobial therapy is not appropriate for all patients with intra-abdominal infections.

In uncomplicated IAIs, when the focus of infection is treated effectively by surgical excision of the involved tissue, the administration of antibiotics is unnecessary beyond prophylaxis [175].

In complicated IAIs, when infectious process proceeds beyond the organ, causing either localized peritonitis (intra-abdominal abscess), or diffuse peritonitis antimicrobial therapy is mandatory.

The choice of antimicrobial regimen depends on the source of intra-abdominal infection, risk factors for specific microorganisms and resistance patterns and clinical patient's condition (Recommendation 1 C).

The principles of empiric antibiotic treatment should be defined according to the most frequently isolated germs, always taking into consideration the local trend of antibiotic resistance.

The major pathogens involved in community-acquired IAIs are Enterobacteriaceae, streptococci and anaerobes. The main resistance problem is represented by ESBL producers Enterobacteriaceae, even today frequently found in community acquired infections.

Many factors can raise the risk of selection of ESBL but prior exposition to antibiotics (mainly third generation cephalosporins) and comorbidities that make frequent the exposure of patients to multiple antibiotic treatments, are the most significant [1,176,177].

Many others factors can contribute to the severity of an intra-abdominal infection and to a patient's risk for a poor outcome, like patient age, underlying co-morbidities, extent of infection, nutritional status and the success of initial source control procedures. Dividing patients with intra-abdominal infections into lower and higher risk categories is not always simple, but attempting to assess a patient's risk of treatment failure is essential to optimize a treatment plan. In this context adding a standardized evaluation of the clinical condition, represented by the sepsis grading, may be extremely helpful.

In fact in critically ill patients the possibility that the normal flora may be modified and that the IAI could be caused by several unexpected pathogens and by more resistant flora must be considered. In these patients antimicrobial regimens with broader spectrum of activity are recommended.

Therefore in a stable and low risk patient a simpler antibiotic choice, not including ESBL in the spectrum of activity is correct, while in critical and high risk patients any antibiotic regimen must take into account the risk of ESBL.

The available therapeutic options for the treatment of ESBL-associated infections are limited by drug resistance conferred by the ESBLs. The frequently observed co-resistances include various antibiotic classes (fluoroquinolones, aminoglycosides, tetracyclines, and trimethoprim/sulfamethoxazole). Carbapenems, stable against hydrolyzing activity of ESBLs, are considered as the drug of choice for the treatment of these infections. Tigecycline and polymyxins have a strong in vitro antimicrobial activity against ESBL-producing bacteria, and the first should be considered a reasonable alternative. This is particularly true from an epidemiological point of view; in fact today any large hospital should implement carbapenems-sparing stewardship programs to control the spread of carbapenemase producing gram negative bacteria.

Although in the prospective French survey by Montravers and coll, a higher percentage of isolation of *Enterococcus faecalis* in non surviving patients was reported (23% versus 9%) [35], empirical treatment against Enterococci and has not been generally recommended for patients with community-acquired IAI. In fact in several clinical trials comparing different therapeutic options inclusion/exclusion of agents with enterococcal coverage provides no impact in outcomes for patients with community-acquired infections [178,179].

In the setting of community acquired IAIs, antimicrobial therapy for enterococci should be considered on a patient-by-patient basis, mainly in high risk patients, in immunocompromised patients and in patients with valvular heart disease or prosthetic materials [180].

Methicillin resistant *Staphylococcus aureus* (MRSA) is not commonly isolated from patients with community-acquired intra-abdominal infection. Therefore empirical treatment against MRSA is not recommended in this setting.

Normally empiric antifungal therapy for *Candida* is not recommended for adult and pediatric patients with community acquired intra-abdominal infection with the exclusion of immunocompromised patients (because of neutropenia, and receipt of immunosuppressive agents, including glucocorticosteroids, chemotherapeutic agents, and immunomodulators) and in patients recently exposed to broad spectrum antimicrobials. However, considering the aforementioned high morality rate of candida peritonitis [38], considering an antifungal coverage in critically ill patients should be correct.

Community-acquired IAIs may be managed with either single or multiple antimicrobial regimens, in relation to the need to ensure a spectrum of antimicrobial activity more or less wide.

Beta-lactam/beta-lactamase inhibitor combinations have an in vitro activity against gram-positive, gram-negative and anaerobe organisms [181,182] and are still reliable option for the empiric treatment of IAIs [183]. However, the increasing resistance of *Enterobacteriaceae* reported in the last decade also among community-acquired infections restricts their empirical use to patients without risk factor for resistances [184].

In the past Cephalosporins have been often used in the treatment of intra-abdominal infections. Among third generation cephalosporins both subgroups with poor activity against *Pseudomonas aeruginosa* and with activity against *Pseudomonas aeruginosa* (cefepime and ceftazidime) have been used in the treatment of IAIs in association with metronidazole. Both cephalosporins have acquired resistance in enterobacteriaceae and intrinsic resistance in Enterococci [185-188]. In light of the emerging concern of ESBL producing enterobacteriaceae species due to selection pressure by increase use of cephalosporins, the routinely use of all cephalosporins should be discouraged.

Aztreonam is a parenteral synthetic beta-lactam antibiotic and the first monobactam to be marketed. Aztreonam exhibits potent and specific activity in vitro against a wide spectrum of Gram-negative aerobic pathogens including *Pseudomonas aeruginosa* but its use is burdened by the same problems of resistances to cephalosporins.

Carbapenems have a spectrum of antimicrobial activity that includes Gram-positives (except MDR resistant gram positive cocci) and Gram-negative aerobic and anaerobic pathogens. They are the preferred antimicrobial agents for ESBL and AmpC-producing organisms; however, their widespread use in outbreaks and endemic regions of these organisms has led to increased rates of carbapenem-resistant *P. aeruginosa* and *Acinetobacter sp.* In addition, the selection of intrinsically carbapenem-resistant organisms such as *Stenotrophomonas maltophilia* and vancomycin-resistant *Enterococcus faecium* can be seen [189].

Group 1 carbapenems includes ertapenem, a once a day carbapenem that shares the activity of imipenem and meropenem against most species, including extended-spectrum beta-lactamase (ESBL) - producing pathogens, but is not active against *Pseudomonas spp.* and *Enterococcus* [190,191].

Group 2 includes imipenem/cilastatin, meropenem and doripenem, that share activity against non-fermentative gram-negative bacilli. Slightly higher in-vitro activity against some strains of Pseudomonas sp. has been reported with doripenem in registrative trials [192].

Also fluoroquinolones have been widely used in the last years for the treatment of IAIs, because of their excellent activity against aerobic Gram-negative bacteria and tissue penetration. In addition all the fluoroquinolones are rapidly and almost completely absorbed from the gastrointestinal tract [193,194]. The combination of ciprofloxacin/metronidazole has been one of the most commonly used regimens for the treatment of patients with complicated IAIs in the last years. The last quinolone developed, Moxifloxacin, has shown activity against a wide range of aerobic Gram-positive and Gram-negative [195]. Compared with ciprofloxacin, moxifloxacin has enhanced activity against Gram-positive bacteria with a decrease in activity against Gram-negative bacteria [196]. Among quinolones moxifloxacin seems to be effective also against *Bacterioides fragilis*, suggesting that it may be effective without antianaerobic agents [197-199].

However, in recent years, the prevalence of resistance between Enterobacteriaceae and non-fermentative gram-negative bacilli has been so high as to make their use in empirical regimen not recommended.

Aminoglycosides are particularly active against aerobic Gram-negative bacteria and act synergistically against certain Gram-positive organisms. They are effective against *Pseudomonas aeruginosa* but not effective against anaerobic bacteria. The aminoglycosides may not be optimal for-the treatment of abscesses or intra-abdominal infections due to their low penetration in acidic environments [200]. Therefore they are not recommended for the routine empiric treatment of community-acquired IAIs and may be reserved for patients with allergies to b-lactam agents [1].

Tigecycline is a parenteral glycylcycline antibiotic derived from minocycline. It is the first representative of the glycylcycline class of antibacterial agents to be marketed for clinical use [201,202]. Tigecycline has no activity in vitro against *P. aeruginosa* and *P. mirabilis* but represents a significant treatment option for complicated IAIs due to its favorable in vitro activity against anaerobic organisms, Enterococci, several ESBL-producing *Enterobacteriaceae* and carbapenemase-producing *Enterobacteriaceae, Acinetobacter sp.* and *Stenotrophomonas maltophilia* [203-206].

The use of tigecycline in the abdominal infections is particularly attractive in view of its pharmacokinetics/pharmacodynamics properties. In fact the drug is eliminated by active biliary secretion, able to determinate very high biliary and fecal concentrations [207]. A study finalized to the determination of tissue and corresponding serum concentration of tigecycline at selected time points in several different body sites, performed in 104 subjects undergoing surgical or medical procedures, showed that concentration, expressed as the ratio of AUC0-24 was extremely high for bile [208].

Moreover a PD analysis based on the data of microbiological surveys, performed by the Montecarlo simulation, demonstrated a predicted cumulative response (PCR) fraction for Tigeciclyne in peritonitis over 95% for *E. coli* and *Enterococcus* and over 75% for *Klebsiella spp, Enterobacter spp* and *A. baumannii* [209]. Tigecycline (TGC) has demonstrated non-inferiority in terms of clinical efficacy and safety versus imipenem/cilastatin and combination regimen of Ceftriaxone/metronidazole in Phase 3 clinical trials for complicated intra-abdominal infection [210,211].

But the greater significance of the use of tigecycline in empirical antibiotic regimens for IAIs is related to the possibility of saving carbapenems prescriptions. From an epidemiological point of view tigecycline should be a qualified therapeutic option in a carbapenems-sparing stewardship programs, as extended-spectrum b-lactamases become widely disseminated among the endogenous gut *Enterobacteriaceae.*

Distinguishing antimicrobial regimens according to the clinical patient's severity, the presumed pathogens and risk factors for major resistance patterns, the presumed/identified source of infection it is possible to standardize the empirical approach to the main clinical condition related to IAIs.

In appendices 1, 2, 3, 4 are summarized the antimicrobial regimens for extrabiliary community-acquired IAIs, recommended by WSES consensus conference.

Since the causative pathogens and the related resistance patterns can not easily be predicted (higher-risk patients), cultures from the site of infection must be always obtained (Recommendation 1 B).

Although the absence of impact of bacteriological cultures has been documented, especially in appendicitis, in this era of the broad spread of resistant microorganisms such as nosocomial and community extended-spectrum b-lactamase (ESBL) Enterobacteriaceae, carbapenemase producing gram negatives, b lactam- and vancomycin resistant enterococci (VRE), the threat of resistance is a source of major concern for clinicians. Therefore the results of the microbiological analyses have great importance for the therapeutic strategy of every patient, in particular in the adaptation of the initial antibiotic treatment, and at the same time are of paramount importance to ensure adequacy of empirical antimicrobial treatment.

The habit of considering the microbiological diagnosis useless is probably responsible for the relative scarcity of microbiological data and the variability of results of the few studies appropriate to emphasize the changes in resistance in IAI patients.

Cultures should be performed at least from intra-abdominal samples from surgery or interventional drainage procedures, providing sufficient volume (at least 1 mL of fluid or tissue, preferably more) and sending them to the laboratory using an appropriate transport system.

Biliary Community-Acquired Intra-Abdominal infections

Source control

Recent guidelines have been published for the management of acute cholecystitis and acute cholangitis [212-214].

Cholecystitis

Laparoscopic cholecystectomy has been accepted as an effective and safe treatment for acute cholecystitis (Recommendation 1 A).

Laparoscopic cholecystectomy versus open cholecystectomy question has been extensively investigated. Beginning in the early 1990s, techniques and indications for laparoscopic management of the acutely inflamed gallbladder were discussed and laparoscopic cholecystectomy is now accepted as being safe for acute cholecystitis.

Many RCTs have demonstrated that laparoscopic cholecystectomy is effective and safe for acute cholecystitis [215-220].

In the Johansson and coll. randomized clinical trial there were no significant differences beetwen laparoscopic cholecystectomy and open cholecystectomy, in rate of postoperative complications, pain score at discharge and sick leave.

Seventy patients who met the criteria for acute cholecystitis were randomized to open or laparoscopic cholecystectomy. In eight patients a laparoscopic procedure was converted to open cholecystectomy. Median operating time was 90 (range 30-155) and 80 (range 50-170) min in the laparoscopic and open groups respectively ($P = 0.040$). The direct medical costs were equivalent in the two groups. Although median postoperative hospital stay was 2 days in each group, it was significantly shorter in the laparoscopic group ($P = 0.011$).

In the Kiviluoto and coll. randomized clinical trial there were no deaths or bile-duct lesions in either group, but the postoperative complication rate was significantly ($p = 0.0048$) higher in the open cholecystectomy than in the laparoscopic cholecystectomy group: seven (23%) patients had major and six (19%) minor complications after OC, whereas only one (3%) minor complication occurred after LC. The postoperative hospital stay was significantly shorter in the LC than the OC group ($p = 0.0063$).

Early laparoscopic cholecystectomy during acute cholecystitis appears safe and shortens the total hospital stay when it is compared with delayed laparoscopic cholecystectomy (Recommendation 1 A).

The most important innovation in the surgical treatment of acute gallstone cholecystitis (AGC) concerns timing.

Several RCTs and meta-analyses [221-224] have showed that, compared with delayed laparoscopic cholecystectomy, early laparoscopic cholecystectomy for acute cholecystitis reduces the total length of hospital stay and the risk of readmissions attributable to recurrent acute cholecystitis. It is a more cost-effective approach for the management of acute cholecystitis.

In the Gurusamy and coll. meta-analysis [221] there was no significant difference between early and delayed groups in terms of bile duct injury or conversion to open cholecystectomy. The total hospital stay was shorter by 4 days for early laparoscopic cholecystectomy.

In Siddiqui and coll. meta-analysis [222] there was no significant difference in conversion rates and postoperative complications between early and delayed groups. Operation time was significantly reduced with delayed cholecystectomy. The total hospital stay was significantly reduced with early cholecystectomy.

In order to analyze whether delay from onset of symptoms was related to the conversion rate in patients with a acute cholecystitis, a retrospective case note review of patients undergoing emergency cholecystectomy in a single institution between January 2002 and December 2005 was published on 2007 [225]. Early intervention for acute cholecystitis (preferably within 2 days of onset of symptoms) was most likely to result in successful laparoscopic cholecystectomy; increasing delay was associated with conversion to open surgery.

The use of percutaneous cholecystostomy in critically ill patients with acute cholecystitis is both safe and effective (Recommendation 2 B).

There are no randomized studies evaluating the outcome of percutaneous cholecystostomy vs. cholecystectomy. It is not possible to make definitive recommendations regarding treatment by PC or cholecystectomy in elderly or critically ill patients with acute cholecystitis. The use of percutaneous cholecystostomy in critically ill patients with acute cholecystitis is both safe and effective.

Whenever possible, percutaneous cholecystostomy should be followed by laparoscopic cholecystectomy.

A systematic electronic database search was performed on the subject of percutaneous cholecystostomy (PC) in the elderly population [226].

Successful intervention was seen in 85.6% of patients with acute cholecystitis. A total of 40% of patients treated with PC were later cholecystectomized, with a mortality rate of 1.96%. Procedure mortality was 0.36%, but 30-day mortality rates were 15.4% in patients treated with PC and 4.5% in those treated with acute cholecystectomy ($P < 0.001$).

Early diagnosis of gallbladder perforation and immediate surgical intervention may decrease morbidity and mortality (Recommendation 1 C).

Gallbladder perforation is an unusual initial presentation of gallbladder disease. Early diagnosis of gallbladder perforation and immediate surgical intervention are of prime importance in decreasing morbidity and mortality associated with this condition.

It is rarely diagnosed preoperatively. Late operative intervention is associated with increased morbidity, mortality, number of ICU admissions, and long postoperative hospital stays [227-230].

Cholangitis

Biliary drainage is a radical method to relieve cholestasis, a cause of acute cholangitis, and takes a central part in the treatment of acute cholangitis.

Biliary drainage can be achieved by three different procedures:

- Endoscopic
- Percutaneous transhepatic
- Open drainage

It has been reported that when no appropriate biliary drainage was available 20-30 years ago, the mortality of acute cholangitis with conservative treatment was extremely high. There has been no randomized controlled trial (RCT) comparing conservative treatment and biliary drainage. However, many patients with acute cholangitis cannot be treated by conservative treatment alone [231,232].

Endoscopic drainage is safer and more effective than open drainage. (Recommendation 1 A).

A randomized controlled trial (RCT) was conducted to compare endoscopic and open drainage in 82 patients with severe acute cholangitis with hypotension and disturbed consciousness. This RCT demonstrated that the morbidity and mortality of endoscopic naso-biliary drainage (ENBD) + endoscopic sphincterotomy (EST; $n = 41$) were significantly lower than those of T-tube drainage under laparotomy ($n = 41$). The Authors concluded that morbidity and mortality of endoscopic naso-biliary drainage (ENBD) + endoscopic sphincterotomy are lower than those of T-tube drainage under laparotomy [233].

Endoscopic modalities currently are favored over percutaneous procedures because of a lower risk of complication. There is no RCT comparing endoscopic and percutaneous drainage (Recommendation 2 C).

Considering the rare occurrence of serious complications such as intraperitoneal hemorrhage and biliary peritonitis, and the shorter duration of hospitalization, endoscopic drainage is preferred whenever it is available and applicable [234-237].

Open drainage should only be used in patients for whom endoscopic or percutaneous transhepatic drainage is contraindicated or those in whom it has been unsuccessfully performed. (Recommendation 2 C).

There is no RCT comparing open drainage and endoscopic or percutaneous drainage [238].

Antimicrobial therapy for biliary infections

Antibiotics are always recommended in complicated cholecystitis and in delayed treatment of uncomplicated cholecystitis.

In uncomplicated cholecystitis, when the focus of infection is treated effectively by cholecystectomy, the administration of antibiotics is unnecessary beyond prophylaxis.

Patients with an infected focus that can be eradicated effectively by surgical intervention can potentially be treated with only 24 hours of antimicrobial prophylaxis.

The most important factors for antimicrobial drug selection in biliary infections are antimicrobial activity against causative bacteria, clinical patient's condition and biliary levels of the antimicrobial agents (Recommendation 1 B).

Knowledge of the secretion of antibiotics into bile and of their efficacy should be helpful in choosing the best therapeutic regimen (Recommendation 1 C).

Organisms most often isolated in biliary infections are the gram-negative aerobes, *Escherichia coli* and *Klebsiella pneumonia* and anaerobes, especially *Bacteroides fragilis.* Activity against enterococci is not required since their pathogenicity in biliary tract infections remains unclear [239-241].

The efficacy of antibiotics in the treatment of biliary infections depends on effective biliary antibiotic concentrations [242-245].

It has been debated whether antimicrobials with good biliary penetration should be recommended for biliary infections. However, there are no clinical or experimental data to strongly support the recommendation of antimicrobials with excellent biliary penetration for these patients. Other important factors include the antimicrobial potency of individual compounds, and the effect of bile on antibacterial activity [246].

Penicillins are still frequently used in biliary infections. Aminopenicillins such as amoxicillin are excreted unchanged in the bile. In patients with normal function of biliary tract, amoxicillin bile concentrations are higher than the serum concentrations (3 rates higher than the concentrations in plasma).

Fluoroquinolones have excellent bioavailability; they are excreted by renal, hepatic and biliary excretion. Ciprofloxacin biliary concentrations are generally higher then the concentrations in the plasma (28 to 45 rates higher than the concentrations in plasma). Besides, ciprofloxacin has been proven to reach high biliary concentrations also in patients with obstruction due to the anticipated secretion of quinolone by biliary epithelium. An alternative to amoxicillin/clavulanate, ciprofloxacin plus metronidazole may be indicated for biliary infections, in no critically ill patient and in absence of risk factors for resistance patterns.

Piperacillin is the penicillin with highest rate of bile excretion (25% in active form). Bile concentrations are up to 60 rates higher than the concentrations in plasma. The combination of piperacillin with tazobactam further extends its spectrum. However tazobactam pharmacokinetics is different from piperacillin pharmacokinetics and during a regular therapy regimen employing piperacillin/tazobactam combination, tazobactam reaches effective concentrations in the bile only during the first 3 hours following its administration.

Glicilcyclines such as tigecycline have a broad spectrum of activity and a very good availability in the bladder wall and bile. Tigecycline is a very good antimicrobial option in biliary infections.

Also for biliary intra-abdominal infections WSES consensus conference distinguished antimicrobial regimens according to the clinical patient's condition and the risk factors for resistance patterns.

In appendices 5, 6, 7, 8 are summarized the antimicrobial regimens for biliary community-acquired intra-abdominal infections, recommended by WSES consensus conference.

Hospital-acquired intra-abdominal infections

Hospital-acquired intra-abdominal infections are infections not present on admission that become evident 48 hours or more after admission in patients hospitalized for a reason other than intra-abdominal infection [247].

Both post-operative and non post-operative nosocomial intra-abdominal infections are associated with increased mortality due to underlying patient health status and increased likelihood of infection caused by MDR organisms [248-255].

The main clinical differences between the patients with community-acquired intra-abdominal infections and patients with nosocomial intra-abdominal infections are [35]:

- higher proportion of underlying disease
- severity criteria at the time of diagnosis for nosocomial cases

The most common cause of postoperative peritonitis is anastomotic failure/leak.

In few instances of postoperative peritonitis, the anastomosis may be intact; however, the patient may remain sick because of residual peritonitis. Among them is the inadequate drainage of the initial septic focus, in which the surgeon failed to drain completely, or more commonly, the peritoneum does not have the sufficient defense capacity to control the problem.

Hospital acquired, non-postoperative IAIs, which arise in patients hospitalized for reasons unrelated to abdominal pathology, portend a particularly poor prognosis.

Diagnosis is often delayed due to both a low index of suspicion, poor underlying health status, and altered sensorium.

Non-postoperative nosocomial intra-abdominal infections are frequently characterized as severe infections diagnosed lately in fragile patients [254].

Prospective analysis of patients operated for secondary non-postoperative nosocomial intra-abdominal infections collected in 176 French study centers was published 2004 [254].

When compared with CAI patients, Non-PostopNAI patients presented:

- increased interval between admission to the surgical ward and operation
- increased proportions of underlying diseases

In non-PostopNAI patients, increased proportions of therapeutic failure and of fatalities were observed [254].

Unlike previous studies, recent studies observed no difference in incidence of prognosis between community-acquired and nosocomial intra-abdominal infections.

Riché and coll. [45] have prospectively studied a cohort of 180 consecutive patients operated on for generalized peritonitis.

There were 24 deaths among the 112 patients with community-acquired peritonitis (21% mortality rate) and 11 deaths among the 68 patients with postoperative peritonitis (16% mortality rate). Survival rates at day 30 were not statistically different for community-acquired and postoperative peritonitis. The proportion of patients operated less than 24 hours after the onset of symptoms was not different between community-acquired and postoperative peritonitis (54% *vs.* 49%, respectively; $P = 0.61$).

In the Inui and coll. [256] study, 452 patients, 234 (51.8%) had CIAIs and 218 (48.2%) had NIAIs, treated at a single urban academic hospital over 8 years (June 1999-June 2007) were retrospectively reviewed.

When patients with appendicitis were excluded, there was no difference in mortality or complications between patients with CIAIs and NIAIs.

Source control represents a key component of success in therapy of sepsis. It includes drainage of infected fluids, debridement of infected soft tissues, removal of infected devices or foreign bodies, and finally, definite measures to correct anatomic derangement resulting in ongoing microbial contamination and to restore optimal function.

Recommendations have low grade due to the difficulty to perform appropriate randomized clinical trials in this respect.

Percutaneous abscess drainage should be the primary procedure to treat postoperative localized intra-abdominal abscess without signs of generalized peritonitis (Recommendation 2 C).

Some retrospective studies in the surgery and radiology literature have documented the effectiveness of percutaneous drainage to treat postoperative localized intra-abdominal abscess [257-259].

Source control should be obtained as early as possible after the diagnosis of postoperative intra-abdominal peritonitis has been confirmed. Inability to control the septic source is associated significantly with increase in mortality (Recommendation 1 C).

Inability to control the septic source is associated significantly with increase in mortality.

Delaying relaparotomy for more than 24 h or the presence of organ failure result in higher mortality in post-operative intra-abdominal infections.

The value of physical tests and laboratory parameters in diagnosing abdominal sepsis is limited. CT-scanning revealed the highest diagnostic accuracy. Early relaparotomy appears to be the most reasonable option to treat postoperative peritonitis [260].

Re-laparotomy strategy

Some patients are prone to persisting intra-abdominal infection regardless of eradication of the source of infection and timely relaparotomy provides the only surgical option that significantly improves outcome.

In these cases single operation may not be sufficient to achieve source control, thus re-exploration is necessary [261-263].

The decision to and when to perform a relaparotomy in secondary peritonitis is largely subjective and based on professional experience. Factors indicative of progressive or persistent organ failure during early post-operative follow-up are the best indicators for ongoing infection and associated positive findings at relaparotomy [264-266].

Three methods of local mechanical management of abdominal sepsis following initial laparotomy for source control are currently debated:

(1) Open-abdomen
(2) planned relaparotomy
(3) on-demand relaparotomy

On demand relaparotomy may be considered the preferred surgical strategy in patients with severe peritonitis because it has a substantial reduction in relaparotomies, health care utilization, and medical costs. (Recommendation 1 A)

In 2007 van Ruler and coll. [267] published a randomized, clinical trial comparing on-Demand Vs Planned Relaparotomy strategy in patients with severe peritonitis.

In the van Ruler trial a total of 232 patients with severe intra-abdominal infections (116 on-demand and 116 planned) were randomized.

In planned relaparotomy group, relaparotomies were performed every 36 to 48 hours after the index laparotomy to inspect, drain, lavage, and perform other necessary abdominal interventions for residual peritonitis or new infectious focus.

In on-Demand relaparotomy group, relaparotomies were only performed in patients with clinical deterioration or lack of clinical improvement with a likely intra-abdominal cause.

Patients in the on-demand relaparotomy group did not have a significantly lower rate of adverse outcomes compared with patients in the planned relaparotomy group but did have a substantial reduction in relaparotomies, health care utilization, and medical costs.

Patients in the on-demand group had shorter median intensive care unit stays (7 vs 11 days; $P = .001$) and shorter median hospital stays (27 vs 35 days; $P = .008$). Direct medical costs per patient were reduced by 23% using the on-demand strategy.

Some studies have investigated open abdomen in intra-abdominal infections and generated great interest and hope [268-270].

In 2007 a randomized study by Robledo and coll. [271] compared open with closed "on demand" management of severe peritonitis.

During a 24-month period, 40 patients with SSP were admitted for treatment. Although the difference in the mortality rate (55% vs. 30%) did not reach statistical significance ($p < 0.05$; chi-square and Fisher exact test), the relative risk and odds ratio for death were 1.83 and 2.85 times higher in open abdomen patients group. This clinical finding, as evidenced by the clear tendency toward a more favorable outcome for patients in closed open group, led to termination of the study at the first interim analysis.

This randomized study from a single institution demonstrates that closed management of the abdomen may be a more rational approach after operative treatment of SSP and questions the recent enthusiasm for the open alternative, which has been based on observational studies. However in this study, the "open abdomen" was managed with a non-absorbable polypropylene mesh, without topical negative pressure.

Antimicrobial treatment of hospital-acquired intra-abdominal infections

Hospital-acquired IAIs are among the most difficult infections to diagnose early and treat effectively.

A successful outcome depends on early diagnosis, rapid and appropriate surgical intervention, and the selection of effective antimicrobial regimens.

Hospital acquired infections are commonly caused by larger and more resistant flora, and for these infections, complex multidrug regimens are always recommended (Recommendation 1 B).

The threat of antimicrobial resistance has been identified as one of the major challenges in the management of complicated IAIs and was already discussed in the previous chapter.

In order to describe the differences in microbiological and resistance patterns between community-acquired and nosocomial intra-abdominal infections a prospective, observational multicentric study (EBIIA) was completed in French [35]. From January to July 2005, patients undergoing surgery/interventional drainage for IAIs with a positive microbiological culture were included by 25 French centers. A total of 829 microorganisms were cultured.

In this study the number of peritoneal microorganisms per sample was ≥3 in 34% and 54% of cases, respectively, for community-acquired and nosocomial infections ($P < 0.001$). The distribution of the microorganisms differed according to the nosocomial or community origin of the infection but not according to their location (data not shown). In nosocomial patients, increased proportions of *Enterococcus faecalis* (33% versus 19% in community-acquired patients; $P < 0.05$) and Pseudomonas aeruginosa strains (13% versus 5% in community-acquired patients; $P < 0.01$) were observed. Conversely, in nosocomial patients, decreased proportions of *Escherichia coli* (52% versus 72% in community-acquired patients, $P < 0.001$) and streptococci strains were reported (31% versus 50% in community-acquired patients, $P < 0.01$).

Therefore the inclusion of anti-enterococcal drugs in any empirical antibiotic regimens in severe nosocomial IAIs and/or in patients with well known risk factors, seems appropriate, mainly if directed against *E. faecalis*.

Empiric therapy directed against vancomycin-resistant *Enterococcus faecium* is not recommended unless the patient is at very high risk for an infection due to this organism, such as a liver transplant recipient with an intra-abdominal infection originating in the hepatobiliary tree or a patient known to be colonized with vancomycin-resistant *E. faecium*.

Enterococcus infections are difficult to treat because of both intrinsic and acquired resistance to many antibiotics.

Enterococci are intrinsically resistant to many penicillins, and all cephalosporins with the possible exception of ceftobiprole and ceftaroline, currently undergoing clinical evaluation. Besides Enterococci have acquired resistance to many other classes of antibiotics, to which the organisms are not intrinsically resistant, including fluoroquinolones, aminoglycosides, and penicillins. Many strains of *E. faecalis* are susceptible to certain penicillins and glycopeptides; however, some strains of *E. faecium* may be resistant to these agents [272].

Vancomycin-resistant *Enterococcus* (VRE) infections have been associated with increased morbidity and mortality [273,274].

Many factors can increase the risk of colonization with VRE. These include previous antibiotic therapy (the number and duration of antibiotics received) prolonged hospitalization, hospitalization in an intensive care unit severity of illness, invasive procedures and devices, gastrointestinal surgery, transplantation, proximity to another VRE-positive patient [275].

Affected patients usually have multiple and relevant co-morbidities, with prolonged hospital stay and received long courses of broad spectrum antibiotics.

In the survey of Montravers and coworkers no differences in frequency of isolation of Candida spp were identified in community or hospital acquired IAIs, and the overall prevalence was under 5%, in contrast with other observations, especially those related to patients with recurrent gastrointestinal perforation/anastomotic leakage [276,277].

Although the epidemiological role of Candida spp in nosocomial peritonitis is not yet defined, the clinical role is significant, because Candidal isolation is normally associated to a poor prognosis.

The same study group on 2006 published an elegant retrospective, case-control study conducted in critically ill patients admitted to 17 French ICUs where the yielding of Candida spp from peritoneal specimen was a variable independently associated to mortality in the setting of nosocomial peritonitis [37].

More recently Montravers and coll. reported a mortality rate of 38% in a prospective cohort of 93 patients admitted to ICU with candidal peritonitis [38].

Therefore, like for Enterococci, the inclusion of an anticandidal drug in the empiric regimen of severe nosocomial acquired IAIs, seems appropriate as confirmed by IDSA guidelines [1].

The recently published IDSA guidelines for the treatment of invasive candidiasis [278] don't comprise a chapter specifically dedicated to candidal peritonitis. However the expert panels generically favor the use of echinocandins as first line empirical therapy in severely ill patients, recommending fluconazole for less severe conditions.

Therefore, transferring this concept to the context of IAIs we might advise the proscription of echinocandins as first line treatment in severe nosocomial IAIs. The IDSA guidelines also recommend the transition from an echinocandin to fluconazole for patients clinically stable and who have isolates of *Candida spp* susceptible to fluconazole; so the final recommendation would be to start with an echinocandin and to de-escalate to fluconazole as soon as possible on a clinical or microbiological basis.

In appendices 9,10 are summarized the antimicrobial regimens for hospital-acquired intra-abdominal infections, recommended by WSES consensus conference.

Conclusions

The timing and adequacy of source control is the most important issue in the management of intra-abdominal sepsis, because an inadequate and late operation may have a negative effect on the outcome.

Concomitant adequate empiric antimicrobial therapy further influences patients' morbidity and mortality. Inappropriate antibiotic therapy of intra-abdominal infections may result in poor patient outcome and the selection of an appropriate agent is a real challenge because of the emerging resistance of target organisms to commonly prescribed antibiotics.

It is demonstrated that a strategy of early goal-directed therapy decreases the in-hospital mortality of patients who are taken to the emergency department in septic shock. An organized approach to the haemodynamic support to sepsis includes use of fluid resuscitation, vasopressor therapy and inotropic therapy.

A multidisciplinary approach to the management of critically ill patients may be an important factor in the quality of care.

Appendices

Appendix 1. Antimicrobial therapy for community-acquired extrabiliary IAI in no critically ill patient, in absence of risk factors for ESBL

Community-acquired extrabiliary IAI

No critically ill patient

No risk factors for ESBL

AMOXICILLIN/CLAVULANATE

Daily schedula: 2.2 g every 6 hours (Infusion time 2 hours)

OR (Allergy to beta-lactams):

CIPROFLOXACIN

Daily schedula: 400 mg every 8 hours (Infusion time 30 min)

+

METRONIDAZOLE

Daily schedula: 500 mg every 6 hours (Infusion time 1 hour)

Appendix 2. Antimicrobial therapy for community-acquired extrabiliary IAI in no critically ill patient, in presence of risk factors for ESBL

Community-acquired extrabiliary IAI

No critically ill patient

Risk factors for ESBL

ERTAPENEM

Daily schedula: 1 g every 24 hours (Infusion time 2 hours)

OR

TIGECYCLINE

Daily schedula: 100 mg LD then 50 mg every 24 hours (Infusion time 2 hours)

Appendix 3. Antimicrobial therapy for community-acquired extrabiliary IAI in critically ill patient, in absence of risk factors for ESBL

Community-acquired extrabiliary IAI

Critically ill patient (± SEVERE SEPSIS)

No risk factors for ESBL

PIPERACILLIN/TAZOBACTAM

Daily schedula: 8/2 g LD then 16/2 g/die by continuous infusion or

4.5 g every 6 hours (infusion time 4 hours)

Appendix 4. Antimicrobial therapy for community-acquired extrabiliary IAI in critically ill patient, in presence of risk factors for ESBL

Community-acquired IAI

Critically ill patient (± SEVERE SEPSIS)

Risk factors for ESBL

MEROPENEM

Daily schedula: 500 mg every 6 hours (Infusion time 6 hours)

OR

IMIPENEM

Daily schedula: 500 mg every 4 hours (Infusion time 3 hours)

+/-
FLUCONAZOLE
Daily schedula: 600 mg LD then 400 mg every 24 hours (Infusion time 2 hours)

Appendix 5. Antimicrobial therapy for biliary IAI in no critically ill patient, in absence of risk factors for ESBL
Community-acquired biliary IAI
No critically ill patient
No risk factors for ESBL
AMOXICILLIN/CLAVULANATE
Daily schedula: 2.2 g every 6 hours (Infusion time 2 hours)
OR (Allergy to beta-lactams)
CIPROFLOXACIN
Daily schedula: 400 mg every 8 hours (Infusion time 30 min)
+
METRONIDAZOLE
Daily schedula: 500 mg every 6 hours (Infusion time 1 hour)

Appendix 6. Antimicrobial therapy for biliary IAI in no critically ill patient, in presence of risk factors for ESBL
Community-acquired biliary IAI
No critically ill patient
Risk factors for ESBL
TIGECYCLINE
Daily schedula: 100 mg LD then 50 mg every 12 hours (Infusion time 2 hours)

Appendix 7. Antimicrobial therapy for biliary IAI in critically ill patient, in absence of risk factors for ESBL
Community-acquired biliary IAI
Critically ill patient (± SEVERE SEPSIS)
No risk factors for ESBL
PIPERACILLIN/TAZOBACTAM
Daily schedula: 8/2 g LD then 16/2 g/die by continuous infusion or
4.5 g every 6 hours (infusion time 4 hours)

Appendix 8. Antimicrobial therapy for biliary IAI in critically ill patient, in presence of risk factors for ESBL
Community-acquired biliary IAI
Critically ill patient (SEVERE SEPSIS)
Risk factors for ESBL
PIPERACILLIN
Daily schedula: 8 g by LD then 16 g by continuous infusion or
4 g every 6 hours (Infusion time 4 hours)
+
TIGECYCLINE
Daily schedula: 100 mg LD then 50 mg every 12 hours (Infusion time 2 hours)
+/-
FLUCONAZOLE
Daily schedula: 600 mg LD then 400 mg every 24 hours (Infusion time 2 hours)

Appendix 9. Antimicrobial therapy for hospital-acquired IAI in no critically ill patient
Hospital acquired IAI
No critically ill patient (< SEVERE SEPSIS)
Risk factors for MDR pathogens
PIPERACILLIN
Daily schedula: 8 g by LD then 16 g by continuous infusion or
4 g every 6 hours (Infusion time 4 hours)
+
TIGECYCLINE
Daily schedula: 100 mg LD then 50 mg every 12 h (Infusion Time: 2 hours)
+
FLUCONAZOLE
Daily Schedula: 600 mg LD then 400 mg every 24 h (Infusion time: 2 hours)

Appendix 10. Antimicrobial therapy for hospital-acquired IAI in critically ill patient
Hospital-acquired extrabiliary IAI
Critically ill patient (±SEVERE SEPSIS)
Risk factors for MDR pathogens
PIPERACILLIN
Daily schedula: 8 g by LD then 16 g by continuous infusion or
4 g every 6 hours (Infusion time 4 hours)
+
TIGECYCLINE
Daily schedula: 100 mg LD then 50 mg every 12 h (Infusion Time: 2 hours)
+
ECHINOCANDIN
caspofungin (loading dose of 70 mg, then 50 mg daily),
anidulafungin (loading dose of 200 mg, then 100 mg daily),
micafungin (100 mg daily)
OR
MEROPENEM
Daily Schedula: 500 mg every 6 h (Infusion time: 6 hours)
IMIPENEM
Daily Schedula: 500 mg every 4 h (Infusion time: 3 hours)
DORIPENEM
Daily Schedula: 500 mg every 8 h (Infusion time: 4 hours)
+
TEICOPLANIN

Daily Schedula: LD 12 mg/kg/12 h for 3 doses then 6 mg/kg every 12 h (with TDM corrections - PD target 20-30 mg/L)

Daily schedula: 16 g by continuous infusion or

4 g every 6 hours (infusion time 4 hours)

+

ECHINOCANDIN

caspofungin (loading dose of 70 mg, then 50 mg daily),

anidulafungin (loading dose of 200 mg, then 100 mg daily),

micafungin (100 mg daily)

Author details

[1]Department of Surgery, Macerata Hospital, Italy. [2]Clinic of Infectious Diseases, Department of Internal Medicine Geriatrics and Nephrologic Diseases, St Orsola-Malpighi University Hospital, Bologna, Italy. [3]Department of Primary Care & Emergency Medicine, Kyoto University Graduate School of Medicine, Japan. [4]Institute of Clinical Pharmacology and Toxicology, Azienda Ospedaliera Universitaria Santa Maria Misericordia, Department of Experimental and Clinical Pathology and Medicine, University of Udine, Italy. [5]Department of Surgery, Radboud University Nijmegen Medical Centre, The Netherlands. [6]Department of Surgery, "Mazzoni" Hospital, Ascoli Piceno Italy. [7]Department of Surgical Sciences San Gerardo Hospital, Monza, University of Milano-Bicocca, Italy. [8]Department of Surgery, University of Ancona, Italy. [9]Department of General and Transplant surgery, St Orsola-Malpighi University Hospital, Bologna, Italy. [10]Department of Surgery, "Ospedali Riuniti" Hospital, Bergamo, Italy. [11]Department of Surgery, Helsinki University Central Hospital, Finland. [12]Department of Surgery, Denver Health Medical Center, USA. [13]Department of Surgery, University of Texas Health Science Center, Houston, USA. [14]Emergency Surgery Department, University of São Paulo, Brazil.

Authors' contributions

MS, PV designed the study. MS, CT partecipated in collection and assembly of data. MS, PV, KK, GG wrote the manuscript. All authors read and approved the final manuscript.

Competing interests

The authors declare that they have no competing interests.

References

1. Solomkin JS, Mazuski JE, Bradley JS, Rodvold KA, Goldstein EJ, Baron EJ, O'Neill PJ, Chow AW, Dellinger EP, Eachempati SR, Gorbach S, Hilfiker M, May AK, Nathens AB, Sawyer RG, Bartlett JG: **Diagnosis and management of complicated intra-abdominal infection in adults and children: guidelines by the Surgical Infection Society and the Infectious Diseases Society of America.** *Clin Infect Dis* 2010, **15,50(2)**:133-6.
2. Guyatt G, Gutterman D, Baumann MH, Addrizzo-Harris D, Hylek EM, Phillips B, Raskob G, Lewis SZ, Schunemann H: **Grading strength of recommendations and quality of evidence in clinical guidelines: Report from an American College of Chest Physicians task force.** *Chest* 2006, **129**:174-181.
3. Brozek JL, Akl EA, Jaeschke R, Lang DM, Bossuyt P, Glasziou P, Helfand M, Ueffing E, Alonso-Coello P, Meerpohl J, Phillips B, Horvath AR, Bousquet J, Guyatt GH, Schunemann HJ: **Grading quality of evidence and strength of recommendations in clinical practice guidelines: Part 2 of 3. The GRADE approach to grading quality of evidence about diagnostic tests and strategies.** *Allergy* 2009, **64**:1109-1116.
4. Moore LJ, Moore FA, Jones SL, Xu J, Bass BL: **Sepsis in general surgery: a deadly complication.** *Am J Surg* 2009, **198(6)**:868-74.
5. Moore LJ, Moore FA, Todd SR, Jones SL, Turner KL, Bass BL: **Sepsis in general surgery: the 2005-2007 national surgical quality improvement program perspective.** *Arch Surg* 2010, **145(7)**:695-700.
6. Dellinger RP, Levy MM, Carlet JM, Bion J, Parker MM, Jaeschke R, Reinhart K, Angus DC, Brun-Buisson C, Beale R, Calandra T, Dhainaut JF, Gerlach H, Harvey M, Marini JJ, Marshall J, Ranieri M, Ramsay G, Sevransky J, Thompson BT, Townsend S, Vender JS, Zimmerman JL, Vincent JL, International Surviving Sepsis Campaign Guidelines Committee; American Association of Critical-Care Nurses; American College of Chest Physicians; American College of Emergency Physicians; Canadian Critical Care Society; European Society of Clinical Microbiology and Infectious Diseases; European Society of Intensive Care Medicine; European Respiratory Society; International Sepsis Forum; Japanese Association for Acute Medicine; Japanese Society of Intensive Care Medicine; Society of Critical Care Medicine; Society of Hospital Medicine; Surgical Infection Society; World Federation of Societies of Intensive and Critical Care Medicine: **Surviving Sepsis Campaign: international guidelines for management of severe sepsis and septic shock: 2008.** *Crit Care Med* 2008, **36(1)**:296-327.
7. Bone RC, Balk RA, Cerra FB, Dellinger RP, Fein AM, Knaus WA, Schein RM, Sibbald WJ, American College of Chest Physicians/Society of Critical Care Medicine Consensus Conference: **Definitions for sepsis and organ failure and guidlines for the use of innovative therapies in sepsis.** *Chest* 1992, **101**:1644-1655.
8. Calandra T: **Pathogenesis of septic shock: implications for prevention and treatment.** *J Chemother* 2001, **13(Spec No 1(1))**:173-80, Review.
9. Bochud PY, Calandra T: **Pathogenesis of sepsis: new concepts and implications for future treatment.** *BMJ 2003* **326**:262-6.
10. Dinarello CA: **Proinfiammatory and anti-infiammatory cytokines as mediators in the pathogenesis of septic shock.** *Chest* 1997, **112**:321S-329S.
11. Rivers E, Nguyen B, Havstad S, Ressler J, Muzzin A, Knoblich B, Peterson E, Tomlanovich M, Early Goal-Directed Therapy Collaborative Group: **Early goal-directed therapy in the treatment of severe sepsis and septic shock.** *N Eng J Med* 2001, **345**:1368-1377.
12. Vincent JL, Biston P, Devriendt J, Brasseur A, De Backer D: **Dopamine versus norepinephrine: is one better?** *Minerva Anestesiol* 2009, **75(5)**:333-337.
13. Hollenberg SM: **Vasopressor support in septic shock.** *Chest* 2007, **132(5)**:1678-1687.
14. Bellomo R, Chapman M, Finfer S, Hickling K, Myburgh J: **Low-dose dopamine in patients with early renal dysfunction: A placebo-controlled randomised trial. Australian and New Zealand Intensive Care Society (ANZICS) Clinical Trials Group.** *Lancet* 2000, **356**:2139-2143.
15. Kellum J, Decker J: **Use of dopamine in acute renal failure: A meta-analysis.** *Crit Care Med* 2001, **29**:1526-1531.
16. Hesselvik JF, Brodin B: **Low dose norepinephrine in patients with septic shock and oliguria: effects on afterload, urine flow, and oxygen transport.** *Crit Care Med* 1989, **17**:179-180.
17. Meadows D, Edwards JD, Wilkins RG, Nightingale P: **Reversal of intractable septic shock with norepinephrine therapy.** *Crit Care Med* 1988, **16**:663-667.
18. Martin C, Papazian L, Perrin G, Saux P, Gouin F: **Norepinephrine or dopamine for the treatment of hyperdynamic septic shock.** *Chest* 1993, **103**:1826-1831.
19. Patel GP, Grahe JS, Sperry M, Singla S, Elpern E, Lateef O, Balk RA: **Efficacy and safety of dopamine versus norepinephrine in the management of septic shock.** *Shock* 2010, **33(4)**:375-80.
20. Flancbaum L, Dick M, Dasta J, Sinha R, Choban P: **A dose-response study of phenylephrine in critically ill, septic surgical patients.** *Eur J Clin Pharmacol* 1997, **51**:461-465.
21. De Backer D, Creteur J, Silva E, Vincent JL: **Effects of dopamine, norepinephrine, and epinephrine on the splanchnic circulation in septic shock: which is best?** *Crit Care Med* 2003, **31(6)**:1659-67.
22. Hollenberg SM, Ahrens TS, Annane D, Astiz ME, Chalfin DB, Dasta JF, Heard SO, Martin C, Napolitano LM, Susla GM, Totaro R, Vincent JL, Zanotti-Cavazzoni S: **Practice parameters for hemodynamic support of sepsis in adult patients: 2004 update.** *Crit Care Med* 2004, **32**:1928-1948.
23. Annane D, Vignon P, Renault A, Bollaert PE, Charpentier C, Martin C, Troché G, Ricard JD, Nitenberg G, Papazian L, Azoulay E, Bellissant E, CATS Study Group: **Norepinephrine plus dobutamine versus epinephrine alone for management of septic shock: a randomised trial.** *Lancet* 2007, **370(9588)**:676-84.
24. Holmes CL, Patel BM, Russell JA, Walley KR: **Physiology of vasopressin relevant to management of septic shock.** *Chest* 2001, **120(3)**:989-1002.

25. Russell JA, Walley KR, Singer J, Gordon AC, Hébert PC, Cooper DJ, Holmes CL, Mehta S, Granton JT, Storms MM, Cook DJ, Presneill JJ, Ayers D, VASST Investigators: **Vasopressin versus norepinephrine infusion in patients with septic shock.** *N Engl J Med* 2008, **358(9)**:877-87.
26. Azzarello G, Lanteri R, Rapisarda C, Santangelo M, Racalbuto A, Minutolo V, Di Cataldo A, Licata A: **Ultrasound-guided percutaneous treatment of abdominal collections.** *Chir Ital* 2009, **61(3)**:337-340.
27. Gazelle GS, Mueller PR: **Abdominal abscess: Imaging and intervention.** *Radiol Clin North Am* 1994, **32**:913-932.
28. VanSonnenberg E, Ferrucci JT, Mueller PR, Wittenberg J, Simeone JF: **Percutaneous drainage of abscesses and fluid collections: Technique, results, and applications.** *Radiology* 1982, **142**:1-10.
29. Bouali K, Magotteaux P, Jadot A, Saive C, Lombard R, Weerts J, Dallemagne B, Jehaes C, Delforge M, Fontaine F: **Percutaneous catheter drainage of abdominal abscess after abdominal surgery: Results in 121 cases.** *J Belg Radiol* 1993, **76**:11-14.
30. VanSonnenberg E, Wing VW, Casola G, Coons HG, Nakamoto SK, Mueller PR, Ferrucci JT Jr, Halasz NA, Simeone JF: **Temporizing effect of percutaneous drainage of complicated abscesses in critically ill patients.** *Am J Roentgenol* 1984, **142**:821-826.
31. Bufalari A, Giustozzi G, Moggi L: **Postoperative intra-abdominal abscesses: Percutaneous versus surgical treatment.** *Acta Chir Belg* 1996, **96(5)**:197-200.
32. VanSonnenberg E, Mueller PR, Ferrucci JT Jr: **Percutaneous drainage of 250 abdominal abscesses and fluid collections. I. Results, failures, and complications.** *Radiology* 1984, **151**:337-341.
33. Jaffe TA, Nelson RC, DeLong D, Paulson EK: **Practice Patterns in Percutaneous Image-guided Intra-abdominal Abscess Drainage: Survey of Academic and Private Practice Centres.** *Radiology* 2004, **233(3)**:750-6.
34. Shani V, Muchtar E, Kariv G, Robenshtok E, Leibovici L: **Systematic review and meta-analysis of the efficacy of appropriate empiric antibiotic therapy for sepsis.** *Antimicrob Agents Chemother* 2010, **54(11)**:4851-63.
35. Montravers P, Lepape A, Dubreuil L, Gauzit R, Pean Y, Benchimol D, Dupont H: **Clinical and microbiological profiles of community-acquired and nosocomial intra-abdominal infections: results of the French prospective, observational EBIIA study.** *J Antimicrob Chemother* 2009, **63(4)**:785-94.
36. Swenson BR, Metzger R, Hedrick TL, McElearney ST, Evans HL, Smith RL, Chong TW, Popovsky KA, Pruett TL, Sawyer RG: **Choosing antibiotics for intra-abdominal infections: what do we mean by "high risk"?** *Surg Infect (Larchmt)* 2009, **10(1)**:29-39.
37. Montravers P, Dupont H, Gauzit R, Veber B, Auboyer C, Blin P, Hennequin C, Martin C: **Candida as a risk factor for mortality in peritonitis.** *Crit Care Med* 2006, **34(3)**:646-52.
38. Montravers P, Mira JP, Gangneux JP, Leroy O, Lortholary O, the AmarCand study group: **A multicentre study of antifungal strategies and outcome of Candida spp. peritonitis in intensive-care units.** *Clin Microbiol Infect* 2010.
39. Lumb J: **Carbapenems in the treatment of intra-abdominal infection. Report from the 20th European Congress of Clinical Microbiology and Infectious Diseases. Vienna, Austria, 10-13 April 2010.** *Future Microbiol* 2010, **5(8)**:1165-6.
40. Hawser SP, Bouchillon SK, Hoban DJ, Badal RE, Cantón R, Baquero F: **Incidence and antimicrobial susceptibility of Escherichia coli and Klebsiella pneumoniae with extended-spectrum beta-lactamases in community- and hospital-associated intra-abdominal infections in Europe: results of the 2008 Study for Monitoring Antimicrobial Resistance Trends (SMART).** *Antimicrob Agents Chemother* 2010, **54(7)**:3043-6.
41. Coque TM, Baquero F, Canton R: **Increasing prevalence of ESBL-producing Enterobacteriaceae in Europe.** *Euro Surveill* 2008, **13(47)**[http://www.eurosurveillance.org/ViewArticle.aspx?ArticleId=19044].
42. Vatopoulos A: **High rates of metallo-beta-lactamase-producing Klebsiella neumoniae in Greece - a review of the current evidence.** *Euro Surveill* 2008, **13(4)**.
43. Ho J, Tambyah PA, Paterson DL: **Multiresistant Gram-negative infections: a global perspective.** *Curr Opin Infect Dis* 2010, **23(6)**:546-53.
44. Ho J, Tambyah PA, Paterson DL: **Multiresistant Gram-negative infections: a global perspective.** *Curr Opin Infect Dis* 2010, **23(6)**:546-53.
45. Riché FC, Dray X, Laisné MJ, Matéo J, Raskine L, Sanson-Le Pors MJ, Payen D, Valleur P, Cholley BP: **Factors associated with septic shock and mortality in generalized peritonitis: Comparison between community-acquired and postoperative peritonitis.** *Crit Care* 2009, **13(3)**:R99.
46. Pea F, Viale P, Furlanut M: **Antimicrobial therapy in critically ill patients: a review of pathophysiological conditions responsible for altered disposition and pharmacokinetic variability.** *Clin Pharmacokinet* 2005, **44**:1009-1034.
47. Pea F, Viale P: **Bench-to-bedside review: Appropriate antibiotic therapy in severe sepsis and septic shock–does the dose matter?** *Crit Care* 2009, **13(3)**:214.
48. Ho J, Tambyah PA, Paterson DL: **Multiresistant Gram-negative infections: a global perspective.** *Curr Opin Infect Dis* 2010, **23(6)**:546-53.
49. Pea F, Brollo L, Viale P, Pavan F, Furlanut M: **Teicoplanin therapeutic drug monitoring in critically ill patients: a retrospective study emphasizing the importance of a loading dose.** *J Antimicrob Chemother* 2003, **51(4)**:971-5.
50. Pea F, Viale P: **The antimicrobial therapy puzzle: could pharmacokinetic-pharmacodynamic relationships be helpful in addressing the issue of appropriate pneumonia treatment in critically ill patients?** *Clin Infect Dis* 2006, **42(12)**:1764-71.
51. Craig WA: **Basic pharmacodynamics of antibacterials with clinical applications to the use of beta-lactams, glycopeptides, and linezolid.** *Infect Dis Clin North Am* 2003, **17(3)**:479-501.
52. Lorente L, Jiménez A, Martín MM, *et al*: **Clinical cure of ventilator-associated pneumonia treated with piperacillin/tazobactam administered by continuous or intermittent infusion.** *Int J Antimicrob Agents* 2009, **33(5)**:464-8.
53. Lorente L, Lorenzo L, Martín MM, Jiménez A, Mora ML: **Meropenem by continuous versus intermittent infusion in ventilator-associated pneumonia due to gram-negative bacilli.** *Ann Pharmacother* 2006, **40(2)**:219-23.
54. Roberts JA, Lipman J, Blot S, Rello J: **Better outcomes through continuous infusion of time-dependent antibiotics to critically ill patients?** *Curr Opin Crit Care* 2008, **14(4)**:390-6.
55. Mueller EW, Boucher BA: **The use of extended-interval aminoglycoside dosing strategies for the treatment of moderate-to-severe infections encountered in critically ill surgical patients.** *Surg Infect (Larchmt)* 2009, **10(6)**:563-70.
56. Chakraborty A, Roy S, Loeffler J, Chaves RL: **Comparison of the pharmacokinetics, safety and tolerability of daptomycin in healthy adult volunteers following intravenous administration by 30 min infusion or 2 min injection.** *J Antimicrob Chemother* 2009, **64(1)**:151-8.
57. Menichetti F, Sganga G: **Definition and classification of intra-abdominal infections.** *J Chemother* 2009, , **Suppl 1**: 3-4.
58. Malangoni MA, Inui T: **Peritonitis - the Western experience.** *World J Emerg Surg* 2006, **1**:25.
59. Pieracci FM, Barie PS: **Management of severe sepsis of abdominal origin.** *Scand J Surg* 2007, **96(3)**:184-96.
60. Osborn TM, Nguyen HB, Rivers EP: **Emergency medicine and the surviving sepsis campaign: an international approach to managing severe sepsis and septic shock.** *Ann Emerg Med* 2005, **46(3)**:228-31.
61. Esteban A, Frutos-Vivar F, Ferguson ND, Peñuelas O, Lorente JA, Gordo F, Honrubia T, Algora A, Bustos A, García G, Diaz-Regañón IR, de Luna RR: **Sepsis incidence and outcome: contrasting the intensive care unit with the hospital ward.** *Crit Care Med* 2007, **35(5)**:1284-9.
62. Emmi V, Sganga G: **Diagnosis of intra-abdominal infections: clinical findings and imaging.** *Infez Med* 2008, , **Suppl 1**: 19-30.
63. Bartolozzi C: **Imaging and invasive techniques for diagnosis and treatment of surgical infections.** *Surg Infect (Larchmt)* 2006, **7(Suppl 2)**: S97-9.
64. Foinant M, Lipiecka E, Buc E, Boire JY, Schmidt J, Garcier JM, Pezet D, Boyer L: **Impact of computed tomography on patient's care in non-traumatic acute abdomen: 90 patients.** *J Radiol* 2007, **88(4)**:559-566.
65. Emmi V, Sganga G: **Clinical diagnosis of intra-abdominal infections.** *J Chemother* 2009, **21(Suppl 1)**:12-8.
66. Puylaert JB, van der Zant FM, Rijke AM: **Sonography and the acute abdomen: practical considerations.** *Am J Roentgenol* 1997, **168(1)**:179-86.
67. Doria AS, Moineddin R, Kellenberger CJ, Epelman M, Beyene J, Schuh S, Babyn PS, Dick PT: **US or CT for diagnosis of appendicitis in children and adults? A meta-analysis.** *Radiology* 2006, **241**:83-94.
68. TJ, Park KG, Steele RJ, Chung SS, Li AK: **A randomized trial of nonoperative treatment for perforated peptic ulcer.** *N Engl J Med* 1989, **320**:970-973.

69. Boey J, Lee NW, Koo J, Lam PH, Wong J, Ong GB: **Immediate definitive surgery for perforated duodenal ulcers: a prospective controlled trial.** *Ann Surg* 1982, **196**:338-344.
70. Millat B, Fingerhut A, Borie F: **Surgical treatment of complicated duodenal ulcers: controlled trials.** *World J Surg* 2000, **24**:299-306.
71. Crisp E: **Cases of perforation of the stomach with deductions therefrom relative to the character and treatment of that lesion.** *Lancet* **1843(2)**:639.
72. Wangensteen OH: **Nonoperative treatment of localized perforations of the duodenum.** *Minn Med* 1935, **18**:477-480.
73. Taylor H: **Peptic ulcer perforation treated without operation.** *Lancet* 1946, **2**:441-444.
74. Crofts TJ, Park KG, Steele RJ, Chung SS, Li AK: **A randomized trial of nonoperative treatment for perforated peptic ulcer.** *N Engl J Med* 1989, **320**:970-973.
75. Bucher P, Oulhaci W, Morel P, Ris F, Huber O: **Results of conservative treatment for perforated gastroduodenal ulcers in patients not eligible for surgical repair.** *Swiss Med Wkly* 2007, **137**:337-340.
76. Sogne B, Jean F, Foulatier O, Khalil H, Scotté M: **Non operative treatment for perforated peptic ulcer: results of a prospective study.** *Ann Chir* 2004, **129**:578-582.
77. Crofts TJ, Park KG, Steele RJ, Chung SS, Li AK: **A randomized trial of nonoperative treatment for perforated peptic ulcer.** *N Engl J Med* 1989, **320**:970-973.
78. Bucher P, Oulhaci W, Morel P, Ris F, Huber O: **Results of conservative treatment for perforated gastroduodenal ulcers in patients not eligible for surgical repair.** *Swiss Med Wkly* 2007, **137**:337-340.
79. Sogne B, Jean F, Foulatier O, Khalil H, Scotté M: **Non operative treatment for perforated peptic ulcer: results of a prospective study.** *Ann Chir* 2004, **129**:578-582.
80. Boey J, Choi SKI, Poon A, *et al*: **Risk stratification in perforated duodenal ulcers.** *Ann Surg* 1987, **205**:22-26.
81. Crofts TJ, Park KG, Steele RJ, Chung SS, Li AK: **A randomized trial of nonoperative treatment for perforated peptic ulcer.** *N Engl J Med* 1989, **320**:970-973.
82. Sogne B, Jean F, Foulatier O, Khalil H, Scotté M: **Non operative treatment for perforated peptic ulcer: results of a prospective study.** *Ann Chir* 2004, **129**:578-5827.
83. Svanes C, Lie RT, Svanes K, Lie SA, Soreide O: **Adverse effects of delayed treatment for perforated peptic ulcer.** *Ann Surg* 1994, **220(2)**:168-75.
84. Boey J, Lee NW, Koo J, Lam PH, Wong J, Ong GB: **Immediate definitive surgery for perforated duodenal ulcers: a prospective controlled trial.** *Ann Surg* 1982, **196**:338-344.
85. Tanphiphat C, Tanprayoon T, Nathalong A: **Surgical treatment of perforated duodenal ulcer: A prospective trial between simple closure and definitive surgery.** *Br J Surg* 1985, **72**:370.
86. Christiansen J, Andersen OB, Bonnesen T, Baekgaard N: **Perforated duodenal ulcer managed by simple closure versus closure and proximal gastric vagotomy.** *Br J Surg* 1987, **74(4)**:286-7.
87. Hay JM, Lacaine F, Kohlmann G, Fingerhut A: **Immediate definitive surgery for perforated duodenal ulcer does not increase operative mortality: a prospective controlled trial.** *World J Surg* 1988, **12(5)**:705-9.
88. Mikulicz J: **Ueber Laparotomie bei Magen und Darmperforation.** *Samml Klin Vort Leipzig* 1885, **262**:2307.
89. Cellan-Jones CJ: **A rapid method of treatment in perforated duodenal ulcer.** *BMJ* 1929, 1076-1077.
90. Graham RR: **The treatment of perforated duodenal ulcers.** *Surg Gynecol Obstet* 1937, 235-238.
91. Lau WY, Leung KL, Kwong KH, Davey IC, Robertson C, Dawson JJ, Chung SC, Li AK: **A randomized study comparing laparoscopic versus open repair of perforated peptic ulcer using suture or sutureless technique.** *Ann Surg* 1996, **224**:131-138.
92. Boey J, Lee NW, Koo J, Lam PH, Wong J, Ong GB: **Immediate definitive surgery for perforated duodenal ulcers: a prospective controlled trial.** *Ann Surg* 1982, **196**:338-344.
93. Tanphiphat C, Tanprayoon T, Nathalong A: **Surgical treatment of perforated duodenal ulcer: A prospective trial between simple closure and definitive surgery.** *Br J Surg* 1985, **72**:370.
94. Christiansen J, Andersen OB, Bonnesen T, Baekgaard N: **Perforated duodenal ulcer managed by simple closure versus closure and proximal gastric vagotomy.** *Br J Surg* 1987, **74(4)**:286-7.
95. Hay JM, Lacaine F, Kohlmann G, Fingerhut A: **Immediate definitive surgery for perforated duodenal ulcer does not increase operative mortality: a prospective controlled trial.** *World J Surg* 1988, **12(5)**:705-9.
96. Ng EK, Lam YH, Sung JJ, Yung MY, To KF, Chan AC, Lee DW, Law BK, Lau JY, Ling TK, Lau WY, Chung SC: **Eradication of Helicobacter pylori prevents recurrence of ulcer after simple closure of duodenal ulcer perforation: randomized controlled trial.** *Ann Surg* 2000, **231(2)**:153-8.
97. Haberer Von, Zur H: **Therapie akuter Geschwursperforationen des Magens und Duodenums in die freie Bauchhohle.** *Wien Klin Wochnschr* 1919, **32**:413.
98. Sarath Chandra SS, Kumar SS: **Definitive or conservative surgery for perforated gastric ulcer? An unresolved problem.** *Int J Surg* 2009, **7**:136-139.
99. Turner WW Jr, Thompson WM Jr, Thal ER: **Perforated gastric ulcers. A plea for management by simple closures.** *Arch Surg* 1988, **123(8)**:960-4.
100. Wysocki A, Biesiada Z, Beben P, Budzynski A: **Perforated gastric ulcer.** *Dig Surg* 2000, **17**:132-7.
101. Tsugawa K, Koyanagi N, Hashizume M, Tomikawa M, Akahoshi K, Ayukawa K, *et al*: **The therapeutic strategies in performing emergency surgery for gastroduodenal ulcer perforation in 130 patients over 70 years of age.** *Hepatogastroenterology* 2001, **48(37)**:156-62.
102. Sanabria A, Villegas MI, Morales Uribe CH: **Laparoscopic repair for perforated peptic ulcer disease.** *Cochrane Database of Systematic Reviews* 2010, **Issue 4.**
103. Lau H: **Laparoscopic repair of perforated peptic ulcer: a meta-analysis.** *Surg Endosc* 2004, **18(7)**:1013-21.
104. Lau WY, Leung KL, Kwong KH, Davey IC, Robertson C, Dawson JJ, Chung SC, Li AK: **A randomized study comparing laparoscopic versus open repair of perforated peptic ulcer using suture or sutureless technique.** *Annals of Surgery* 1996, **224**:131-8.
105. Siu WT, Leong HT, Law BK, Chau CH, Li AC, Fung KH, Tai YP, Li MK: **Laparoscopic repair for perforated peptic ulcer: a randomized controlled trial.** *Annals of Surgery* 2002, **235**:313-9.
106. Bertleff MJ, Halm JA, Bemelman WA, van der Ham AC, van der Harst E, Oei HI, Smulders JF, Steyerberg EW, Lange JF: **Randomized clinical trial of laparoscopic versus open repair of the perforated peptic ulcer: the LAMA Trial.** *World Journal of Surgery* 2009, **33**:1368-73.
107. Gertsch P, Choe LWC, Yuen ST, Chau KY, Lauder IJ: **Long term survival after gastrectomy for advanced bleeding or perforated gastric carcinoma.** *Eur J Surg* 1996, **162**:723-727.
108. Lehnert T, Buhl K, Dueck M, Hinz U, Herfarth C: **Two-stage radical gastrectomy for perforated gastric cancer.** *Eur J Surg Oncol* 2000, **26**:780-784.
109. Ozmen MM, Zulfikaroglu B, Kece C, Aslar AK, Ozalp N, Koc M: **Factors influencing mortality in spontaneous gastric tumour perforations.** *J Int Med Res* 2002, **30**:180-184.
110. So JBY, Yam A, Cheah WK, Kum CK, Goh PM: **Risk factors related to operative mortality and morbidity in patients undergoing emergency gastrectomy.** *Br J Surg* 2000, **87**:1702-1707.
111. Roviello F, Simone R, Marrelli D, *et al*: **Perforated gastric carcinoma: a report of 10 cases and review of the literature.** *World J Surg Oncol* 2006, **4**:19-24.
112. Jwo S, Chien R, Chao T, *et al*: **Clinicopathological features, surgical management, and disease outcome of perforated gastric cancer.** *J Surg Oncol* 2005, **91**:219-25.
113. Adachi Y, Mori M, Maehara Y, *et al*: **Surgical results of perforated gastric carcinoma: an analysis of 155 Japanese patients.** *Am J Gastroenterol* 1997, **92**:516-8.
114. Lehnert T, Buhl K, Dueck M, *et al*: **Two-stage radical gastrectomy for perforated gastric cancer.** *Eur J Surg Oncol* 2000, **26**:780-4.
115. Ayite A, Dosseh DE, Tekou HA, James K: **Surgical treatment of singl non traumatic perforation of small bowel: excision-suture or resection-anastomosis.** *Ann Chir* 2005, **131(2)**:91-5, (EL 3b).
116. Kirkpatrick AW, Baxter KA, Simons RK, Germann E, Lucas CE, Ledgerwood AM: **Intra-abdominal complications after surgical repair of small bowel injuries: an international reiew.** *J Trauma* 2003, **55(3)**:399-406.
117. Kirkpatrick AW, Baxter KA, Simons RK, Germann E, Lucas CE, Ledgerwood AM: **Intra-abdominal complications after surgical repair of small bowel injuries: an international reiew.** *J Trauma* 2003, **55(3)**:399-406.

118. Ayite A, Dosseh DE, Tekou HA, James K: **Surgical treatment of single non traumatic perforation of small bowel: excision-suture or resection-anastomosis.** *Ann Chir* 2005, **131(2)**:91-5, (EL 3b).
119. Kirkpatrick AW, Baxter KA, Simons RK, Germann E, Lucas CE, Ledgerwood AM: **Intra-abdominal complications after surgical repair of small bowel injuries: an international reiew.** *J Trauma* 2003, **55(3)**:399-406.
120. Kirkpatrick AW, Baxter KA, Simons RK, Germann E, Lucas CE, Ledgerwood AM: **Intra-abdominal complications after surgical repair of small bowel injuries: an international reiew.** *J Trauma* 2003, **55(3)**:399-406.
121. De Graaf JS, van Goor H, Blechrodt RP: **Primary small bowel anastomosis in generalized peritonitis.** *Eur j Surg* 1996, **162(1)**:55-8.
122. Sinha R, Sharma N, Joshi M: **Laparoscopic repair of small bowel perforation.** *JSLS* 2005, **9**:399-402.
123. Hansson J, Körner U, Khorram-Manesh A, Solberg A, Lundholm K: **Randomized clinical trial of antibiotic therapy versus appendicectomy as primary treatment of acute appendicitis in unselected patients.** *Br J Surg* 2009, **96**:473-481.
124. Styrud J, Eriksson S, Nilsson I, Ahlberg G, Haapaniemi S, Neovius G, Rex L, Badume I, Granström L: **Appendectomy versus antibiotic treatment in acute appendicitis. A prospective multicenter randomized controlled trial.** *World J Surg* 2006, **30**:1033-1037.
125. Eriksson S, Granström L: **Randomized controlled trial of appendicectomy versus antibiotic therapy for acute appendicitis.** *Br J Surg* 1995, **82**:166-169.
126. Varadhan KK, Humes DJ, Neal KR, Lobo DN: **Antibiotic therapy versus appendectomy for acute appendicitis: a meta-analysis.** *World J Surg* 2010, **34**:199-209.
127. Taylor M, Emil S, Nguyen N, Ndiforchu F: **Emergent vs urgent appendectomy in children: a study of outcomes.** *J Pediatr Surg* 2005, **40**:1912-1915.
128. Ditillo MF, Dziura JD, Rabinovici R: **Is it safe to delay appendectomy in adults with acute appendicitis?** *Ann Surg* 2006, **244**:656-660.
129. Sauerland S, Lefering R, Neugebauer EA: **Laparoscopic versus open surgery for suspected appendicitis.** *Cochrane Database Syst Rev* 2002, CD001546.
130. Faiz O, Clark J, Brown T, Bottle A, Antoniou A, Farrands P, Darzi A, Aylin P: **Traditional and laparoscopic appendectomy in adults: outcomes in English NHS hospitals between 1996 and 2006.** *Ann Surg* 2008, **248**:800-806.
131. Sporn E, Petroski GF, Mancini GJ, Astudillo JA, Miedema BW, Thaler K: **Laparoscopic appendectomy–is it worth the cost? Trend analysis in the US from 2000 to 2005.** *J Am Coll Surg* 2009, **208**:179-185.
132. Oliak D, Yamini D, Udani VM, Lewis RJ, Arnell T, Vargas H, Stamos MJ: **Initial nonoperative management for periappendiceal abscess.** *Dis Colon Rectum* 2001, **44**:936-941.
133. Brown CV, Abrishami M, Muller M, Velmahos GC: **Appendiceal abscess: immediate operation or percutaneous drainage?** *Am Surg* 2003, **69**:829-832.
134. Andersson RE, Petzold MG: **Nonsurgical treatment of appendiceal abscess or phlegmon: a systematic review and meta-analysis.** *Ann Surg* 2007, **246**:741-748.
135. Corfield L: **Interval appendicectomy after appendiceal mass or abscess in adults: what is "best practice"?** *Surg Today* 2007, **37**:1-4.
136. Kaminski A, Liu IL, Applebaum H, Lee SL, Haigh PI: **Routine interval appendectomy is not justified after initial nonoperative treatment of acute appendicitis.** *Arch Surg* 2005, **140**:897-901.
137. Rafferty J, Shellito P, Hyman NH, Buie WD: **Standards Committee of American Society of Colon and Rectal Surgeons: Practice parameters for sigmoid diverticulitis.** *Dis Colon Rectum* 2006, **49**:939-944.
138. Wong WD, Wexner SD, Lowry A, Vernava A, Burnstein M, Denstman F, Fazio V, Kerner B, Moore R, Oliver G, Peters W, Ross T, Senatore P, Simmang C: **Practice parameters for the treatment of sigmoid diverticulitis–supporting documentation. The Standards Task Force. The American Society of Colon and Rectal Surgeons.** *Dis Colon Rectum* 2000, **43**:290-297.
139. Patient Care Committee of the Society for Surgery of the Alimentary Tract (SSAT): **Surgical treatment of diverticulitis.** *J Gastrointest Surg* 1999, **3**:212-213.
140. Stollman NH, Raskin JB: **Diagnosis and management of diverticular disease of the colon in adults. Ad Hoc Practice Parameters Committee of the American College of Gastroenterology.** *Am J Gastroenterol* 1999, **94**:3110-3121.
141. Köhler L, Sauerland S, Neugebauer E: **Diagnosis and treatment of diverticular disease: results of a consensus development conference. The Scientific Committee of the European Association for Endoscopic Surgery.** *Surg Endosc* 1999, **13**:430-436.
142. Hinchey EJ, Schaal PG, Richards GK: **Treatment of perforated diverticular disease of the colon.** *Adv Surg* 1978, **12**:85-109.
143. Ambrosetti P, Jenny A, Becker C, Terrier TF, Morel P: **Acute left colonic diverticulitis–compared performance of computed tomography and water-soluble contrast enema: prospective evaluation of 420 patients.** *Dis Colon Rectum* 2000, **43**:1363-1367.
144. Stollman N, Raskin JB: **Diverticular disease of the colon.** *Lancet* 2004, **363**:631-639.
145. Jacobs DO: **Clinical practice. Diverticulitis.** *N Engl J Med* 2007, **357**:2057-2066.
146. Broderick-Villa G, Burchette RJ, Collins JC, Abbas MA, Haigh PI: **Hospitalization for acute diverticulitis does not mandate routine elective colectomy.** *Arch Surg* 2005, **140**:576-581.
147. Mueller MH, Glatzle J, Kasparek MS, Becker HD, Jehle EC, Zittel TT, Kreis ME: **Long-term outcome of conservative treatment in patients with diverticulitis of the sigmoid colon.** *Eur J Gastroenterol Hepatol* 2005, **17**:649-654.
148. Ambrosetti P, Robert J, Witzig JA, Mirescu D, de Gautard R, Borst F, Rohner A: **Incidence, outcome, and proposed management of isolated abscesses complicating acute left-sided colonic diverticulitis: a prospective study of 140 patients.** *Dis Colon Rectum* 1992, **35**:1072-1076.
149. Siewert B, Tye G, Kruskal J, Sosna J, Opelka F, Raptopoulos V, Goldberg SN: **Impact of CT-guided drainage in the treatment of diverticular abscesses: size matters.** *AJR Am J Roentgenol* 2006, **186**:680-686, [Erratum, AJR Am J Roentgenol 2007; 189:512.].
150. Kumar RR, Kim JT, Haukoos JS, Macias LH, Dixon MR, Stamos MJ, Konyalian VR: **Factors affecting the successful management of intra-abdominal abscesses with antibiotics and the need for percutaneous drainage.** *Dis Colon Rectum* 2006, **49**:183-189.
151. McKee RF, Deignan RW, Krukowski ZH: **Radiological investigation in acute diverticulitis.** *Br J Surg* 1993, **80**:560-565.
152. Padidar AM, Jeffrey RB Jr, Mindelzun RE, Dolph JF: **Differentiating sigmoid diverticulitis from carcinoma on CT scans: mesenteric inflammation suggests diverticulitis.** *AJR Am J Roentgenol* 1994, **163**:81-83.
153. Stabile BE, Puccio E, vanSonnenberg E, Neff CC: **Preoperative percutaneous drainage of diverticular abscesses.** *Am J Surg* 1990, **159**:99-104.
154. Kaiser AM, Jiang JK, Lake JP, Ault G, Artinyan A, Gonzalez-Ruiz C, Essani R, Beart RW Jr: **The management of complicated diverticulitis and the role of computed tomography.** *Am J Gastroenterol* 2005, **100**:910-917.
155. Biondo S, Parés D, Martí-Ragué J, Kreisler E, Fraccalvieri D, Jaurrieta E: **Acute colonic diverticulitis in patients under 50 years of age.** *Br J Surg* 2002, **89**:1137-1141.
156. Schoetz DJ: **Diverticular disease of the colon: a century-old problem.** *Dis Colon Rectum* 1999, **42**:703-709.
157. Thaler K, Baig MK, Berho M, Weiss EG, Nogueras JJ, Arnaud JP, Wexner SD, Bergamaschi R: **Determinants of recurrence after sigmoid resection for uncomplicated diverticulitis.** *Dis Colon Rectum* 2003, **46**:385-388.
158. Schwandner O, Farke S, Fischer F, Eckmann C, Schiedeck TH, Bruch HP: **Laparoscopic colectomy for recurrent and complicated diverticulitis: a prospective study of 396 patients.** *Langenbecks Arch Surg* 2004, **389**:97-103.
159. Guller U, Jain N, Hervey S, Purves H, Pictoobon R: **Laparoscopic vs. open colectomy: outcomes comparison based on large nationwide databases.** *Arch Surg* 2003, **138**:1179-1186.
160. Dwivedi A, Chahin F, Agrawal S, Chau WY, Tootla A, Tootla F, Silva YJ: **Laparoscopic colectomy vs. open colectomy for sigmoid diverticular disease.** *Dis Colon Rectum* 2002, **45**:1309-1314.
161. Tuech JJ, Pessaux P, Rouge C, Regenet N, Bergamaschi R, Arnaud JP: **Laparoscopic vs. open colectomy for sigmoid diverticulitis: a prospective comparative study in the elderly.** *Surg Endosc* 2000, **14**:1031-1033.
162. Bartus CM, Lipof T, Sarwar CM, Vignati PV, Johnson KH, Sardella WV, Cohen JL: **Colovesicle fistula: not a contraindication to elective laparoscopic colectomy.** *Dis Colon Rectum* 2005, **48**:233-236.

163. Chapman J, Davies M, Wolff B, Dozois E, Tessier D, Harrington J, Larson D: **Complicated diverticulitis: is it time to rethink the rules?** *Ann Surg* 2005, **242**:576-581.
164. Ordoñez CA, Puyana JC: **Management of peritonitis in the critically ill patient.** *Surg Clin North Am* 2006, **86**:1323-1349.
165. Blot S, De Waele JJ: **Critical issues in the clinical management of complicated intra-abdominal infections.** *Drugs* 2005, **65**:1611-1620.
166. Belmonte C, Klas JV, Perez JJ, *et al*: **The Hartmann procedure. First choice or last resort in diverticular disease?** *Arch Surg* 1996, **131**:612-615.
167. Rothenberger DA, Wiltz O: **Surgery for complicated diverticulitis.** *Surg Clin North Am* 1993, **73**:975-992.
168. Constantinides VA, Tekkis PP, Athanasiou T, Aziz O, Purkayastha S, Remzi FH, Fazio VW, Aydin N, Darzi A, Senapati A: **Primary resection with anastomosis vs. Hartmann's procedure in nonelective surgery for acute colonic diverticulitis: a systematic review.** *Dis Colon Rectum* 2006, **49**:966-981.
169. Vermeulen J, Coene PPLO, van Hout NM, van der Harst E, Mannaerts GHH, Weidema WF, Lange JF: **Restoration of bowel continuity after surgery for acute perforated diverticulitis: should Hartmann's procedure be considered a one-stage procedure?** *Colorectal Dis* 2009, **11**:619-624.
170. Nugent KP, Daniels P, Stewart B, Patankar R, Johnson CD: **Quality of life in stoma patients.** *Dis Colon Rectum* 1999, **42**:1569-1574.
171. Vermeulen J, Gosselink MP, Busschbach JJ, Lange JF: **Avoiding or reversing Hartmann's procedure provides improved quality of life after perforated diverticulitis.** *J Gastrointest Surg* 2010, **14**:651-657.
172. Salem L, Flum DR: **Primary anastomosis or Hartmann's procedure for patients with diverticular peritonitis? A systematic review.** *Dis Colon Rectum* 2004, **47**:1953-1964.
173. Blair NP, Germann E: **Surgical management of acute sigmoid diverticulitis.** *Am J Surg* 2002, **183**:525-528.
174. Lee EC, Murray JJ, Coller JA, Roberts PL, Schoetz DJ Jr: **Intraoperative colonic lavage in nonelective surgery for diverticular disease.** *Dis Colon Rectum* 1997, **40**:669-674.
175. Solomkin JS, Mazuski JE, Baron EJ, Sawyer RG, Nathens AB, DiPiro JT, Buchman T, Dellinger EP, Jernigan J, Gorbach S, Chow AW, Bartlett J, Infectious Diseases Society of America: **Guidelines for the selection of anti-infective agents for complicated intra-abdominal infections.** *Clin Infect Dis* 2003, **15,37(8)**:997-1005.
176. Weigelt JA: **Empiric treatment options in the management of complicated intra-abdominal infections.** *Cleve Clin J Med* 2007, **74(Suppl 4)**:S29-37.
177. Oteo J, Pérez-Vázquez M, Campos J: **Extended-spectrum [beta]-lactamase producing Escherichia coli: changing epidemiology and clinical impact.** *Curr Opin Infect Dis* 2010, **23(4)**:320-6, Review.
178. Solomkin JS, Yellin AE, Rotstein OD, Christou NV, Dellinger EP, Tellado JM, Malafaia O, Fernandez A, Choe KA, Carides A, Satishchandran V, Teppler H, Protocol 017 Study Group: **Ertapenem versus piperacillin/tazobactam in the treatment of complicated intraabdominal infections: results of a double-blind,randomized comparative phase III trial.** *Ann Surg* 2003, **237(2)**:235-45.
179. Malangoni MA, Song J, Herrington J, Choudhri S, Pertel P: **Randomized controlled trial of moxifloxacin compared with piperacillin-tazobactam and amoxicillin-clavulanate for the treatment of complicated intra-abdominal infections.** *Ann Surg* 2006, **244(2)**:204-11.
180. Mazuski JE: **Antimicrobial treatment for intra-abdominal infections.** *Expert Opin Pharmacother* 2007, **8(17)**:2933-45.
181. Powell LL, Wilson SE: **The role of beta-lactam antimicrobials as single agents in treatment of intra-abdominal infection.** *Surg Infect (Larchmt)* 2000, **1(1)**:57-63.
182. Lode HM: **Rational antibiotic therapy and the position of ampicillin/ sulbactam.** *Int J Antimicrob Agents* 2008, **32(1)**:10-28.
183. Gin A, Dilay L, Karlowsky JA, Walkty A, Rubinstein E, Zhanel GG: **Piperacillin-tazobactam: A beta-lactam/beta-lactamase inhibitor combination.** *Expert Rev Anti Infect Ther* 2007, **5(3)**:365-383.
184. Al-Hasan MN, Lahr BD, Eckel-Passow JE, Baddour LM: **Antimicrobial resistance trends of Escherichia coli bloodstream isolates: A population-based study, 1998-2007.** *J Antimicrob Chemother* 2009, **64(1)**:169-174.
185. Paterson DL, Bonomo RA: **Extended-Spectrum ß-Lactamases: A Clinical Update.** *Clin Microbiol Rev* 2005, **18(4)**:657-686.
186. Paterson DL: **Resistance in gram-negative bacteria: Enterobacteriaceae.** *Am J Infect Control* 2006, **34(5 Suppl 1)**:S20-8.
187. Murray BE: **The life and times of the Enterococcus.** *Clin Microbiol Rev* 1990, **3**:45-65.
188. Garbino J, Villiger P, Caviezel A, Matulionyte R, Uckay I, Morel P, Lew D: **A randomized prospective study of cefepime plus metronidazole with imipenem-cilastatin in the treatment of intra-abdominal infections.** *Infection* 2007, **35(3)**:161-166.
189. Ho J, Tambyah PA, Paterson DL: **Multiresistant Gram-negative infections: a global perspective.** *Curr Opin Infect Dis* 2010, **23(6)**:546-53.
190. Hammond ML: **Ertapenem: A Group 1 carbapenem with distinct antibacterial and pharmacological properties.** *J Antimicrob Chemother* 2004, **53(Suppl 2)**:ii7-9.
191. Falagas ME, Peppas G, Makris GC, Karageorgopoulos DE, Matthaiou DK: **Meta-analysis: Ertapenem for complicated intra-abdominal infections.** *Aliment Pharmacol Ther* 2008, **27(10)**:919-931.
192. Chahine EB, Ferrill MJ, Poulakos MN: **Doripenem: A new carbapenem antibiotic.** *Am J Health Syst Pharm* 2010, **67(23)**:2015-24.
193. Borcherding SM, Stevens R, Nicholas RA, Corley CR, Self T: **Quinolones: A practical review of clinical uses, dosing considerations, and drug interactions.** *J Fam Pract* 1996, **42**:69-78.
194. Falagas ME, Matthaiou DK, Bliziotis IA: **Systematic review: Fluoroquinolones for the treatment of intra-abdominal surgical infections.** *Aliment Pharmacol Ther* 2007, **25(2)**:123-131.
195. Weiss G, Reimnitz P, Hampel B, Muehlhofer E, Lippert H, AIDA Study Group: **Moxifloxacin for the treatment of patients with complicated intra-abdominal infections (the AIDA Study).** *J Chemother* 2009, **21(2)**:170-180.
196. Stein GE: **Pharmacokinetics and pharmacodynamics of newer fluoroquinolones.** *Clin Infect Dis* 1996, **23(suppl 1)**:S19-24.
197. Edmiston CE, Krepel CJ, Seabrook GR, Somberg LR, Nakeeb A, Cambria RA, Towne JB: **In vitro activities of moxifloxacin against 900 aerobic and anaerobic surgical isolates from patients with intra-abdominal and diabetic foot infections.** *Antimicrob Agents Chemother* 2004, **48(3)**:1012-1016.
198. Goldstein EJ, Citron DM, Warren YA, Tyrrell KL, Merriam CV, Fernandez H: **In vitro activity of moxifloxacin against 923 anaerobes isolated from human intra-abdominal infections.** *Antimicrob Agents Chemother* 2006, **50(1)**:148-155.
199. Solomkin J, Zhao YP, Ma EL, Chen MJ, Hampel B: **DRAGON Study Team.** *Int J Antimicrob Agents* 2009, **34(5)**:439-445.
200. Wagner C, Sauermann R, Joukhadar C: **Principles of antibiotic penetration into abscess fluid.** *Pharmacology* 2006, **78(1)**:1-10.
201. Bradford PA: **Tigecycline: A first in class glycylcycline.** *Clin Microbiol Newsl* 2004, **26**:163-168.
202. Townsend ML, Pound MW, Drew RH: **Tigecycline in the treatment of complicated intra-abdominal and complicated skin and skin structure infections.** *Ther Clin Risk Manag* 2007, **3(6)**:1059-1070.
203. Boucher HW, Wennersten CB, Eliopoulos GM: **In vitro activities of the glycylcycline GAR-936 against gram-positive bacteria.** *Antimicrob Agents Chemother* 2000, **44**:2225-2229.
204. Papaparaskevas J, Tzouvelekis LS, Tsakris A, Pittaras TE, Legakis NJ, Hellenic Tigecycline Study Group: **In vitro activity of tigecycline against 2423 clinical isolates and comparison of the available interpretation breakpoints.** *Diagn Microbiol Infect Dis* 2010, **66(2)**:187-194.
205. Giamarellou H, Poulakou G: **Multidrug-resistant Gram-negative infections: What are the treatment options?** *Drugs* 2009, **69(14)**:1879-1901.
206. Hirsch EB, Tam VH: **Detection and treatment options for Klebsiella pneumoniae carbapenemases (KPCs): an emerging cause of multidrug-resistant infection.** *J Antimicrob Chemother* 2010, **65(6)**:1119-25.
207. Hoffmann M, DeMaio W, Jordan RA, Talaat R, Harper D, Speth J, Scatina J: **Metabolism, excretion, and pharmacokinetics of [14C]tigecycline, a first-in-class glycylcycline antibiotic, after intravenous infusion to healthy male subjects.** *Drug Metab Dispos* 2007, **35(9)**:1543-53.
208. Rodvold KA, Gotfried MH, Cwik M, Korth-Bradley JM, Dukart G, Ellis-Grosse EJ: **Serum, tissue and body fluid concentrations of tigecycline after a single 100 mg dose.** *J Antimicrob Chemother* 2006, **58(6)**:1221-9.
209. Eagye KJ, Kuti JL, Dowzicky M, Nicolau DP: **Empiric therapy for secondary peritonitis: a pharmacodynamic analysis of cefepime, ceftazidime, ceftriaxone, imipenem, levofloxacin, piperacillin/tazobactam, and tigecycline using Monte Carlo simulation.** *Clin Ther* 2007, **29(5)**:889-99.

210. Babinchak T, Ellis-Grosse E, Dartois N, Rose GM, Loh E, Tigecycline 301 Study Group: **The efficacy and safety of tigecycline for the treatment of complicated intra-abdominal infections: analysis of pooled clinical trial data.** *Clin Infect Dis* 2005, **41(Suppl 5)**:S354-67.
211. Towfigh S, Pasternak J, Poirier A, Leister H, Babinchak T: **A multicentre, open-label, randomized comparative study of tigecycline versus ceftriaxone sodium plus metronidazole for the treatment of hospitalized subjects with complicated intra-abdominal infections.** *Clin Microbiol Infect* 2010, **16(8)**:1274-81.
212. Yoshida M, Takada T, Kawarada Y, *et al*: **Antimicrobial therapy for acute cholecystitis: Tokyo Guidelines.** *J Hepatobiliary Pancreat Surg* 2007, **14**:83-90.
213. Takada T, Kawarada Y, Nimura Y, *et al*: **Background: Tokyo Guidelines for the management of acute cholangitis and cholecystitis.** *J Hepatobiliary Pancreat Surg* 2007, **14**:1-10.
214. Mayumi T, Takada T, Kawarada Y, *et al*: **Results of the Tokyo Consensus Meeting Tokyo Guidelines.** *J Hepatobiliary Pancreat Surg* 2007, **14**:114-21.
215. Kiviluoto T, Sirén J, Luukkonen P, Kivilaakso E: **Randomised trial of laparoscopic versus open cholecystectomy for acute and gangrenous cholecystitis.** *Lancet* 1998, **351(9099)**:321-5.
216. Johansson M, Thune A, Nelvin L, Stiernstam M, Westman B, Lundell L: **Randomized clinical trial of open versus laparoscopic cholecystectomy in the treatment of acute cholecystitis.** *Br J Surg* 2005, **92(1)**:44-9.
217. Kum CK, Goh PMY, Isaac JR, Tekant Y, Ngoi SS: **Laparoscopic cholecystectomy for acute cholecystitis.** *Br J Surg* 1994, **81**:1651-1654.
218. Chau CH, Tang CN, Siu WT, Ha JP, Li MK: **Laparoscopic cholecystectomy versus open cholecystectomy in elderly patients with acute cholecystitis: retrospective study.** *Hong Kong Med* 2002, **J8**:394-399.
219. Pessaux P, Regenet N, Tuech JJ, Rouge C, Bergamaschi R, Arnaud JP: **Laparoscopic versus open cholecystectomy: a prospective comparative study in the elderly with acute cholecystitis.** *Surg Laparosc Endosc Percutan Tech* 2001, **11**:252-255.
220. Lujan JA, Parrilla P, Robles R, Marin P, Torralba JA, Garcia-Ayllon J: **Laparoscopic chole cystectomy vs open cholecystectomy in the treatment of acute cholecystitis: a prospective study.** *Arch Surg* 1998, **133**:173-175.
221. Gurusamy K, Samraj K, Gluud C, Wilson E, Davidson BR: **Meta-analysis of randomized controlled trials on the safety and effectiveness of early versus delayed laparoscopic cholecystectomy for acute cholecystitis.** *Br J Surg* 2010, **97(2)**:141-50.
222. Siddiqui T, MacDonald A, Chong PS, Jenkins JT: **Early versus delayed laparoscopic cholecystectomy for acute cholecystitis: a meta-analysis of randomized clinical trials.** *Am J Surg* 2008, **195(1)**:40-7.
223. Lau H, Lo CY, Patil NG, Yuen WK: **Early versus delayed-interval laparoscopic cholecystectomy for acute cholecystitis: a meta-analysis.** *Surg Endosc* 2006, **20(1)**:82-7.
224. Papi C, Catarci M, D'Ambrosio L, Gili L, Koch M, Grassi GB, Capurso L: **Timing of cholecystectomy for acute calculous cholecystitis: a meta-analysis.** *Am J Gastroenterol* 2004, **99(1)**:147-55.
225. Hadad SM, Vaidya JS, Baker L, Koh HC, Heron TP, Hussain K, Thompson AM: **Delay from symptom onset increases the conversion rate in laparoscopic cholecystectomy for acute cholecystitis.** *World J Surg* 2007, **31(6)**:1298-01, discussion 1302-3.
226. Winbladh A, Gullstrand P, Svanvik J, Sandström P: **Systematic review of cholecystostomy as a treatment option in acute cholecystitis.** *HPB (Oxford)* 2009, **11(3)**:183-93.
227. Menakuru SR, Kaman L, Behera A, Singh R, Katariya RN: **Current management of gall bladder perforations.** *ANZ J Surg* 2004, **74**:843-846.
228. Roslyn JJ, Thompson JE Jr, Darvin H, DenBesten L: **Risk factors for gallbladder perforation.** *Am J Gastroenterol* 1987, **82**:636-640.
229. Ong CL, Wong TH, Rauff A: **Acute gall bladder perforation-a dilemma in early diagnosis.** *Gut* 1991, **32**:956-958.
230. Stefanidis D, Sirinek KR, Bingener J: **Gallbladder perforation: risk factors and outcome.** *J Surg Res* 2006, **131(2)**:204-8, Epub 2006 Jan 18.
231. O'Connor MJ, Schwartz ML, McQuarrie DG, Sumer HW: **Acute bacterial cholangitis: an analysis of clinical manifestation.** *Arch Surg* 1982, **117**:437-41, 2.
232. Welch JP, Donaldson GA: **The urgency of diagnosis and surgical treatment of acute suppurative cholangitis.** *Am J Surg* 1976, **131**:527-32.
233. Lai EC, Mok FP, Tan ES, Lo CM, Fan ST, You KT, Wong J: **Endoscopic biliary drainage for severe acute cholangitis.** *N Engl J Med* 1992, **24**:1582-6.
234. Lee DWH, Chung SCS: **Biliary infection.** *Baillieres Clin Gastroenterol* 1997, **11**:707-24.
235. Lipsett PA, Pitt HA: **Acute cholangitis.** *Surg Clin North Am* 1990, **70**:1297-312.
236. Hanau LH, Steigbigel NH: **Acute cholangitis.** *Infect Dis Clin North Am* 2000, **14**:521-46.
237. Lee JG: **Diagnosis and management of acute cholangitis.** *Nat Rev Gastroenterol Hepatol* 2009, **6(9)**:533-41.
238. Saltzstein EC, Peacock JB, Mercer LC: **Early operation for acute biliary tract stone disease.** *Surgery* 1983, **94**:704-8.
239. Westphal JF, Brogard JM: **Biliary tract infections: a guide to drug treatment.** *Drugs* 1999, **57(1)**:81-91.
240. Jarvinen H: **Biliary bacteremia at various stages of acute cholecystitis.** *Acta Chir Scand* 1980, **146**:427-30.
241. Westphal J, Brogard J: **Biliary tract infections: a guide to drug treatment.** *Drugs* 1999, **57**:81-91.
242. Sinanan M: **Acute cholangitis.** *Infect Dis Clin North Am* 1992, **6**:571-99.
243. Blenkharn J, Habib N, Mok D, John L, McPherson G, Gibson R, *et al*: **Decreased biliary excretion of piperacillin after percutaneous relief of extrahepatic obstructive jaundice.** *Antimicrob Agents Chemother* 1985, **28**:778-80.
244. van den Hazel S, De Vries X, Speelman P, Dankert J, Tytgat G, Huibregtse K, *et al*: **Biliary excretion of ciprofloxacin and piperacillin in the obstructed biliary tract.** *Antimicrob Agents Chemother* 1996, **40**:2658-60.
245. Levi J, Martinez O, Malinin T, Zeppa R, Livingstone A, Hutson D, *et al*: **Decreased biliary excretion of cefamandole after percutaneous biliary decompression in patients with total common bile duct obstruction.** *Antimicrob Agents Chemother* 1984, **26**:944-6.
246. Tanaka A, Takada T, Kawarada Y, Nimura Y, Yoshida M, Miura F, Hirota M, Wada K, Mayumi T, Gomi H, Solomkin JS, Strasberg SM, Pitt HA, Belghiti J, de Santibanes E, Padbury R, Chen MF, Belli G, Ker CG, Hilvano SC, Fan ST, Liau KH: **Antimicrobial therapy for acute cholangitis: Tokyo Guidelines.** *J Hepatobiliary Pancreat Surg* 2007, **14(1)**:59-67, Epub 2007 Jan 30.
247. Pacelli F, Doglietto GB, Alfieri S, *et al*: **Prognosis in intraabdominal infection. Multivariate analysis in 604 patients.** *Arch Surg* 1996, **131**:641-645.
248. Roehrborn A, Thomas L, Potreck O, Ebener C, Ohmann C, Goretzki P, Röher H: **The microbiology of postoperative peritonitis.** *Clin Infect Dis* 2001, **33**:1513-1519.
249. Torer N, Yorganci K, Elker D, Sayek I: **Prognostic factors of the mortality of postoperative intraabdominal infections.** *Infection* 2010.
250. Mulier S, Penninckx F, Verwaest C, Filez L, Aerts R, Fieuws S, Lauwers P: **Factors affecting ortality in generalized postoperative peritonitis: multivariate analysis in 96 patients.** *World J Surg* 2003, **27(4)**:379-84.
251. Khamphommala L, Parc Y, Bennis M, Ollivier JM, Dehni N, Tiret E, Parc R: **Results of an aggressive surgical approach in the management of postoperative peritonitis.** *ANZ J Surg* 2008, **78(10)**:881-8.
252. Parc Y, Frileux P, Schmitt G, Dehni N, Ollivier JM, Parc R: **Management of postoperative peritonitis after anterior resection: experience from a referral intensive care unit.** *Dis Colon Rectum* 2000, **43(5)**:579-587.
253. Bohnen J, Boulanger M, Meakins JL, McLean AP: **Prognosis in generalized peritonitis. Relation to cause and risk factors.** *Arch Surg* 1983, **118(3)**:285-90.
254. Montravers P, Chalfine A, Gauzit R, Lepape A, Pierre Marmuse J, Vouillot C, Martin C: **Clinical and therapeutic features of nonpostoperative nosocomial intra-abdominal infections.** *Ann Surg* 2004, **239(3)**:409-16.
255. Ordoñez CA, Puyana JC: **Management of peritonitis in the critically ill patient.** *Surg Clin North Am* 2006, **86(6)**:1323-49.
256. Inui T, Haridas M, Claridge JA, Malangoni MA: **Mortality for intra-abdominal infection is associated with intrinsic risk factors rather than the source of infection.** *Surgery* 2009, **146(4)**:654-61, discussion 661-2.ct;146 (4):654-61; discussion 661-2.
257. Theisen J, Bartels H, Weiss W, Berger H, Stein HJ, Siewert JR: **Current concepts of percutaneous abscess drainage in postoperative retention.** *J Gastrointest Surg* 2005, **9(2)**:280-3.
258. Khurrum Baig M, Hua Zhao R, Batista O, Uriburu JP, Singh JJ, Weiss EG, Nogueras JJ, Wexner SD: **Percutaneous postoperative intra-abdominal abscess drainage after elective colorectal surgery.** *Tech Coloproctol* 2002, **6(3)**:159-64.

259. Benoist S, Panis Y, Pannegeon V, Soyer P, Watrin T, Boudiaf M, Valleur P: **Can failure of percutaneous drainage of postoperative abdominal abscesses be predicted?** *Am J Surg* 2002, **184(2)**:148-53.
260. Koperna T, Schulz F: **Prognosis and treatment of peritonitis. Do we need new scoring systems?** *Arch Surg* 1996, **131(2)**:180-6.
261. Koperna T, Schulz F: **Relaparotomy in peritonitis: prognosis and treatment of patients with persisting intraabdominal infection.** *World J Surg* 2000, **24(1)**:32-7.
262. Farthmann EH, Schoffel U: **Principles and limitations of operative management of intraabdominal infections.** *World J Surg* 1990, **14(2)**:210-217.
263. Hutchins RR, Gunning MP, Lucas DN, Allen-Mersh TG, Soni NC: **Relaparotomy for suspected intraperitoneal sepsis after abdominal surgery.** *World J Surg* 2004, **28(2)**:137-41.
264. van Ruler O, Lamme B, Gouma DJ, Reitsma JB, Boermeester MA: **Variables associated with positive findings at relaparotomy in patients with secondary peritonitis.** *Crit Care Med* 2007, **35(2)**:468-76.
265. Hutchins RR, Gunning MP, Lucas DN, Allen-Mersh TG, Soni NC: **Relaparotomy for suspected intraperitoneal sepsis after abdominal surgery.** *World J Surg* 2004, **28(2)**:137-41.
266. Lamme B, Mahler CW, van Ruler O, Gouma DJ, Reitsma JB, Boermeester MA: **Clinical predictors of ongoing infection in secondary peritonitis: systematic review.** *World J Surg* 2006, **30(12)**:2170-81.
267. van Ruler O, Mahler CW, Boer KR, Reuland EA, Gooszen HG, Opmeer BC, de Graaf PW, Lamme B, Gerhards MF, Steller EP, van Till JW, de Borgie CJ, Gouma DJ, Reitsma JB, Boermeester MA, Dutch Peritonitis Study Group: **Comparison of on-demand vs planned relaparotomy strategy in patients with severe peritonitis: a randomized trial.** *JAMA* 2007, **298(8)**:865-72.
268. Amin AI, Shaikh IA: **Topical negative pressure in managing severe peritonitis: a positive contribution?** *World J Gastroenterol* 2009, **15(27)**:3394-7.
269. Adkins AL, Robbins J, Villalba M, Bendick P, Shanley CJ: **Open abdomen management of intra-abdominal sepsis.** *Am Surg* 2004, **70**:137-140.
270. Schein M: **Planned reoperations and open management in critical intra-abdominal infections: prospective experience in 52 cases.** *World J Surg* 1991, **15**:537-545.
271. Robledo FA, Luque-de-León E, Suárez R, Sánchez P, de-la-Fuente M, Vargas A, Mier J: **Open versus closed management of the abdomen in the surgical treatment of severe secondary peritonitis: a randomized clinical trial.** *Surg Infect Larchmt* 2007, **8(1)**:63-72.
272. Linden PK: **Optimizing therapy for vancomycin-resistant Enterococci (VRE).** *Semin Respir Crit Care Med* 2007, **28**:632-645.
273. Chou YY, Lin TY, Lin JC, Wang NC, Peng MY, Chang FY: **Vancomycin-resistant enterococcal bacteremia: Comparison of clinical features and outcome between Enterococcus faecium and Enterococcus faecalis.** *J Microbiol Immunol Infect* 2008, **41(2)**:124-129.
274. Jean SS, Fang CT, Wang HK, Hsueh PR, Chang SC, Luh KT: **Invasive infections due to vancomycin-resistant Enterococci in adult patients.** *J Microbiol Immunol Infect* 2001, **34**:281-286.
275. Noskin GA: **Vancomycin-resistant Enterococci: Clinical, microbiologic, and epidemiologic features.** *J Lab Clin Med* 1997, **130**:14-20.
276. Blot SI, Vandewoude KH, De Waele JJ: **Candida peritonitis.** *Curr Opin Crit Care* 2007, **13(2)**:195-199.
277. Senn L, Eggimann P, Ksontini R, Pascual A, Demartines N, Bille J, Calandra T, Marchetti O: **Caspofungin for prevention of intra-abdominal candidiasis in high-risk surgical patients.** *Intensive Care Med* 2009, **35(5)**:903-908.
278. Pappas PG, Kauffman CA, Andes D, Benjamin DK Jr, Calandra TF, Edwards JE Jr, Filler SG, Fisher JF, Kullberg BJ, Ostrosky-Zeichner L, Reboli AC, Rex JH, Walsh TJ, Sobel JD, Infectious Diseases Society of America: **Clinical practice guidelines for the management of candidiasis: 2009 update by the Infectious Diseases Society of America.** *Clin Infect Dis* 2009, **1;48(5)**:503-35.

2

Oesophageal injuries: Position paper, WSES, 2013

Rao R Ivatury[1*], Frederick A Moore[2], Walter Biffl[3], Ari Leppeniemi[4], Luca Ansaloni[5], Fausto Catena[6], Andrew Peitzman[7] and Ernest E Moore[8]

Abstract

The oesophagus is a difficult challenge for the surgeon because of its lack of serosal covering, the tenuous, segmental blood supply and the common delay in the diagnosis of injury. Early diagnosis is the key to successful management. Recent introduction of newer, minimally invasive techniques have provided management alternatives for both the normal and the diseased organ that is injured with both early and delayed diagnosis.

Surgical anatomy

The oesophagus is a long, muscular organ that begins at the pharyngooesophageal junction at the level of the sixth cervical vertebra. It ends at the gastrooesophageal junction. The area of its origin at the cricopharyngeus muscle is an area of potential injury by the endoscopist or the neophyte anesthesiologist. Passing into the thorax, the oesophagus and the trachea traverse the superior mediastinum behind the great vessels and with a slight curve passes behind the left mainstem bronchus. From this point, the oesophagus curves to the right in the posterior mediastinum, curves back to the left behind the pericardium and crosses the thoracic aorta. Lying anterior to the thoracic aorta, it reaches the abdomen through the oesophageal hiatus of the diaphragm. There is no serosal covering for the structure. The outer layers are composed entirely of longitudinal and circular muscle fibers with squamous epithelium as the mucosal lining. The blood supply is segmental and is derived from branches of the inferior thyroid, bronchial, intercostal arteries and the aorta. Venous drainage is through submucosal channels into a perioesophageal plexus which eventually enters into the inferior thyroid and vertebral veins in the neck, the azygos and hemiazygos veins in the thorax and the left gastric vein in the abdomen.

Introduction

Oesophageal perforation is a potentially life-threatening clinical situation with a high morbidity and a mortality. The clinical symptoms and signs are non-specific. The relative paucity of experience at any given center makes the diagnosis difficult and often delayed. There are no randomized studies, no class I evidence for diagnostic and management precepts. However, multiple series reported in the literature allow some strong recommendations.

Review of literature

Oesophageal perforation is slightly more common in males [1-7] in their sixties.

Iatrogenic perforation is the most common cause of injury. The incidence is small, less than 0.5%, when all the procedures on the oesophagus are considered. Sclerotherapy of oesophageal varices, nasogastric tubes and improperly placed Sengstaken- Blakemore tubes have been known to produce oesophageal perforation. Oesophageal "stents", temperature probes, repeated attempts at endotracheal intubation, impacted foreign bodies, both sharp and blunt, may all cause oesophageal injury. Blast injury and spontaneous rupture of the oesophagus are secondary to a sudden rise in intraluminal pressure and occur usually at the lower end of the oesophagus. Oesophageal trauma has been reported as a complication following anti-reflux procedures, pneumonectomy, truncal vagotomy (an incidence of 0.5%) and rarely, during anterior cervical spinal fusion Blunt oesophageal injury is exceedingly rare and often is missed. The predominant site of rupture is in the cervical and upper thoracic location (82.3%), and associated tracheooesophageal fistulas were noted in 28 patients in one series. Penetrating objects, usually GSW, injure the oesophagus more commonly than does blunt mechanism. It is not a very frequent injury. In a large multi-center study from the AAST, Asensio [3] collected 405 patients from 34 trauma centers over 10.5 years. Ingestion injury to the oesophagus may occur with caustic liquids [8], especially in

* Correspondence: raoivatury@gmail.com
[1]Surgery, Virginia Commonwealth University Health System, Richmond, VA, USA
Full list of author information is available at the end of the article

children by cleaners, battery liquids and solutions used in industrial operations. Acids cause coagulative tissue necrosis with a lower risk of penetration while alkalis tend to be more palatable and cause liquefactive necrosis that rapidly becomes transmural. The amount, viscosity and concentration of the agent and the duration of contact between the caustic agent and the oesophageal mucosa determine the depth and extent of the injury.

Diagnosis

The clinical symptomatology is non-specific early after perforation. Radiologic clues are subtle and may easily be missed. Consequently, delayed diagnosis of oesophageal perforation is extremely frequent. This is especially true in non-endoscopic iatrogenic trauma and after spontaneous perforation. In the AAST study [3], delayed diagnosis after penetrating trauma occurred in about 50% of patients reaching the operating room.

Pain, usually located in the chest with cervical perforations and perhaps referred to the abdomen with thoracic perforations, is a frequent complaint by patients with oesophageal perforation, occurring in 70% to 90% of patients. Pain preceded by repeated episodes of vomiting is a particularly important history that needs to be elicited. Dyspnea is the second common symptom, especially with thoracic perforations and infrequently is seen with cervical or abdominal perforations. Subcutaneous emphysema and crepitus are seen frequently with cervical perforations. Dysphonia, hoarseness, cervical dysphagia and subcutaneous emphysema are encountered in various combinations in this group of patients. There is sometimes acute abdominal or epigastric pain in patients with perforation of the gastro oesophageal junction. Notably, perforations rarely manifest with hematemesis or other signs of gastrointestinal bleeding, including melena [1-7].

Plain radiographs

The radiologic findings that are suggestive of the diagnosis are free air in the soft tissues of the neck, and retropharyngeal or retro tracheal swelling. Chest radiographs may reveal free mediastinal or cervical air, mediastinal widening, pneumothorax, or, in delayed cases, pulmonary infiltrates.

Contrast studies

Contrast oesophagography is indicated to confirm the diagnosis, localize the site of perforation and define the presence or absence of associated oesophageal pathology. In combined oesophageal and tracheal injuries or where there is suspicion of an abnormal oesophago-tracheobronchial communication, thin barium is the agent of choice. Free perforations into the pleura or the mediastinum (the presence of pneumomediastinum or pneumothorax) are best demonstrated by gastrografin. Once a gross extravasation is ruled out, a fluoroscopic study with thin barium is the next step to rule out a small perforation that may have been overlooked by the gastrografin study [1,2].

Endoscopy

Endoscopy has a limited application as the *only* investigation. In instances of blunt or penetrating trauma where the patient is rushed to the operating room for control of other injuries, intraoperative oesophagoscopy may be employed to rule out gross oesophageal injury. Subtle perforations may be missed, especially by flexible endoscopy. In patients with a suspicion of oesophageal injury after external trauma, triple endoscopy (laryngoscopy, oesophagoscopy and bronchoscopy) is indicated. Injury to one of these structures should raise the suspicion of injury to the adjacent organs. The same principles are recommended for transmediastinal missile wounds as well as cervical penetrating wounds. The sensitivity and specificity of endoscopy in the diagnosis of oesophageal injury are unknown, but definitely are related to operator experience. The combination of contrast studies and endoscopy are accurate in more than 90% of patients. Intra-operative endoscopy while palpating the esophagus near the penetrating tract and insufflation of air looking for air-leak are useful techniques. Perforations caused by the endoscopist during oesophagoscopy are usually promptly suspected.

Miscellaneous diagnostic methods

CT, in addition, may show collection of air or fluid in the mediastinum, pleural effusions, pneumopericardium and pneumoperitoneum as important diagnostic findings in these patients. The tract of the bullet in proximity to the esophagus gives another clue. The site of perforation and the degree of containment may also be noted. Tube thoracostomy for a hydrothorax with the demonstration of a continuous air leak not in synchrony with respiration may suggest an oesophageal injury. Increased levels of amylase in chest tube fluid in the appropriate clinical scenario is highly suggestive of oesophageal perforation [1-7]. Operative exploration is a useful diagnostic modality. Especially in patients with pressing indications for surgical exploration (hemorrhage, vascular injury), the oesophagus must be inspected in proximity injuries and operatively explored in the region of the penetrating wound. Adjunctive methods at exploration include instillation of saline or dye (methylene blue) intraluminally with manual compression of the organ to exclude a leak. The same purpose may be achieved by filling the operative field with saline and vigorously injecting air into the oesophagus to demonstrate an air leak. As mentioned earlier, intra-operative endoscopy is a useful option.

Management

The choice of approach depends on the following factors: 1. the anatomic location of the perforation, 2. the time interval between the onset of perforation and the initiation of treatment, 3. whether the injury is contained or free, 4. the severity of illness of the patient, 5. the mechanism of injury and 6. Whether the oesophagus is normal or there is an associated lesion [1,3,5,6].

Injuries to the cervical oesophagus

The management of cervical oesophageal perforation depends on the mechanism of injury. Neck exploration is performed through a left neck incision along the anterior border of the sternocleidomastoid muscle with medial retraction of the carotid vessels. Adequate mobilization behind the trachea and palpation of the nasogastric tube facilitate identification of the oesophagus. The recurrent laryngeal nerve needs to be protected in the dissection and frequently may be palpated or visualized. The oesophageal perforation is identified either by direct visualization or with the help of intraluminal saline or dye. The perforation is repaired in one or two layers. Neither the number of suture layers nor the type of suture material (absorbable or non-absorbable) seem to influence the incidence of fistulization after the repair. If the operative exploration is delayed, suturing may be difficult because of extensive inflammation in the area. In either instance (early or delayed operation), wide drainage is the key to success. Closed suction drains (Jackson- Pratt) usually are preferred. Broad-spectrum antibiotics (usually a synthetic penicillin) are commenced and continued peri-operatively. The drains are left for a period of 5–7 days. Most surgeons recommend a contrast study before the removal of the drain, because of the frequent occurrence of fistula without clinical symptomatology. Nutritional support may be delivered during this period by a nasogastric tube.

Cervical oesophageal fistulas are reported in 10% to 28% of cases after oesophageal repair. The factors that contribute to this complication include inadequate debridement, oesophageal devascularization, tension on the suture line and associated infection. Adequate drainage, exclusion of distal obstruction and maintenance of nutritional support are the cornerstones of fistula management and the majority of them heal with time [1,5].

Combined tracheo-oesophageal injuries: Combined tracheo-oesophageal trauma poses special problems: they are distinctly uncommon and thus may lead to management errors, they produce unique technical problems and may lead to complex complications in the remote postoperative period. Nearly always due to gun-shot injury, energy transfer; e.g., close range SGW vs. jacketed 32 caliber bullets determines the outcome. Feliciano and colleagues [3], based on an 11-year experience of 23 patients, recommend the following principles: 1. the addition of tracheostomy to a simple repair of the trachea may actually lead to a higher infectious morbidity in terms of pneumonia, mediastinal abscesses and wound infections. 2. For extensive oesophageal injuries in the cervical area, a cervical oesophagostomy, side or end, should be considered at the initial operation. 3. Sternocleidomastoid or, preferably, strap muscle interposition should be employed between tracheal and oesophageal repairs as well as to cover carotid artery repairs. It must be remembered that the sternocleidomastoid has a segmental blood supply in thirds and the upper (from occipital artery) and the middle (from the superior thyroid artery) are more reliable for flap creation. And 4. Drainage of combined cervical injuries should be directed anteriorly and through the contralateral neck if a carotid artery injury is present.

Injuries to the thoracic oesophagus

Iatrogenic and trauma related perforations

Non-operative management: A conservative, non-surgical approach occasionally is recommended for thoracic oesophageal perforations in selected patients. The perforation has to be contained for eligibility for non-operative management. Santos and Frater [8] described a system of "transoesophageal irrigation of the mediastinum" as a method of conservative management in patients with a delayed diagnosis of spontaneous rupture. The authors reported excellent results (7 of 8 survived) with a Levin tube placed in the oesophagus proximal to the tear, a chest-tube placed in proximity to the oesophagus, constant irrigation through the Levin tube and continuous suction to the chest tube: a method that ensured constant, mediastinal irrigation. Others used mediastinal irrigation by a transnasal catheter. Percutaneous drainage of pleural effusions, collections or abscesses [9], temporary endoscopic oesophageal stents [10-12] to seal oesophageal leakage and to recover gastrointestinal continuity are being recommended in selected patients. Use of endoscopic clips for perforation closure, endoscopic vacuum sponge therapy are being introduced recently to aid successful drainage and healing of oesophageal perforation or anastomotic insufficiency [2].

For instance, Fischer [13] reported in 2006 nonoperative treatment of 15 benign oesophageal perforations after endoscopic procedures with self-expandable covered metal stents. Seven patients (group 1) underwent stent insertion with an average time delay of 45 minutes. In 8 patients (group 2), the median delay was 123 hours. All patients in group 1 had an uneventful recovery and left hospital 5 days (range, 3 to 9) after stent insertion. One patient in group 2 (1 of 8) died of pneumonia after 6 days. In the other 7 cases, perforations healed successfully after stent placement, but the clinical course was generally complicated with sepsis and multiple organ failure. The average hospital stay was 44 days (range, 15 to 70).

Linden [9] described 43 procedures on the oesophagus with a 30-day or in-hospital mortality of 7.0% and an overall morbidity of 47%. Most acute thoracic oesophageal perforations were treated with primary repair with a low mortality rate of 5%. Most delayed perforations were treated with T-tube repair and had a mortality rate of 8.7%. The complication rate was much lower in the in the group repaired within 24 hours.

Freeman [10] reported on 17 patients treated with silicone-coated stents placed endoscopically utilizing general anesthesia and fluoroscopy with adequate drainage of infected areas. Leak occlusion was confirmed by oesophagogram in 16 patients (94%). Fourteen patients (82%) were able to initiate oral nutrition within 72 hours of stent placement. One patient (6%) experienced a continued leak after stent placement and underwent operative repair. Stent migration requiring repositioning (2) or replacement (2) occurred in 3 patients (18%). All stents were removed at a mean of 52 +/- 20 days after placement. Hospital length of stay for patients treated with oesophageal stent placement was 8 +/- 9 days (median, 5). In another variation of non-operative treatment, Linden [9] used T-tube repair in delayed perforations with a mortality rate of 8.7%. In another recent series (12), 14 consecutive patients with spontaneous oesophageal perforation were treated with coated self-expandable stent and a debridement procedure (three patients by thoracotomy, four by thoracoscopy, three by tube drainage, and two patients with no drainage). Eight patients had one stent, while six patients needed one or more additional stents to achieve source control. Two patients (14%) died during the in-hospital stay, both of them having received more than one stent. Eight patients had one stent, while six patients needed one or more additional stents to achieve source control. Fourteen percent of patients who underwent stenting within 24 hours to stent placement were in septic shock compared with 86% of patients with a delay of more than 24 hours.

In a recent review, Kuppusamy [11] described 81 consecutive patients with acute oesophageal perforation. 48 patients (59%) were managed operatively, 33 (41%) nonoperatively, and 10 patients with hybrid approaches involving a combination of surgical and interventional techniques; 57 patients (70%) were treated <24 hours and 24 (30%) received treatment >24 hours after perforation. LOS was lower in the early-treatment group; however, there was no difference in complications or mortality. Nonoperative therapy increased from 0% to 75% over time. Nonsurgical therapy was more common in referred cases (48% vs 30%) and in the >24 hours treatment group (46% vs 38%). Over the period of study, there were decreases in complications (50% to 33%) and LOS (18.5 to 8.5 days). Mortality for the entire series involved 3 patients (4%): 2 operative and 1 nonoperative. The author concluded that referral to a tertiary care center, treatment within 24 hours, an experienced surgical management team using a diversified approach can expect to shorten LOS and limit complications and mortality.

Surgical intervention is indicated if the patient should worsen on conservative treatment or should develop a mediastinal abscess or empyema. The presence or the development of pneumothorax, pneumoperitoneum, systemic signs of sepsis or shock are contraindications for a nonoperative approach. Non-operative treatment should also be used when the perforation is related to an inoperable malignant stricture. Patient outcome depends mainly on the proper treatment of mediastinal and pleural contamination. Indications for percutaneous drainage or more extensive drainage by surgical intervention should be considered carefully if there is gross contamination [1,11].

Operative management: Operative repair is the treatment of choice for free perforations. This is true for injuries diagnosed both early (< 24 hours) and late (> 24 hours.) The operative approach consists of thoracotomy on the side of the leak (left thoracotomy for lower oesophageal injury and right thoracotomy for upper oesophageal injury), exposure of the oesophagus and thorough debridement of all necrotic tissue. The perforation is identified and closed. In penetrating trauma, multiple perforation are not uncommon and should be looked for diligently. The choice of suture material for closure of the perforation is variable between surgeons, as is the necessity for a two-layered closure with an inner absorbable and outer nonabsorbable sutures. A pleural flap or various neighboring structures (diaphragm, intercostal muscle, vascularized or a free graft of pericardium, extracostal chest wall muscle, omentum or a pedicled jejunal segment) may be used as a "buttress" to the repair... In the lower thoracic area, the gastric fundus has been used as an onlay type of patch by enlarging the oesophageal hiatus and bringing the gastric fundus to the perforation. Drainage of the area extensively, usually with large caliber chest tubes placed in the vicinity of the oesophageal repair, is the most important part of treatment. Primary repair of oesophageal perforation is possible, especially in patients admitted to the hospital within 24 hours of the event. However, multiple recent studies found that mortality risk was not related to wait time exceeding 24 Hours. When repair is attempted in iatrogenic cases with a stricture distal to the perforation, a myotomy might be indicated and the defect covered with a fundoplication. Repair over a T-tube is an alternative treatment that allows for a controlled esophago-cutaneous fistula to be established. This allows healing to take place without contamination [9]. The T-tube can be removed in most patients after 4–6 weeks, and the fistula will eventually close.

With recent advances in video endoscopy, identification and repair of oesophageal perforation by Video Assisted Thoracic Surgery (VATS) has been reported. The future will determine if this modality will enable an earlier, more efficient recognition of oesophageal injury.

Treatment of delayed recognition of the perforation: Oesophageal exclusion and other adjunctive techniques: The problems of delayed treatment involve extensive mediastinitis, necrosis of the oesophageal wall and the difficulty of effectively closing the perforation, even with various buttressing methods. Even when repair is technically feasible, subsequent breakdown of the repair is the rule rather than the exception. It is in such patients that "exclusion" procedures were previously recommended. The rationale for this approach is to exclude the repair from the rest of the oesophagus and allow it to heal while nutritional support is maintained by intravenous or enteral route. The decision to perform exclusion or repair depends on the local findings at thoracotomy as well as the time delay between perforation and operative treatment. In several series, exclusion procedures generally were reserved for a delay in treatment of more than 48 hours.

The principles of exclusion procedures are: 1. to divert the oesophagus from above, 2. to prevent gastric reflux from below and 3. To drain the area widely, usually by tube thoracostomy and 4. Feeding jejunostomy.

1. Diversion from above: by a long T-Tube with the side arm brought out through the perforation and the chest wall to divert the saliva and achieve a controlled fistula. Other techniques described included a lateral cervical oesophagostomy by making an opening in the cervical oesophagus and suturing the opening to the skin. The oesophagus distal to the ostomy may be closed or stapled. 2. Diversion from below: Some authors recommended looping the distal oesophagus with a prolene suture that is brought out of the abdomen along with a gastrostomy. After the oesophageal perforation healed, the Prolene suture was removed, without laparotomy, restoring oesophageal continuity [14].

The problem of exclusion-diversion procedures is that the majority of these patients require a secondary procedure to restore continuity of the GI tract after the fistula had healed. These procedures involve a colon or gastric interposition, depending on the surgeon's preference. In many instances, the exclusion becomes permanent. Oesophageal exclusion is now reserved for the very poor risk patient who cannot tolerate any major surgical procedures.

Perforation with pre-existing pathology: *Oesophageal Resection:* Emergency resection of the perforated oesophagus is undoubtedly the treatment of choice when there is associated distal obstruction. The results of oesophagectomy for simple or delayed perforations with or without associated oesophageal disease have been poor in most series. A more optimistic evaluation of emergency oesophagectomy for oesophageal disruption was reported by Orringer and Stirling [15]. A diverse group of 24 patients was presented including 20 with preexisting oesophageal diseases (chronic strictures, achalasia, reflux esophagitis, carcinoma, diffuse oesophageal spasm and monilial esophagitis). Forty-five percent of the patients had a delay of > 3 days prior to oesophagectomy. Alimentary tract continuity was restored in 13 of the 24 by oesophagogastric anastomosis. In 11 patients, the oesophagus was resected preserving as much of the normal esophagus as possible. The proximal oesophagus was then delivered into the neck, tunnelled in front of the clavicle and the end was constructed as an ostomy on the chest wall. The authors felt that the risk of oesophageal resection in these patients was less than that from repair or exclusion procedures.

Recent series of oesophageal injury: Eroglu [16] performed a retrospective clinical review of 44 patients treated for oesophageal perforation in 2009. Perforation occurred in the cervical oesophagus in 14 patients (32%), thoracic oesophagus in 18 patients (40%), and abdominal oesophagus in 12 patients (27%). The perforation was treated by primary closure in 23 patients (52%), resection in 7 patients (16%), and nonsurgical therapy in 14 patients (32%). In the surgically treated group, the mortality rate was 3 of 30 patients (10%). 2 of 14 patients (14.3%) died in the conservatively managed group. Four of the 14 nonsurgical patients were inserted with covered self-expandable stents. Describing a single surgeon experience, Kiernan et al. [17] reported on 48 patients with a survival of 96% with early surgical treatment. Even when the diagnosis was delayed > 24 hours, hospital survival was 82.6%, increasing to 92.3% when treated with surgery. The authors recommended aggressive, definitive surgery for thoracic oesophageal perforations and reserved conservative, medical therapy in patients with 'microperforations' with no continuing leak.

Richardson [18] summarized the results of aggressive surgical management for oesophageal perforation. All were treated by operative repairs, buttressed with muscle or pleura. Sternocleidomastoid muscle was used to buttress or primarily close the defects in the neck, and a flap of diaphragm was often used for thoracic perforation. Patients with perforated cancer or severe underlying disease had an oesophagectomy. With these techniques, 50 of 64 patients underwent preservation of the oesophagus after closure of the perforation and 14 underwent resection. The leak rate was 17%, but all healed. One patient treated with primary closure died (1.5% mortality) and only 1 patient required subsequent oesophagectomy.

Vallböhmer [19] described an institutional experience of 44 patients over a period of 12 years. Iatrogenic injury was the most frequent cause of oesophageal perforation. Eight patients (18%) underwent conservative treatment with cessation of oral intake, antibiotics, and parenteral nutrition. Twelve (27%) patients received an endoscopic stent implantation. Surgical therapy was performed in 24 (55%) patients with suturing of the lesion in nine patients, oesophagectomy with delayed reconstruction in 14 patients, and resection of the distal oesophagus and gastrectomy in one patient. The hospital mortality rate was 6.8% (3 of 44 patients): one patient with an iatrogenic perforation after conservative treatment, and two patients after surgery (one with Boerhaave syndrome, one with iatrogenic rupture). No death occurred in the 25 patients when the diagnosis was made in less than 24 hours. When it was delayed, 19% of 16 patients died (P = 0.05).

Keeling et al. [20] in 2010 retrospectively reviewed all cases of oesophageal perforation from 1997 through 2008 at Emory University. Among 91 patients, the perforation was iatrogenic in 50 (52%), spontaneous in 23 (24%), and idiopathic in 22 (23%). The authors concluded that the overall mortality from oesophageal perforation can be less than 10%. Primary repair should be considered as first-line treatment when appropriate even in patients who present more than 24 hours after perforation. Non- operative management, in appropriate patients, can be used in selected patients. Similar results were recorded by the Houston group [21] and two recent meta-analyses [22,23].

Results and prognostic considerations

In the multi-institutional series reported by Asensio [4], a logistic regression of 346 patients reaching the O.R. after penetrating trauma established that a delay in preoperative evaluation, AAST organ injury score > 2 and resection and diversion were independent factors for increased oesophagus-related complications. The prognosis appears to be much improved with modern approaches to diagnosis and critical care but is still high with delayed diagnosis and treatment. Emphasis should be placed on early diagnosis of injury and careful selection of operative versus non-operative treatment by experienced clinicians. The excellent results with nonoperative management of iatrogenic injuries mask the potential life-threatening complications of pathologic lesions, and trauma is in between.

Recommendations

We recommend a strong suspicion for oesophageal injury in the appropriate clinical situation of potential injury to the organ and aggressive pursuit of diagnosis to be made within 12 to 24 hours. CT scanning is a useful diagnostic modality in cases of suspected perforation.

We recommend prompt surgical exposure and closure of oesophageal perforation in layers with adequate drainage of the area and antibiotic therapy. In cervical oesophageal injuries with associated tracheal or vascular repairs, these should be separated from the oesophageal repair by sternocleidomastoid or strap muscle interposition.

We recommend that the treatment of the injured oesophagus be given by clinicians experienced in the endoscopic or surgical management of the organ, ideally in a tertiary center with multispecialty availability by experienced clinicians.

We suggest non-operative management of small perforations diagnosed within 24–48 hours in a stable patient with no mediastinitis or empyema.

In non-trauma injuries, that are initially missed and/or present in a delayed fashion, the initial management of sepsis by resuscitation, antibiotics and chest drainage is the priority. A variety of techniques including stents, t-tubes and clipping are available and should be individualized to the clinical situation and patient. These patients need nutritional supplementation, preferably enteral, while the oesophagus heals. We suggest careful observation of these patients for signs of escalating septic complications and prompt surgical intervention, should these occur.

We suggest oesophageal resection by experienced surgeons for perforation of the diseased organ and planned reconstruction of esophago-gastric continuity.

Competing interests
The authors declare that they have no competing interests.

Authors' contributions
"RRI drafted the manuscript. FAM, WB, AL, LA, FC, AP, EEM reviewed the draft and made corrections and revisions". All authors read and approved the final manuscript.

Author details
[1]Surgery, Virginia Commonwealth University Health System, Richmond, VA, USA. [2]Acute Care Surgery, University of Florida, Gainesville, FL, USA. [3]Surgery, Denver Health Medical Center, University of Colorado School of Medicine, 777 Bannock St., MC 0206, Denver, CO 80204, USA. [4]Surgery, Meilahti Hospital, Haartmaninkatu 4, P.O. Box: 34000029 Helsinki, Finland. [5]Surgery I, Papa Giovanni XXIII Hospital, Piazza OMS 1, 24127 Bergamo, Italy. [6]Department of Emergency Surgery, Parma University Hospital, Parma, Italy. [7]Department of CSurgery, University of Pittsburgh, Pittsburgh, USA. [8]University of Colorado Denver, Denver, CO 80206, USA.

References

1. Attar S, Hankins JR, Sutter CM: **Esophageal perforation: a therapeutic challenge.** *Ann Thorac Surg* 1990, **50:**45.
2. Soreidel JA, Asgaust V: **Scand J trauma Esophageal perforation: diagnostic work-up and clinical decision-making in the first 24 hours.** *Resusc Emerg Med* 2011, **19:**66.
3. Feliciano DV, Bitondo CG, Mattox KL, *et al*: **Combined tracheoesophageal injuries.** *Am J Surg* 1985, **150:**710–715.

4. Asensio JA, Chahwan S, Forno W, *et al*: **Penetrating Esophageal injuries: multicenter study of the American Association for the Surgery of Trauma.** *Trauma* 2001, **50:**289–296.
5. Sepesi B, Raymond DP, Peters JH: **Esophageal perforation: surgical, endoscopic and medical management strategies.** *Curr Opin Gastroenterol* 2010, **26:**379–383.
6. Abbas G, Schuchert MJ, Pettiford BL, Pennathur A, Landreneau J, Luketich JD, Landreneau RJ: **Contemporaneous management of Esophageal perforation.** *Surgery* 2009, **146:**749–755.
7. Bhatia P, Fortin D, Inculet RI, Malthaner RA: **Current concepts in the management of Esophageal perforations: a twenty-seven year Canadian experience.** *Ann Thorac Surg* 2011, **92:**209–215.
8. Santos GH, Frater RW: **Transesophageal irrigation for the treatment of mediastinitis produced by Esophageal rupture.** *J Thorac Cardiovasc Surg* 1986, **91**(1):57–62.
9. Linden PA: **Modified T-tube repair of delayed esophageal perforation results in a low mortality rate similar to that seen with acute perforations.** *Ann Thorac Surg* 2007, **83**(3):1129–1133.
10. Freeman RK: **Esophageal stent placement for the treatment of iatrogenic intrathoracic Esophageal perforation.** *Ann Thorac Surg* 2007, **83**(6):2003–2007.
11. Kuppusamy MK: **Evolving management strategies in Esophageal perforation: surgeons using nonoperative techniques to improve outcomes.** *J Am Coll Surg* 2011, **213**(1):164–171.
12. Koivukangas V, Biancari F, Meriläinen S, Ala-Kokko T, Saarnio J: **Esophageal stenting for spontaneous Esophageal perforation.** *J Trauma Acute Care Surg* 2012, **73**(4):1011–1013.
13. Fischer A: **Nonoperative treatment of 15 benign Esophageal perforations with self-expandable covered metal stents.** *Ann Thorac Surg* 2006, **81**(2):467–472.
14. Urschel HC Jr, Razzuk MA, Wood RE, *et al*: **Improved management of Esophageal perforation: exclusion and diversion in continuity.** *Ann Surg* 1974, **179**(5):587–591.
15. Orringer MB, Stirling MC: **Esophagectomy for Esophageal disruption.** *Ann Thorac Surg* 1990, **49:**35–4216.
16. Eroglu A: **Current management of Esophageal perforation: 20 years experience.** *Dis Esophagus* 2009, **22**(4):374–380.
17. Kiernan PD, Sheridan MJ, Hettrick V, Vaughan B, Graling P: **Thoracic Esophageal perforation: one surgeon's experience.** *Dis Esophageal* 2006, **19**(1):24–30.
18. Richardson JD: **Management of Esophageal perforations: the value of aggressive surgical treatment.** *Am J Surg* 2005, **190**(2):161–165.
19. Vallböhmer D: **Options in the management of Esophageal perforation: analysis over a 12-year period.** *Dis Esophagus* 2010, **23**(3):185–190.
20. Keeling WB, Miller DL, Lam GT, Kilgo P, Miller JI, Mansour KA: **Force SD: Low mortality after treatment for Esophageal perforation: a single-center experience.** *Ann Thorac Surg* 2010, **90**(5):1669–1673.
21. Wu JT, Mattox KL, Wall MJ, Wall MJ JR: **Esophageal perforations: new perspectives and treatment paradigms.** *J Trauma* 2007, **63**(5):1173–1184.
22. Hasimoto CN, Cataneo C, Eldib R, Thomazi R, Pereira RS, Minossi JG, Cataneo AJ: **Efficacy of surgical versus conservative treatment in Esophageal perforation: a systematic review of case series studies.** *Acta Cir Bras* 2013, **28**(4):266–271.
23. Biancari F, D'Andrea V, Paone R, Di Marco C, Savino G, Koivukangas V, Saarnio J, Lucenteforte E: **Current treatment and outcome of Esophageal perforations in adults: systematic review and meta-analysis of 75 studies.** *World J Surg* 2013, **37**(5):1051–1059.

3

The value of C-reactive protein and lactate in the acute abdomen in the emergency department

Zainna C Meyer*, Jennifer MJ Schreinemakers and Lijckle van der Laan

Abstract

Case presentation: This report describes the presentation of three critically ill patients with non-traumatic acute abdominal pain and increased concentrations of the biomarkers C-reactive protein (CRP) and lactate. In these three patients an exploratory laparotomy was carried out. Remarkably, the laparotomy showed no intra-abdominal abnormalities. We discuss the usefulness of these biomarkers in practice and their influence on establishing a diagnose and making a decision to perform an intervention.

Conclusion: We conclude that biomarkers lactate and CRP in patients with acute abdominal pain should only be used in adjunct to the history and clinical findings, as they are not specific and can be misleading in establishing a diagnosis. In addition, relying on these biomarkers may contribute to more diagnostic examinations and/or unnecessary invasive interventions (for example laparotomy).

Keywords: Acute abdomen, C-reactive protein, Lactate

Background

Diagnosing patients who present in the emergency department with acute abdominal pain can be challenging. In addition to history taking and physical examination, clinicians often use laboratory tests and radiological examinations to exclude diagnoses that can mimic acute abdominal pain for example pneumonia. Physicians in the emergency department often base their decisions for consultation of the surgeon for a laparotomy on clinical presentation combined with biochemical abnormalities. Examples of those biochemical parameters are high concentrations of C-reactive protein (CRP) or lactate concentrations [1,2]. The question remains if these parameters are reliable to diagnose an acute abdomen. The pitfall of relying on laboratory values could lead to over treatment or under treatment.

This report presents three patients with non-traumatic acute abdominal pain and abnormal C-reactive protein and/or lactate concentrations with a negative laparotomy. Furthermore, we discuss the usefulness of these markers in practice and their contribution to establish a diagnosis by means of interventions in the emergency department.

* Correspondence: zienalove@hotmail.com
Department of Surgery, Amphia Hospital, Breda, the Netherlands

Case presentation

First case

Our first case was of a 65 years-old man who presented in the emergency department (ED) of our tertiary health care institute with acute abdominal pain which irradiated to the back in combination with hypotension. He was recently admitted into an orthopedic ward for two days with lumbar pain due to discopathy of all lumbar vertebrae with signs of spondylodicitis. Suspicion of an aneurysm of the abdominal aorta raised at presentation and a CT-scan was made. No acute pathology was seen except a dilatation of the stomach and small intestine. Laboratory results showed a leucocytes count of $8.4 \cdot 10^9$/L (normal reference value: 4–10 $\cdot 10^9$/L), CRP concentration of 661 mg/L (0.8-2 mg/L), creatinine level of 548 μmol/L (45–100 μmol/L) with a glomerular filtration rate of 9 mL/min/1.73 m^2 and a lactate level of 3.9 mmol/L (<1.8 mmol/L). Additional conventional chest X-rays was also made without pathological findings. Based on the clinical presentation and laboratory results we performed a laparotomy, which showed no abnormalities. He was admitted into the Intensive Care Unit (ICU) for pulmonary and cardiovascular support.

During the first five days of admission he was septic and required cardiovascular and pulmonary support. Continuous Venovenous Hemofiltration (CVVH) for acute kidney failure was started. The first blood cultures showed a staphylococcus aureus. At that time, the patient was treated with Tobramycine and Cefotaxim as prophylaxis for ventilator-associated pneumonia in combination with Orabase protective paste. A Positron Emission Tomography- Computed Tomography scan (PET-CT scan) and several CT-scans were performed, but did not show a focus.

After a stay on the ICU of one month with several complications he stabilized and was discharged. Complications included re-intubation, a central venous line infection with Enterococcus Faecium, an ischemic cerebrovascular accident in the left fronto-occipital region, an ileus and a segmental ischemic colitis with deep ulcers in the transverse colon. The lactate levels and CRP concentrations decreased to near normal values (Figure 1). Within a few days on the ward he developed a pneumosepsis, which was treated with Augmentin. When the patient deteriorated he was abstained from further treatment after consultation with patient and family. He deceased within 24 hours.

Second case

The second patient was a 60 years-old woman. She presented in the ED with acute intense pain in the lower abdomen. One day earlier she started vomiting. Within the last six months she had several attacks of abdominal pain. The medical history included a laparoscopic cholecystectomy. On physical examination she had a tachycardia and was tachypnoeic. The lower abdomen was tender and a mass was palpated. A rectal and vaginal exam showed no abnormalities. Laboratory results demonstrated a leucocytes count of $18.1 \cdot 10^9$/L, CRP 4 mmol/L and no abnormal kidney or liver function parameters. Arterial gas showed a pH of 7.71 (normal ref. values: 7.35-7.45), pCO_2 of 1.7 kPa (4.7-6.4 kPa), pO_2 15.2 kPa (10.0-13.3 kPa), bicarbonate 4 mmol/L (22–29 mmol/L), base excess of −21.6 mmol/L (−3.0-3.0 mmol/L) and lactate level 6.7 mmol/L. Abdominal ultrasonography and conventional chest X-rays showed no abnormalities except a bladder retention which was treated.

Based on clinical and laboratory findings, a laparotomy was performed with the differential diagnosis of acute mesenterial ischemia. The laparotomy was negative for mesenterial ischemia, but bladder retention of more than one liter was found despite earlier treatment with an urinary catheter.

Postoperatively, the patient was admitted into the ICU and the lactate levels increased till 10 mmol/L and thereafter decreased to normal values (Figure 2). The CRP followed the same pattern (Figure 2). She was hemodynamically stable with low dosage of vasoactive medication and had mechanical ventilation support for a short period. Also, she developed acute kidney failure. Spontaneous mild correction of renal failure was seen within some days with a normal urine production of 60 ml/hour after administration of Furosemide. Abdominal pains in the right lower abdomen without a focus remained her main complain. After 3 days she was discharged from the ICU.

Complementary diagnostic examination by means of a gastroscopy showed a mild gastritis. A new abdominal ultrasonography showed no pathological findings.

During the stay on the internal medicine ward a spontaneous recovery of kidney failure was seen and constipation was successfully treated with Movicolon (a polyethylene glycol preparation; PEG 3350). Her abdominal pain decreased but was not totally over. After 11 days of admission, she was discharged.

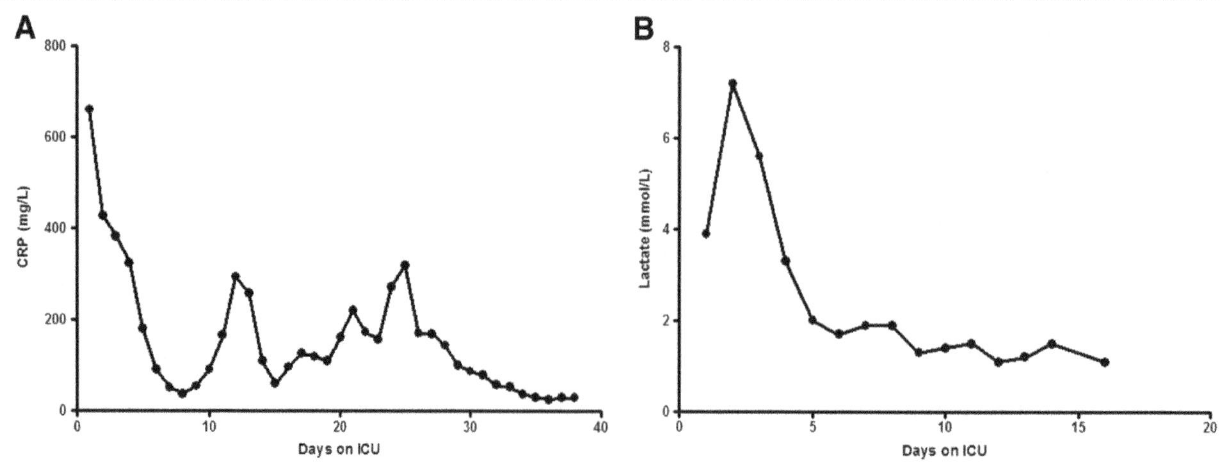

Figure 1 C-reactive protein and lactate concentrations over time of the first case. ***A*** C-reactive protein concentrations and ***B*** Lactate concentrations. C-reactive protein levels and lactate concentrations decreased to near normal values during the ICU stay.

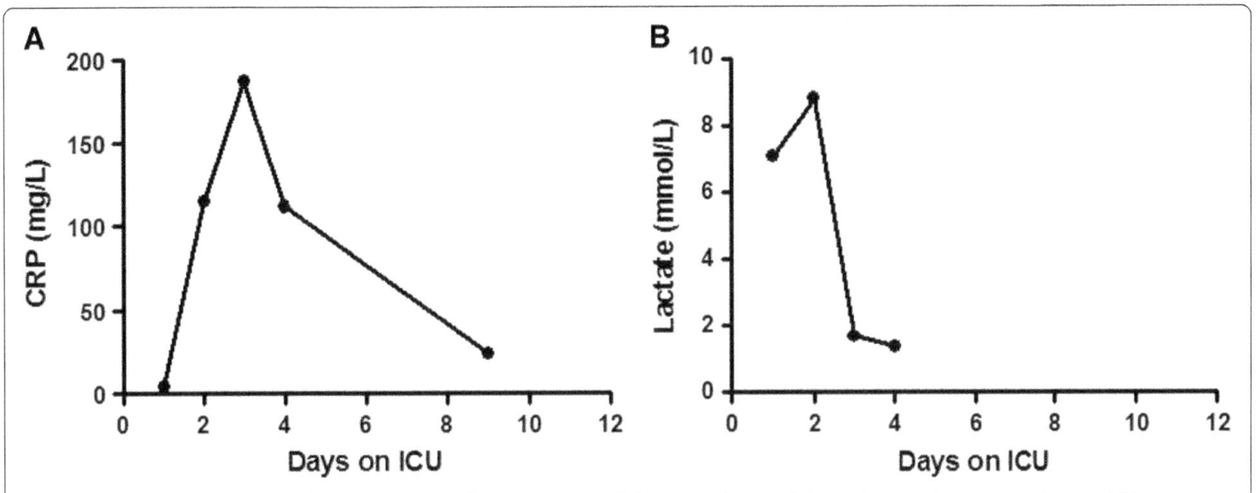

Figure 2 C-reactive protein and lactate concentrations over time of the second case. A C-reactive protein concentrations and B Lactate concentrations **A** C-reactive protein concentrations and **B** Lactate concentrations**.** After admittance into the ICU, the lactate levels increased till 10 mmol/L and thereafter decreased to normal values. The C-reactive protein levels follow the same pattern.

Third case

The third patient was a 68 years-old male which presented in the ED with a productive cough, sore throat and perspiration at night without a fever. Furthermore he developed a generalized rash. He recently spent time abroad (Finland) for construction work. Clinical features at the ED showed petechial rash on the face, extremities and abdomen. Furthermore, an enlarged submandibular lymph node was palpated. Examination of the abdomen was normal without tenderness. Laboratory results demonstrated a thrombocytes count of $20{\cdot}10^9$/L (normal ref. values: 150-400$10^9$/L), hemoglobin concentration of 9.1 mmol/L, leucocytes count of 6.6 mmol/L, CRP 9 mmol/L, bilirubine 24 µmol/L (0.0-20.0 µmol/L), alanine transaminase 212 U/L (0–45 U/L), aspartate transaminase 340 U/L (0–35 U/L), lactate dehydrogenase 677 U/L (,<248 U/L) alkaline phosphatase 684 U/L (0–115 U/L) and gamma-glutamyl transferase 265 U/L (0-55U/L). He was admitted into the internal medicine ward for further analysis of thrombocytopenia and liver failure.

Complementary diagnostic examination of the bone marrow demonstrated an increase in small lymfoide T-cells. Serology for viruses was negative. Conventional chest X-rays showed peribronchial changes like seen in COPD without other pathologic signs. Abdominal ultrasonography demonstrated a hepatomegaly, a small liver hemangioma and a thickened gallbladder wall without gallstones or signs of cholecystitis. Based on these findings the diagnosis for viral infection or auto-immune disease was made.

On the seventh day after admission he developed a fever of 38 °C without any complaints. The same generalized petechial was observed without abdominal tenderness. Laboratory results showed further liver failure and no signs of infection. Because of a fever (>39 °C), a CT-thorax and abdomen were made which showed a small consolidation in the right dorsal lung sinus, ascitis and infiltrative changes in mesenterium with air bubbles. It was suggested that these findings might indicate a bile-induced peritonitis. Antibiotics by means of Augmentin were started and a surgeon was consulted. Considering that the patient had no abdominal pain and no tenderness during physical examination, the team agreed to a conservative treatment. During the day and night the patient deteriorated with abnormal breathing, tachycardia of 110 beats per minute and jaundice without abdominal complaints or tenderness. New laboratory findings showed an increased lactate level with deterioration of liver tests (Figure 3). He was admitted into the ICU with the diagnosis abdominal sepsis with high lactate concentrations (lactate 15.1 mmol/L). The surgeon was consulted again based on a suspicion of intestinal pneumatosis due to acute mesenterial ischemia by means of high lactate levels, although no abdominal pain or abnormal physical examination was seen. A diagnostic laparotomy was performed. No pathological findings were observed except serosangulent fluids. He returned to the ICU.

On the ICU the patient remained hemodynamically unstable with high doses of inotropics and vasoactive medications. He had no abdominal pain and a normal physical examination. All cultures of blood, urine, sputum, ascitis and perioperative fluids were negative for infection. Nevertheless, broad spectrums of antibiotics were administered (Tobramycine, Augmentin and Doxycicline). CVVH was started due to acute kidney failure. During the next days the patient remained septic with high lactate concentrations, liver failure and kidney failure, disseminated intravascular coagulation accompanied with bleeding of the eyes and mucous membranes. Based on all the clinical findings, multi organ failure and

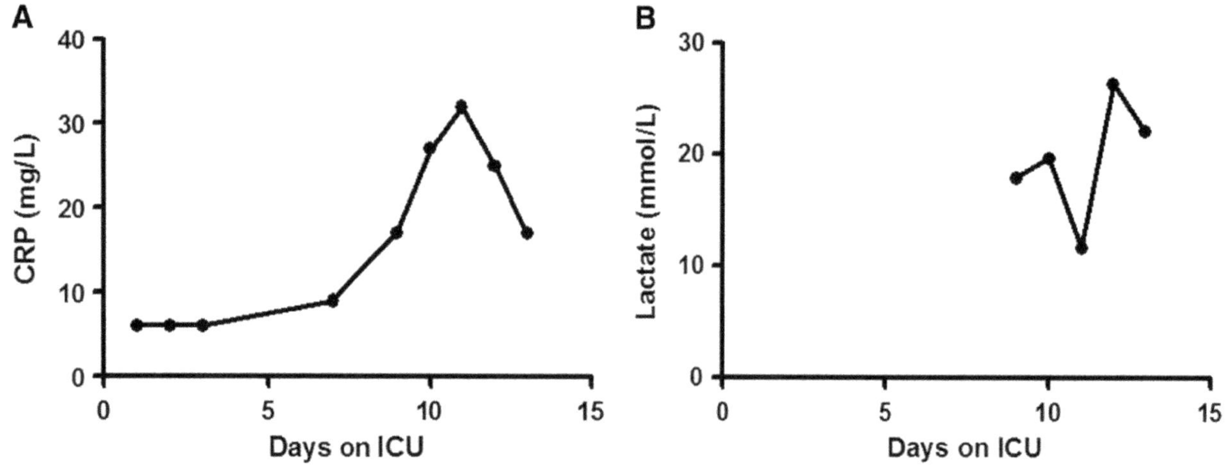

Figure 3 C-reactive protein and lactate concentrations over time of the third case. ***A*** C-reactive protein concentrations and ***B*** Lactate concentrations. During admission both C-reactive protein as lactate levels increased over time.

inability to stabilize him, further treatment was stopped. He died 13 days after admission.

Discussion

Although some biomarkers like lactate and C-reactive protein can be useful in the diagnosis of an acute abdomen, these cases demonstrate that these parameters can mislead the physician and contribute to more diagnostic examinations or unnecessary invasive interventions like a laparotomy.

As described in all cases the main suspicion was acute mesenteric ischemia. This is a complex disease with a high mortality rate [3]. Until now, no reliable parameters to help diagnose such serious disease have been found and a search to identify this factor continues. One of the markers that are frequently used is plasma lactate concentration. An increase of lactate levels indicates an anaerobe glucogenesis and therefore it is a parameter for inadequate perfusion, oxygenation and an estimate of tissue oxygen deficiency. Increased plasma lactate concentrations were observed in patients with mesenteric ischemia with a sensitivity of 100% and a specificity of 42% [3]. Yet, another study on patient with an acute abdomen and increased lactate levels in the ED, showed a sensitivity of 75% and specificity 39% when using lactate concentrations for the diagnosis of acute mesenteric ischemia [4]. On the other hand the study of Lange et. al. [3] showed that elevation in lactate concentration can be due to other conditions as well. For example general bacterial peritonitis and in about 50% of the cases with strangulated intestinal obstructions [3].

Furthermore, other conditions correlated with high lactate concentrations are (septic) shock, diabetic ketoacidosis, liver coma, renal failure and acute pancreatitis. When other conditions have been excluded, an increased lactate level often may indicate an emergency abdominal condition. Some authors recommend an laparotomy in all patients with abdominal complaints and a raised plasma lactate level when other conditions correlated with increased lactate levels have been excluded [3]. However, we believe that this matter is more subtle as we observe that lactate levels are being used as a parameter only for acute mesenterial ischemia. Our third case is an example of a patient without abdominal pain but with high lactate levels, probably due to liver failure. Based on the lactate levels, an unnecessary invasive diagnostic intervention, a laparotomy was performed. As a study concluded, the determination of lactate concentrations has no better sensitivity in establishing the diagnosis of patient with acute abdomen compared to clinical findings and normal laboratory examination [4].

Another biomarker often used in the emergency department to aid in the diagnosis of an acute abdomen is the C-reactive protein (CRP). Most studies have focused mainly on the use of this parameter in establishing the diagnosis of appendicitis. Few studies have assessed its diagnostic role in the general conditions describing acute abdominal pain. The diagnostic value of CRP in the overall patient with acute abdominal pain showed a sensitivity of 79%, specificity of 64% and global accuracy of 73% for predicting subsequent hospitalization using a cut-off value for positive test of >5 mg/L [2]. More recently, Salem et. al. [5] reviewed the diagnostic value of CRP in true surgical patients with acute abdominal pain in the ED. They concluded that CRP alone is not useful in differentiating between surgical causes of acute abdomen or self-limiting condition [5]. In addition, CRP can neither differentiate between surgical conditions requiring intervention from those who can be treated non-operatively [5]. In conclusion, these studies confirm the difficulty to diagnose an acute abdomen and assessing the need for a laparotomy as in our cases. Although high CRP levels or increase in CRP concentrations are seen in combination with abdominal complaints, it does not directly mean that a surgical complication should be the problem.

When CRP is compared with lactate, one study concluded that CRP is as a poor marker for the diagnosis of an acute abdomen considering that its activation is later in the onset of the disease compared to lactate or Interleukin-6 (IL-6) [1,5]. Patient with severe sepsis and those with sepsis on the ED with an acute abdomen can superiorly be differentiated by levels IL-6 and lactate [1]. But this study only included patients with sepsis or shock.

From our cases and a review of literature it is clear that we need more reliable markers to help establishing a fast and reliable diagnosis of patients with acute abdominal pain. Recently, the newer biomarker procalcitonin (PCT) showed to be a reliable marker to differentiate bacterial from nonbacterial infection or noninfectious inflammation with high accuracy [6]. Prospective studies on the use of PCT as screening test for appendicitis on the ED showed that this marker may only be useful in identifying patients with complicated (severe) appendicitis [7,8]. Furthermore, procalcitonin has also been proven to be helpful during the diagnosis or exclusion of acute mesenterial ischemia, intestinal ischemia or necrosis in acute bowel obstruction and abdominal sepsis [9-11]. Its use may be considered as additional tool to improve clinical decision making and appropriate therapy.

Imaging modalities have proven to be valuable adjuncts in diagnosis patients with acute abdominal pain. In one patient the CT-scan revealed no abnormalities and neither did the following laparotomy. The third patient did not have abdominal pain and the CT-scan showed potential bile peritonitis. The critical illness of the patient with abnormal increase in CRP and lactate concentration pushed the surgeons to perform a laparotomy, again without abnormalities. Perhaps, it should be recommended that all patients with acute abdominal pain and increased CRP and/or lactate levels should additionally undergo a CT-scan [12]. Even though it is known that a CT-scan is not completely reliable, a biphasic CT angiography has been reported with a sensitivity of approximately 90% for the diagnosis of mesenteric ischemia independent of the underlying pathology [13,14]. In addition, the CT scan can also provide alternative diagnoses for patients with an acute abdomen [13].

Conclusion

These cases demonstrate that although biomarkers CRP and lactate can be useful in the diagnosis of an acute abdomen, they are not specific and can be misleading in establishing a diagnosis. In addition, relying on these biomarkers may contribute to more diagnostic examinations and/or unnecessary invasive interventions (e.g. laparotomy). We conclude that lactate levels and CRP concentrations in patients with acute abdominal pain should only be used in adjunction to the history and clinical findings and perhaps to a CT-scan as well.

Consent

Written informed consent was obtained from all patients or next of kin of the patients for publication of this Case report. A copy of the written consent is available for review by the Editor-in-Chief of this Journal.

Abbreviations

CRP: C-reactive Protein; ED: Emergency Department; ICU: Intensive Care Unit; CVVH: Continuous Venovenous Hemofiltration; CT-scan: Computed Tomography scan; PET-CT scan: Position Emission Tomography-Computed Tomography scan; PCT: Procalcitonin.

Competing interests

The authors declare that they have no competing interests.

Author's contributions

ZM acquired data for the case report, interpreted the data, drafted the manuscript and has given approval for the final version. JM and LL interpreted the data, revised the manuscript critically for important intellectual content. All authors read and approved the version to be published.

References

1. Ravishankaran P, Shah AM, Bhat R: **Correlation of interleukin-6, serum lactate, and C-reactive protein to inflammation, complication, and outcome during the surgical course of patients with acute abdomen.** *J Interferon Cytokine Res* 2011, **31**:685–690.
2. Chi CH, Shiesh SC, Chen KW, Wu MH, Lin XZ: **C-reactive protein for the evaluation of acute abdominal pain.** *Am J Emerg Med* 1996, **14**:254–256.
3. Lange H, Jackel R: **Usefulness of plasma lactate concentration in the diagnosis of acute abdominal disease.** *Eur J Surg* 1994, **160**:381–384.
4. Vahl AC, Out NJ, Kapteijn BA, Koomen AR: **Nothing gained from the determinations of plasma lactate levels in the evaluation of a patient with acute abdomen.** *Ned Tijdschr Geneeskd* 1998, **142**:901–904
5. Salem TA, Molloy RG, O'Dwyer PJ: **Prospective study on the role of C-reactive protein (CRP) in patients with an acute abdomen.** *Ann R Coll Surg Engl* 2007, **89**:233–237.
6. Becker KL, Snider R, Nylen ES: **Procalcitonin assay in systemic inflammation, infection, and sepsis: clinical utility and limitations.** *Crit Care Med* 2008, **36**:941–952.
7. Sand M, Trullen XV, Bechara FG, Pala XF, Sand D, Landgrafe G, Mann B: **A prospective bicenter study investigating the diagnostic value of procalcitonin in patients with acute appendicitis.** *Eur Surg Res* 2009, **43**:291–297.
8. Wu JY, Chen HC, Lee SH, Chan RC: *Lee CC.* Chang SS: Diagnostic Role of Procalcitonin in Patients with Suspected Appendicitis. World J Surg; 2012 [Epub ahead of print].
9. Markogiannakis H, Memos N, Messaris E, Dardamanis D, Larentzakis A, Papanikolaou D, Zografos GC, Manouras A: **Predictive value of procalcitonin for bowel ischemia and necrosis in bowel obstruction.** *Surgery* 2011, **149**:394–403.
10. Rau B, Kruger CM, Schilling MK: **Procalcitonin: improved biochemical severity stratification and postoperative monitoring in severe abdominal inflammation and sepsis.** *Langenbecks Arch Surg* 2004, **389**:134–144.

4

Complicated intra-abdominal infections in a worldwide context

Massimo Sartelli[1*], Fausto Catena[2], Luca Ansaloni[3], Ernest Moore[4], Mark Malangoni[5], George Velmahos[6], Raul Coimbra[7], Kaoru Koike[8], Ari Leppaniemi[9], Walter Biffl[4], Zsolt Balogh[10], Cino Bendinelli[10], Sanjay Gupta[11], Yoram Kluger[12], Ferdinando Agresta[13], Salomone Di Saverio[14], Gregorio Tugnoli[14], Elio Jovine[15], Carlos Ordonez[16], Carlos Augusto Gomes[17], Gerson Alves Pereira Junior[18], Kuo-Ching Yuan[19], Miklosh Bala[20], Miroslav P Peev[6], Yunfeng Cui[21], Sanjay Marwah[22], Sanoop Zachariah[23], Boris Sakakushev[24,25], Victor Kong[26], Adamu Ahmed[27], Ashraf Abbas[28], Ricardo Alessandro Teixeira Gonsaga[29], Gianluca Guercioni[30], Nereo Vettoretto[31], Elia Poiasina[3], Offir Ben-Ishay[12], Rafael Díaz-Nieto[32], Damien Massalou[33], Matej Skrovina[34], Ihor Gerych[35], Goran Augustin[36], Jakub Kenig[37], Vladimir Khokha[38], Cristian Tranà[39], Kenneth Yuh Yen Kok[40], Alain Chichom Mefire[41], Jae Gil Lee[42], Suk-Kyung Hong[43], Helmut Alfredo Segovia Lohse[44], Wagih Ghnnam[45], Alfredo Verni[46], Varut Lohsiriwat[47], Boonying Siribumrungwong[48], Alberto Tavares[49], Gianluca Baiocchi[50], Koray Das[51], Julien Jarry[52], Maurice Zida[53], Norio Sato[8], Kiyoshi Murata[54], Tomohisa Shoko[55], Takayuki Irahara[56], Ahmed O Hamedelneel[57], Noel Naidoo[58], Abdul Rashid Kayode Adesunkanmi[59], Yoshiro Kobe[60], AK Attri[11], Rajeev Sharma[11], Federico Coccolini[3], Tamer El Zalabany[61], Khalid Al Khalifa[61], Juan Sanjuan[16], Rita Barnabé[15] and Wataru Ishii[62]

Abstract

Despite advances in diagnosis, surgery, and antimicrobial therapy, mortality rates associated with complicated intra-abdominal infections remain exceedingly high. The World Society of Emergency Surgery (WSES) has designed the CIAOW study in order to describe the clinical, microbiological, and management-related profiles of both community- and healthcare-acquired complicated intra-abdominal infections in a worldwide context. The CIAOW study (Complicated Intra-Abdominal infection Observational Worldwide Study) is a multicenter observational study currently underway in 57 medical institutions worldwide. The study includes patients undergoing surgery or interventional drainage to address complicated intra-abdominal infections. This preliminary report includes all data from almost the first two months of the six-month study period. Patients who met inclusion criteria with either community-acquired or healthcare-associated complicated intra-abdominal infections (IAIs) were included in the study. 702 patients with a mean age of 49.2 years (range 18–98) were enrolled in the study. 272 patients (38.7%) were women and 430 (62.3%) were men. Among these patients, 615 (87.6%) were affected by community-acquired IAIs while the remaining 87 (12.4%) suffered from healthcare-associated infections. Generalized peritonitis was observed in 304 patients (43.3%), whereas localized peritonitis or abscesses was registered in 398 (57.7%) patients. The overall mortality rate was 10.1% (71/702). The final results of the CIAOW Study will be published following the conclusion of the study period in March 2013.

* Correspondence: m.sartelli@virgilio.it
[1]Department of Surgery, Macerata Hospital, Macerata, Italy
Full list of author information is available at the end of the article

Introduction

Intra-abdominal infections (IAIs) include a wide spectrum of pathological conditions, ranging from uncomplicated appendicitis to fecal peritonitis [1].

From a clinical perspective, IAIs are classified in two major categories: complicated and uncomplicated.

In uncomplicated IAIs, the infectious process only involves a single organ and does not spread to the peritoneum. Patients with such infections can be managed with either surgical resection or antibiotics. When the focus of infection is treated effectively by surgical excision, 24-hour perioperative prophylaxis is typically sufficient. Patients with less severe intra-abdominal infections, including acute diverticulitis and certain forms of acute appendicitis, may be treated non-operatively.

In complicated IAIs, the infectious process extends beyond a singularly affected organ, and causes either localized peritonitis or diffuse peritonitis. The treatment of patients with complicated intra-abdominal infections involves both source control and antibiotic therapy.

Intra-abdominal infections are further classified in two groups: community-acquired intra-abdominal infections (CA-IAIs) and healthcare-associated intra-abdominal infections (HA-IAIs). CA-IAIs are acquired directly in the community while HA-IAIs develop in hospitalized patients or residents of long-term healthcare facilities. HA-IAIs are associated with higher rates of mortality due to the patients' poorer underlying health and an increased likelihood of infection by multi-drug resistant microorganisms.

Source control encompasses all measures undertaken to eliminate the source of infection and to control ongoing contamination.

The most common source of infection in community-acquired intra-abdominal infections is the appendix, followed by the colon, and then the stomach. Dehiscence complicates 5-10% of intra-abdominal bowel anastomoses and is associated with high rates of mortality [2].

Ultrasound- and CT-guided percutaneous drainage of abdominal and extra-peritoneal abscesses have proven to be safe and effective in select patients [3-10].

Surgery is the most important therapeutic recourse for controlling intra-abdominal infections.

Generally, the choice of the procedure depends on the anatomical source of infection, on the degree of peritoneal inflammation, on the generalized septic response and on the patient's general conditions.

Patients suffering from severe peritonitis are prone to persisting intra-abdominal sepsis, even when the source of infection has been neutralized. Timely re-laparotomy is the only possible known surgical recourse, capable to significantly improve patient outcome in these cases.

In the event of secondary peritonitis, the decision and timing of re-laparotomy is largely subjective and is often based on a surgeon's professional experience. Factors indicative of progressive or persistent organ failure during early postoperative follow-up analysis are the strongest indicators of ongoing infection and suggest positive findings upon re-laparotomy [11-13].

Three methods of localized, mechanical management of abdominal sepsis following the initial laparotomy, which was performed for purposes of source control, are currently debated within the medical community: open-abdomen, planned re-laparotomy and on-demand re-laparotomy

Antimicrobial therapy plays an integral role in the management of intra-abdominal infections, especially in critically ill patients requiring immediate empiric antibiotic therapy.

Empiric antibiotic therapy accounts for the most frequently isolated microorganisms as well as any local trends of antibiotic resistance.

The major pathogens involved in community-acquired intra-abdominal infections are Enterobacteriaceae and anaerobic microbes (especially B. fragilis).

An antimicrobial-based approach to treating intra-abdominal infections involves a delicate balance between the optimization of empirical therapy, which has been shown to improve clinical outcomes, and the reduction of excessive antimicrobial use, which has been proven to increase the rate of emergence of antimicrobial-resistant strains.

The threat of antimicrobial resistance is one of the major challenges associated with the antimicrobial management of complicated intra-abdominal infections.

The recent and rapid spread of serine carbapenemases in Klebsiella pneumoniae (KPC) has become an important concern when administering antimicrobial therapy in hospitals worldwide [14].

The growing emergence of multidrug-resistant bacteria and the limited availability of new antibiotics to counteract them has brought about an impending crisis with alarming implications (especially regarding gram-negative microorganisms).

Methods

Aim

The purpose of the study is to describe the clinical, microbiological, and treatment profiles of both community-associated and healthcare-acquired complicated intra-abdominal infections (IAIs) in a worldwide context.

Patients older than 18 years with both community-acquired and healthcare-associated intra-abdominal infections will be included in the database.

In Europe, the CIAO Study has recently ended, concluding a six-month, multicenter observational study across twenty European countries. The study's findings have recently been published [15].

Given the promising results of the CIAO Study, the World Society of Emergency Surgery (WSES) has designed a prospective observational study investigating the management of complicated intra-abdominal infections in a worldwide context.

Study population

The CIAOW study (Complicated Intra-Abdominal infection Observational Worldwide Study) is a multicenter observational study currently underway in 57 medical institutions worldwide. The study includes patients undergoing surgery or interventional drainage to address complicated IAIs.

Medical institutions from each continent participate in the study. The geographical distribution of the participating centers is represented in Figure 1.

Study design

The study does not attempt to change or modify the laboratory or clinical practices of the participating physicians, and neither informed consent nor formal approval by an Ethics Committee has been required.

The study meets the standards outlined in the Declaration of Helsinki and Good Epidemiological Practices.

The study is monitored by the coordination center, which investigates and verifies missing or unclear data submitted to the central database. It is performed under the direct supervision of the board of directors of WSES.

Data collection

In each center, the coordinator collects and compiles data in an online case report system.These data include the following: (i) patient and disease characteristics, i.e., demographic data, type of infection (community- or healthcare-acquired), severity criteria, previous curative antibiotic therapy administered in the 7 days preceding surgery; (ii) origin of infection and surgical procedures performed; and (iii) microbiological data, i.e., identification of bacteria and microbial pathogens within the peritoneal fluid, the presence of yeasts (if applicable), and the antibiotic susceptibilities of bacterial isolates.

The primary endpoints include the following:

- Clinical profiles of intra-abdominal infections
- Epidemiological profiles (epidemiology of the microorganisms isolated from intra-abdominal samples and these organisms' resistance to antibiotics)
- Management profiles

Statistical analysis

At the end of the six-month study period statistical comparisons will be performed using the Student's t-test, $\chi 2$ analysis, or the Kruskall–Wallis/Wilcoxon tests, as dictated by the natural parameters of the data. Statistical significance will be defined as a P-value less than 0.05 ($P < 0.05$). Multivariate analysis will be carried out by means of stepwise logistic regressions in order to assess the predictive factors of mortality during hospitalization. Adjusted odds ratios (OR) and their 95% confidence intervals (CI) will also be included.

Inclusion criteria

- Patients older than 18 years
- Community- and healthcare-acquired complicated intra-abdominal infections

Exclusion criteria

- Age under 18 years old
- Pancreatitis
- Primary peritonitis.

Preliminary results

Patients

This preliminary report includes all data from the first two months of the six-month study period.

702 patients with a mean age of 49.2 years (range 18–98) were enrolled in the study. 272 patients (38.7%) were women and 430 (62.3%) were men. Among these patients, 615 (87.6%) were affected by community-acquired IAIs while the remaining 87 (12.4%) suffered from healthcare-associated infections.

304 patients (43.3%) were affected by generalized peritonitis while 398 (57.7%) suffered from localized peritonitis or abscesses.

112 patients (15.9%) were admitted in critical condition (severe sepsis, septic shock).

Source control

The various sources of infection are outlined in Table 1. The most frequent source of infection was acute appendicitis. 243 cases were attributable to this condition.

The most frequently performed procedure employed to address complicated appendicitis was the open appendectomy. 136 patients (55.9%) admitted for complicated appendicitis underwent open appendectomies: 95 patients (69.8%) for localized infection or abscesses and 41 patients (31.2%) for generalized peritonitis. A laparoscopic appendectomy was performed on 93 patients (39.4%) presenting with complicated acute appendicitis, 82 (88.2%) and 11 (11.8%) of whom underwent the procedure for localized peritonitis/abscesses and generalized peritonitis, respectively. Open colonic resection was performed on 1 patient to address complicated appendicitis. In the other cases of complicated appendicitis, conservative treatment (percutaneous drainage, surgical drainage,

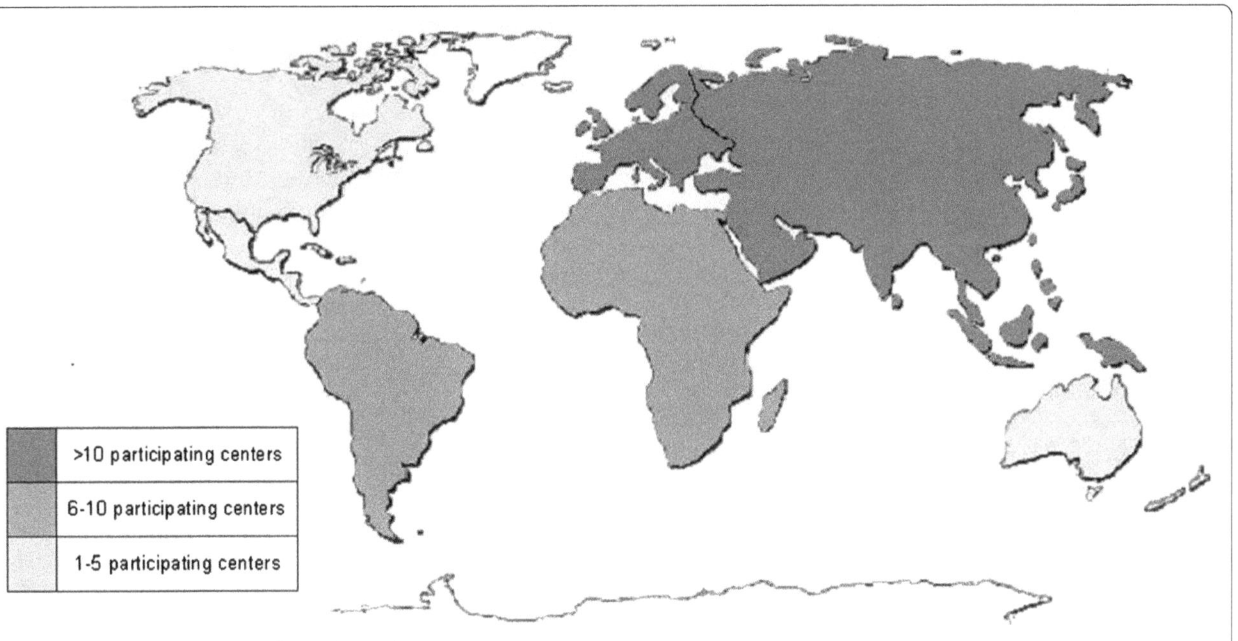

Figure 1 Participating centers for each continent.

and non-operative treatment) was performed. 7 (3%) patients underwent percutaneous drainage to address appendicular abscesses.

For patients with complicated acute cholecystitis (104 cases), the most frequently performed procedure to address cholecystitis was the open cholecystectomy. 53 cholecystitis patients (51%) underwent this procedure. A laparoscopic cholecystectomy was performed on 27 patients (26%). In the remaining cases, conservative treatment methods (percutaneous drainage, non-operative treatment) were alternatively employed.

Among the patients with complicated diverticulitis (40) the Hartmann resection was the most frequently performed procedure. 12 patients (30%) underwent a Hartmann resection. All these resections were open procedures. 8 of these patients underwent a Hartmann resection for generalized peritonitis, while the remaining 4 underwent the same procedure for localized peritonitis or abscesses.

Colo-rectal resection was performed in 11 cases (27.5%) (4 with and 7 without stoma protection).

The other patients received conservative treatment (percutaneous drainage, non-operative treatment, surgical drainage and stoma). Only two (5%) underwent laparoscopic lavage and drainage.

Of the 100 patients with gastro-duodenal perforations, the most frequent surgical procedure was gastro-duodenal suture. It was performed in 91 patients (91%): 85 patients underwent open gastro-duodenal suture and 6 patients underwent laparoscopic gastro-duodenal suture. Four (4%) patients underwent gastro-duodenal resection. The remaining patients (5%) received conservative treatment (non-operative treatment, surgical drainage).

Among the 53 patients with small bowel perforations, 35 underwent open small bowel resection (79.5%) and one (4.5%) underwent laparoscopic small bowel resection. Fourteen patients were treated by stoma. Two patients were treated by open drainage

Among the 38 patients with colonic non-diverticular perforation, 15 patients (66%) underwent open Hartmann resection, 1 patient (2.6%) underwent laparoscopic Hartmann resection, 9 (25%) underwent open resection with anastomosis and without stoma protection, and 4 underwent open resection with stoma protection (10.5%).

Microbiology

Intraperitoneal specimens were collected from 415 (59.1%) patients.

Intraperitoneal specimens were isolated from 336 of the 615 patients with community-acquired intra-abdominal infections (54.6%). Among the remaining 87 patients with healthcare-associated intra-abdominal infections, intraperitoneal specimens were collected from 79 patients (90.9%).

The major pathogens involved in intra-abdominal infections were found to be Enterobacteriaceae.

The aerobic bacteria identified in samples of peritoneal fluid are reported in Table 2.

According to CIAOW Study data, ESBL producers were the most commonly identified drug-resistant microorganism involved in IAIs.

Table 1 Source of infection

Source of infection	Patients N 702 (100%)
Appendicitis	243 (34.6%)
Cholecystitis	104 (14.8%)
Post-operative	53 (7.5%)
Colonic non diverticular perforation	38 (5.4%)
Gastroduodenal perforations	100 (14.2%)
Diverticulitis	40 (5.7%)
Small bowel perforation	53 (7.5%)
Others	52 (7.4%)
PID	8 (1.1%)
Post traumatic perforation	11 (1.6%)

1 identified isolate of Klebsiella pneumoniae proved resistant to Carbapenems.

Among the identified aerobic gram-negative isolates, there were 25 isolates of Pseudomonas aeruginosa, comprising 5.5% of all identified aerobic bacteria isolates.

Among the identified aerobic gram-positive bacteria, Enterococci (E. faecalis and E. faecium) were the most prevalent, representing 10.5% of all aerobic isolates, 3 glycopeptide-resistant Enterococci were identified; 2 were glycopeptide-resistant Enterococcus faecalis isolates and 1 was glycopeptide-resistant Enterococcus faecium isolates.

Tests for anaerobes were conducted for 168 patients.

52 anaerobes were observed. The most frequently identified anaerobic pathogen was Bacteroides. 39 Bacteroides isolates were observed during the course of the study.

Additionally, 36 Candida isolates were collectively identified. 30 were Candida albicans and 6 were non-albicans Candida.

Outcome

The overall mortality rate was 10.1% (71/702).

68 patients (9.7%) were admitted to the intensive care unit in the early recovery phase immediately following surgery.

90 patients (12.8%) ultimately required additional surgeries; 54% of these underwent relaparotomies "on-demand", 28.9% underwent open abdomen procedures.

According to univariate statistical analysis, a critical clinical condition (severe sepsis and septic shock) upon hospital admission was the most significant risk factor for death; indeed, the rate of patient mortality was 36.6% (41/112) among critically ill patients (patients presenting with septic shock and severe sepsis upon admission), but the mortality rate was only 5.1% (30/590) for clinically stable patients ($p < 0.0001$).

For patients with generalized peritonitis, the mortality rate was 18% (55/304) while patients with localized peritonitis or abscesses demonstrated a mortality rate of only 4% (16/398) ($p < 0,001$).

The immediate post-operative clinical course was a significant parameter for predicting mortality: the rate of patient mortality was 54.9% (51/93) among critically ill patients (patients presenting with septic shock and severe sepsis upon the immediate post-operative course), but the mortality rate was only 3.3% (20/609) for clinically stable patients ($p < 0.0001$).

Table 2 Aerobic bacteria identified in peritoneal fluid

Total	**455 (100%)**
Aerobic gram-negative bacteria	**352**
Escherichia coli	226(49.7%)
(Escherichia coli resistant to third generation cephalosporins)	37 (8.1%)
Klebsiella pneuumoniae	53 (11.6%)
(Klebsiella pneumoniae resistant to third generation cephalosporins)	13 (2.9%)
Klebsiella oxytoca	3 (0.7%)
Enterobacter	10 (2.2%)
Proteus	13 (2.9%)
Pseudomonas	25 (5.5%)
Others	22 (4.8%)
Aerobic gram-positive bacteria	**103**
Enterococcus faecalis	27 (5.9%)
Enterococcus faecium	21 (4.6%)
Staphylococcus Aureus	11 (2.4%)
Streptococcus spp.	29 (6.5%)
Others	15 (3.3%)

Preliminary statistical analyses were performed using MedCalc® statistical software.

Conclusion

Complicated intra-abdominal infections remain an important cause of morbidity with poor clinical prognoses.

The purpose of the CIAOW Study is to describe the epidemiological, clinical, microbiological, and treatment profiles of both community-acquired and healthcare-acquired complicated intra-abdominal infections (IAIs) based on the data collected over a six-month period (October 2012 to March 2013) from 56 medical institutions Worldwide.

The final results of the CIAOW Study will be published following the conclusion of the study period in March 2013.

Competing interests

The authors declare that they have no competing interests.

Authors' contributions

MS designed the study and wrote the manuscript. All authors read and approved the final manuscript.

Author details

[1]Department of Surgery, Macerata Hospital, Macerata, Italy. [2]Emergency Surgery, Maggiore Parma Hospital, Parma, Italy. [3]Department of General Surgery, Ospedali Riuniti, Bergamo, Italy. [4]Department of Surgery, Denver Health Medical Center, Denver, CO, USA. [5]American Board of Surgery, Philadelphia, PA, USA. [6]Harvard Medical School, Division of Trauma, Emergency Surgery and Surgical Critical Care Massachusetts General Hospital, Boston, MA, USA. [7]Department of Surgery, UC San Diego Health System, San Diego, CA, USA. [8]Department of Primary Care & Emergency Medicine, Kyoto University Graduate School of Medicine, Kyoto, Japan. [9]Department of Abdominal Surgery, University Hospital Meilahti, Helsinki, Finland. [10]Department of Surgery, University of Newcastle, Newcastle, NSW, Australia. [11]Department of Surgery, Govt Medical College and Hospital, Chandigarh, India. [12]Department of General Surgery, Rambam Health Care Campus, Haifa, Israel. [13]Department of Surgery, Adria Hospital, Adria, Italy. [14]Trauma Surgery Unit, Maggiore Hospital, Bologna, Italy. [15]Department of Surgery, Maggiore Hospital, Bologna, Italy. [16]Department of Surgery, Universidad del Valle, Fundacion Valle del Lili, Cali, Colombia. [17]Department of Surgery, Monte Sinai Hospital, Juiz de Fora, Brazil. [18]Emergency Unit, Department of Surgery, Ribeirão Preto, Brazil. [19]Department of Surgery, Chang Gung Memorial Hospital, Taoyuan, Taiwan. [20]Department of General Surgery, Hadassah Medical Center, Jerusalem, Israel. [21]Department of Surgery, Tianjin Nankai Hospital, Nankai Clinical School of Medicine, Tianjin Medical University, Tianjin, China. [22]Department of Surgery, Pt BDS Post-graduate Institute of Medical Sciences, Rohtak, India. [23]Department of Surgery, MOSC medical college, Cochin, India. [24]First Clinic of General Surgery, University Hospital /UMBAL/ St George Plovdiv, Plovdiv, Bulgaria. [25]General Surgery Clinic, Medical University/University Hospital St.George, Plovdiv, Bulgaria. [26]Department of Surgery, Edendale Hospital, Pietermaritzburg, Republic of South Africa. [27]Department of Surgery, Ahmadu Bello University Teaching Hospital Zaria, Kaduna, Nigeria. [28]Department of Surgery, Mansoura University Hospital, Mansoura, Egypt. [29]Department of Surgery, Faculdades Integradas Padre Albino, Catanduva, Brazil. [30]Department of Surgery, Mazzoni Hospital, Ascoli Piceno, Italy. [31]Department of Surgery, Mellini Hospital, Chiari (BS), Italy. [32]Department of General and Digestive Surgery, Virgen de la Victoria, University Hospital, Malaga, Spain. [33]Department of General Surgery and Surgical Oncology, Université de Nice Sophia-Antipolis, Universitary Hospital of Nice, Nice, France. [34]Department of Surgery, Hospital and Oncological Centre, Novy Jicin, Czech Republic. [35]Department of General Surgery, Lviv Emergency Hospital, Lviv, Ukraine. [36]Department of Surgery, University Hospital Center Zagreb, Zagreb, Croatia. [37]3rd Department of General Surger Jagiellonian Univeristy, Narutowicz Hospital, Krakow, Poland. [38]Department of Surgery, Mozyr City Hospital, Mozyr, Belarus. [39]Department of Surgery, Ancona University, Ancona, Italy. [40]Department of Surgery, Ripas Hospital, Bandar Seri Begawan, Brunei. [41]Clinical Sciences, Regional Hospitals Limbe and Buea, Limbe, Cameroon. [42]Department of Surgery, Severance Hospital, Yonsei University College of Medicine, Seoul, Republic of Korea. [43]Division of Trauma and Surgical Critical Care, Department of Surgery, University of Ulsan, Seoul, Republic of Korea. [44]II Cátedra de Clínica Quirúrgica, Hospital de Clínicas, Asuncion, Paraguay. [45]Department of Surgery, Khamis Mushayt General Hospital, Khamis Mushayt, Saudi Arabia. [46]Department of Surgery, Cutral Co Clinic, Neuquen, Argentina. [47]Department of Surgery, Faculty of Medicine Siriraj Hospital, Bangkok, Thailand. [48]Department of Surgery, Thammasat University Hospital, Pathumthani, Thailand. [49]Department of Surgery, Hospital Regional de Alta Especialidad del Bajio, Leon, Mexico. [50]Department of Clinical and Experimental Sciences, Brescia University, Brescia, Italy. [51]General Surgery, Adana Numune Training and Research Hospital, Adana, Turkey. [52]Visceral Surgery, Military Hospital Desgenettes, Lyon, France. [53]Visceral Surgery, Teaching Hospital Yalgado Ouedraogo, Ouagadougou, Burkina Faso. [54]Department of Acute and Critical care medicine, Tokyo Medical and Dental University, Tokyo, Japan. [55]The Shock Trauma and Emergency Medical Center, Matsudo City Hospital, Chiba, Japan. [56]Emergency and Critical Care Center of Nippon Medical School, Tama-Nagayama Hospital, Tokyo, Japan. [57]Department of Surgery, Our Lady of Lourdes Hospital, Drogheda, Ireland. [58]Department of Surgery, Port Shepstone Hospital, Port Shepstone, South Africa. [59]Department of Surgery, College of Health Sciences, Obafemi Awolowo University Hospital, Ile-Ife, Nigeria. [60]Department of Emergency and Critical Care Medicine, Chiba University Hospital, Chiba, Japan. [61]Department of Surgery, Bahrain Defence Force Hospital, Manama, Bahrain. [62]Department of Emergency Medicine, Kyoto Second Red Cross Hospital, Kyoto, Japan.

References

1. Sartelli M, Viale P, Koike K, Pea F, Tumietto F, van Goor H, Guercioni G, Nespoli A, Tranà C, Catena F, Ansaloni L, Leppaniemi A, Biffl W, Moore FA, Poggetti R, Pinna AD, Moore EE, WSES consensus conference: **Guidelines for first-line management of intra-abdominal infections.** *World J Emerg Surg* 2011, **6**:2.
2. Sartelli M: **A focus on intra-abdominal infections.** *World J Emerg Surg.* 2010, **5**:9.
3. Azzarello G, Lanteri R, Rapisarda C, Santangelo M, Racalbuto A, Minutolo V, Di Cataldo A, Licata A: **Ultrasound-guided percutaneous treatment of abdominal collections.** *Chir Ital* 2009, **61**:337–340.
4. Gazelle GS, Mueller PR: **Abdominal abscess: Imaging and intervention.** *Radiol Clin North Am* 1994, **32**:913–932.
5. VanSonnenberg E, Ferrucci JT, Mueller PR, Wittenberg J, Simeone JF: **Percutaneous drainage of abscesses and fluid collections: Technique, results, and applications.** *Radiology* 1982, **142**:1–10.
6. Bouali K, Magotteaux P, Jadot A, Saive C, Lombard R, Weerts J, Dallemagne B, Jehaes C, Delforge M, Fontaine F: **Percutaneous catheter drainage of abdominal abscess after abdominal surgery: Results in 121 cases.** *J Belg Radiol* 1993, **76**:11–14.
7. VanSonnenberg E, Wing VW, Casola G, Coons HG, Nakamoto SK, Mueller PR, Ferrucci JT Jr, Halasz NA, Simeone JF: **Temporizing effect of percutaneous drainage of complicated abscesses in critically ill patients.** *Am J Roentgenol* 1984, **142**:821–826.
8. Bufalari A, Giustozzi G, Moggi L: **Postoperative intra-abdominal abscesses: Percutaneous versus surgical treatment.** *Acta Chir Belg* 1996, **96**(5):197–200.
9. VanSonnenberg E, Mueller PR, Ferrucci JT Jr: **Percutaneous drainage of 250 abdominal abscesses and fluid collections. I. Results, failures, and complications.** *Radiology* 1984, **151**:337–341.
10. Jaffe TA, Nelson RC, DeLong D, Paulson EK: **Practice Patterns in Percutaneous Image-guided Intra-abdominal Abscess Drainage: Survey of Academic and Private Practice Centres.** *Radiology* 2004, **233**:750–756.
11. van Ruler O, Lamme B, Gouma DJ, Reitsma JB, Boermeester MA: **Variables associated with positive findings at relaparotomy in patients with secondary peritonitis.** *Crit Care Med* 2007, **35**(2):468–476.

12. Hutchins RR, Gunning MP, Lucas DN, Allen-Mersh TG, Soni NC: **Relaparotomy for suspected intraperitoneal sepsis after abdominal surgery.** *World J Surg* 2004, **28**(2):137–141.
13. Lamme B, Mahler CW, van Ruler O, Gouma DJ, Reitsma JB, Boermeester MA: **Clinical predictors of ongoing infection in secondary peritonitis: systematic review.** *World J Surg* 2006, **30**(12):2170–2181.
14. Hawser SP, Bouchillon SK, Lascols C, Hackel M, Hoban DJ, Badal RE, Woodford N, Livermore DM: **Susceptibility of Klebsiella pneumoniae isolates from intra-abdominal infections and molecular characterization of ertapenem-resistant isolates.** *Antimicrob Agents Chemother* 2011, **55**(8):3917–3921.
15. Sartelli M, Catena F, Ansaloni L, Leppaniemi A, Taviloglu K, Goor H, Viale P, Lazzareschi DV, Coccolini F, Corbella D, Werra C, Marrelli D, Colizza S, Scibè R, Alis H, Torer N, Navarro S, Sakakushev B, Massalou D, Augustin G, Catani M, Kauhanen S, Pletinckx P, Kenig J, Saverio S, Jovine E, Guercioni G, Skrovina M, Diaz-Nieto R, Ferrero A, *et al*: **Complicated intra-abdominal infections in Europe: a comprehensive review of the CIAO study.** *World J Emerg Surg* 2012, **7**(1):36.

5

Anorectal avulsion: an exceptional rectal trauma

Karim Ibn majdoub Hassani*, Said Ait laalim, El Bachir Benjelloun, Imane Toughrai and Khalid Mazaz

Abstract

Anorectal avulsion is an exceptional rectal trauma in which the anus and sphincter no longer join the perineum and are pulled upward. As a result, they ventrally follow levator ani muscles. We present a rare case of a 29-years old patient who was admitted in a pelvic trauma context; presenting a complete complex anorectal avulsion. The treatment included a primary repair of the rectum and a diverting colostomy so as to prevent sepsis. Closure of the protective sigmoidostomy was performed seven months after the accident and the evolution was marked by an anal stenosis requiring iterative dilatations.

Keywords: Anorectal avulsion, Rectal trauma, Surgical management

Introduction

Anorectal avulsion is an exceptional rectal trauma. In this kind of lesions, the anus and sphincter no longer join the perineum and are pulled upward. They are in addition ventrally following levator ani muscles. The management of this kind of lesions remains a matter of great debate. Early repair of the rectum, diverting colostomy, wound debridement, distal rectal wash-out are the most important procedures that help prevent sepsis. In addition, the colostomy closure can only be performed after pelvic rehabilitation in order to prevent transitory incontinence.

Observation

A 29-years-old patient was admitted to the emergency room (ER) of the University hospital Hassan II of Fez after having an accident which resulted in a severe pelvic trauma. When the patient was admitted to the ER, he was agitated but conscious and hemodynamically stable with slightly discolored conjunctives. The physical examination revealed a pulse rate of 90 beat per minute, a blood pressure of 110/80 mmHg, but there was no fever. Abdominal examination showed minimal tenderness in the hypogastria with a distended bladder. Urologic examination revealed urethral bleeding with a large scrotal scar. The perineal exam showed a big substance loss with complete anorectal avulsion due to the contraction of the elevator ani muscle (Figure 1). Laboratory data showed a white-blood cell count of 10 900/mm3, serum hemoglobin concentration of 10,4 g/dl with a normal blood platelet level (390,000/mm3), a blood urea of 0.45 g/l and a creatinine level of 10 mg/L. Hemostasis laboratory data, chemistry and serum lipase were within normal limits. So, being hemodynamic stable, the patient underwent chest X-ray. The latter was normal. The pelvic X-ray showed a right ischio pubic rami fracture (Figure 2). A contrast-enhanced computed tomography (CT) was performed and therefore showed a pelvic trauma with right ischio pubic rami fracture (Figure 3) as well as a fracture in the right transverse process of L5 and S1 sacral wing. CT scan also showed a right bladder effusion extending to the retro peritoneal area. Furthermore, there was a large inguinal hematoma measuring 10 x 4 cm and fusing along the right thigh. It was therefore associated with symphysis emphysematous soft tissue extending down to the scrotum the thing that resulted in a right scrotal pneumatocele (Figure 4). There was also free air in the perineum, the perirectal space and the right lateral abdominal wal (Figures 5, 6). No free abdominal fluid or air was detected. The patient was taken to the operating room. Suprapubic cyst catheter was placed. During the perineal exam, the anorectal stump was hardly recognized among the injured tissues for it was retracted upward and ventrally making the distance between the anal canal and the perineal skin about 6 cm (Figure 7). A rectal washout was performed. Necrosectomy with several debridements as well as presacral irrigation were realized. The anorectal mucosa was closed at first; then the torn ends of the

* Correspondence: ibnmajdoubkarim@gmail.com
Department of Surgery, School of Medicine and Pharmacy of Fez, Sidi Mohammed Ben Abdellah University, BP: 1893; Km2.200, Route de Sidi Hrazem, Fez 30000, Morocco

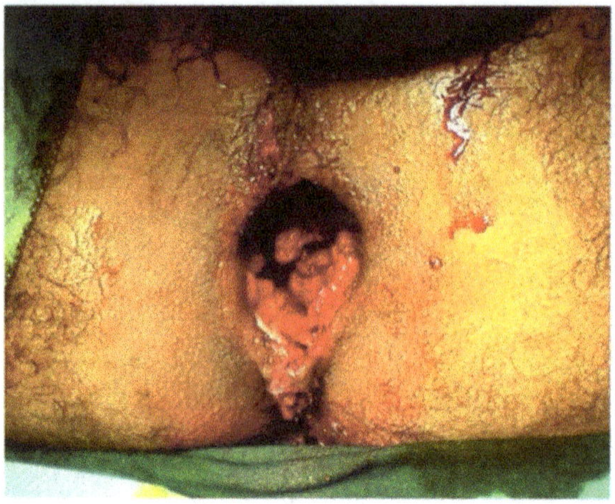

Figure 1 Inspection of the perineum showing a big loss of substance with complete avulsion of anorectal complex.

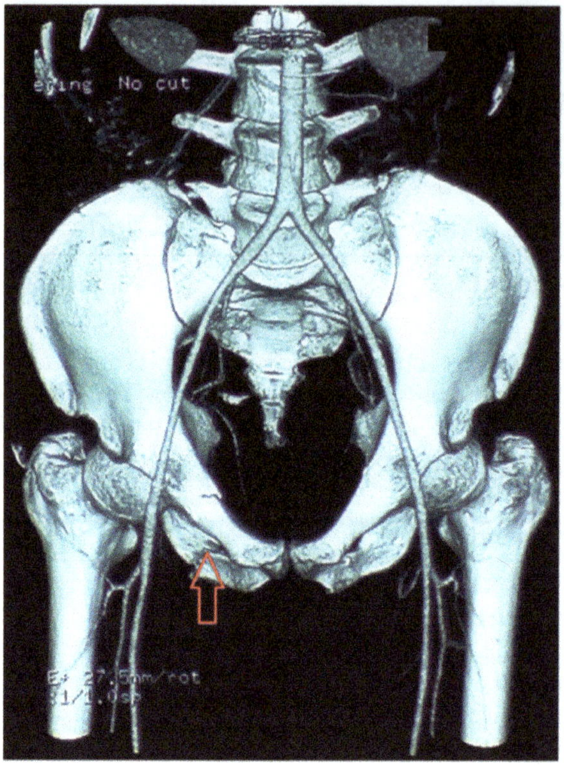

Figure 3 Computed tomography (CT) showing a right ischio pubic rami fracture.

external sphincter were identified and sutured accurately. Presacral drainage was placed in the ischio rectal area by a passive drain and delbet lames (Figure 8). Finally the perineal skin was closed using good mattress sutures to build up the perineal body. A sigmoid loop colostomy was performed through an elective laparotomy in the left iliac fossa. As far as the treatment is concerned, the patient was given an antibiotic regimen consisting of ciprofloxacin and metronidazole for two weeks. The postoperative course was unremarkable. Drainage was removed at the fifth day after surgery. Conservative treatment was undertaken for spine and rib fracture. Anorectal Manometry was performed six months after surgery. The latter did not show any physiologic dysfunction except the length

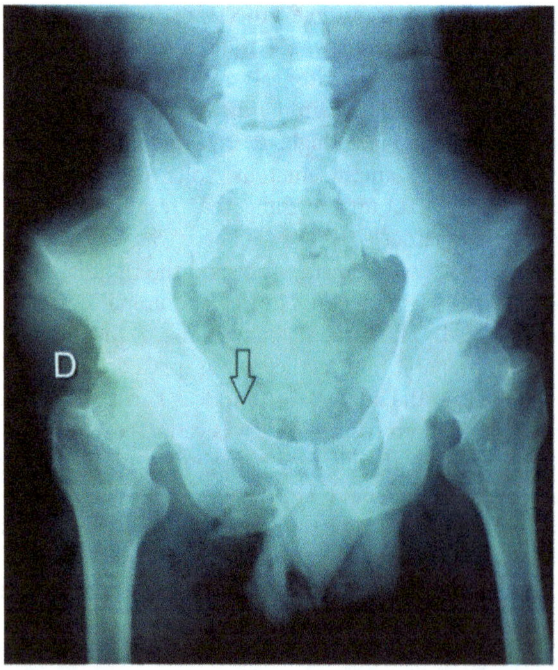

Figure 2 Pelvic X-ray showing a right ischio pubic rami fracture.

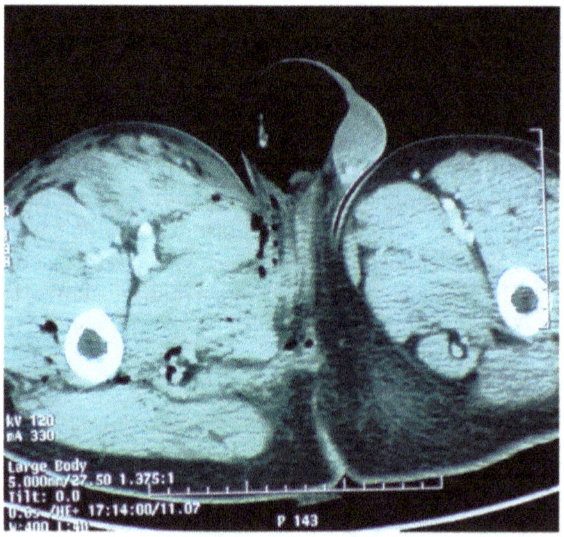

Figure 4 CT showing a right scrotal Pneumatocele.

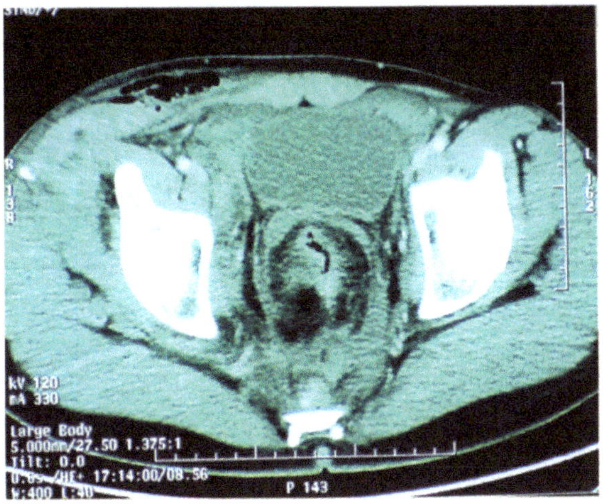

Figure 5 CT showing free air in perirectal space and in the right lateral abdominal wall.

of the anal canal which was reduced to less than 2 cm (Figure 9). Sigmoidostomy closure was performed seven months after the surgery. Unfortunately, the evolution was marked by anal stenosis which required iterative dilatations. Nowadays, during 9 months of follow up, the patient is free of any symptoms since the very last dilatation.

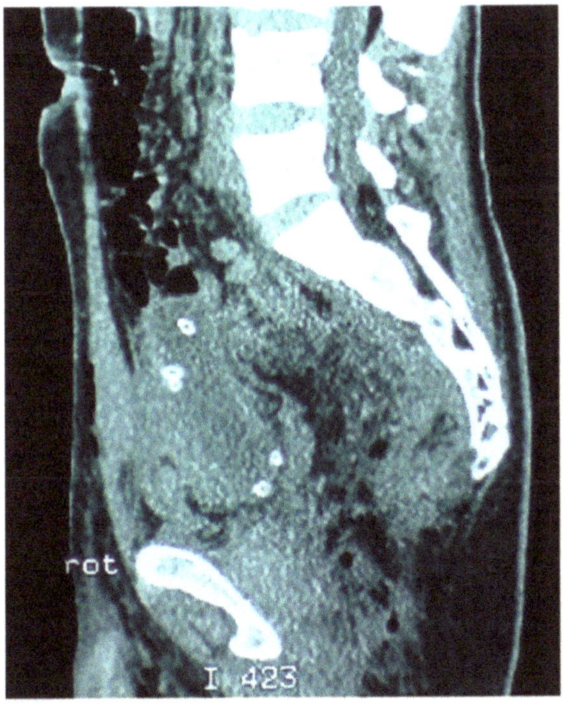

Figure 6 Coronal coupe showing the anorectal avulsion with free air in the perirectal space.

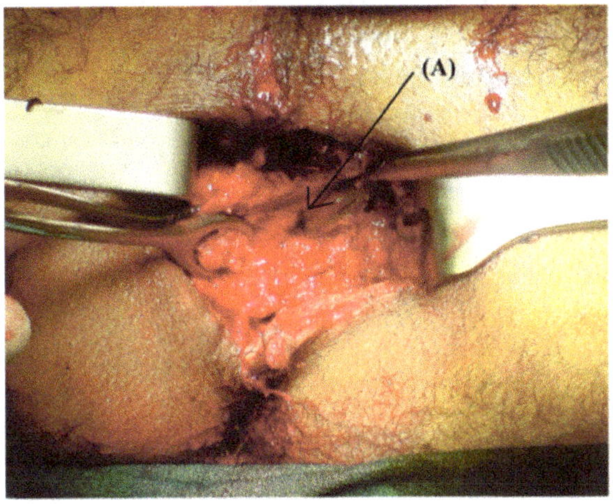

Figure 7 The perineum examination showing anorectal stump retracted upward and ventrally (A: rectal lumen).

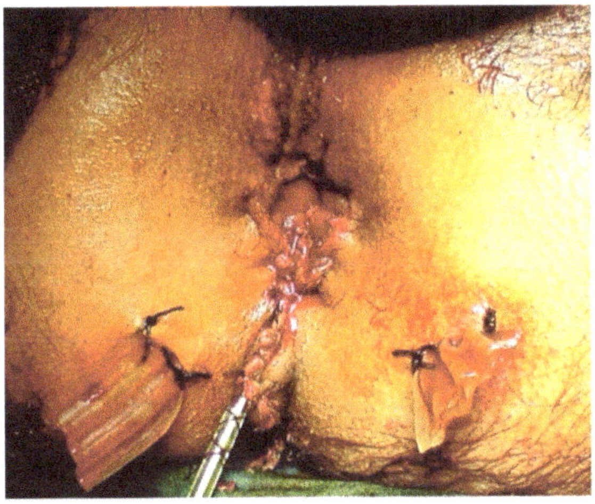

Figure 8 Perineal skin closed with presacral drainage.

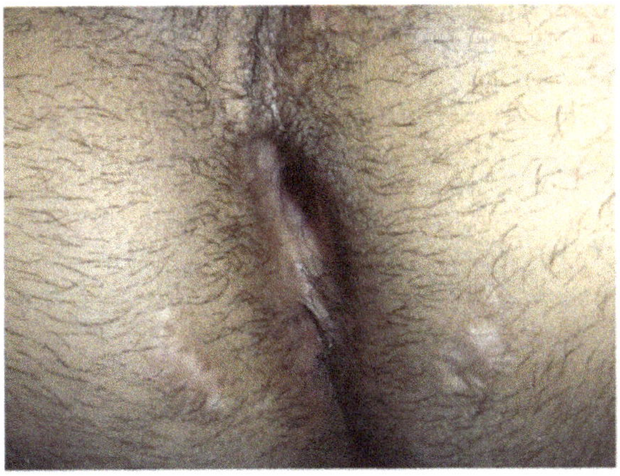

Figure 9 Final aspect of the anal margin six months after anorectal repair.

Table 1 Reported cases of anorectal avulsion

Authors	Year	Title	Management of the anorectal avulsion
Mathieson, A. J et al.	1965	Rupture of the posterior urethra and avulsion of the rectum and anus as a complication of fracture of the pelvis	Primary repair + presacral drainage + sigmoid loop colostomy
Sharma D. et al	2000	Anorectal avulsion: an unusual rectal injury	Primary repair + presacral drainage + sigmoid loop colostomy
Terrosu G. et al	2011	Anal avulsion caused by abdominal crush injury	Anal reimplantation + pelvic drainage tubes + loop transverse colostomy
Rispoli C. et al.	2012	Anorectal avulsion: Management of a rare rectal trauma	Direct suture not possible sigmoid loop colostomy + presacral drainage + anoperineal reparation 10 weeks later
R. M. Gomesa et al	2013	Anorectal avulsion: report of a rare case of rectal injury	diverting sigmoid loop colostomy (primary repair not possible)

Discussion

Although there are similarities between colonic injuries and rectal ones, there are also differences which are unique to the rectum. Approximately 80% of rectal injuries are attributable to firearms and less than 3% are secondary to stab or impalement etiologies. Less than 10% of rectal injuries are blunt by nature as a result of falls, motor vehicle accidents or pelvic fractures [1]. While the management of rectal injuries has changed over the last few years, optimal treatment remains a matter of great debate. The anorectal avulsion is a particular case of rectal injuries. It's a very rare rectal trauma. After reviewing the literature, we found out that the first case of post traumatic anorectal avulsion was reported in 1965 by Mathieson et al. [2]. During the following years, only few case reports were described (Table 1) [3-6]. In this kind of lesions, the anus and sphincter no longer join the perineum and are pulled upward and thus ventrally follow levator ani muscles. In addition, their treatment is controversial and not standardized [7]. A multidisciplinary approach is mandatory involving general surgeons, anesthetists and rehabilitators [8,9]. The main difficulties encountered when treating these lesions are: to prevent sepsis and keep good anal sphincter functions at the same time. Management strategies described in the literature include diverting sigmoidostomy, presacral drainage, direct suture repair of the rectal laceration and irrigation of the rectum. In 1989, Burch et al. [10] recommended fecal diversion and presacral drainage for rectal injury management. The primary repair of a rectal lesion should be always tried if local conditions allow it. This was the case of our patient in which direct suture was difficult to perform but was still possible. Presacral drainage is believed to prevent perirectal infections due to fecal contamination and has been used widely to reduce abscess formation in extraperitoneal rectal trauma. This evidence derives mainly by war injury [7], but some authors [9,11,12] demonstrated no difference in infection rates associated with civilian rectal trauma caused by low velocity injury. Diverting colostomy has been demonstrated safe and effective in reducing the infection rate associated with rectal trauma 8 and a valid tool to perform rectal wash-out. However, in a study by Gonzales [13], fourteen patients suffering from non-destructive penetrating extraperitoneal rectal injuries were treated without fecal diversion or direct suture repair. Infectious complications didn't occur in any of these patients. Furthermore, Navsaria and colleagues concluded from their retrospective review that extraperitoneal rectal injuries caused by low-velocity penetrating trauma could be treated only by fecal diversion [9]. Although there are controversies concerning the colostomy type, the drainage method, the need for distal washout, and the need to repair the rectal wound, most trauma surgeons as it is the case with our surgical tream, would agree about the need for diversion and drainage in the management of extraperitoneal rectal injuries in addition to primary repair of rectal lesion which should always be tried if local conditions allow it [14,15].

Consent

Written informed consent was obtained from the patient for publication of this Case report and any accompanying images.

Competing interests

All authors declare no competing interests.

Authors' contributions

KIM and SA participated in writing the case report and revising the draft, IT took the photos E B and KM participated in the follow up. All authors read and approved the final manuscript.

Authors' information

School of Medicine And Pharmacy of Fez, Sidi Mohammed Ben Abdellah University Department of Surgery, University hospital HASSAN II, BP: 1893; Km2.200, Route de Sidi Hrazem; FEZ 30000, MOROCCO.

Acknowledgements

The authors would like to thank the patient for his written consent and permission to present this case report. They would also like to thank Miss Ibn Majdoub Hassani Soukaina (Master : Multilingual Specialized Translation, Faculty of Arts and Humanities Sais-Fez /Sidi Mohamed Ben Abdellah University) for her help in editing and correcting this manuscript.

References

1. Cintron JR: *Colon and rectum trauma.* www.fascrs.org/physicians/education/core_subjects/2006/colon_rectal_trauma/.
2. Mathieson AJM, Mann TS: **Rupture of the posterior urethra and avulsion of the rectum and anus as a complication of fracture of the pelvis.** *Brit J Surg* 1965, **52:**309.
3. Sharma D, Rahman H, Mandloi KC, Saxena A, Raina VK, Kapoor JP: **Anorectal avulsion: an unusual rectal injury.** *Digestive Surg* 2000, **17:**193–194. PubMed: 10781991.
4. Terrosu G, Rossetto A, Kocjancic E, Rossitti P, Bresadola V: **Anal avulsion caused by abdominal crush injury.** *Tech in Coloproctology* 2011, **15:**465–468 [PubMed: 21556880].
5. Rispoli C, Andreuccetti J, Iannone L, *et al*: **Anorectal avulsion: management of a rare rectal trauma.** *Int J Surg Case Rep* 2012, **3:**319–321.
6. Gomesa RM, Kudchadkara J, Araujob E, Gundawarc T: **Anorectal avulsion: report of a rare case of rectal injury, letter to the editor.** *Ann Gastroenterology* 2013, **26:**1.
7. Velmahos GC, Gomez H, Falabella A, Demetriades D: **Operative management of civilian rectal gunshot wounds: simpler is better.** *World J Surg* 2000, **24**(1):114–118. PubMed: 10594214.
8. Cleary RK, Pomerantz RA, Lampman RM: **Colon and rectal injuries.** *Dis Colon and Rectum* 2006, **49**(8):1203–1222. PubMed: 16858663.
9. Navsaria PH, Edu S, Nicol AJ: **Civilian extraperitoneal rectal gunshot wounds: surgical management made simpler.** *World J Surg* 2007, **31**(6):1345–1351. PubMed: 17457641.
10. Burch MD JM, Feliciano MD DV, Mattox MD KL: **Colostomy and drainage for civilian rectal injuries: is that all?** *Ann Surg* 1989, **209**(5):600–610. discussion 610-1.
11. Gonzalez RP, Falimirski ME, Holevar MR: **The role of presacral drainage in the management of penetrating rectal injuries.** *J Trauma* 1998, **45**(4):656–661. PubMed: 9783600.
12. Armstrong RG, Schmitt HJ Jr, Patterson LT: **Combat wounds of the extraperitoneal rectum.** *Surgery* 1973, **74:**570–574. PubMed: 4729222.
13. Gonzalez RP, Phelan H 3rd, Hassan M, Ellis CN, Rodning CB: **Is fecal diversion necessary for nondestructive penetrating extraperitoneal rectal injuries ?** *J Trauma* 2006, **61**(4):815–819.
14. Burch JM, Feliciano DV, Mattox KL: **Colostomy and drainage for civilian rectal injuries: is that all?** *Ann Surg* 1989, **209**(5):600–610.
15. Ivatury RR, Licata J, Gunduz Y, Rao P, Stahl WM: **Management options in penetrating rectal injuries.** *Am Surg* 1991, **57**(1):50–55.

6

Appendicular perforation at the base of the caecum, a rare operative challenge in acute appendicitis

Chee Siong Wong* and Syed Altaf Naqvi

Abstract

Background: Acute appendicitis is the most common acute surgical condition of the abdomen. Diagnosis is made based on full clinical history and examination as well as supported by a routine blood investigation and urine test. Prompt diagnosis and surgical referral may reduce the risk of perforation and prevent complications. The mortality rate of non-perforated appendicitis is less than 1 percent. Perforated appendicitis is associated with a higher mortality rate - as high as five percent and may be particularly more in extreme of age group attributed to delay in clinical presentation or diagnosis in the younger group and multiple co-morbidities in the elderly group. The aetiology is unknown. It may be linked with lack of fibre, familial tendency, or viral infection. It may be precipitated by faecaliths. The commonest site of the appendix is retrocaecal.

Case Report: We report a case of a 46 year old male who was admitted under the surgical service in Mid-Western Regional Hospital, Limerick with suspected appendicitis which turned out to be a perforated caecum, a rare complication of an acute appendicitis. We performed a literature review comparing two main approaches - right hemicolectomy and primary closure with omental patch - discuss and highlight their differences as well as a guide to its management.

Conclusion: There are limited studies to compare these two surgical options in the literature. A larger prospective study is needed to compare both approaches and long term outcome.

Background

Acute appendicitis remains the most common reason for intervention in acute abdominal pain. Diagnosis is made based on full clinical history and examination as well as supported by a routine blood investigation and urine test. It is a common condition can be difficult in making a diagnosis when the clinical picture is borderline suggestive of acute appendicitis. Especially in children, acute Meckel's diverticulitis must be kept in mind, as the clinical picture is indistinguishable from acute appendicitis. Perforation of a large bowel is associated with severe acute appendicitis but further surgical management of this condition uncommonly described in the literature. We highlighted this question and performed a literature review to compare two possible surgical approaches faced by surgeons.

* Correspondence: cswmichael@yahoo.co.uk
Department of Surgery, Mid Western Regional Hospital, Dooradoyle, Co. Limerick, Ireland

Case Report

A 46 year old man presented with a day history of sudden onset of right iliac fossa pain associated with nausea, fever, and anorexia. No urinary and bowel symptoms. There was no significant past surgical or medical history. No history of recent travel and family history of colitis or inflammatory bowel disease. On physical examination, his temperature was 39.4 degree Celsius, pulse rate 91 beats per minute, blood pressure 159/80 mmHg, respiratory rate 20. His abdomen was not distended but tender in the right iliac fossa with some voluntary guarding. No rebound tenderness was elicited on examination. Rovsing's sign was positive.

Full blood count shows elevated WBC $19.91 \times 10^9/L$, Hb 13.7 g/dl, Platelet 242 $10^9/L$. Na 137 mmol/L, K 3.8 mmol/L, urea 4.8 mmol/L, creatinine 92 mmol/L, amylase 24 IU/L. Urine Microscopy - negative for urinary tract infection, leucocytes < 10/ul and red cell < 10/ul.

Plain film of Abdomen and Chest X-Ray were not remarkable (Figure 1 and 2). Diagnosis of acute appendicitis was made clinically and the patient was consented for an open appendicectomy under general anaesthesia.

Operation: Intravenous antibiotics were commenced pre-operatively. An extended McBurney's or grid iron incision was made. Dissection of the appendix was carried out with some difficulties and approximately 50 mls of pus found in the peritoneal cavity around the appendix. There was a large 3 × 3 cm caecum perforation seen at the base of the appendix (Figure 3). Macroscopically, appendix was perforated and gangrenous. Perforation at the base of caecum was repaired with an absorbable suture and the omental patch was used to cover the caecum (Figure 4). A thorough washout with warm saline and bethidine solution was carried out to prevent gross peritoneal contamination. A corrugated drain was inserted. The abdominal incision was closed by a mass closure technique using loop PDS 2/0 and absorbable sutures to subcutaneous tissue and staples to skin.

Post operative progress. Inflammatory markers were responding with intravenous antibiotic. No further spiking temperature. The drain was removed postoperative day 5 and patient was discharged the next day. The histolopathology of the appendix showed acutely inflamed appendix with periappendiceal abscess formation. The epithelium shows reactive/reparative changes. No malignancy is seen.

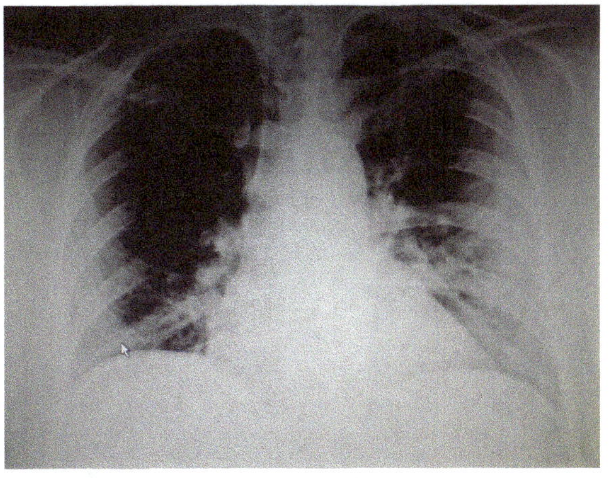

Figure 2 Normal erect chest x-ray. No air under the diaphragm.

Discussion

Appendicitis perforations, commonly occur at the tip of the appendix, are associated with the presence of a faecolith on CT scan and not the anatomical location of the appendix (retrocaecal appendix) as previously

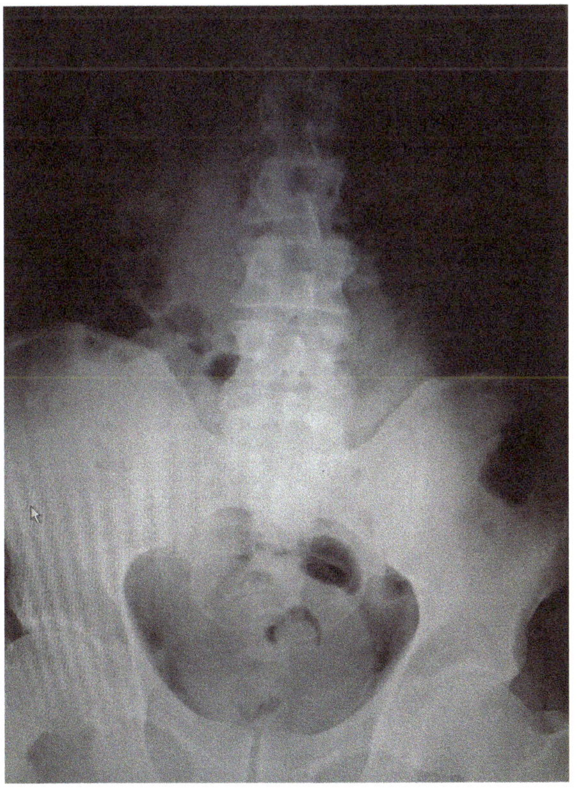

Figure 1 Normal plain film of the abdomen.

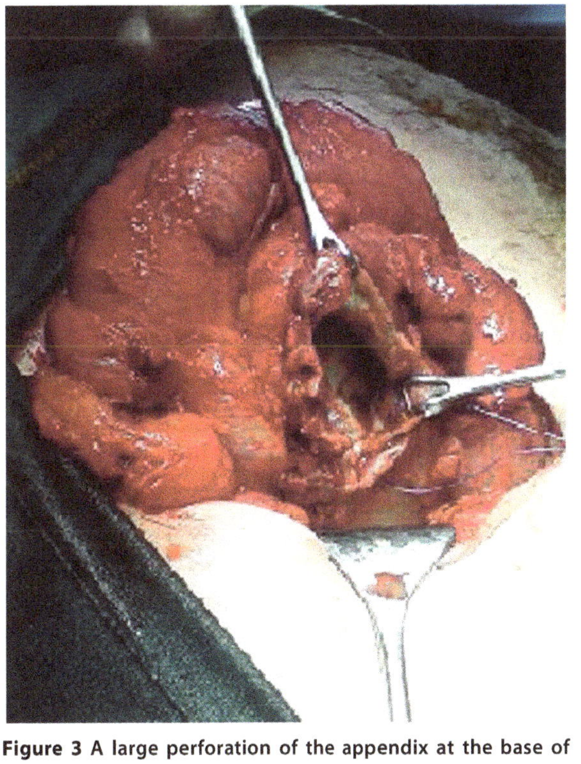

Figure 3 A large perforation of the appendix at the base of the caecum.

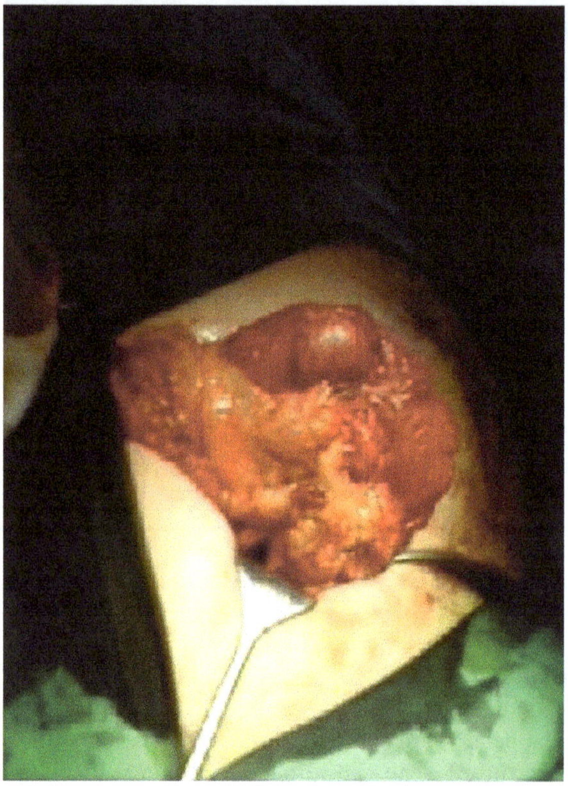

Figure 4 The perforation was oversewn and omentum was used to cover the defect on the caecum.

thought [1]. Perforation of caecum is an uncommon differential diagnosis for an acute appendicitis. Other possible causes of caecum perforation include perforated right diverticulitis [2,3], caecal tumor, and rarely associated with foreign body [4,5], in burn patient [6], tuberculosis infection [7] and following caesarean section [8,9] or iatrogenic endoscopic procedure had been reported. Surgery for colonic perforation is associated with high morbidity and mortality rates.

While omental patch repair is a common surgical approach to management of stomach and duodenum perforation, there are only few reports in the literature that compare two very different surgical approaches - omental patch with primary repair vs right hemicolectomy. In the presence of an uncomplicated perforation, absence of severe infection, and well controlled localized haemostasis - a less invasive surgical approach with post operative intravenous antibiotics would be the management of choice.

Right hemicolectomy carries a higher morbidity and mortality but it is generally recommended only in selected cases - severe inflammation, torsion, haemorrhage, and inflammatory mass or caecal neoplasm found intraoperatively [10]. The presence of severe appendicitis; or caecum appears necrotic in some cases warrants right hemicolectomy to be performed.

A caecum perforation is a very rare identity and so far only nine case reports have been published (Table 1). The most frequent operation for perforated caecum is right hemicolectomy although some surgeons might advocate oversewn the perforation is equally adequate in repairing the defect. The advantages of the latter are associated with shorter length of hospital stay, less blood loss, easier haemostasis control, and lower risk of anastomosis breakdown. However, there is no clinical data yet to support this hypothesis.

Although right hemicolectomy may be the conventional approach in some cases of caecal perforation, however, in a highly contaminated case as such in this scenario would have a significantly higher postoperative complication likely secondary to infection or systemic septicaemia. Therefore, the decision for a primary repair of the perforation was carried out.

Conclusion

A primary hemicolectomy in perforated lesion of the caecum is recommended but there have been no recent studies comparing this approach with primary caecum

Table 1 Various similar case reports and their surgical approaches

Author (Year) [Ref]	Case Reports
Jain et al (2010) [7]	Primary tubercular caecal perforation and a right hemicolectomy with ileostomy was performed
Cole et al (2009) [11]	A perforated caecal diverticulum and a right hemicolectomy was carried out
Papapolychroniadis et al (2004) [2]	Two cases of perforated caecum diverticulum and right hemicolectomy was carried out on both cases
Mauvais et al (1999) [3]	Perforated caecum due to diverticulitis on post operative findings. However author did not discuss further on surgical approach
Vitali et al (1998) [12]	Caecal perforated diverticulitis but did not mention of its surgical approach
Mosca et al (1997) [13]	A case of perforated caecum diverticulitis and right hemicolectomy was carried out
Ghoneim et al (1995) [6]	Caecal perforation in burn patient was treated using a right hemicolectomy
Dorfman et al (1990) [14]	Reported five cases of perforated caecal diverticulitis. Two cases were treated with a right hemicolectomy
Wesch et al (1980) [8]	Two cases of perforation of the cecum following caesarean section. The perforation is oversewn

repair with omental patch. A larger prospective study is needed to compare both approaches and long term outcome.

Authors' contributions

MW drafted the manuscript, searched the literature and the findings, manuscript writing & editing and submission of the manuscript. SAN critically reviewed the manuscript. Both authors read and approved the final manuscript submission.

Competing interests

The authors declare that they have no competing interests.

References

1. Herscu G, Kong A, Russell D, Tran CL, Varela JE, Cohen A, Stamos MJ: **Retrocecal appendix location and perforation at presentation.** *Am Surg* 2006, **72(10)**:890-3.
2. Papapolychroniadis C, Kaimakis D, Fotiadis P, Karamanlis E, Stefopoulou M, Kouskouras K, Dimitriadis A, Harlaftis N: **Perforated diverticulum of the caecum. A difficult preoperative diagnosis. Report of 2 cases and review of the literature.** *Neumann U, Tech Coloproctol* 2004, **8(Suppl 1)**:s116-8.
3. Mauvais F, Benoist S, Panis Y, Chafaï N, Valleur P: **Three cases of diverticular perforation of the caecum and ascending colon.** *Ann Chir* 1999, **53(1)**:89-91.
4. Fielitz J, Ehlert HG: **Perforation of the cecum by a toothpick–a rare differential acute appendicitis diagnosis. Case report and review of the literature.** *Chirurg* 2000, **71(11)**:1405-8.
5. Renner K, Holzer B, Hochwarter G, Weihsbeck E, Schiessel R: **Dig Surg.** *Needle perforation of the appendix* 2000, **17(4)**:413-4.
6. Ghoneim IE, Bang RL: **Caecal perforation in a burn patient.** *Burns* 1995, **21(8)**:619-21.
7. Jain DK, Aggarwal G, Lubana PS, Moses S, Joshi N: **Primary tubercular caecal perforation: a rare clinical entity.** *BMC Surg* 2010, **10**:12.
8. Wesch G, Ehrlich G, Storz LW, Wiest W: **Two cases of perforation of the cecum following caesarean section.** *Geburtshilfe Frauenheilkd* 1980, **40(2)**:116-20.
9. Durai R, Linsell J: **Caecal perforation following a caesarean section.** *Br J Hosp Med (Lond)* 2011, **72(5)**:290-1.
10. Kumar Susim, Fitzmaurice JGerard, O'Donnell EMark, Brown Robin: **Acute right iliac fossa pain: not always appendicitis or a caecal tumour: two case reports.** *Cases J* 2009, **2**:88.
11. Cole M, Ayantunde AA, Payne J: **Caecal diverticulitis presenting as acute appendicitis: a case report.** *World J Emerg Surg* 2009, **4**:29.
12. Vitali V, Di Vito A, Menno P: **A rare case of a perforated diverticulum of the cecum.** *Minerva Chir* 1998, **53(6)**:531-4.
13. Mosca F, Stracqualursi A, Piazza D, Zappalà O, Lanzafame S, Latteri F: **A rare case of acute abdomen: perforated acute diverticulitis of the cecum.** *G Chir* 1997, **18(8-9)**:421-5.
14. Dorfman S, Barboza R, Finol F, Cardozo J: **Single diverticulum of perforated cecum. Report of 5 cases.** *Rev Esp Enferm Dig* 1990, **77(2)**:147-8.

7

Methylene Blue injection via superior mesenteric artery microcatheter for focused enterectomy in the treatment of a bleeding small intestinal arteriovenous malformation

James Frydman[1*], Hany Bahouth[1], Maxim Leiderman[2], Amos Ofer[2] and Yoram Kluger[1]

Abstract

Introduction: Obscure gastrointestinal bleeding from the small intestine may present the Acute Care Surgeon with a formidable diagnostic and therapeutic challenge. Despite the current array of diagnostic studies, localization of the causative pathology may be elusive, especially when the bleeding is intermittent. When a small intestinal arteriovenous malformation is the responsible lesion, a technique combining super-selective angiography with intra-operative methylene blue injection and focused enterectomy has been described in a number of case series. The current case report utilizes this same approach with emphasis on computed tomography angiography representing a key first step in the diagnostic algorithm.

Case report: In this case report, we describe the diagnosis and treatment of obscure gastrointestinal bleeding emanating from an arteriovenous malformation in the small intestine of a 52 year old male. After an extensive work-up including upper and lower endoscopy, double balloon enteroscopy and capsule endoscopy, he was referred for computed tomography angiography. Though he was not actively bleeding, a jejunal arteriovenous malformation was localized on imaging. This prompted directed transfemoral angiography, placement of a super-selective microcatheter in the 4th jejunal arterial branch, intra-operative methylene blue injection and focused enterectomy with pathological confirmation. The patient was found to be free of gastrointestinal bleeding on 6 month follow-up.

Conclusions: A step-wise, rational diagnostic approach should be utilized in the evaluation of obscure gastrointestinal bleeding. In the non-actively bleeding patient, computed tomography angiogram may facilitate the diagnosis of a small intestinal arteriovenous malformation. Methylene blue injection via a super-selective angiographic microcatheter may then allow for focused enterectomy.

Keywords: Obscure gastrointestinal bleeding, Computed tomography angiography, Super-selective angiography, Intra-operative methylene blue injection

* Correspondence: j_frydman@rambam.health.gov.il
[1]Department of General Surgery, Rambam Health Care Campus, P.O. B 9602, 31096 Haifa, Israel
Full list of author information is available at the end of the article

Introduction

Gastrointestinal (GI)bleeding from the small intestine remains a formidable diagnostic and therapeutic challenge for the Acute Care Surgeon. This is secondary to its length and mobility, as well as relative inaccessibility [1]. While the stomach, duodenum, and colon are comparatively fixed in location and evaluable by means of conventional upper and lower endoscopy, the diagnosis of bleeding from the jejunum and ileum may require a series of alternative tests. This may include, but not limited to, small bowel enteroscopy, double balloon enteroscopy, capsule endoscopy, nuclear medicine bleeding scan, computed tomography angiography (CTA), invasive angiography, or exploratory laparotomy with intraoperative enteroscopy.

In a landmark paper in 1978, Fogler and Golembe described the injection of methylene blue through direct cannulation of the superior mesenteric artery in the operating theater, guided by preoperative angiographic findings of an arteriovenous malformation (AVM) in the proximal jejunum. A segment of small bowel measuring 10 cm which *cleared* the blue dye rapidly while the color remained in proximal and distal segments was presumed to contain the pathological AVM. Though this was not demonstrated on pathology, the patient remained free of GI bleeding on 6 month follow-up [2].

From this highly invasive and non-selective approach, several refinements on this technique have been pioneered over the years to result in a less invasive and more focused surgical resection in the treatment of GI bleeding from the small intestine [3-8]. In this report, we describe how pathological findings on CTA in a non-actively, obscure GIB patient prompted super-selective angiographic catheter placement and, ultimately, limited enterectomy directed by intra-operative methylene blue injection.

Case report

The patient is a 52 year-old male with past medical history significant for coronary artery disease, hyperlipidemia, gout and obesity. He had undergone cardiac catheterization and stent placement 4 years ago and continued on anti-platelet therapy with aspirin and Plavix. Two years prior to current presentation, he underwent work-up for melanotic stools with upper, lower and capsule endoscopy. He was diagnosed at that time with duodenitis, attributed to Arcoxia, a COX-2 inhibitor he had been prescribed for treatment of gouty arthritis, with likely synergistic effect due to concomitant aspirin intake. Past surgical history was notable for laparoscopic sleeve gastrectomy earlier this year with resultant 35 kilogram weight loss.

His current presentation was marked by intermittent melanotic stools, fall in hemoglobin to a low of 7.3 g/dl and orthostatic symptoms. He was resuscitated and required a blood transfusion. Nasogastric tube placement did not reveal evidence of bleeding. Further work-up included upper and lower endoscopy which failed to reveal the source of bleeding. Capsule endoscopy, however, showed active bleeding localized to the jejunum, which prompted small bowel enteroscopy, which failed to show pathology to a depth of 160 cm. This was followed by double balloon enterosopy to a depth of 2m reaching the ileum. Again, this was negative for any responsible lesions. At this time, we elected to perform CTA of the abdomen both to exclude a mass lesion and attempt to localize a possible AVM. Of note, the patient was not experiencing any active bleeding at this time.

In the selected cut from his CTA (Figure 1), an ectatic, antimesenteric blood vessel was noted adjacent to a loop of jejunum in the left side of the abdomen. This appeared to be an anomalous AVM as evidenced by early filling of an associated vein on arterial phase. Also notable was the finding of replaced left *and* right hepatic arteries. Given the CTA findings, he was referred for angioembolization. During this procedure, the visualized fourth jejunal branch from the superior mesenteric artery appeared to give rise to the AVM seen on CTA (Figure 2). This was cannulated distally with a super-selective 2.7 Fr microcatheter, but the lesion was not amenable to embolization given robust collateralization. The decision was made to leave the micro-angiocatheter in-situ to facilitate intraoperative

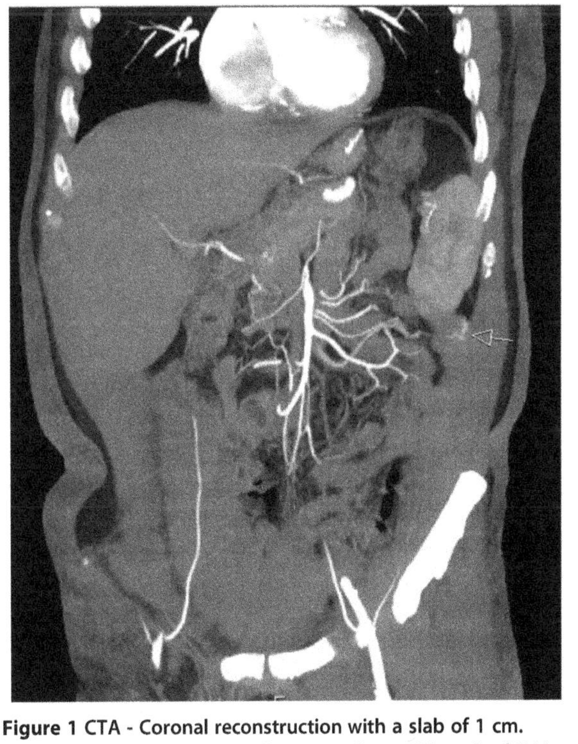

Figure 1 CTA - Coronal reconstruction with a slab of 1 cm. Abnormal vessel (AVM) (arrow) from a small jejunal branch of SMA.

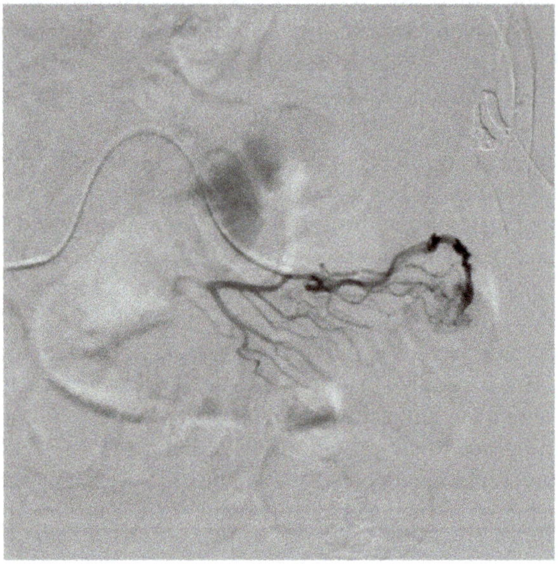

Figure 2 **Transfemoral angiography - selective injection of 4th jejunal branch through a 2.7 Fr microcatheter.**

identification of the small intestinal AVM. The sheath and catheter were secured at the groin entry site, 2500 units of heparin were administered intravenously and the patient was transported directly to the operating theater.

A limited midline incision was utilized to gain access into the peritoneal cavity and expose the small intestine. Two mL of dilute methylene blue were then injected via the super-selective angiographic microcatheter, immediately staining a 10 cm segment of the distal jejunum and corresponding mesentery (Figure 3). A segmental small bowel resection was performed. The patient had an unremarkable post-operative course and pathology demonstrated angiodysplasia in the small bowel segment with clean margins. At 6 month telephone follow-up the patient is doing well and denies any further episodes of melena.

Discussion

Obscure GI bleeding has been defined as bleeding which persists or recurs after upper and lower endoscopy and radiographic evaluation of the small bowel. Comprising up to 5% of cases of GI bleeding with 75% of them localizing to the small intestine [9], these patients may require multiple blood transfusions and be subject to a battery of repeat diagnostic studies before definitive diagnosis is accomplished. The most likely etiologies are broken down by age group. In patients younger than 40, the most likely lesions include Meckel's diverticulum, inflammatory bowel disease, or a small bowel tumor such as a gastrointestinal stromal tumor (GIST), lymphoma, carcinoid, polyp or adenocarcinoma. In contrary, patients older than 40 are most likely to have bleeding

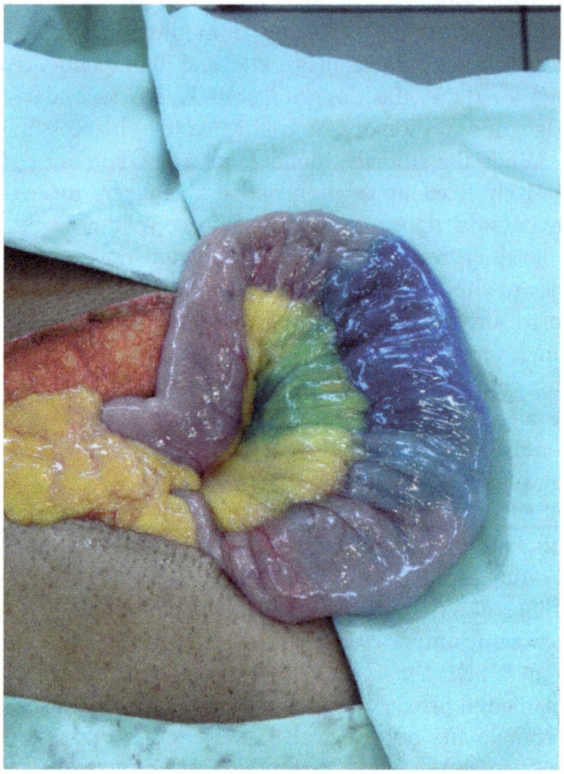

Figure 3 **Intraoperative demonstration of methylene blue staining of affected small bowel segment containing the AVM.**

from vascular anomalies, erosions or NSAID-related ulcerations. Overall, vascular lesions comprise 40% of all causes [10].

Two years after Fogler and Golembe's description of open cannulation of the superior mesenteric artery, Athanasoulis and colleagues in 1980 described the placement of super-selective angiographic catheters and intraoperative methylene blue injection to localize and treat two patients with AVMs and one with ulcerations in the small intestine [3]. Refinements on the technique have been described in subsequent reports which have paralleled advancement in angiographic methods, including provocative angiography with fibrinolytic agents [4-8].

From these reports, several guiding principles can be elucidated. When the AVM is localized on angiography, the most distal arterial tributary should be cannulated by a microcatheter and safely secured for transport. This can be done in the angiography suite or a hybrid operating theater. Following this the small bowel must be exposed either via a limited midline laparotomy or laparoscopy *before* injection of methylene blue. The limited segment of small bowel, usually 10cm or less is readily identified and resected with pathological confirmation. Clinical success is confirmed by long-term follow up.

After a careful review of the literature, this report represents the first case in the utilization of CTA in the diagnosis of a non-actively bleeding small bowel AVM which then enabled focused angiography and subsequent limited enterectomy. The CTA demonstrated the abnormality in the left-sided, proximal jejunum which corresponded to the 4th jejunal branch by transfemoral angiography. Not only did this spare the patient additional contrast load, it may have not been localized, or required provocative angiography, with its inherent risks, if not for the pathological finding on CTA. As the quality of the CTA has improved with new generation scanner technology, this diagnostic study should be considered in the work-up of the non-actively, obscure GI bleeding patients, with a focus on small bowel lesions and AVMs. Further study is warranted to truly gauge its sensitivity and specificity in this patient population.

Consent

Written informed consent was obtained from the patient for publication of this Case Report and any accompanying images. A copy of the written consent is available for review by the Editor-in-Chief of this journal.

Competing interests

The authors do not have any financial or non-financial competing interests to declare.

Authors' contributions

Study concept and design: JF, HB, YK. Acquisition of data: JF, HB, ML, AO. Analysis of data: JF, HB, ML, AO, YK. Drafting of manuscript: JF. Critical revision of manuscript: YK. Study supervision: AO, YK. All authors read and approved the final manuscript.

Author details

[1]Department of General Surgery, Rambam Health Care Campus, P.O. B 9602, 31096 Haifa, Israel. [2]Depatment of Radiology, Rambam Health Care Campus, P.O. B 9602, 31096 Haifa, Israel.

References

1. Lau WY, Wong SY, Ngan H, Fan ST, Wong KK: **Intra-operative localization of bleeding small intestinal lesions.** *Br J Surg* 1988, **75:**249–251.
2. Fogler R, Golembe E: **Methylene blue injection: An intraoperative guide in small bowel resection for arteriovenous malformation.** *Arch Surg* 1978, **113:**194–195.
3. Athanasoulis CA, Moncure AC, Greenfield AJ, Ryan JA, Dodson TF: **Intraoperative localization of small bowel bleeding sites with combined use of angiographic methods and methylene blue injection.** *Surgery* 1980, **87**(1):77–84.
4. McDonald ML, Farnell MB, Stanson AW, Ress AM: **Preoperative highly selective catheter localization of occult small-intestinal hemorrhage with methylene blue dye.** *Arch Surg* 1995, **130:**106–108.
5. Schechter S, Deorchis D, Bass J, Marcoux DA: **Angiographic selective methylene blue staining of an occult small-bowel arteriovenous malformation.** *Am Surg* 2002, **68:**15–17.
6. Stauffer JA, Shaddix KK, Achem SR, Stark M, Adelson A, Metzger PP, Landmann RG: **Intra-operative use of super-selective or highly selective angiography with methylene blue injection to localize arterial-venous malformation.** *Colorectal Dis* 2011, **13**(4):e65–e66.
7. Gifford SM, Peck MA, Reyes AM, Lundy JB: **Methylene blue enteric mapping for intraoperative localization in obscure small bowel hemorrhage: report of a new technique and literature review.** *J Gastrointest Surg* 2012, **16:**2177–2181.
8. Pai M, Frampton AE, Virk JS, Nehru N, Kyriakides C, Limongelli P, Jackson JE, Jiao LR: **Preoperative super selective mesenteric angiography and methylene blue injection for localization of obscure gastrointestinal bleeding.** *JAMA Surg* 2013, **148**(7):665–668.
9. Tee HP, Kaffes AJ: **Non-small-bowel lesions encountered during double-balloon enteroscopy performed for obscure gastrointestinal bleeding.** *World J Gastroenterol* 2010, **16**(15):1885–1889.
10. Raju GS, Gerson L, Das A, Lewis B: **American Gastroenterological Association (AGA) institute medical position statement on obscure gastrointestinal bleeding.** *Gastroenterology* 2007, **133**(5):1694–1696.

8

Surgical pathology and the diagnosis of invasive visceral yeast infection

Paola Di Carlo[1*], Gaetano Di Vita[2], Giuliana Guadagnino[1], Gianfranco Cocorullo[3], Francesco D'Arpa[3], Giuseppe Salamone[3], Buscemi Salvatore[2], Gaspare Gulotta[3] and Daniela Cabibi[1]

Abstract

Invasive mycoses are life-threatening opportunistic infections that have recently emerged as a cause of morbidity and mortality following general and gastrointestinal surgery.
Candida species are the main fungal strains of gut flora. Gastrointestinal tract surgery might lead to mucosal disruption and cause *Candida* spp. to disseminate in the bloodstream.
Here we report and discuss the peculiar clinical and morphological presentation of two cases of gastrointestinal *Candida albicans* lesions in patients who underwent abdominal surgery.
Although in the majority of cases reported in the literature, diagnosis was made on the basis of microbiological criteria, we suggest that morphological features of fungi in histological sections of appropriate surgical specimens could help to detect the degree of yeast colonization and identify patients at risk of developing severe abdominal *Candida* infection.
Better prevention and early antifungal treatments are highlighted, and relevant scientific literature is reviewed.

Keywords: Surgical pathology, Gastrointestinal candidiasis, Diagnosis

Introduction

Invasive mycoses are important healthcare-associated infections, and have become an increasingly frequent problem in immunocompromised and severely ill patients [1]. Medical progress, which has resulted in a growing number of invasive procedures, new dimensions in aggressive immunosuppressive and immunomodulatory treatments and widespread use of broad-spectrum antibiotics, is the main catalyst for this development [1-3].

Invasive fungal infections, *Candida* species in particular, are the fourth most common cause of nosocomial bloodstream infections, and are associated with high morbidity and mortality in critically-ill patients, particularly those who have recently undergone extensive gastro-abdominal surgery [4].

Several studies conducted over the last two decades have shown that gastrointestinal surgeries are associated with an increased risk of fungemia, and patients admitted to surgical intensive care units (ICUs) are considered to have a greater risk of developing it [3,4].

Candida spp. are the main fungal strains of gut flora. Gastrointestinal tract surgery might lead to mucosal disruption and cause *Candida* spp. to disseminate through the bloodstream.

Lastly, despite a strong index of suspicion in high-risk subjects such as patients who require surgical re-intervention, and international guidelines on the use of antifungal prophylaxis, the incidence and severity of candidiasis in post-surgical patients appears significant. Moreover, isolated species show virulence factors and exhibit varying levels of susceptibility to antifungal drugs [1,5,6].

In the present study, we report two cases of *Candida albicans* infection identified in abdominal specimens from patients who had undergone gastro-abdominal surgery.

* Correspondence: paola.dicarlo@unipa.it
[1]Department of Sciences for Health Promotion and Mother-Child Care "G. D'Alessandro", University of Palermo, Via del Vespro 127, I- 90127 Palermo, Italy
Full list of author information is available at the end of the article

Case presentation

First case

In December 2012, a 54 year-old woman of Italian origin and nationality presented to the general surgery and emergency unit of the "P. Giaccone" Teaching Hospital in Palermo, Italy, with severe epigastric left-upper-quadrant pain that was progressive and burning.

Her medical history was significant for hypertension, asthma and rectal cancer surgery ($T_1N_0M_0$) involving low anterior resection with total mesorectal excision and end to end anastomosis in October 2012. Recovery from surgery was hampered by recurrent episodes of fever but no specific infectious agent was detected; in view of this, the patient showed clinical improvement after empirical treatment with fluconazole.

Physical examination revealed a soft abdomen with positive bowel sounds, and tenderness to palpation in the left upper quadrant. Rectal examination was guaiac-negative, and a complete blood count indicated leukocytosis with left shift. CT scan of abdomen showed a gastric dilatation, marked thickening of the anterior wall and necrotic areas within.

An exploratory upper laparotomy confirmed acute gastric dilatation and necrosis of the anterior surface of the stomach. A "sleeve" gastrectomy to ablate the necrotic area was performed and a feeding jejunostomy.

The gastric wall appeared very thin and totally necrotic upon macroscopic examination by the pathologist. No layers or structures were identifiable on histological examination, but numerous fungal yeasts were identified inside the necrotic areas with PAS and Gomori Silvermthenamina stains (Figure 1).

Culture of the intra-operative surgical specimen confirmed the presence of *Candida albicans.*

Yeast isolates were identified to the species level by conventional morphological and biochemical methods, as previously reported [3,7,8].

The yeast isolate was susceptible to fluconazole and echinocandin, according to CLSI cut off values [9,10]. It is noteworthy that blood cultures were negative.

Echinocandin (70 mg on the first day, i.e., day 103, followed by 50 mg/day) was administered parenterally for a total of 14 days, followed by maintenance therapy with 400 mg of oral fluconazole per day.

The patient was discharged in stable condition and antifungal therapy was continued in an outpatient setting. She has been doing well since then.

Second case

In January 2013, a 62 year-old woman of Italian origin and nationality with BMI of 35 kg/m^2, presented to the general surgery and emergency unit of the "P. Giaccone" Teaching Hospital in Palermo, Italy, with complicated midline incisional hernia, nausea, vomiting and abdominal distension.

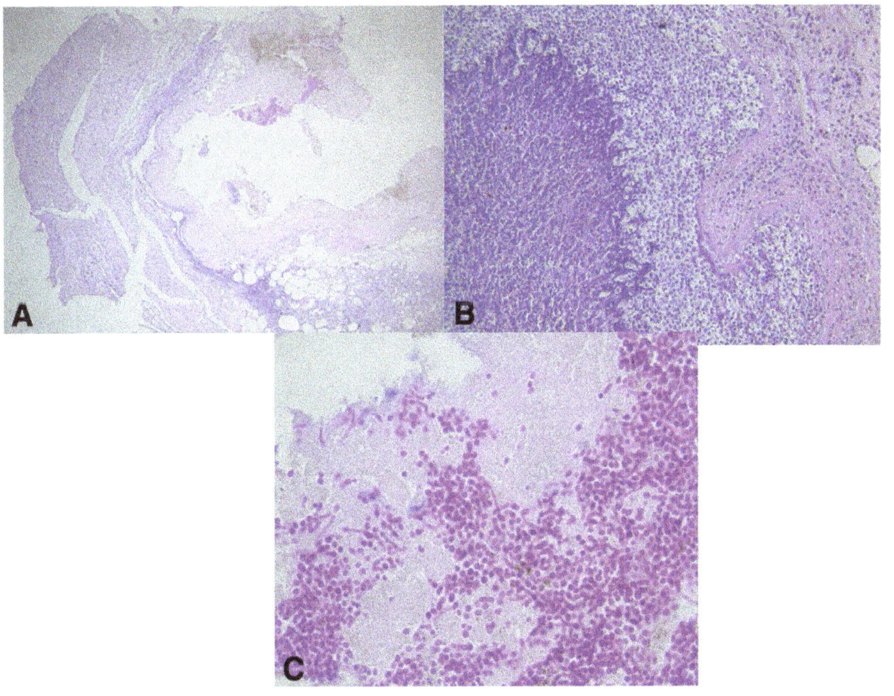

Figure 1 Histological section. A) Very thin and totally necrotic gastric wall. **B, C)** Numerous fungal yeasts were present. PAS stain **(A)** ×100; **(B)** ×200; **(C)** ×400.

Her initial vital signs were notable for a temperature of 38°C, respiratory rate of 22 breaths per minute, heart rate of 110 beats per minute and blood pressure of 90/60 mmHg. She was suffering from severe abdominal pain and breathing difficulties. On clinical examination, she presented a tender abdomen, ulcerated skin with associated necrosis and dry skin.

Her past medical history showed three caesarean sections, treatment for arterial hypertension, COPD and a diagnosis of type II diabetes mellitus (DM) about 15 years previously, treated with insulin.

Emergency surgery was required, and surgical exploration showed a congested, edematous and necrotic strangulated intestinal tract. The section of necrotic intestine was removed and ileo-ileostomy was performed. The surgery was successful, without additional complications, and an abdominal subcutaneous drain was inserted. The surgical specimen was sent to the Pathology Laboratory for histological examination.

During the postoperative period, the patient remained febrile but two routine blood cultures were negative.

Furthermore, histological examination of both the skin and the small bowel specimens using special histochemical stains (PAS, Gomori Silvermethenamine) showed severe inflammation and massive areas of necrosis containing fungal spores and numerous budding hyphae (Figure 2).

Some yeasts were present across vessel walls of the small bowel, suggesting systemic blood dissemination (Figure 2C).

These findings were in keeping with culture results of intraoperative specimens and serial drainage fluids, showing fluconazole-resistant *Candida albicans*, susceptible to echinocandin according to CLSI cut off values [8].

Echinocandin (70 mg on the first day, i.e., day 103, followed by 50 mg/day) was administered parenterally for a total of 21 days.

The patient's clinical conditions improved, fever disappeared and she was subsequently discharged in a good clinical state.

Discussion

We have reported two cases of abdominal surgery patients who developed systemic candidiasis, and whose clinical symptoms improved following the initiation of therapy with 70/50 mg/day echinocandin. Oral thrush and esophageal candidiasis are the most common manifestations of Candida infection in the GI tract, with only occasional involvement of the colon and rectum. Despite the high concentration of *Candida* spp. in the lower GI tract, infection does not occur under normal circumstances, owing to innate defense mechanisms.

In this manuscript, we have described abdominal lesions due to *Candida albicans* infection. In a previous

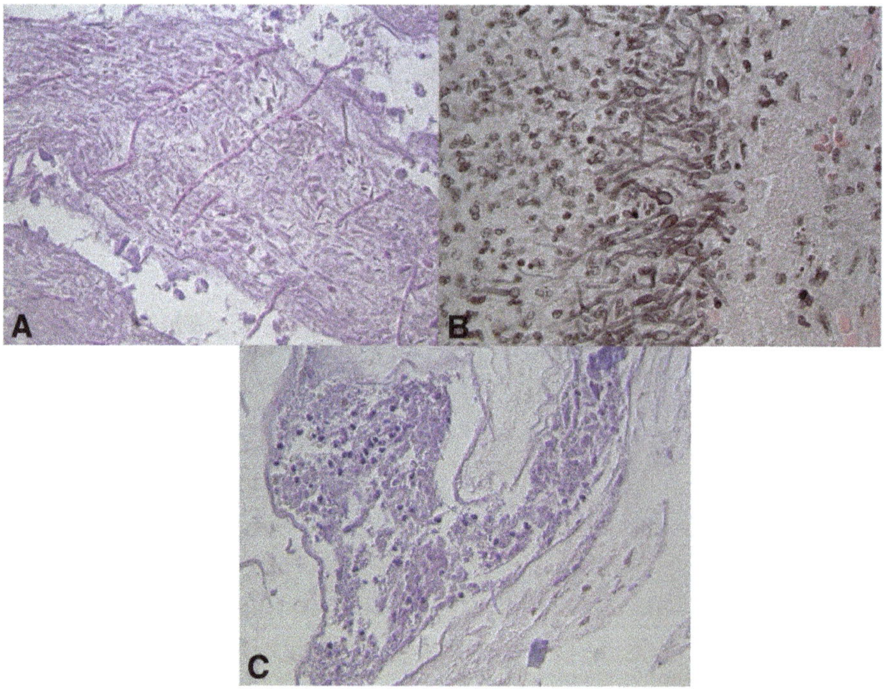

Figure 2 Histological section. A) Necrotic tissue from the cutaneous specimen, with fungal hyphae. **B-C)** Hyphae in the small bowel specimen. In **C** some of them appear to cross the vessel wall. PAS stain **(A)** ×200; GMS stain **(B)** ×400, PAS stain **(C)** ×200.

case report, we described a vegetating gastric *Candida albicans* lesion in an immunocompetent patient, endoscopically simulating a neoplasia [11]. This study reports two new cases of abdominal fungal infection in patients who had undergone abdominal surgery.

Gastrointestinal candida lesions remain difficult to diagnose because of the prevalence of colonization without accompanying infection, non-specific symptoms, and variable presentation.

In our two cases, despite blood cultures being negative for yeast, the histological analysis, performed with special histochemical stains, and culture of specimens or drainage fluid allowed us to identify it.

Although new, rapid and sensitive methods for diagnosing invasive fungal disease are available [12], histopathologic examination remains one of the major diagnostic tools in mycology because it permits rapid, presumptive identification of fungal infections [13,14].

Newer fungal, invasive visceral candidiasis and multidrug-resistant bacteria involving hollow gastrointestinal viscera are emerging pathologies for abdominal surgery [11,14,15].

Minali et al. reported that stomach candidiasis was seen in 0.96% of upper intestinal endoscopies [16]. Furthermore, Gupta described a fatal case of gastric perforation where biopsy revealed fungal hyphae [17].

In our patients' case, systemic echinocandin treatment led to a substantial improvement in their clinical condition and a favorable outcome, despite the presence of several risk factors such as diabetes and/or re-intervention.

In the first case, fever disappeared with antifungal treatment after rectal cancer surgery was suggestive of fungemia and the authors hypothesized that fungal flora which normally colonize the gastric mucosa may overgrow under certain conditions, resulting in mucosal lesions of the digestive tract, in different sites and regardless of the site of surgery [18].

In fact, our patient had undergone rectal resection for neoplasm, but surgical re-intervention was required after 2 months for necrosis of the stomach, when diffuse yeasts were observed.

In the second case, where the reason for surgery was a complicated incisional hernia, we believe that the presence of candida was due to a superinfection in intestinal tissue which had undergone necrotic degeneration due to mechanical reasons. However, the cutaneous abscess adjacent to the complicated incisional hernia where numerous hyphae were also observed, could be a primary abscess due to disseminated intestinal fungal overgrowth. In both cases, early detection of *Candida albicans* by culture and histology permitted us to start the correct therapeutic approach with echinocandin, which led to a rapid improvement in the patients' clinical condition.

In one study by Ears et al., gut mycosis was observed in 109 (4.35%) out of 2517 cases studied from 1960–1964 [19].

In Japan, Tsukamoto et al. reported that gut mycosis was present in 196 (5.9%) out of 3,339 cases recorded from 1971 to 1983 [20]. In these reports, the most commonly-affected organ was the esophagus, followed by the stomach, the small intestine and the large intestine [17,20].

Although the presence of *Candida* spp.in intra-abdominal specimens is associated with increased mortality in certain subgroups of patients, both of our patients with *Candida albicans* involvement had a favorable outcome after echinocandin treatment.

The use of Echinocandins is justified by their poor ability to develop resistance, which makes these molecules notably effective and reliable. Current guidelines recommend them for the treatment of targeted candidemia [2,6,21].

Previous studies have demonstrated the importance of echinocandin in patients who have recently undergone abdominal surgery, who present recurrent gastrointestinal perforations, anastomotic failure, are ventilated, hospitalized for more than 3 days, treated with broad-spectrum antibiotics and who have a CVC inserted [22,23].

Further studies are needed to define the sensitivity and specificity of this assay to diagnose fungal infection prior to the existence of other clinical or laboratory indications of invasive fungal infection.

Conclusions

Three interesting findings emerge from these case reports. Firstly, the clinical recognition and effective management of fungal infections in surgical settings is challenging and the strategy to reduce damages needs a multistep diagnostic approach to establish a certain diagnosis.

Secondly, the study underlines the importance of culture and histological examination of surgical specimens, which could detect the presence of fungi even when blood cultures are negative.

Finally, histological examination allows us to observe the quantity and the morphological aspects of budding hyphae which can suggest a real overgrowth and a pathogenic role. More consideration needs to be given to selecting the appropriate antifungal agent for high-risk surgical patients.

Consent

Written informed consent was obtained from patients for publication of these Case Reports and any accompanying images. A copy of the written consent is available for review by the Editor-in-Chief of this journal.

Abbreviations
Candida spp.: *Candida* species; GMS: Gomori methenamine silver stain; PAS: Periodic acid Schiff stain.

Competing interests
The authors declare that they have no competing interests.

Authors' contributions
PDC and GDV participated in the conception, design of the study and sequence alignment, and drafted the manuscript. DC carried out the histopathological studies. GG, FDA, GS, BS and GC participated in the clinical and surgical management. All the authors have read and approved the final manuscript.

Author details
[1]Department of Sciences for Health Promotion and Mother-Child Care "G. D'Alessandro", University of Palermo, Via del Vespro 127, I- 90127 Palermo, Italy. [2]Department of Surgery and Oncology Sciences, General Surgery Unit, University of Study of Palermo, Italy, Via del Vespro 127, I- 90127 Palermo, Italy. [3]Department of General Surgery, Urgency and Organ Transplantation, University of Palermo, Via del Vespro 127, I- 90127 Palermo, Italy.

References

1. Chahoud J, Kanafani ZA, Kanj SS: **Management of candidaemia and invasive candidiasis in critically ill patients.** *Int J Antimicrob Agents* 2013, **8**:134–139.
2. Sartelli M, Catena F, Ansaloni L, Moore E, Malangoni M, Velmahos G, Coimbra R, Koike K, Leppaniemi A, Biffl W, Balogh Z, Bendinelli C, Gupta S, Kluger Y, Agresta F, Di Saverio S, Tugnoli G, Jovine E, Ordonez C, Augusto Gomes C, Pereira GA, Yuan KC, Bala M, Peev MP, Cui Y, Marwah S, Zachariah S, Sakakushev B, Kong V, Ahmed A, *et al*: **Complicated intra-abdominal infections in a worldwide context: an observational prospective study (CIAOW Study).** *World J Emerg Surg* 2013, **8**:1.
3. Di Carlo P, Pantuso G, Cusimano A, D'Arpa F, Giammanco A, Gulotta G, Latteri AM, Madonia S, Salamone G, Mammina C: **Two cases of monomicrobial intraabdominal abscesses due to KPC-3 *Klebsiella pneumoniae* ST258 clone.** *BMC Gastroenterol* 2011, **11**:103.
4. Tortorano AM, Peman J, Bernhardt H, Klingspor L, Kibbler CC, Faure O, Biraghi E, Canton E, Zimmermann K, Seaton S, Grillot R, ECMM Working Group on Candidaemia: **Epidemiology of candidaemia in Europe: results of 28-month European Confederation of Medical Mycology (ECMM) hospital-based surveillance study.** *Eur J Clin Microbiol Infect Dis* 2004, **23**:317–322.
5. Ables AZ, Blumer NA, Valainis GT, Godenick MT, Kajdasz DK, Palesch YY: **Fluconazole prophylaxis of severe Candida infection in trauma and postsurgical patients: a prospective, double-blind, randomized, placebo-controlled trial.** *Infect Dis Clin Pract* 2000, **9**:169–175.
6. Sartelli M, Viale P, Koike K, Pea F, Tumietto F, van Goor H, Guercioni G, Nespoli A, Tranà C, Catena F, Ansaloni L, Leppaniemi A, Biffl W, Moore FA, Poggetti R, Pinna AD, Moore EE: **WSES consensus conference: Guidelines for first-line management of intra-abdominal infections.** *World J Emerg Surg* 2011, **6**:2.
7. Chiarini A, Palmeri A, Amato T, Immordino R, Di Stefano S, Giammanco A: **Detection of Bacterial and Yeast Species with the Bactec 9120 Automated System with Routine Use of Aerobic, Anaerobic, and Fungal Media.** *J Clin Microbiol* 2008, **46**:4029–4033.
8. Spreghini E, Maida CM, Milici ME, Scalise G, Barchiesi F: **Posaconazole Activity against *Candida glabrata* after Exposure to Caspofungin or Amphotericin B.** *Antimicrob Agents Chemother* 2008, **52**:513–517.
9. Clinical and Laboratory Standards Institute: *Clinical and Laboratory Standards Institute, 2008a. Reference method for broth dilution antifungal susceptibility testing of yeasts, third ed., Approved standard M27-A3.* Wayne, PA: Clinical and Laboratory Standards Institute; 2008a.
10. Pfaller MA, Messer SA, Woosley LN, Jones RN, Castanheira M: **Echinocandin and triazole antifungal susceptibility profiles of opportunistic yeast and mould clinical isolates (2010–2011): Application of new CLSI clinical breakpoints and epidemiological cutoff values to characterize geographic and temporal trends of antifungal resistance.** *J Clin Microbiol* 2013, **29**:308–313.
11. Mansueto P, Pisciotta G, Tomasello G, Cabibi D, Seidita A, D'Alcamo A, Patti AM, Sprini D, Carroccio A, Rini GB, Fede GD: **Malignant tumor-like gastric lesion due to Candida albicans in a diabetic patient treated with cyclosporin: a case report and review of the literature.** *Clin Exp Med* 2012, **12**:201–205.
12. Ohrmalm C, Eriksson R, Jobs M, Simonson M, Strømme M, Bondeson K, Herrmann B, Melhus A, Blomberg J: **Variation-tolerant capture and multiplex detection of nucleic acids: application to detection of microbes.** *J Clin Microbiol* 2012, **50**:3208–3215.
13. Sangoi AR, Rogers WM, Longacre TA, Montoya JG, Baron EJ, Banaei N: **Challenges and pitfalls of morphologic identification of fungal infections in histologic and cytologic specimens: a ten-year retrospective review at a single institution.** *Am J Clin Pathol* 2009, **131**:364–375.
14. Watts JC: **Surgical pathology and the diagnosis of infectious diseases.** *Am J Clin Pathol* 1994, **102**:711–712.
15. Vikram HR, Smilack JD, Leighton JA, Crowell MD, De Petris G: **Emergence of gastrointestinal basidiobolomycosis in the United States, with a review of worldwide cases.** *Clin Infect Dis* 2012, **54**:1685–1691.
16. Di Carlo P, Gulotta G, Casuccio A, Pantuso G, Raineri M, Farulla CA, Bonventre S, Guadagnino G, Ingrassia D, Cocorullo G, Mammina C, Giarratano A: **KPC - 3 Klebsiella pneumoniae ST258 clone infection in postoperative abdominal surgery patients in an intensive care setting: analysis of a case series of 30 patients.** *BMC Anesthesiol* 2013, **13**:13–29.
17. Minali G, Teruzzi V, Butti G, Frigerio G, Rossini A: **Gastric candidiasis: an endoscopic and a histological study in 26 patients.** *Gastrointestinal endoscopy* 1982, **28**:59–61.
18. Gupta N: **A rare cause of gastric perforation-Candida infection: a case report and review of the literature.** *J Clin Diagn Res* 2012, **6**:1564–1565.
19. Holzknecht BJ, Thorup J, Arendrup MC, Andersen SE, Steensen M, Hesselfeldt P, Nielsen JM, Knudsen JD: **Decreasing candidaemia rate in abdominal surgery patients after introduction of fluconazole prophylaxis.** *Clin Microbiol Infect* 2011, **17**:1372–1380.
20. Ears P, Goldstein M, Sherlock P: **Candida infections of the gastrointestinal tract.** *Medicine* 1972, **51**:367–379.
21. Tsukamoto H: **Clinicopathological studies on fungal infections of the digestive tract.** *Jpn J Gastroenterol* 1986, **83**:2341–2350.
22. Ullmann AJ, Cornely OA, Donnelly JP, Akova M, Arendrup MC, Arikan-Akdagli S, Bassetti M, Bille J, Calandra T, Castagnola E, Garbino J, Groll AH, Herbrecht R, Hope WW, Jensen HE, Kullberg BJ, Lass-Flörl C, Lortholary O, Meersseman W, Petrikkos G, Richardson MD, Roilides E, Verweij PE, Viscoli C, Cuenca-Estrella M, ESCMID Fungal Infection Study Group: **ESCMID* guideline for the diagnosis and management of Candida diseases 2012: developing European guidelines in clinical microbiology and infectious diseases.** *Clin Microbiol Infect* 2012, **18**:1–8.
23. Senn L, Eggimann P, Ksontini R, Pascual A, Demartines N, Bille J, Calandra T, Marchetti O: **Caspofungin for prevention of intra-abdominal candidiasis in high-risk surgical patients.** *Intensive Care Med* 2009, **35**:903–908.

Successful open abdomen treatment for multiple ischemic duodenal perforated ulcers in dermatomyositis

Roberta Villa[1,2], Stefano Costa[1], Sibilla Focchi[1,2], Carlo Corbellini[1,2], Massimo Vigorelli[1] and Ettore Contessini Avesani[1,2*]

Abstract

Introduction: Dermatomyositis is an autoimmune disease characterized by proximal myopathy, cutaneous Gottron papules and heliotrope rash; intestinal involvement associated to acute vasculitis is less common but could be a life-threatening condition.

Methods: A 21-year-old woman, affected by dermatomyositis, presented to our attention with a three-day story of severe abdominal pain, no bowel movement and biliary vomit. She was diagnosed with acute abdomen. A CT scan with bowel contrast demonstrated the presence of a leakage from the retroperitoneal aspect of duodenum. The surgical and clinical management in the light of literature review is presented.

Results: Our first approach consisted in primary repair of the duodenal perforation with omentopexy. Post-operative course was complicated by hemorrhage. A reintervention showed a new perforation associated with multiple ischemic intestinal areas. We performed a gastroenteric anastomosis with functional exclusion of the damaged duodenum and positioning of drainages to create a biliary fistula. A nutritional enteric tube and an open abdomen vacuum-assisted closure system to monitor the fistula creation and to prevent abdominal contamination and collections were positioned. To reduce the amount of biliary leakage, a percutaneous transhepatic biliary drainage was placed, with progressive fistula flow disappearance in four months.

Conclusions: In patients with dermatomyositis, when clinical findings and symptoms suggest abdominal vasculitis, it is very important to be aware of the risk of bowel and particularly duodenal perforations. Open abdomen treatment favors control of contamination by gastrointestinal contents, offers temporary abdominal closure, helps ICU care and delays definitive surgery.

Keywords: Dermatomyositis, Duodenal perforations, Retroperitoneal air, Intestinal ischemia, Acute abdomen, Emergency surgery, Open abdomen

Background

Dermatomyositis (DM) is an autoimmune disease characterized by cutaneous heliotropic rash, Gottron papules and proximal myopathy associated to dysphagia, dysphonia, Raynaud phenomenon, fatigue and non-erosive inflammatory polyarthritis [1]. Vasculitis of the gastrointestinal tract is a life threatening complication, potential cause of hemorrhage and perforation [2].

We performed a literature review by searching on PubMed (keywords: dermatomyositis, acute vasculitis, ischemic perforation, bowel perforation, emergency surgery): only few cases of bowel perforation associated to dermatomyositis are described in literature, and surgical approach is not always mentioned or specified [2-19]. In literature gastroenteric vasculitic manifestations of DM are often associated to the juvenile form [20] of the disease, affecting children in 95.1% and adults in 4,9% of cases, with clinical onset before 16 years old. To our knowledge, in literature, are reported 18 articles describing 35 cases of bowel perforation and only two cases

* Correspondence: ettore.contessini@unimi.it
[1]Department of General and Emergency Surgery, Fondazione IRCCS Ca' Granda Ospedale Maggiore Policlinico, Milan, Italy
[2]Faculty of Medicine, Università degli Studi di Milano, Milano, Italy

related to adult patients (Table 1) [2-19]. Major sites of perforation are the esophagus (5,5%), the stomach (2,8%), the duodenum (25%), the ileum (2,8%), the right colon (17.1%), the transverse colon (2,8%), the sigmoid colon (2,8%) and the gastrointestinal tract with no specific site description (41,2%). Reported mortality rate is 14,3%, principally due to encephalic vasculitis and septic complications.

We report the case of a 21-year-old patient affected by DM presenting with rapid onset acute abdomen associated to severe vasculitis and complicated duodenal perforation, and discuss the surgical and clinical management in the light of literature review.

Case report

A 21-year-old female diagnosed with DM in 2008, on treatment with prednisone and cyclosporine with moderate disease activity until December 2012, presented to our Emergency Department (ED) with a three day history of diffuse, acute abdominal pain, no bowel movement and biliary vomit. She underwent laparoscopic cholecystectomy in 2010 for symptomatic calculosis. The patient was admitted to our Department with a bowel perforation suspect. An oral follow-through was negative but a CT scan with oral contrast demonstrated a small leakage from the posterior aspect of the third duodenal portion (Figure 1). An emergency laparotomy was performed, with intraoperative finding of multiple ischemic vasculitic lesions of the small bowel, retroperitoneal perforation of the third duodenal portion and a minimum local biliary contamination. The lesion was sutured with omentopexy and an abdominal drainage was placed. After surgery, the patient was transferred to Intensive Care Unit (ICU) for postoperative monitoring. Her clinical course, in the following two days, was complicated by acute hemorrhage. She underwent, therefore, a second operation due to the bleeding from a small branch of the anterior pancreaticoduodenal artery. A new ischemic perforation in the same duodenal region was recognized and multiple small ischemic areas involving the entire small bowel were observed. A gastroenteric anastomosis was performed, excluding the duodenum. Two drainages were placed near the perforated site to drain any possible biliary fistula. A nasoenteral feeding tube was then positioned. To manage the

Table 1 Intestinal perforation in dermatomyositis, literature review

Author	N° of cases	Site of perforation	Treatment	Outcome
Zarbalian Y et al. 2013 [10]	1	Right colon	Right hemicolectomy	Uneventful
Mamyrova G et al. 2007 [9]	2	Right colon	Right hemicolectomy	Uneventful
		Duodenum	Unknown	Left hemicolectomy for left colon perforation
Morita Y et al. 2007 [3]	1	Duodenum	Primary suture repair	Uneventful
Chiu SK et al. 2007 [11]	1	Duodenum	Not described	Uneventful
Chen G et al. 2005 [12]	1	Occult perforation	Exploratory laparotomy	Fatal sepsis
Wang IJ et al. 2001 [5]	1	Duodenum	Not described	Uneventful
Suwa A et al. 1997 [8]	1	Right colon	Right hemicolectomy	Uneventful
Lin W et al. 1995 [2]	1	Sigmoid colon	Total colectomy	Fatal sepsis
Ghayad E et al. 1993 [13]	1	Colon	Not described	Not described
Niizawa M et al. 1991 [7]	1	Right colon	Right hemicolectomy	Uneventful
Downey EC et al. 1988 [14]	4	Esophago-colonic	Suture, resection and drainage	Not described
Miller LC et al. 1987 [15]	10	Esophago-colonic	Not described	Fatal sepsis
Schullinger JN et al. 1985 [16]	4	Duodenum, esophagus and colon	Partial gastrectomy, drainage	Uneventful
		Duodenum	Partial gastrectomy	Uneventful
		Stomach	Partial gastrectomy	Uneventful
		Transverse colon	Colostomy	Fatal vascular cerebral complications
Magill HL et al. 1984 [4]	2	Duodenum	Not described	Not described
Thompson JW et al. 1984 [6]	1	Esophagus	Debridement and drainage	Uneventful
Kaplinsky et al. 1978 [17]	1	Duodenum	Non described	Not described
Koiunderliev et al. 1975 [18]	1	Small bowel	Segmentary resection	Uneventful
Bureau et al. 1958 [19]	1	Duodenum	Exploratory laparotomy	Fatal sepsis

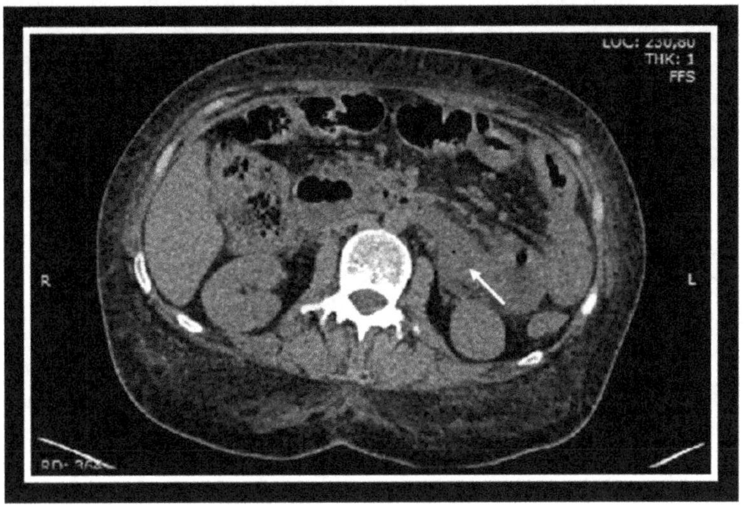

Figure 1 Abdominal computed tomography (CT) scan showed free retroperitoneal air (arrow), suspected for a small leakage from the posterior aspect of the third duodenal portion.

potential perforation risk of the duodenal and ileal ulcerations caused by acute vasculitis, to preserve the abdominal cavity from intraperitoneal collections and to create a guided biliary fistula, an open abdomen treatment with negative pressure system was placed; we positioned a temporary fascial mesh to preserve the fascia and prevent its retraction. Two weeks after the second surgical procedure a percutaneous transhepatic biliary drainage (PTBD) was placed to reduce the flow of the peritoneal biliary fistula.

We changed the negative pressure dressing every 3–4 days, washing the peritoneal cavity and tightening the fascial mesh. The negative pressure system was very useful and effective because of the large amount of biliary leakage and bowel contamination caused by multiple ischemic ulcers in the second and third portion of the duodenum, otherwise this condition was not manageable with the use of simple drains. After two months, the open abdomen treatment was suspended, the fascial mesh was removed and the fascia was primarily closed. Afterward, we removed the PTBD and the abdominal drain following the execution of abdominal X-ray with oral contrast, demonstrating absence of residual duodenal biliary leakage after four months.

During her ICU stay, the patient presented signs of renal vasculitis, therefore she underwent cycles of continuous veno-venous hemodialysis (CCVHD), plasmapheresis and intravenous immunoglobulin (IVIG), showing clear improvement of her renal function and negative immunological test. Low molecular weight heparin (LMWH) treatment was complicated by heparin induced thrombocytopenia (HIT) with low platelet (PLT) count (99.000/μm^3). Argatroban was administered obtaining progressive increase in PLT count (354.000/μm^3). Three months after surgery she had seizures with MRI scan positive for vasculitic diffuse encephalic lesions, treated with levetiracetam and metilprendisone. During hospitalization we observed nasal regurgitation of fluids, nasal speech and hoarseness probably due to loss of pharyngoesophageal muscle tone and increase and reduction in hepatic stasis values of unknown origin. After 8 months of follow-up, no signs or symptoms of abdominal disease were reported.

DM is an autoimmune disease characterized by cutaneous heliotropic rash, Gottron papules and proximal myopathy associated to dysphagia, dysphonia, Raynaud phenomenon, fatigue and non-erosive inflammatory polyarthritis [1]. Vasculitis of the gastrointestinal tract is a life threatening complication, more frequently observed in children than in adults [3]. It may vary from segmental bowel edema to ulcerations, gangrene and perforation [2]. The classic clinical findings may be masked by corticosteroids therapy and the radiographic investigations may be negative even in presence of bowel perforation, as the lesion may be very small, retroperitoneal, self sealed or well contained by the adjacent structures. Extraluminal air can be observed in 50–70% of patients [21]. Many cases involve the duodenum and particularly the third portion and its retroperitoneal aspect [3-5,9,11,16,17,19]. Other typical sites of perforation are the esophagus [6,14-16], the cecum, and the right and left colon in their retroperitoneal portion [2,7-10,13]. Histopathological findings are related to acute arteriopathy, with arterial and venous intimal hyperplasia and occlusion of vessels by fibrin thrombi. Chronic vasculopathy is characterized by reduction or complete occlusion of multiple small and medium arteries, subintimal foam cells, fibromixoid neointimal expansion and significant luminal compromise and infiltration of macrophages through the muscle layers into the intima [9,22]. In younger patients systemic vasculitis with specific involvement of renal and encephalic system can be observed. Radiological features of vasculitis include widespread thickening of mucosal fold and irregularity of small intestine, giving rise to a "stacked coin" appearance [1]. When clinical findings and symptoms suggest possible abdominal vasculitis in a young subject known for DM, it is very important to consider bowel and particularly retroperitoneal perforation. In order to manage this difficult clinical and surgical condition it is mandatory to consider the medical complexity of this disease and the necessity to treat the patient with a specific therapy to control the acute vasculitic process conditioning damage to multiple organs such as respiratory, renal and encephalic system, causing septic shock, renal failure and encephalitis. In this case, during the recovery, we had to manage gastroenteric, renal and encephalic vasculitic complications. The patient underwent three cycles of CCVHD, plasmapheresis and IVIG, multiple antibiotic coverage and careful steroid management. Her course was also complicated by heparin-induced thrombocytopenia during treatment with LMWH to prevent thromboembolism; treatment with argatroban permitted a progressive platelet count improvement. Her recovery was also complicated by dysphagia for both solids and liquids, caused by loss of pharyngoesophageal muscle tone and encephalic vasculitis, which started with seizures and was treated with levetiracetam and metilprednisolone.

Surgical treatment is not standardized because of the rarity and variety of the gastrointestinal DM presentations that can affect the entire gastrointestinal tract. In literature we found few descriptions of ischemic gastrointestinal perforation in DM. Surgical treatments and outcomes reported were anecdotic and varied, including resection of the affected tract or sutures of the lesions (Table 1). High recurrence of reintervention for anastomotic dehiscence or new perforations was observed. The use of negative pressure treatment was never reported. Open abdomen treatment allows the reduction of contamination by gastrointestinal contents decreasing the risk of abdominal collections, favors rapid evidence of hemorrhage permitting a prompt control of the bleeding source, offers temporary abdominal closure, helps ICU care and delays definitive surgery [23,24]. In this case we performed an open abdomen treatment to better remove the losses and control possible sources of new perforations, without needing of bowel resection. The mesh-mediated fascial traction technique combined with negative pressure treatment allowed to preserve the fascia, and to obtain the fascial primarily closure. As reported in literature, achievement of fascial closure has significant implications for the recovery of the patients, reducing ICU and hospital length of stay, and need for surgical reconstruction of the abdominal wall [25]. We had to perform a bowel deviation because of the critical ischemic vasculitis of the duodenum. To reduce the amount of biliary leakage and to obtain a faster outcome, we positioned a PTBD. Using this composite technique progressive fistula flow reduction was obtained, allowing abdominal closure after two months and PTBD removal after four months.

Conclusions

When clinical findings and symptoms suggest possible abdominal vasculitis in a young subject known for DM, it is very important to consider bowel and particularly duodenal perforation. We found very helpful CT scan with oral contrast to support diagnosis and we had to face the more life-threatening condition of multiple ischemic intestinal ulcerations conditioning duodenal multiple perforations. To manage this challenging condition we used open abdomen treatment with exclusion of the duodenal ischemic perforated tract through a gastroenteroanastomosis and PTBD with the creation of a guided fistula to decrease the flow and obtaining progressive healing with improvement of patient's general conditions. This surgical treatment must always be accompanied by DM specific medical treatment to avoid further vasculitic complications and to obtain control of the disease activity.

Consent

Written informed consent was obtained from the patient for publication of this Case report and any accompanying images. A copy of the written consent is available for review by the Editor-in-Chief of this journal.

Abbreviations

CAPS: Anti-phospholipidic catastrophic syndrome; CT: Computed tomography; CVVHD: Continuous veno-venous haemodialysis; DM: Dermatomyositis; ED: Emergency Department; HIT: Heparin induced thrombocytopenia; ICU: Intensive care unit; IVIG: IntraVenous immunoGlobulin; LAC: Lupus anti coaugulant; LMWH: Low molecular weight heparin; MRI: Magnetic resonance imaging; NGT: Naso-gastric tube; PTBD: Percutaneous transhepatic biliary drainage; PLT: Platelet.

Competing interests

The authors declare that they have no competing interests.

Authors' contributions

RV made substantial contributions to acquisition and interpretation of data, was involved in conception and drafting of the manuscript. SC contributed to interpretation of data, was involved in conception, drafting and revision of the manuscript. SF and CC contributed to acquisition of data, drafted the manuscript. MV was involved in revising the manuscript critically for important intellectual content. ECA contributed to interpretation of data, gave final approval of the version to be published. All authors read and approved the final manuscript.

References

1. Ebert EC: **Review article: the gastrointestinal complication of myositis.** *Aliment Pharmacol Ther* 2009, **31**(3):359–365.
2. Lin WY, Wang SJ, Hwang DW, Lan JL, Yeh SH: **Technetium-99 m-Pyrophosphate scintigraphic finding of intestinal perforation in dermatomyositis.** *J Nucl Med* 1995, **36**(9):1615–1617.
3. Morita Y, Sakuta T, Nagasu H, Kuwabara A, Tokuoka Y, Teshigawara S, Horike H, Kashihara N: **Bilateral ureteral stenosis and duodenal perforation in a patient with dermatomyositis.** *Mod Rheumatol* 2007, **17**:54–56.
4. Magill HL, Hixson SD, Whitington G, Igarashi M, Hannissian A: **Duodenal perforation in childhood dermatomyositis.** *Pediatr Radiol* 1984, **14**:28–30.
5. Wang IJ, Hsu WM, Shun CT, Chiang BL, Ni YH: **Juvenile dermatomyositis complicated with vasculitis and duodenal perforation.** *J Formos Med Assoc* 2001, **100**(12):844–846.
6. Thompson JW: **Spontaneous perforation of the esophagus as a manifestation of dermatomyositis.** *Ann Otol Rhinol Laryngol* 1984, **93**:464–467.
7. Niizawa M, Maie O, Asanuma Y, Saito T: **Adult dermatomyositis with angiopathy and cecum perforation and panniculitis.** *Nihon Hifuka Zasshi* 1991, **101**:447–451.
8. Suwa A, Hirakata M, Hama N, Ishiyama K, Amano K, Tanaka H, Fujimaki J, Mimori T, Inada S, Akizuki M: **An adult case of dermatmyositis complicated with cecum perforation and panniculitis.** *Nihon Rinsho Gakkai Kaishi* 1997, **20**:60–66.
9. Mamyrova G, Kleiner DE, James-Newton L, Shaham B, Miller FW, Rider LG: **Late-onset gastrointestinal pain in juvenile dermatomyositis as a manifestation of ischemic ulceration from chronic endarteropathy.** *Arthritis Rheum* 2007, **57**:881–884.
10. Zarbalian Y, von Rosenvince EC, Twadell W, Mikdashi J: **Recurrent pneumatosis intestinalis in a patient with dermatomyositis.** *BMJ Case Rep* 2013, **23**:2013.
11. Chiu SK, Yang YH, Wang LC, Chiang BL: **Ten-year experience of juvenile dermatomyositis: a retrospective study.** *J Microbiol Immunol Infect* 2007, **40**(1):68–73.
12. Chen GY, Liu MF, Lee YJJ, Chen WC: **Combination of massive mucinosis, dermatomyositis, pyoderma gangrenosum-like ulcer, bullae and fatal intestinal vasculopathy in a young female.** *Eur J Dermatol* 2005, **15**(5):396–400.
13. Ghayad E, Tohme A, Ingea H: **Digestive manifestastions of juvenile dermatomyositis. A case report and review of the literature.** *J Med Liban* 1993, **41**(4):240–243.
14. Downey EC Jr, Woolley MM, Hanson V: **Required surgical theraphy in the pediatric patient with dermatomyositis.** *Arch Surg* 1988, **123**(9):1117–1120.
15. Miller LC, Michael AF, Kim Y: **Childhood dermatomyositis. Clinical course and long-term follow-up.** *Clin Pediatr (Phila)* 1987, **26**(11):561–566.
16. Shullinger JN, Jacobs JC, Berdon WE: **Diagnosis and management of gastrointestinal perforations in childhood dermatomyositis with particular reference to perforations of the duodenum.** *J Pediatr Surg* 1985, **20**(5):521–524.
17. Kaplinsky N, Hod C, Gal-Semo R, Frankl O: **Spontaneous duodenal perforation during fulminant dermatomyositis.** *J Am Med Womens Assoc* 1978, **33**(5):213–214.
18. Koiunderliev P, Slavkov N: **Case of an acute form of dermatomyositis with visceral changes complicated by small intestine perforation.** *Khirurgiia (Sofiia)* 1975, **28**(1):79–80.
19. Bureau Y, Jerry, Barriere, Feve: **Acute dermatomyositis: fatal duodenal perforation during treatment with cortansyl.** *Bull Soc Fr Dermatol Syphiligr* 1958, **65**(3):327–328.
20. Neto NS, Goldenstein-Schainberg C: **Juvenile dermatomyositis: review and update of the pathogenesis and treatment.** *Bras J Rheumatol* 2010, **50**(3):299–312.
21. Smerud MJ, Johnson CD, Stephens DH: **Diagnosis of bowel infarction: a comparison of plain films and CT scans in 23 cases.** *AJR Am J Roentgenol* 1990, **154**:99–103.
22. Marvi U, Chung L, Fiorentino DF: **Clinical presentation and evaluation of dermatomyositis.** *Indian J Dermatol* 2012, **57**:375–381.
23. Kritayakirana K, M Maggio P, Brundage S, Purtill MA, Staudenmayer K, A Spain D: **Outcomes and complications of open abdomen technique for managing non-trauma patients.** *J Emerg Trauma Shock* 2010, **3**(2):118–122.
24. Kushimoto S, Miyauchi M, Yokota H, Kawai M: **Damage control surgery and open abdominal management: recent advances and our approach.** *J Nippon Med Sch* 2009, **76**:280–290.
25. Navsaria P, Nicol A, Hudson D, Cockwill J, Smith J: **Negative pressure wound therapy management of the "open abdomen" following trauma: a prospective study and systematic review.** *World J Emerg Surg* 2013, **8**(1):4.

10

Emergency presentation of the gastric cancer; prognosis and implications for service planning

Peter Vasas*, Tom Wiggins, Asif Chaudry, Catherine Bryant and Frances S Hughes

Abstract

Aims: To compare emergency and elective presentation of gastric cancer by mode of clinical presentation, initial stage, intervention and prognosis.

Methods: Data were collected prospectively for all cases of gastric cancer presenting to a tertiary referral centre between 2003 and 2010. This was stratified by emergency and elective presentation and was analysed for mode of presentation, initial stage and outcome. Statistical analysis was performed using unpaired t-test and Chi^2 test.

Results: A total of 291 patients presented: Forty-two (14.43%) were emergencies and 249 (85.57%) elective presentations. Analysis of the emergency cohort showed 25 patients presented with obstruction (59.52%), 15 presented with haematemesis (35.71%) and 2 with perforation (4.76%).

Eighteen of the emergency patients (45%) presented with stage 4 disease compared to 60 (25.42%) in the elective group ($p < 0.005$). Fourteen of the emergency patients were treated with curative intent (33.3%) compared with 130 (55.56%) in the elective group ($p < 0.01$). Over 6 years only 2 patients needed operation within 24 hours of presentation.

Overall survival at one year for emergency patients was 48.3% compared to 63.4% in elective patients ($p < 0.05$). There were no survivors from the emergency group after 3 years but 32.46% of the elective patients survived ($p < 0.02$). Elective presentation with disease stage 1A-3B had a two year survival rate of 54.95% compared to only 20% in the emergency group ($p < 0.05$). Of patients who underwent operative intervention 67.44% of patients who presented electively survived to 2 years. This compared to just 25% presenting as emergencies ($p < 0.001$).

Conclusions: Emergency presentation of gastric cancer is rare; is associated with higher stage of disease at presentation and lower rates of operability. The necessity to perform emergency operation within 24 hours is exceedingly rare. Emergency presentation is a marker of poor long term outcome for equivalent cancer stage in non-advanced (stages 1A-3B) disease.

Introduction

Gastric cancer is the second most common cause of cancer death worldwide [1], being responsible for 650 000 deaths annually. In the UK in 2007, there were 5,236 deaths from stomach cancer, making it the seventh most common cause of cancer death and responsible for over 3% of all cancer related mortality [2]. In 2007 the age-standardised rate of gastric carcinoma in the UK was 5.7 per 100 000 population.

The majority of the patients present with non-acute symptoms but gastric cancer can also manifest as an emergency with haematemesis, visceral perforation, or gastric outlet obstruction. Emergency presentation of gastric cancer has been shown to have an influence on overall survival, which is independent to any other factors. Blackshaw et al. [3] showed that patients presenting as an emergency had a median survival of 6 months, compared to 12 months for patients referred as an outpatient. Therefore, although emergency presentation is relatively rare, it may significantly affect prognosis.

Recent advances in diagnostic tools and new oncological treatments may improve the overall outcome of gastric carcinoma, but emergency presentation continues to be associated with higher stage of disease at presentation and lower rates of operability. The majority of the peer-reviewed papers report 10-25 patients in the emergency group [4-7].

* Correspondence: vasasdr@gmail.com
Academic Surgical Department, Barts and the London NHS Trust, Whitechapel, London (E1 1BB), United Kingdom

Perforated gastric cancer is rare accounting for 0.3-3% of gastric cancer cases [6-8], but gastric cancer is present in 10-16% of patients presenting with gastric perforation [9]. Only one-third of cases of perforated gastric cancer are diagnosed pre-operatively [7]. The diagnosis of gastric cancer is usually confirmed by post-operative histological examination. A two-staged procedural approach is sometimes used for the treatment of perforated gastric carcinoma; the first procedure controls the perforation and treats peritonitis, followed by a second procedure involving definitive gastrectomy with appropriate lymph node dissection [10,11].

Minor bleeding is a well-known characteristic of gastric cancer, often causing chronic microcytic hypochromic anaemia, prompting gastroscopy. However, gastric cancer can also present with major bleeding in up to 5% of patients [12]. These patients may require blood transfusion to prevent haemodynamic compromise. Endoscopic therapy can be used to control bleeding with the use of injection of adrenaline to the tumour base, argon plasma coagulation or with application of endo-clips [13]. However patients may require surgery for bleeding control if endoscopic measures for haemostasis fail.

Gastric outlet obstruction is more common than other emergency presentations and is usually a sign of locally advanced incurable disease. Traditionally, surgical bypass with gastrojejunostomy or palliative distal gastrectomy were the only therapeutic options to restore the gastric outflow. However increasingly, endoscopic stenting is utilised for to relieve obstruction in gastric cancer [14].

With specialist oesophagogastric surgeons being increasingly based in tertiary referral centres, there have been concerns that specialist surgeons may not be available should emergency surgical intervention be necessary in cases of gastric cancer. This raises the question of how commonly specialist oesophagogastric intervention is necessary in the emergency setting and how hospitals should plan their surgical service.

Aims

This study aims to compare the influence mode of presentation (emergency or elective) has on the outcome of patients with gastric cancer in a deprived inner city area. The frequency with which emergency operative intervention within 24 hours of presentation is necessary will also be established. The study aims to provide suggestion for the service planning; as examine the surgeons sub-specialty training who were involved into the emergency operations.

Patients and methods

Data were collected prospectively from all consecutive cases of gastric cancer patients presenting to the Upper Gastro-Intestinal Multidisciplinary Team at The Royal London Hospital between September 2003 and January 2010. Patient demographics, mode of presentation, disease stage at presentation, interventions and treatment undertaken, complications, hospital stay and survival were retrospectively analysed from the Departmental Database.

All consecutive patients presenting with gastric cancer to The Royal London Hospital or referred for treatment from one of the local diagnostic centres were involved. All of them were discussed at the specialised Multidisciplinary Team meeting; patients requiring urgent intervention often were discussed after initiation of treatment. Patients with stage IV disease or those deemed unfit for resection were diverted to a palliative care pathway. Fit patients with resectable disease were treated with curative intent. Neoadjuvant chemotherapy was considered in all patients with T3 or higher stage of cancer (according to the MAGIC trial) [15].

Emergency presentation was defined as those patients whom required immediate admission for treatment of symptoms (bleeding, perforation or obstruction). Major bleeding was characterised by the requirement of one or more unit of blood transfusion for acute blood loss.

Patients with cancer at the gastro-oesophageal junction were excluded, as were any patients undergoing prophylactic gastrectomy due to hereditary risk of gastric carcinoma.

Data was analysed to investigate the effect of emergency presentation upon the stage of disease at presentation and the proportion of patients treated with curative intent. The number of patients requiring emergency surgical intervention within 24 hours of presentation was recorded. Cumulative survival periods were calculated using the Kaplan-Meier method and differences in survival rates by disease stage were analyzed by COX-regression analysis. Comparison between the emergency and the elective presentations the χ^2 test and Fisher's exact test were used.

Results

Patient demographics and presentation

A total of 291 patients presented to our centre with gastric carcinoma during the 77-month period. Forty-two (14.4%) of these patients presented as an emergency with upper gastrointestinal (GI) bleeding, gastric perforation or gastric outlet obstruction. The remaining 249 patients (85.6%) presented electively via an outpatient referral with non-acute symptoms.

The mean age at presentation was 67 years in the emergency group and 68 in the elective group. From the emergency group twenty-five patients presented with obstruction (59.6%), two patients with perforation (4.8%) and 15 patients presented with upper GI bleeding (35.7%) and 7 of these patients required blood transfusion.

Elective patients presented with lower stage disease, stages 1 and 2 accounting for 37.6% of cases, compared with 23.1% of the emergency cases ($p < 0.05$). Twenty-five percent of elective cases presented with stage 4 disease, compared to 45% of the emergency cases ($p<0.005$).

Interventions and operative procedures

One hundred sixty-nine patients underwent operative intervention (58.1%), the remaining 122 patients had oncological, endoscopic or supportive palliative care.

In the elective group 139 patients out of 249 (55.8%) were treated with curative intent, compared with 15 out of 42 (35.7%) in the emergency group ($P < 0.05$ with χ^2 test).

In the emergency group 13 patients (30.9%) were unfit for any operative intervention and were treated palliatively, 14 patients (33.3%) underwent non-curative procedures (laparotomy with further procedure abandoned due to evidence of malignant spread (n = 3), gastrojejunostomy (n = 6) or non-curative distal gastrectomy (n = 5)). Of emergency cohort patients 11 patients were suitable to undergo distal gastrectomy (26.2%) and total gastrectomy was performed in 4 cases (9.5%).

In the elective group the pre-operative assessment, cross-sectional imaging and laparoscopy identified 106 patients, (42.5%) with unresectable or metastatic disease or patients were unfit to undergo major surgery. A further 9 patients (3.8%) were found to be unresectable at operation, one of these patients underwent local excision. Three patients from the elective group who were suitable for resection declined the operative procedure. The surgical procedures performed are shown in Table 1.

Inpatient stay for patients undergoing operative intervention was similar for both groups. The median postoperative hospital stay for the emergency group was 9.5 days (IQR = 4), compared to 12 days (IQR = 7) in the elective group.

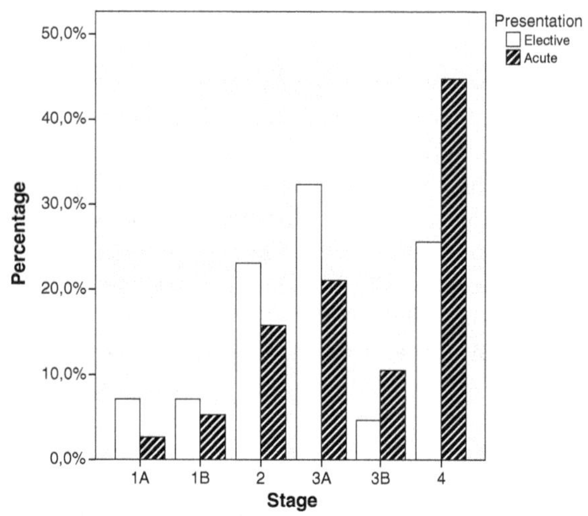

Figure 1 Stage at presentation.

Emergency surgery in the first 24 hours

Three patients required emergency operation within 24 hours of admission. This represents 1% of all presentations, and 7.1% of emergency presentations of gastric carcinoma. In each of these cases the emergency procedure was performed by the On-call General Surgeon (Breast, Colorectal and Hepato-Biliary specialists).

Two patients presented with gastric perforation and underwent emergency laparotomy. One patient was found to have metastatic disease and a palliative distal gastrectomy was performed. The second patient had a perforated gastric ulcer which was biopsied and an omental plug applied. The patient received palliative chemotherapy with no response. Survival for these two patients was 5 and 4 months respectively.

The third patient requiring emergency surgery presented with haematemesis to one of our local District General Hospitals. Although endoscopy confirmed a bleeding gastric ulcer, the haemorrhage could not be controlled endoscopically. The patient proceeded to theatre for laparotomy and a 3 cm ulcer high on the greater curvature was found with a central bleeding vessel. This was under-run and biopsies taken which confirmed adenocarcinoma. The patient made a good recovery and was referred to our centre for definitive oncological management. A total gastrectomy was performed six weeks following his initial presentation, the final histology was T1N0 adenocarcinoma, 0/39 nodes. The patient survived for two years following this procedure.

Emergency procedures after 24 hours

The remaining 39 emergency patients were managed without operative intervention over the first 24 hours. Fifteen patients presented with haematemesis. Nine received endoscopic intervention (injection, Argon-beam laser, heater probe) for bleeding control. Four patients were not actively bleeding at the time of endoscopy, and no further procedure was performed at this time. One patient had a large bleeding polyp removed at endoscopy, and three patients required injection of adrenaline to bleeding ulcerated areas. In one of these patients an endoclip was applied and argon plasma coagulation (APC) successfully performed. In only one case was endoscopic therapy not successful in controlling bleeding and this patient proceeded to theatre as described above. Overall 29 patients had some form of operation after complete staging, often on separate admission.

Patients presenting with gastric outlet obstruction were managed conservatively via nasogastric decompression in the initial period whilst further investigations were undertaken to stage their disease and plan further

Table 1 Operations performed

N = 291		Presentation			
		Elective		Acute	
		Number of patients	%	Number of patients	%
Type of operation	None	109	37.5	13	30.9
	Total gastrectomy	61	20.9	4	9.5
	Distal gastrectomy	69	23.7	16	38
	Gastro-jejunostomy	1	0.3	6	14.3
	Laparotomy/laparoscopy	8	2.7	3	7.1
	Local excision	1	0.3	0	0
	Total	**249**		**42**	

intervention. In 2 cases expanding metal stents were inserted endoscopically allowing oral intake and palliative oncological therapies.

Subsequently 3 out of 42 emergency patients (7.1%) and 44 out of 249 elective patients (17.6%) had neoadjuvant chemotherapy after their initial assessment ($p < 0.05$).

Survival

Overall survival

Twelve patients from the elective group and three patients from the emergency were lost to follow-up.

One year survival for patients presenting as an emergency was 48.3% compared to 63.4% in elective patients (p = <0.02). By 3 years follow-up there were only two survivors from the emergency presentation group (14.3%), while 32.5% of the elective patients survived to 3 years (p = <0.006). The overall survival is shown on the Kaplan Meier plot on Figure 2.

Survival with non-metastatic disease

To examine survival for patients with comparable disease stage between the emergency and elective cohorts, all patients presenting with disease stage 1A-3B were further analysed. In the emergency group twenty-four patients (57.1%) presented with non-metastatic disease and the two year survival rate was 20.0% compared with 54.9% from elective group (189/249 patients). None of the emergency patients were alive after 40 months, while 36% of the elective group were alive at this stage.

The survival of patients with non-metastatic disease is shown in Figure 3.

Survival following curative resections

Of patients presenting as emergency who underwent subsequent resection 25% survived to 2 years. This compared to 67.4% two-year survival from elective group (p = <0.01). Five-year survival for elective patients undergoing operative intervention was 33.3% and there were no survivors in the emergency presentation group after 4 years (Figure 4).

Discussion

Studies have shown that emergency presentation of gastric cancer is associated with higher stage disease and is an independent marker of poor prognosis. [3] Our results reinforce this as emergency patients more often presented with advanced stage disease; 45.0% of emergency patients presenting with stage IV, compared to 25.3% of elective patients (p <0.005), (Figure 1). Only 33.3% of emergency patients had resectable disease (compared to 55.6% of elective patients) (p <0.01). There were no survivors to 4 years follow up in the emergency group whereas 33.3% of operable elective patients survived to 5 years.

It is possible to claim that these results relate to the more advanced stage disease in the emergency group and not the presenting modality. However, when survival data for patients with non-metastatic gastric malignancy (stages 1A-3B) is analysed this shows that despite comparable disease stage, patients who present as an emergency have a worse prognosis and decreased survival. This may be due to the physical insult and the acute physiological deterioration during emergency presentation. Similar results were found when survival was compared for patients undergoing curative procedures. This suggests that emergency presentation could be an independent prognostic factor in gastric cancer. Other contributing factors to improved survival in the elective group may include the increased use of neo-adjuvant chemotherapy, and that patients presenting as an emergency may also be more severely malnourished at time of presentation.

Our results showed that the need for operative intervention within 24 hours of presentation is rare with only 3 patients (<10% of the emergency presentation) during this six-year period requiring emergency surgery. Two of these cases were as a result of gastric perforation, and one was due to bleeding despite attempts to control this via endoscopic therapy. These findings correlate with those of Blackshaw et al, who analysed 116 emergency presentations of gastric cancer between 1995 and 2003,

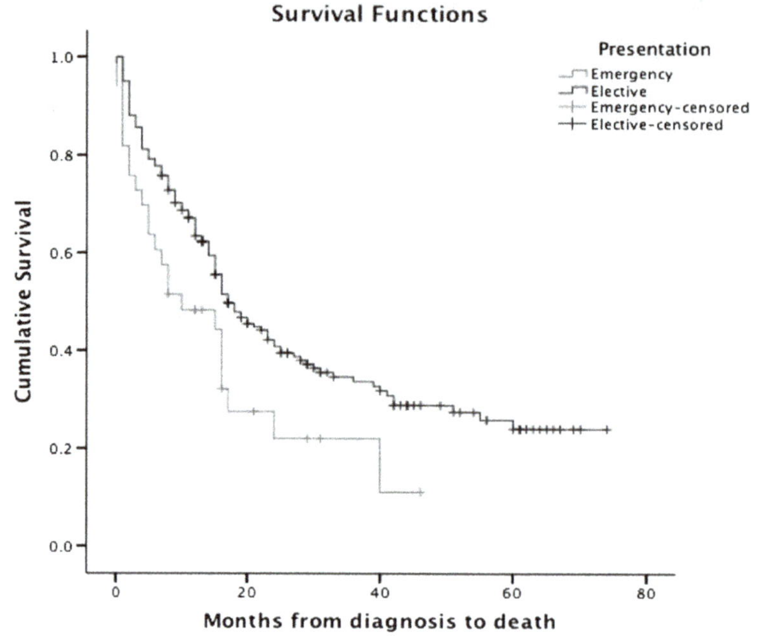

Figure 2 Kaplan-Meier curve showing comparison of survival between patients presenting as an emergency and electively.

and showed that none of these patients required operative intervention within 24 hours of presentation [3].

Centralisation of specialist oesophago-gastric service provision within tertiary referral centres has lead to many District General Hospitals losing their provision for specialist Oesophago-Gastric Surgeons on call. However as shown in this study the need for operative intervention within 24 hours of presentation of gastric carcinoma is exceedingly rare. In only one instance during this six-year series did endoscopic treatment fail to achieve haemostasis. This bleeding ulcer was successfully under-run at a peripheral hospital prior to definitive gastrectomy at our centre once the diagnosis of adenocarcinoma had been confirmed. Perforation of gastric cancer is also rare with a reported incidence rate of 0.3-3% of all cases of gastric carcinoma [6-8].

Performing gastrectomy in the context of gastric perforation and peritonitis presents numerous challenges. Inflammatory changes following peritonitis have lead to reported intra-operative overestimation of local tumour

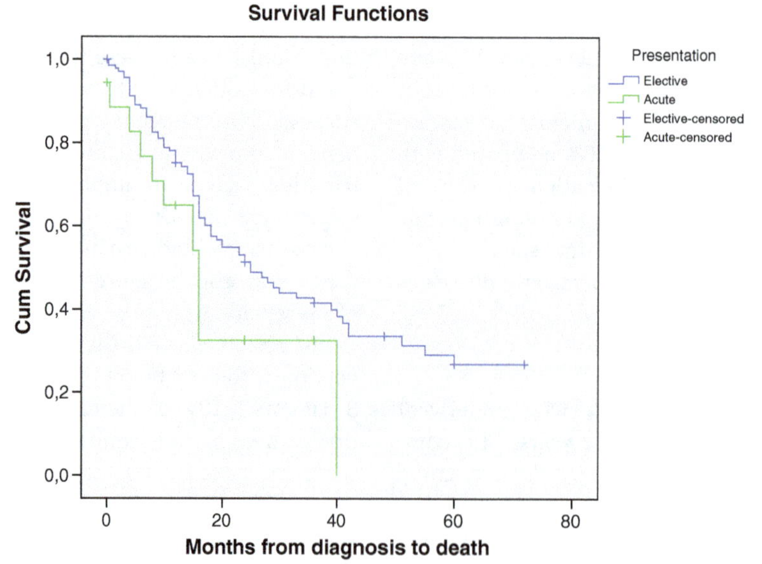

Figure 3 Comparison of survival for patients presenting with disease stage 1A-3B in the emergency and elective presentation groups.

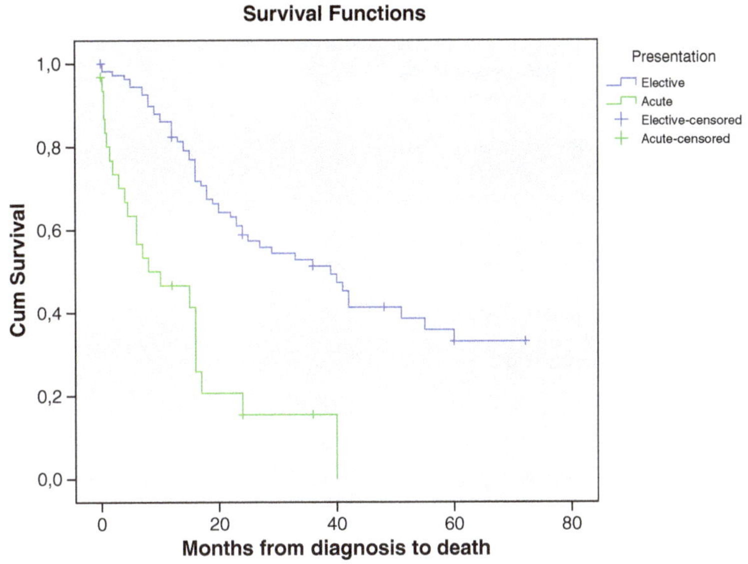

Figure 4 Comparison of survival for patients undergoing operative intervention in the emergency and elective presentation groups.

infiltration and lymph node involvement. [9] Therefore a two-staged approach to dealing with perforated gastric cancer has been proposed as the most suitable method. Lehnert et al recommend that the initial procedure should be directed at the treatment of perforation and peritonitis [9]. This involves either direct closure of the perforation or omental patch application, followed by thorough washout of the peritoneal cavity and drain insertion. Following patient recovery and histological confirmation of malignancy, accurate disease staging can be completed, and a radical oncological operation for gastric cancer or neoadjuvant chemotherapy can be planned as appropriate.

The initial emergency procedure should aim to simply control perforation and relieve peritonitis. Surgeons who are not specialists in Oesophago-gastric surgery could perform this initial procedure and the surgical training should address this question. The period of patient recovery following this emergency intervention would allow transfer to a tertiary referral centre for further assessment and management. Definitive gastrectomy can then be planned where appropriate. This period of planning for radical oncological intervention also allows time for patient optimisation, including nutritional support where necessary. Patients with gastric malignancy are often severely malnourished and a period of pre-operative nutritional optimisation, which is continued post-operatively may reduce complication rates [10].

Conclusion

Emergency surgery within 24 hours of presentation for gastric malignancies is extremely rare. A two-stage approach for management of perforated gastric carcinoma could provide acceptable results and allows patients to be transferred to a tertiary Oesophago-Gastric centre for further assessment prior to definitive treatment; however our observation based on the limited patient number. Our experience shows that emergency lifesaving intervention can be successfully followed by transfer for emergency cancer therapy with reasonable survival. Emergency presentation is usually associated with advanced disease stage and resources should be diverted towards early diagnosis, increasing patient awareness rather than upper GI surgical services on all District General Hospital site.

Competing interests

The authors declare that they have no competing interest.

Authors' contribution

PV: data collection, analysis and conclusions; TW, AC, CB: data collection and processing, FH: study design, paper review. All authors read and approved the final manuscript.

References

1. Fuchs CS, Mayer RJ: **Gastric carcinoma.** *N Engl J Med* 1995, **333**:32–41.
2. Mortality Statistics: *Cause. England and Wales 2007.*: Office for National Statistics; 2009. Ref Type: Report.
3. Blackshaw GR, Stephens MR, Lewis WG, Paris HJ, Barry JD, Edwards P, *et al*: **Prognostic significance of acute presentation with emergency complications of gastric cancer.** *Gastric Cancer* 2004, **7**:91–96.
4. Kasakura Y, Ajani JA, Mochizuki F, Morishita Y, Fujii M, Takayama T: **Outcomes after emergency surgery for gastric perforation or severe bleeding in patients with gastric cancer.** *J Surg Oncol* 2002, **80**:181–185.
5. Kotan C, Sumer A, Baser M, Kiziltan R, Carparlar MA: **An analysis of 13 patients with perforated gastric carcinoma: A surgeon's nightmare?** *World J Emerg Surg* 2008, **3**:17.
6. Roviello F, Rossi S, Marrelli D, de MG, Pedrazzani C, Morgagni P, *et al*: **Perforated gastric carcinoma: a report of 10 cases and review of the literature.** *World J Surg Oncol* 2006, **4**:19.

7. Ozmen MM, Zulfikaroglu B, Kece C, Aslar AK, Ozalp N, Koc M: **Factors influencing mortality in spontaneous gastric tumour perforations.** *J Int Med Res* 2002, **30:**180–184.
8. Kasakura Y, Ajani JA, Fujii M, Mochizuki F, Takayama T: **Management of perforated gastric carcinoma: a report of 16 cases and review of world literature.** *Am Surg* 2002, **68:**434–440.
9. Lehnert T, Buhl K, Dueck M, Hinz U, Herfarth C: **Two-stage radical gastrectomy for perforated gastric cancer.** *Eur J Surg Oncol* 2000, **26:**780–784.
10. Bozzetti F, Gavazzi C, Miceli R, Rossi N, Mariani L, Cozzaglio L, *et al*: **Perioperative total parenteral nutrition in malnourished, gastrointestinal cancer patients: a randomized, clinical trial.** *JPEN J Parenter Enteral Nutr* 2000, **24:**7–14.
11. Ergul E, Gozetlik EO: **Emergency spontaneous gastric perforations: ulcus versus cancer.** *Langenbecks Arch Surg* 2009, **394:**643–646.
12. Fox JG, Hunt PS: **Management of acute bleeding gastric malignancy.** *Aust N Z J Surg* 1993, **63:**462–465.
13. Uchida S, Ishii N, Suzuki S, Uemura M, Suzuki K, Fujita Y: **Endoscopic resection after endoscopic hemostasis for hemorrhagic gastric cancer.** *Hepatogastroenterology* 2010, **57:**1330–1332.
14. Huggett MT, Ghaneh P, Pereira SP: **Drainage and Bypass Procedures for Palliation of Malignant Diseases of the Upper Gastrointestinal Tract.** *Clin Oncol (R Coll Radiol)* 2010.
15. Ng K, Meyerhardt JA, Fuchs CS: **Adjuvant and neoadjuvant approaches in gastric cancer.** *Cancer J* 2007, **13:**168–174.

11

Midgut malrotation first presenting as acute bowel obstruction in adulthood

Okiemute F Emanuwa, Abraham A Ayantunde* and Tony W Davies

Abstract

Malrotation of the midgut is generally regarded as paediatric pathology with the majority of patients presenting in childhood. The diagnosis is rare in adults, which sometimes leads to delay in diagnosis and treatment. A high index of suspicion is therefore required when dealing with patients of any age group with abdominal symptoms. We present a case of a 55-year old man who presented with an acute abdomen with preoperative computed tomography scan and operative findings confirming midgut rotation. The duodenum, small bowel, caecum and appendix were abnormally located, with the presence of classical Ladd's bands. There was no evidence of intestinal volvulus. The patient underwent an emergency laparotomy with an uneventful postoperative recovery. A review of the literature is presented to highlight the rarity of intestinal malrotation and the controversies surrounding its management in the adult population.

Keywords: Midgut malrotation, acute abdomen, Ladd's bands, computed tomography scan, laparoscopy

Introduction

Midgut malrotation is a congenital anomaly in the embryological development of the foetal intestinal rotation. It has been estimated that it affects approximately 1 in 500 live births [1]. However, the true incidence is difficult to determine as a substantial number of cases will go undetected throughout life. The vast majority of the complications associated with midgut malrotation present in the first month of life and 60-85% of cases are diagnosed in this age group [1,2]. It is reported that more than 90% of patients will present by the time of their first birthday [3]. Adult midgut malrotation is very rare and its incidence has been reported to be between 0.0001% and 0.19% [3,4]. Most adult diagnoses of midgut malrotation are made in asymptomatic patients; either on imaging investigations for unrelated conditions or at operations for other pathology. This scenario of incidental diagnosis is becoming increasingly common, particularly with improvements, and increased use, of diagnostic imaging techniques in modern practice. However, there are a small proportion of affected adults who may present with acute or chronic symptoms of intestinal obstruction or intermittent and recurrent abdominal pain. The true diagnosis in this age group is fraught with immense difficulty, especially because the typical presentation is with non-specific symptoms and the fact that adult Surgeons usually have low index of suspicion and may not consider the diagnosis a possibility in the initial evaluation of adult patients with abdominal pain.

We report a case of an adult patient with an acute presentation of midgut malrotation which highlights the dilemmas of preoperative diagnosis, as supported by a review of the literature.

Case report

A 55-year old gentleman was admitted to the Accident and Emergency department with a three day history of acute onset, cramp like abdominal pain. There was associated nausea but no vomiting. Bowels had been opened the day before admission but no flatus had been passed for 24 hours. There were no other associated red flag symptoms. The patient had never experienced similar symptoms and had no previous medical or surgical history.

* Correspondence: biodunayantunde@yahoo.co.uk
Department of Surgery, Queen Mary's Hospital, Frognal Avenue, Sidcup, DA14 6LT, London, UK

On examination, the patient was afebrile and haemodynamically stable. The abdomen was moderately distended with significant tenderness in the central, epigastric and left hypochondrial regions. There was no evidence of peritonitis.

Routine admission blood tests including serum electrolytes, urea, amylase, lactate, liver function tests (LFTs), clotting profile, C-reactive protein (CRP) and an arterial blood gas (ABG) were normal. However, a full blood count (FBC) demonstrated a haemoglobin level of 14.2 g/dl with a slightly raised total white cell count (WCC) of 10.3×10^9 and a neutrophilia of 7.0×10^9.

A chest radiograph did not reveal air under the diaphragm. Abdominal radiograph showed non-dilated gas filled loops of bowel in the central and upper abdominal regions. The diagnosis remained elusive until an emergency computed tomography (CT) scan (Figures 1, 2, 3, 4) was obtained which demonstrated features of malrotation. The duodenum was malpositioned below and to the right of the ascending colon and hepatic flexure. The caecum was located in the left upper quadrant. There were also a few dilated loops of small bowel in the upper abdomen.

The patient was resuscitated with intravenous fluids, analgesia and prepared for an emergency exploratory laparotomy. The findings at operation included dilated small bowel in the upper abdomen, partial torsion and necrosis of the greater omentum, the caecum was on the left side of the abdomen tethered by torted omentum, and loops of small bowel occupying the right paracolic gutter and the right iliac fossa. There were fibrous

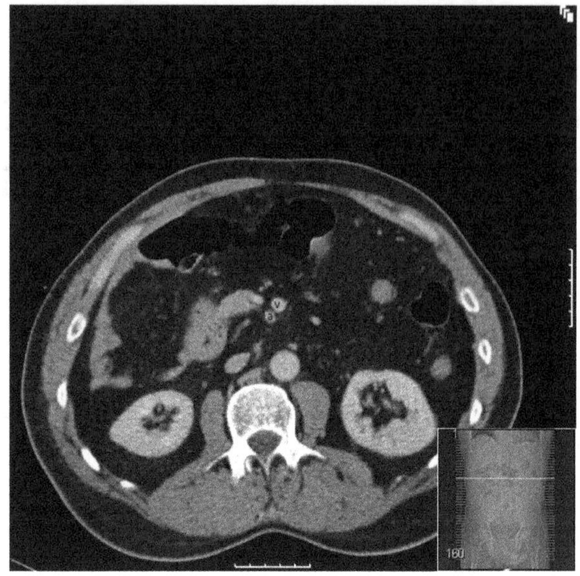

Figure 2 CT scan showing inverse relationship of SMA to SMV (a-artery and v-vein).

bands over the distal part of the duodenum, on the right side of the abdomen, confirming midgut malrotation (Figures 5 & 6).

The twisted, necrotic omentum was excised, the congenital bands were divided and an appendicectomy was carried out. The anatomical malrotation was left uncorrected.

The patient had an uneventful postoperative recovery and was discharged home on the fifth day post- surgery.

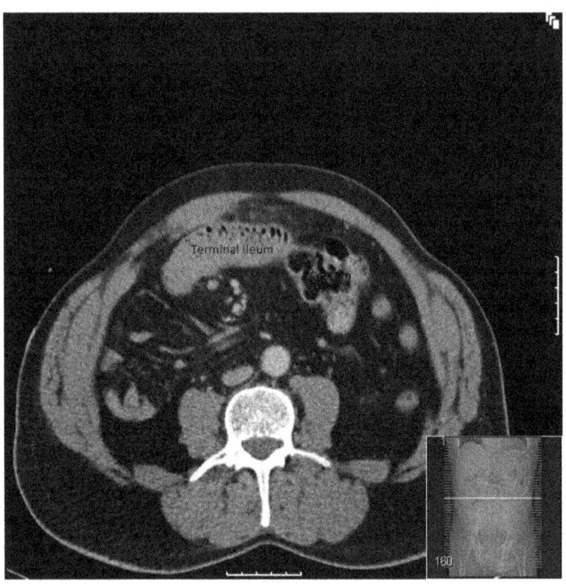

Figure 1 CT scan showing caecum on the left side of the abdomen and terminal ileum entering the caecum from the right side.

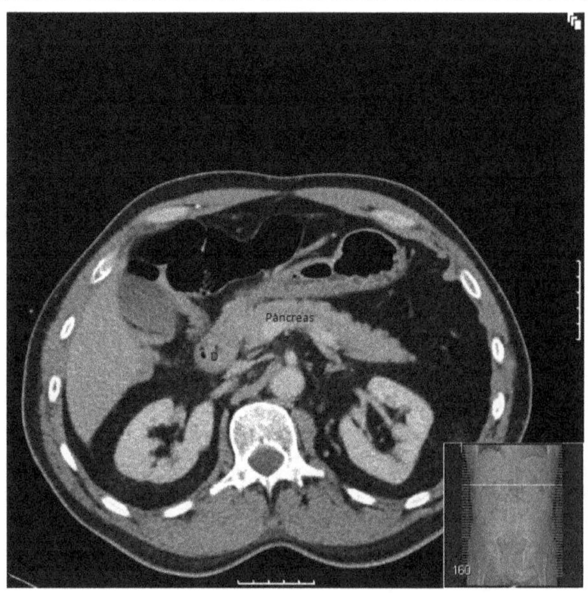

Figure 3 CT scan showing lack of progression of the duodenum across the aorta and the spines (D-duodenum).

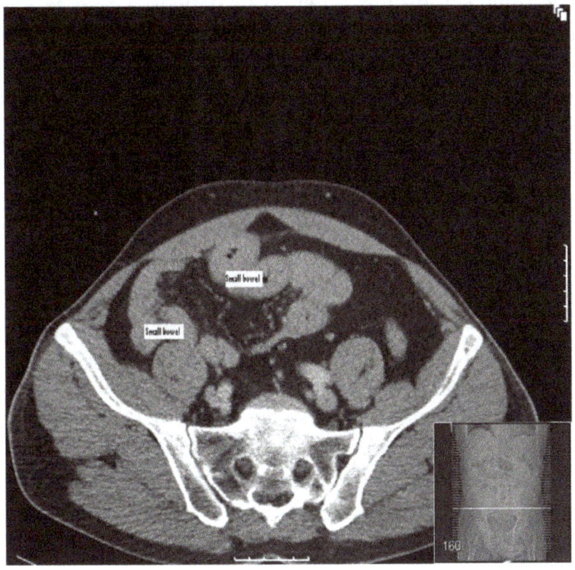

Figure 4 CT scan showing most of the small bowel on the right side of the abdomen.

On follow up he was well and there had been no late complications. He had returned to his premorbid level of function and did not report any symptom recurrence.

Discussion and review of the literature

Initial presentation of symptomatic midgut malrotation is rare in adults. However, a significant number of cases remain quiescent during childhood. Incidental diagnosis may then occur in adulthood; when imaging investigations are carried out for other symptoms or, during surgery for unrelated pathology. It has been reported that the incidence of malrotation in adults is approximately 0.2%. However, it is probable that this rate will rise with future developments in diagnostic imaging. It is difficult to ascertain the true incidence, but evidence from post mortem studies suggest that gut malrotation may affect up to 1 in 6000 [3,4].

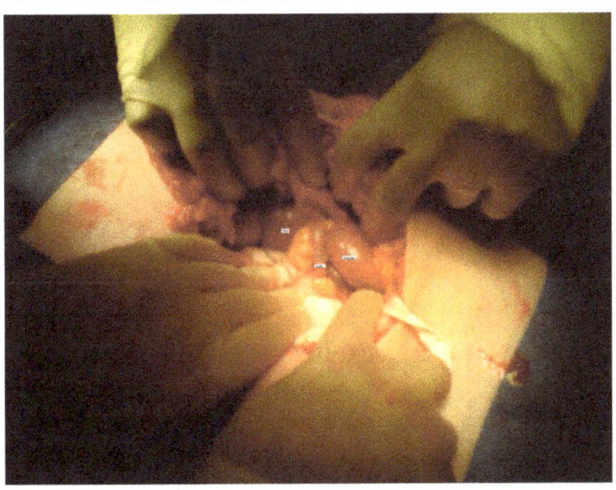

Figure 5 Photograph showing high caecum and appendix located on the left side of the abdomen.

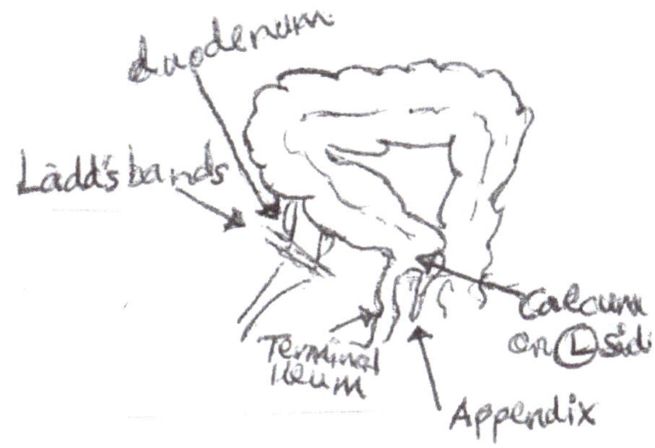

Figure 6 Graphical representation of the intra-operative findings.

Midgut malrotation is broadly considered a deviation from the normal 270 degree counterclockwise rotation of the gut during embryonic development. During week 4 of foetal development, the embryonic gut, consisting of a straight endodermal tube, develops vascular pedicles to be divided into the foregut, midgut and hindgut based on the anatomical blood supply. The midgut is supplied by the superior mesenteric artery (SMA) and by the fifth week of embryonic life, it begins a process of rapid elongation and outgrows the capacity of the abdominal cavity. This leads to a temporary physiological herniation into the umbilical cord at about the sixth week of life with return to the abdominal cavity about 4 to 6 weeks later. During this period, the midgut undergoes a 270 degree counterclockwise rotation around the SMA axis. This process leads to the formation of the duodenal C-loop, placing it behind the SMA in a retroperitoneal position and emerging at the ligament of Treitz. The progressive reduction of the physiological midgut herniation commences at about week 10 of embryonic development. The duodeno-jejunal flexure (DJF) and jejunum to reduce first and lie to the left. The distal small bowel then follows and lies progressively to the right of the abdominal cavity. The descent of the caecum from its higher position in the right upper quadrant forms the latter part of this complex rotational development; it becomes positioned in the right lower abdomen. The ascending colon then assumes a retroperitoneal position, also on the right side. The base of the small bowel mesentery subsequently fuses with the posterior peritoneum in a diagonal fashion, from the ligament of Treitz at the DJF to the caecum, completing the whole process at about the eleventh week of foetal development [1,4-6].

The failure of the normal physiological rotation of the midgut leads to various degrees of anomaly including the entire small bowel remaining on the right side of the abdomen, the caecum, appendix and colon on the left and an absent ligament of Treitz. In addition, the small bowel mesentery may develop a narrow vertical attachment and the peritoneal fibrous bands fixing the duodenum and caecum to the abdominal wall may persist. These congenital bands extend from the right lateral abdominal wall, across the duodenum and attach to the undescended caecum and are known as Ladd's bands [2,4,6,7]. Ladd's bands compress the duodenum and can potentially cause duodenal obstruction. The malrotation of the gut and abnormal location of the caecum produces a narrow superior mesenteric vascular pedicle, as opposed to the normally broadbased small bowel mesentery. This narrow SMA takeoff and lack of posterior peritoneal fusion predispose to subsequent midgut volvulus and obstruction with potential vascular catastrophe [7,8].

Midgut malrotation in adults presents in numerous ways and the symptoms are non-specific. The clinical diagnosis in adolescents and adults is difficult because it is rarely considered on clinical grounds. Many patients remain asymptomatic and the diagnosis is discovered incidentally during investigations or laparotomy for other unrelated problems in adult life. Wang and Welch [4] showed that 24 of 50 patients were clinically asymptomatic in their case series of adolescents and adults with malrotation. Adults with a rotational abnormality of the gut usually present differently to paediatric patients. Two distinct patterns of adult presentations have been reported in the literature: acute and chronic [5,7,9]. Chronic presentation is more common in adults. This is characterised by intermittent crampy abdominal pain, bloating, nausea and vomiting over several months or years. The symptoms may be highly nonspecific. However, the range of clinical presentations, underlines the need for a high index of suspicion of midgut malrotation, when investigating the cause of intermittent and varying abdominal symptomatology in a healthy young adult [5,7]. Dietz et al [5] studied a series of 10 adults with bowel obstruction caused by intestinal malrotation. They reported that 5 adults presented with chronic features and that the duration of symptoms extended to 30 years. Fu et al [7] reported that 6 of 12 patients in their series presented with chronic intermittent abdominal symptoms. Diagnostic delays are common in this group of patients because of the nonspecific nature of the presentations. The pathophysiology of these chronic symptoms may relate to the compression effect of Ladd's bands running from the caecum and ascending colon to the right abdominal wall [5,10].

The other group of symptomatic adults typically present with symptoms of acute bowel obstruction and these patients may or may not report a previous history of abdominal symptoms, as with our patient. These patients may on occasion, have symptoms and signs of an impending abdominal catastrophe. Moldrem et al [9] reported that 48.5% of their thirty-three patients presented with an acute abdomen. Acute presentation may be due to volvulus of the midgut or ileocaecum, reported as the most common cause of bowel obstruction in adults with gut malrotation. Other causes of acute presentation may be related to internal herniation caused by Ladd's bands. There is also a subgroup of acutely presenting adult patients with malrotation. They are identified when affected by other common abdominal diseases. Their unusual intestinal anatomy results in atypical signs and symptoms. These patients may present with localised peritonitis in the right upper quadrant or on the left side of the abdomen if their appendix becomes inflamed. The atypical presentations may lead to confusion, as one common abdominal pathology may mimics another, leading to incorrect diagnosis of conditions such as acute appendicitis, cholecystitis, pancreatitis, perforated peptic ulcer disease and left colonic diverticulitis. Several authors have reported observing atypical presentations of this nature before discovering gut malrotation with abnormal location of the caecum and appendix at surgery [5,7].

We can expect an increase in the incidental diagnosis of gut malrotation with increasing and widespread use of radiological investigations. Diagnostic features of midgut malrotation can be identified using plain abdominal radiograph, ultrasound scan (USS), computed tomography (CT) scan, magnetic resonance imaging (MRI) scan and mesenteric arteriography [9,11]. Conventional plain radiography is neither sensitive nor specific in the diagnosis of gut malrotation although right-sided jejunal markings and the absence of a stool-filled colon in the right lower quadrant may be suggestive, leading to further investigation. Abdominal colour Doppler USS may reveal malposition of the SMA, raising the suspicion of gut malrotation with or without the abnormal location of the hollow viscus [9,11,12]. Characteristic USS findings of midgut volvulus were first described by Pacros et al and include duodenal dilatation with distal tapering and fixed midline bowel and mesentery twisted around the SMA axis. These features classically present as the 'whirlpool' sign [13]. The reported gold standard for diagnosis of gut malrotation is an upper gastrointestinal (UGI) contrast study, particularly in the paediatric age group [5,11,12]. This will generally show the duodenum and duodenojejunal flexure located to the right of the spine. The use of a contrast enema in conjunction with the UGI study has also been advocated as it can be used to demonstrate an abnormally located ileocaecum and right colon. However, contrast study findings may be nonspecific and a normal study does not exclude the possibility of gut malrotation [5,7,10,11].

CT scan with or without UGI contrast study is increasingly used preferentially as it is now considered the investigation of choice; providing diagnostic accuracy of 80% [5,9,11]. CT and MRI scans may show the SMV to be in an anomalous position; posterior and to the left of the SMA. In addition, they may show the abnormal anatomical arrangements of the midgut with the duodenum not crossing the spine. Deviation from the normal positional relationship of SMV and SMA was originally described by Nichols and Li [14] as a useful indicator of the diagnosis of midgut malrotation. However, abnormal orientation of the SMA-SMV relationship is not entirely diagnostic of malrotation; it can also be seen in some patients without the pathology and a proportion of patients with malrotation may have a normal SMA-SMV relationship [11]. Patients with gut malrotation will often have an underdeveloped or absent uncinate process of the pancreas. This is possibly due to the failure of the SMA to migrate to the left of the SMV [9,11]. The CT appearance of midgut volvulus is diagnostic of malrotation. The shortened mesentery allows the small bowel and mesentery to twist and wrap around the narrowed SMA pedicle to create a distinctive 'whirlpool' appearance on CT scan. This pattern was first described by Fisher in a patient with midgut volvulus [15]. It can be detected with both abdominal USS and CT scan. CT scan findings of gut malrotation and small bowel obstruction without volvulus, may show internal herniation secondary to Ladd's bands.

Mesenteric angiography was previously used but is now rarely indicated in the evaluation of malrotation. It has the capacity to demonstrate the abnormal relationship between, and detect the patency of, the mesenteric vasculature. Angiography was used to demonstrate the characteristic corkscrew appearance of a whirling SMA and its branches; the 'barber pole sign' as well as extensive collaterals caused by proximal SMA occlusion [16]. However, its role has been superseded by the CT scan which has the overall advantage of not only detecting the abnormal location of the midgut but also the reversed mesenteric anatomical relationship as well as any other intra-abdominal anomalies associated with malrotation.

Symptomatic midgut malrotation undoubtedly requires surgical intervention although the management of asymptomatic patients is more controversial. Choi et al [17] reviewed 177 patients over a 35-year period. They found that asymptomatic patients had a low risk of intestinal volvulus and therefore advised that routine investigations, screening and elective surgery were not necessary with close follow-up. However, it is increasingly argued that all suitable patients with intestinal malrotation should undergo surgical correction regardless of age as it is impossible to predict which patients will develop catastrophic complications [8]. Several small case series have recommended that elective Ladd's procedure should be performed in all patients with intestinal malrotation. The authors of the studies that include cases of life threatening small bowel ischaemia argue this point particularly strongly [3,5,7,9]. Of course, the operative policy should be based on the presentation and suspected diagnosis; the potential risks of the procedure need to be weighed against the benefits.

The surgical management of intestinal malrotation was first described by William Ladd in 1936 [6] and this remains the mainstay of treatment. The classical Ladd's Procedure consists of 4 parts: division of Ladd's bands overlying the duodenum; widening of the narrowed root of the small bowel mesentery by mobilising the duodenum and division of the adhesions around the SMA to prevent further volvulus; counterclockwise detorsioning of the midgut volvulus if present and appendicectomy to prevent future diagnostic dilemma of an abnormally located appendix [6]. The original Ladd's procedure was described for the paediatric population group and the full components of this procedure may not be offered in the adult group [4-6,9]. Most authors are of the opinion that Ladd's procedure is an adequate treatment for intestinal malrotation. Fu et al [7] reported a complete resolution of symptoms in 9 and near complete resolution in 2 of 11 patients. Dietz et al [5] also reported a complete symptomatic resolution in 8 of their 10 patients treated surgically. Variations of the technique used to manage intestinal malrotation have been introduced to prevent recurrent volvulus. These include re-establishment of the normal gut anatomy by duodenopexy, caecopexy and suture fixation of the ascending colon to the right abdominal wall, in the retroperitoneal position [4,5,18]. We offered a modified procedure to our patient by performing a division of Ladd's bands and an appendicectomy. There was no volvulus and we did not feel that the duodenum needed to be mobilised and straightened in this case. Our patient has been completely symptom free during 12 months of follow up.

There are recent reports of the use of the laparoscopic approach in the surgical treatment of intestinal malrotation. The technique appears to be safe and effective when performed by experienced laparoscopic surgeons, especially in the absence of volvulus [2,7,8,18,19]. Laparoscopic Ladd's procedure in paediatric groups is increasingly reported in the literature. It is becoming more accepted as an initial approach to surgical correction of intestinal malrotation, resulting in shorter hospital stays. There are few reports of this approach in adults. The laparoscopic approach can be technically challenging and conversion to open procedure is common [2,7,8,19]. A few published works have indicated that the laparoscopic approach can be successful in patients with malrotation and midgut volvulus [8,19]. A retrospective analysis of both open and laparoscopic Ladd's procedures by Stanfill et al performed at the Children's Hospital of Illinois, USA noted that short-term results were superior with the laparoscopic approach and can be achieved without any increase in the duration of the operation [20].

Conclusions

Intestinal malrotation is a rare condition but is considered an important cause of bowel obstruction in adults. The diagnosis of malrotation after childhood is difficult and usually not readily considered as the cause of intra-abdominal symptoms. The presentation is usually nonspecific and this often leads to diagnostic and treatment delay with possible bowel ischaemia and necrosis. Evidence of which portends a poor prognosis and death. Therefore, a high index of suspicion needs to be maintained and prompt surgical intervention must be considered in order to prevent an abdominal catastrophe and fatality. There are no reliable means of identifying which group of patients with intestinal malrotation will develop subsequent complications. In the light of this, many authors are now advocating early surgical intervention in the form of a standard and modified Ladd's procedure. There is evidence in the literature that the use of Ladd's procedure or ordinary division of Ladd's bands and adhesiolysis relieves symptoms and in fact, prevents recurrence in the majority of patients.

Patient's consent

Written informed consent was obtained from the patient for publication of this case report and accompanying images. A copy of the written consent is available for review by the Editor-in-Chief of this journal.

Abbreviations

ABGs: Arterial blood gases; CRP: C-reactive protein; CT: Computed tomography; DJF: Duodenal jejunal flexure; FBC: Full blood count; LFTs: Liver function tests; MRI: Magnetic resonance imaging; SMA: Superior mesenteric artery; USS:Ultrasound scan; WCC: White cell count.

Authors' contributions

OFE was involved in postoperative care, conceived the write up, performed the literature search and manuscript preparation.
AAA performed the operation with TWD, involved in the preoperative and postoperative care, conceived the write up, performed the literature search and manuscript preparation.
TWD performed the operation with AAA, involved in the preoperative and postoperative care, conceived the write up, performed the literature search and manuscript preparation.
All authors read and approved the manuscript for submission.

Competing interests

The authors declare that they have no competing interests.

References

1. Torres AM, Ziegler MM: **Malrotation of the intestine.** *World J Surg* 1993, **17**:326-331.
2. Matzke GM, Moir CR, Dozois EJ: **Laparoscopic Ladd procedure for adult malrotation of the midgut with cocoon deformity: report of a case.** *J Laparoendosc Adv Surg Tech A* 2003, **13**:327-329.
3. Von Flue M, Herzog U, Ackermann C, *et al*: **Acute and chronic presentation of intestinal nonrotation in adult.** *Dis Colon Rectum* 1994, **37**:192-198.
4. Wang C, Welch C: **Anomalies of intestinal rotation in adolescents and adults.** *Surgery* 1963, **54**:839-855.
5. Dietz DW, Walsh RM, Grundfest-Broniatowski S, Lavery IC, Fazio VW, Vogt DP: **Intestinal Malrotation: a rare but important cause of bowel obstruction in adults.** *Dis Colon Rectum* 2002, **45(10)**:1381-1386.
6. Ladd WE: **Surgical diseases of the alimentary tract in infants.** *N Engl J Med* 1936, **215**:705-708.
7. Fu T, Tong WD, He YJ, Wen YY, Luo DL, Liu BH: **Surgical management of intestinal malrotation in adults.** *World Journal of Surgery* 2007, **31**:1797-1803.
8. Matzke GM, Dozois EJ, Larson DW, Moir CR: **Surgical management of intestinal malrotation in adults: comparative results for open and laparoscopic Ladd procedures.** *Surg Endosc* 2005, **19**:1416-1419.
9. Moldrem AW, Papaconstantinou H, Broker H, Megison S, Jeyarajah DR: **Late presentation of intestinal malrotation: an argument for elective repair.** *World J Surg* 2008, **32**:1426-1431.
10. Gamblin TC, Stephens RE, Johnson RK, Rothwell M: **Adult malrotation: A case report and review of the literature.** *Current Surgery* 2003, **60(5)**:517-520.
11. Pickhardt PJ, Bhalla S: **Intestinal malrotation in adolescents and adults: spectrum of clinical and imaging features.** *American Journal of Radiology* 2002, **179**:1429-1435.
12. Kapfer SA, Rappold JF: **Intestinal malrotation - not just the paediatric surgeon's problem.** *J Am Coll Surg* 2004, **199**:628-635.
13. Pacros JP, Sann L, Genin G, Tran-Minh VA, Morin de Finfe CH, Foray P, Louis D: **Ultrasound diagnosis of midgut volvulus: the 'whirlpool' sign.** *Paediatr Radiology* 1992, **22**:18-20.
14. Nichols DM, Li DK: **Superior mesenteric vein rotation: a CT sign of midgut malrotation.** *Am J Roentgenol* 1983, **141**:707-708.
15. Fisher JK: **Computer tomographic diagnosis of volvulus in intestinal malrotation.** *Radiology* 1981, **140**:145-146.
16. Hsu CY, Chiba Y, Fukui O, Sasaki Y, Miyashita S: **Counterclockwise barber-pole sign on prenatal three-dimensional power Doppler sonography in a case of duodenal obstruction without intestinal malrotation.** *J Clin Ultrasound Feb* 2004, **32(2)**:86-90.
17. Choi M, Borenstein SH, Hornberger L, Langer JC: **Heterotaxia syndrome: the role of screening for intestinal rotation abnormalities.** *Arch Dis Child* 2005, **90**:13-15.
18. Bax NM, van der Zee DC: **Laparoscopic treatment of intestinal malrotation in children.** *Surg Endosc* 1998, **12(11)**:1314-1316.
19. Kalfa N, Zamfir C, Lopez M, Forgues D, Raux O, Guibal MP, Galifer RB, Allal H: **Conditions required for laparoscopic repair of subacute volvulus of the midgut in neonates with intestinal malrotation: 5 cases.** *Surg Endosc* 2004, **18**:1815-1817.
20. Stanfill AB, Pearl RH, Kalvakuri K, Wallace LJ, Vegunta RK: **Laparoscopic Ladd's Procedure: Treatment of Choice for Midgut Malrotation in Infants and Children.** *J Laparoendosc Adv Surg Tech A* 2010, **20(4)**:369-372.

12

Hartmann's procedure vs loop colostomy in the treatment of obstructive rectosigmoid cancer

Slobodan Krstic[1,2], Vladimir Resanovic[2], Tamara Alempijevic[1,3], Aleksandar Resanovic[4], Ana Sijacki[1,2], Vladimir Djukic[1,2], Zlatibor Loncar[1,2] and Aleksandar Karamarkovic[1,2*]

Abstract

Introduction: Colorectal carcinoma is the most common malignant gastrointestinal tumour. There is still a considerable controversy when it comes to urgent surgical treatment of obstructive carcinoma of the left colon and rectum.

Methods: Seventy-five patients from the randomized trial were followed up. This study was designed as a stratified randomized trial with four stratums according to age and ASA score (older/younger than 60 years and ASA score <>3). Each of the four groups is then divided into two sub-groups according to the operating technique: loop colostomy or Hartmann's procedure.

Results: There were no difference found in hospitalization among the groups (loop colostomy vs. Hartmann's procedure) in the same stratus (P = 0.3192, P = 0.5760, P = 0.9023 respectively), except in the case of doing reconstructive procedure after loop colostomy (P = 0.0049) in the fourth stratum (patients younger than 60 years with ASA score lower than 3). Type of operation had no influence over the blood test values observed on admittance and during hospitalization (P = 0.319, P = 0.871, P = 0.7, P = 0.843, P = 0.52 respectively for the blood values). In terms of surgical and non-surgical complications it has been shown that there is no statistically significant difference between patients treated by two methods. Age, gender, ASA score, type of operation and surgical complications were not singled out as a risk factor for fatal outcome (P = 0.199, P = 0.155, P = 0.764, P = 0.452 and P = 0.724 respectively). The only factors that are singled out as a risk factor for death are the emergence of non-surgical complications and angina pectoris (P = 0.006, P = 0.001).

Conclusions: There is no difference in surgical treatment of large bowel obstruction caused by rectosigmoid carcinoma. Neither of those two methods showed significant advantage in treatment of large bowel obstruction caused by rectosigmoid cancer.

Keywords: Hartmann's procedure, Loop colostomy, Obstructive rectosigmoid cancer, ASA score

Introduction

Colorectal carcinoma is the most common malignant gastrointestinal tumour. Intestinal obstruction is an acute surgical condition. It is believed that about 60% of mechanical bowel obstruction is caused by colorectal tumours, 20% by diverticulosis and about 5% of intestinal obstruction is caused by a colonic volvulus. Despite the significant progress made in the field of screening, prevention and early diagnosis of colorectal cancer, it is known that 20% of patients with these tumours as the first symptom have signs of intestinal obstruction [1-4]. Intestinal obstruction leads towards impaired respiratory function due to reduced diaphragmatic excursions, while the intraluminal microbial proliferation increases the risk of infection [2,3]. Emergency surgery is therefore associated with significant morbidity and mortality in these conditions, which ends, in most cases, by creating a colostomy (temporary or permanent) [1,2,5,6].

There is still a considerable controversy when it comes to urgent surgical treatment of obstructive carcinoma of the left colon and rectum. To resolve this clinical entity there are several possibilities: loop colostomy and subsequent

* Correspondence: smnm@eunet.rs
[1]University of Belgrade, Belgrade, Serbia
[2]Clinic for Emergency Surgery, Emergency center, Clinical centre of Serbia, Belgrade, Serbia
Full list of author information is available at the end of the article

resection (in two or three stages), resection with end colostomy (Hartmann's procedure), and resection and primary anastomosis [7]. The focus of this paper will be on loop colostomy and Hartmann's procedure.

The Association of Coloproctology of Great Britain and Ireland have found that there are four important predictors of outcome: age, ASA score, the need for emergency surgery and Dukes classification [5]. In a poll conducted by the Society of American Gastrointestinal and Endoscopic Surgeons, 67% of surgeons opted for Hartmann's procedure in high-risk patients and 26% of them for loop colostomy [8]. Emergency surgery was identified as an independent risk factor of mortality after surgery, according to the French Association of Surgery investigation. Based on these few studies (only one of them was designed as randomized), there is a recommendation (Consensus conference of the World Society of Emergency Surgery (WSES) and peritoneum and surgery (PnS) society) that Hartmann's procedure should be preferred to loop colostomy (level B recommendation II) [9].

We aimed to evaluate both of these procedures and to show which one is more adequate in case of emergency surgery, using stratified randomized trial. Non-surgical complications and angina pectoris emerged as risk factors for poor outcome, while there was no difference in terms of surgical complications for both surgical procedures.

Material and methods

In this study, 75 patients with obstructive malignant lesion of rectosigmoid carcinoma were included and operated by five experienced surgeons. Patients who had a malignant peritoneal dissemination and patients who were unable to cooperate or who were in poor general health were excluded. Age, gender, hospital stay, surgical and non-surgical complications and blood transfusions (intraoperative and postoperative) were recorded. The aim of the study was to compare two emergency surgical procedures (Hartmann's procedure vs. loop colostomy) used in cases of acute mechanical obstruction caused by rectosigmoid cancer. This study was designed as a stratified randomized trial with four stratums (groups) according to age and ASA score (older/younger than 60 years and ASA score <>3). Each of the four groups is then divided into two sub-groups according to the operating technique: loop colostomy or Hartmann's procedure.

A loop colostomy is mostly performed for creation of a temporary stoma to divert stool away from an area of intestine that has been blocked due to cancer. This surgery brings a loop of bowel through an incision in the abdominal wall. The loop is held in place outside the abdomen by a plastic rod slipped beneath it. An incision is made in the bowel to allow the passage of stool through the loop colostomy. The supporting rod is removed approximately seven to ten days after surgery, when healing has occurred that will prevent the loop of bowel from retracting into the abdomen.

Hartmann's operation or Hartmann's procedure is the surgical resection of the rectosigmoid colon with closure of the rectal stump and formation of an end colostomy. During this procedure, the lesion is removed, the distal bowel closed intraperitoneally and the proximal bowel diverted with a stoma. High ligation of limfo vascular pedicle wasn't mandatory for surgeon due to possible significant bowel distension, although it was performed whenever possible.

Statistical analysis was performed with SPSS 18.0 program. Apart from descriptive statistic methods (mean, standard deviation), we used *t*-test and chi-squared test for quantitative comparisons. $P < 0.05$ was considered statistically significant.

The study was approved by Ethics Committee of the Clinical Center of Serbia, written informed consent was obtained from each human subject and the patients had been operated and postoperatively closely monitored in Emergency center of the Clinical centre of Serbia.

Results

Our study group consisted of 36 men and 39 women, while the mean age was 66.31 ± 12.50 (27 – 99) years. Mean duration of hospitalization in our study group was 10.92 ± 6.85 days (2–35 days). There were no difference found among the groups (loop colostomy vs. Hartmann's procedure) in the same stratus ($P = 0.3192$, $P = 0.5760$, $P = 0.9023$ respectively). The only significant statistic difference in hospitalization was found in the case of doing reconstructive procedure after loop colostomy ($P = 0.0049$) in the fourth stratum (patients younger than 60 years with ASA score lower than 3).

Type of operation had no influence over the blood test values observed on admittance and during hospitalization ($P = 0.319$, $P = 0.871$, $P = 0.7$, $P = 0.843$, $P = 0.52$ respectively for the blood values). In terms of surgical and non-surgical complications it has been shown that there is no statistically significant difference between patients treated by loop colostomy and Hartmann's procedure (Table 1). The amount of transfused blood was without any statistical difference in each of four stratums ($P = 0.689$, $P = 0.848$, $P = 0.495$ $P = 0.687$ respectively). In terms of intraoperative transfusion, we showed that there wasn't any statistical difference ($P = 0.303$, $P = 0.0557$, $P = 0.272$, $P = 0.7183$ respectively). The difference in overall mortality for patients operated by these two techniques was not statistically significant ($P = 0.45$).

Age, gender, ASA score, type of operation and surgical complications were not singled out as a risk factor for fatal outcome ($P = 0.199$, $P = 0.155$, $P = 0.764$, $P = 0.452$ and $P = 0.724$ respectively, Table 2). The only factors that are singled out as a risk factor for death are the emergence of non-surgical complications and angina pectoris

Table 1 Observed characteristics in the function of type of operation

Observed characteristics		Type of operation		
		Loop colostomy	Hartmann's procedure	
Age (X ± SD)		65.68 ± 14.828	66.93 ± 11.020	[b]p = 0.678
Gender	m	12 (42.90%)	23 (50.00%)	[a]p = 0.551
	f	16 (57.10%)	23 (50.00%)	
Randomization groups	> 60 god, ASA ≥ 3	12 (16.20%)	17 (23.00%)	[a]p = 0.265
	> 60 god, ASA < 3	4 (5.4%)	16 (21.60%)	
	< 60 god, ASA ≥ 3	3 (4.10%)	3 (4.10%)	
	< 60 god, ASA < 3	9 (12.20%)	10 (13.50%)	
Surgical complications	Yes	2 (2.7%)	2 (2.7%)	[a]p = 0.579
	No	25 (34.2%)	44 (60.3%)	
Nonsurgical complications	Yes	3 (4.1%)	9 (12.3%)	[a]p = 0.347
	No	24 (32.9%)	37 (50.7%)	

(P = 0.006, P = 0.001). Relative risk for fatal outcome is 1.49 for patients with non-surgical complications and 4 for patients with angina pectoris. Blood transfusion, chronic renal failure and diabetes mellitus have no impact on survival rate (P = 0.427, P = 0.285 and P = 0.81 respectively).

Using the Kaplan-Meier method, we have shown that statistically significant difference exists only between two randomization groups (Figure 1) in terms of intrahospital mortality: older than 60 years with ASA > 3 and younger than 60 years with ASA <3 (P = 0.001).

Discussion

Colorectal cancer is the third most common cancer in the United States, with similar incidence of both men and women. Also, it is the second cause of cancer deaths. Moreover, 53% of all colorectal cancers occur in sygmoid colon and rectum [10]. Recent studies showed that there is an increasing incidence of rectosigmoid and rectal cancer in patients younger than 40 years [11-13].

Colon cancer may be detected in patients with symptoms or may show as a result of screening programme. Despite great progress made in colorectal cancer [CRC} screening, at least 20% of CRC cases is diagnosed on surgical operation due to large bowel obstruction [1-4].

Table 2 Risk factors for fatal outcome

Observed risk factor	P value
Age	P = 0.199
Gender	P = 0.155
ASA score	P = 0.764
Type of operation	P = 0.452
Surgical complications	P = 0.724
Non-surgical complications	P = 0.006
Angina pectoris	P = 0.001

In our study we observed patients presented with large bowel obstruction due to rectosigmoid cancer with no previous data on CRC. Mean duration of hospitalization in our study was 10.92 ± 6.85 days. In the terms of hospitalization, we have showed that there was no significant difference among these groups, except in stratum 4. This difference can be explained by the fact that randomized patients in this group were younger than 60 years and their ASA score was lower than 3. In this stratum (young, healthy and working population) patients underwent reconstructive surgical intervention during the same hospitalization. These patients were operated in a shortest possible time interval because they are relatively young and working population. In this manner, we have tried to minimize recovery period after surgical interventions and to speed up return to work. Comparing Hartmann's procedure (63 patients) with loop colostomy (58 patients), Kronborg showed in his randomized trial that there was significant difference in hospital stay which was shorter in the group treated with Hartmann's procedure [14].

Type of operation had no statistical significant influence on blood test values during the hospitalization. In other words, both surgical procedures had similar blood loss and had no significant impact on the amount of transfused blood. In addition, the rate of surgical and nonsurgical complications showed no statistically significant difference between patients treated by these two techniques. Therefore it can be said that both surgical techniques (loop colostomy and Hartman's technique) are equally good and adequate methods of resolving intestinal obstruction.

In terms of mortality, there weren't any statistical significant difference among all groups, except in the case of older patients with ASA greater than 3. These data are in perfect match with study performed by Kronborg, which has been the only known randomized study so far

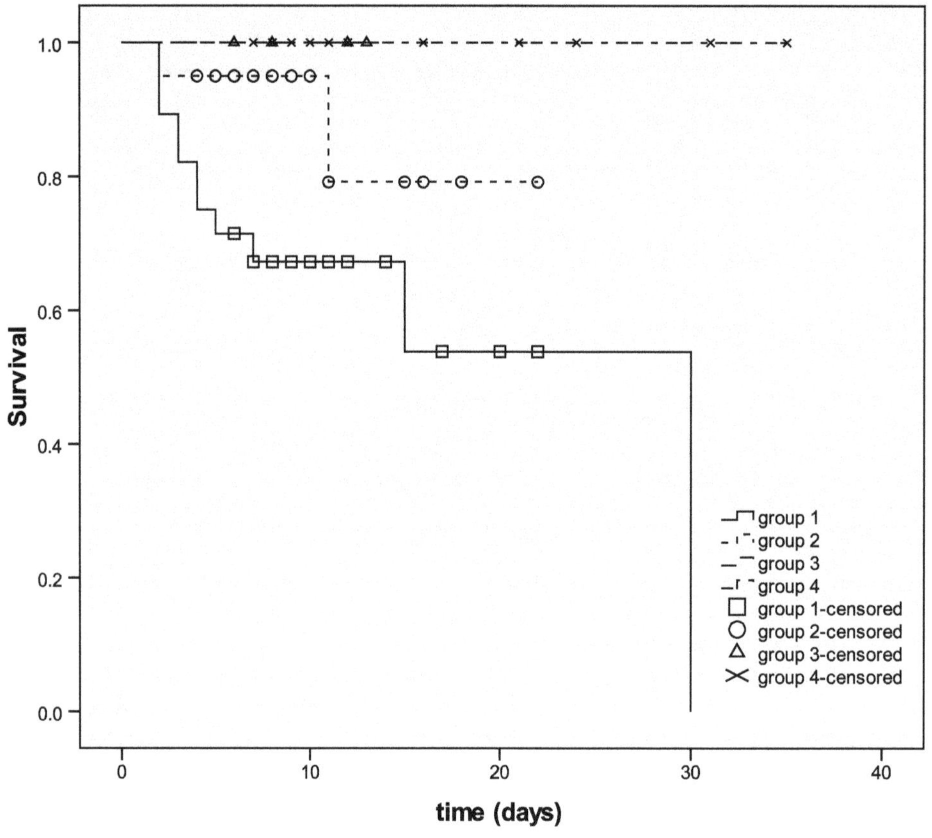

Legend

1. group - older than 60 years and with ASA score greater/equal than 3

2. group - older than 60 years and with ASA score lower than 3

3. group - younger than 60 years and with ASA score greater/equal than 3

4. group - younger than 60 years and with ASA score lower than 3

Figure 1 Intrahospital survival according to randomization groups.

with similar scientific focus. The data obtained in our paper are also in full compliance with Cochrane database review done by DeSalvo et al. [15].

Age, gender, ASA score, type of operation and surgical complications were not singled out as a risk factor for fatal outcome. Non-surgical complications and angina pectoris were the only risk factor for poor outcome. Non-surgical complications are thought primarily to complications from cardiovascular system, which are more common in case of elderly patients with higher values of ASA score.

Using Kaplan Meier analysis of intrahospital mortality, we showed that in only one case there was a highly statistically significant difference between the two randomization groups. It is a group of subjects older than 60 years with ASA score greater than 3 and a group of patients younger than 60 years with ASA score of less than 3. It was the first group where the rate of non-surgical complication was more common, as evidenced by the proven fact that these complications are predictors of poor outcome. Poor outcome is obviously associated with cardiovascular diseases and non-surgical complications.

The results of this study show that there is no difference in surgical treatment of large bowel obstruction caused by rectosigmoid carcinoma. Both methods, loop colostomy and Hartmann's procedure, had similar impact on mortality and hospitalization. Neither of those two methods showed significant advantage in treatment of large bowel obstruction caused by rectosigmoid cancer (mortality and morbidity). The blood loss is similar in both surgical procedures, according to the need for transfusion (intra and postoperative).

Colonic resection and primary anastomosis is a third surgical approach for resolving acute intestinal obstruction caused by rectosigmoid cancer. In the multicentric study by Kube et al. [16] conducted in Germany, 743 patients underwent emergency surgery for obstructive rectosigmoid carcinoma, performed as radical resection. Resection with primary anastomosis has been done in 57.9% cases, resection with anastomosis and protective stoma in 11.7% and Hartmann's procedure in 30.4% patients. In the last group patients were multimorbid, overweight and male. There was no statistical significant diference among those groups regarding morbidity and intrahospital mortality. Also, protective stoma didn't improve the rate of anastomotic leakage. The results of this study showed that Hartmann's procedure should be done in high-risk patients and advanced obstruction. Meyer [17] in his review concluded that Hartmann's procedure remains relevant in high-risk patients operated during the night and weekend, when the most experienced surgeons aren't always available. Furthermore, Jung et al. [18] showed that patients older than 75 years were more likely to undergo Hartmann's procedure even in the case of rectal tumors without colonic obstruction.

According to our findings, Hartmann's procedure is recommended only in older, high risk patients (high ASA score), with advanced and neglected rectosigmoid obstructive tumors and expressed proximal bowel distention. In our study group, 68% of patients were older than 60 years, and most of them presented with neglected rectosygmoid tumors, followed by bowel distention and endangered colon vitality. These patients, with numerous comorbidities, can not be subjected to primary anastomosis after resection, so they underwent Hartmann's procedure and, in addition, high ligation of limfo vascular pedicle.

In the group of patients treated with Hartmann's procedure, we had two patients with wound infection. In the group of patients treated with loop colostomy, two patients had also wound infection as surgical complications. There was no rectal stump dehiscence/leak and no abscess formation and wound dehiscence. As mentioned before, there is no significant difference regarding the rate of surgical complications. When it comes to the non-surgical complications, we showed that they occure more frequently, but again, there is no significant difference according to the type of operation. Myocardial decompensation was the most frequent (50%), followed by pneumonia (33%) and anxiety (17%). Emergence of non-surgical complications singled out as one of the risk factors for poor outcome.

According to recent research, a combination of endoscopy and laparoscopy is an appropriate therapeutic strategy. Placing a preoperative self-expanding metallic stents (SEMS) allows bowel movements and subsequent laparoscopic surgery. Preoperative self-expanding metallic stents insertion does not adversely affect oncological outcomes and patient survival [19]. This approach guarantees a minimum invasiveness, without compromising the effectiveness of treatment. Watt et al. [20] compared the rate of complications after SEMS insertion and emergency surgery for obstructive left colon cancer, while Zhang et al. [21] analyzed 6 retrospective studies and 2 randomized controlled trials (meta analysis) concerning combined endoscopic and surgical approach versus surgery alone. According to their results, there was no statistical significance for permanent rate of colostomy and postoperative mortality (30 days follow-up), although they were lower in SEMS group. Zhao et al. [22] in their report analyzed five randomized controlled trials concerning semielective surgery after SEMS and emergency surgery. They showed that SEMS insertion followed by semielective surgery for obstructive rectosigmoid carcinoma compared to emergency surgery had decreased the rate of postoperative complications, surgical site infections (SSI) and had enhanced the rate of primary anastomosis, which had decreased the rate of colostomy. They didn't detect any statistical significance considering rate of anastomotic leak, primary anastomotic rate and 30 days postoperative mortality.

According to these researches, it can be concluded that SEMS insertion is very promising method that facilitates surgery and provides better oncologic results. However, Liu et al. [23] did the meta-analysis of complications of colonic stenting versus emergency surgery for acute left-sided malignant colonic obstruction. They analyzed Medline, Embase and the Cochrane library in order to evaluate the complications of these procedures. There was no significant difference in hospital death and complications between those two approaches. Unfortunately, this method is still unavailable in our country due to the unfavorable economic situation, but we would like to compare this modern method to older ones.

Conclusion

It can be concluded that Hartmann's procedure (with additional high ligation of limfo vascular pedicle) is better suited to older people because in this manner the tumour is removed, which is quite good if patient can't be ready for next reconstructive operation in a shorter period of time. Loop colostomy could be advised for younger, healthy patients that can be ready for immediate definitive surgery (tumor removal) in a shortest possible period, i.e. two or three weeks. In this case, surgeon on the second operation has better comfort and less bowel inflation facilitates better oncological approach (mandatory high ligation of limfo vascular pedicle) which eventually would very likely improve surgical and oncological results.

Abbreviations

ASA: American Society of Anaestesiologists; CRC: Colorectal cancer; SEMS: Self expanding metallic stents; SSI: Surgical site of infection; GDP: Gross domestic product.

Competing interests

The authors declare that they have no competing interests.

Authors' contributions

SK as lead investigator made substantial contributions to conception and design; VR also made contribution to conception and design of the study, along with collection of data. TA and AR performed the statistical analysis, AS made contribution to the study design. ZL and VD participated in reviewing the manuscript. AK given final approval for publishing of this version. All authors read and approved the final manuscript.

Author details

[1]University of Belgrade, Belgrade, Serbia. [2]Clinic for Emergency Surgery, Emergency center, Clinical centre of Serbia, Belgrade, Serbia. [3]Clinic for Gastroenterology, Clinical Center of Serbia, Belgrade, Serbia. [4]Surgery Department, Medical Center "Bezanijska kosa", Belgrade, Serbia.

References

1. Lee YM, Law WL, Chu KW, Poon RT: **Emergency surgery for obstructing colorectal cancers: a comparison between right-sided and left-sided lesions.** *J Am Coll Surg* 2001, **192:**719–725.
2. Mantion G, Panis Y: *Mortalité et morbidité en chirurgie colo-rectale*. Paris: Rapport de l'Association francaise de chirurgie; 2003:4–28. Arnette éd.
3. Rault A, Collet D, Sa Cunha A, Larroude D, Ndobo'epoy F, Masson B: **Surgical management of obstructed colonic cancer.** *Ann Chir* 2005, **130:**331–335.
4. Umpleby HC, Williamson RCN: **Survival in acute obstructing colorectal carcinoma.** *Dis Colon Rectum* 1984, **27:**299–304.
5. Tekkis PP, Kinsman R, Thompson MR, Stamatakis JD: **The Association of Coloproctology of Great Britain and Ireland study of large bowel obstruction caused by colorectal cancer.** *Ann Surg* 2004, **204:**76–81.
6. Meyer F, Marusch F, Coch A, Meyer L, Fuhrer S, Köckerling F, Lippert H, Gastinger I: **Emergency operation in carcinomas of the left colon: value of Hartmann's procedure.** *Tech Coloproctol* 2004, **8**(Suppl 1):226–229.
7. Villar JM, Martinez AP, Villegas MT, Muffak K, Mansilla A, Garrote D, Ferron JA: **Surgical options for malignant left-sided colonic obstruction.** *Surg Today* 2005, **35:**275–281.
8. Goyal A, Schein M: **Current practices in left-sided colonic emergencies. A survey of US gastrointestinal surgeons.** *Dig Surg* 2001, **18:**399–402.
9. Ansaloni L, Andersson RE, Bazzoli F, Catena F, Cennamo V, Di Saverio S, Fuccio L, Jeekel H, Leppäniemi A, Moore E, Pinna AD, Pisano M, Repici A, Sugarbaker PH, Tuech JJ: **Guidelines in the management of obstructing cancer of the left colon: Consensus conference of the world society of emergency surgery (WSES) and peritoneum and surgery (PnS) society.** *World J Emerg Surg* 2010, **5:**29. doi:10.1186/1749-7922-5-29.
10. American Cancer Society: *Facts and Figures*. Atlanta, Georgia: American Cancer Society; 2006.
11. Meyer JE, Narang T, Schnoll-Sussman FH, Pochapin MB, Christos PJ, Sherr DL: **Increasing incidence of rectal cancer in patients aged younger than 40 years.** *Cancer* 2010, **116:**4354–4359.
12. Pignone M, Rich M, Teutch SM, Berg AO, Lohr KN: **Screening for colorectal cancer in adults at average risk: a summary of the evidence for the U.S. Preventive Services Task Force.** *Ann Intern Med* 2002, **137:**132–141.
13. O'Connell JB, Maggard M, Liu J, Etzioni DA, Livingston EH, Ko CY: **Rates of colon and rectal cancer are increasing in young adults.** *Am Surg* 2003, **69:**866–872.
14. Kronborg O: **Acute obstruction from tumour in the left colon without spread. A randomised trial of emergency colostomy versus resection.** *Int J Colorectal Dis* 1995, **10:**1–5.
15. De Salvo GL, Gava C, Lise M, Pucciarelli S: **Curative surgery for obstruction from primary left colorectal carcinoma: Primary or staged resection?** *Cochrane Database Syst Rev* 2004, **2:**CD002101.
16. Kube R, Granowski D, Stübs P, Mroczkowski P, Ptok H, Schmidt U, Gastinger I, Lippert H, Study group Qualitätssicherung Kolon/Rektum-Karzinome: **Surgical practices for malignant left colonic obstruction in Germany.** *Eur J Surg Oncol* 2010, **36**(1):65–71. doi:10.1016/j.ejso.2009.08.005.
17. Meyer F, Grundmann RT: **Hartmann's procedure for perforated diverticulitis and malignant left-sided colorectal obstruction and perforation.** *Zentralbl Chir* 2011, **136**(1):25–33. doi:10.1055/s-0030-1262753.
18. Jung B, Påhlman L, Johansson R, Nilsson E: **Rectal cancer treatment and outcome in the elderly: an audit based on the Swedish Rectal Cancer Registry 1995-2004.** *BMC Cancer* 2009, **26**(9):68. doi:10.1186/1471-2407-9-68.
19. Tung KL, Cheung HY, Ng LW, Chung CC, Li MK: **Endo-laparoscopic approach versus conventional open surgery in the treatment of obstructing left-sided colon cancer: long-term follow-up of a randomized trial.** *Asian J Endosc Surg* 2013, **6**(2):78–81.
20. Watt AM, Faragher IG, Griffin TT, Rieger NA, Maddern GJ: **Self-expanding metallic stents for relieving malignant colorectal obstruction: a systematic review.** *Ann Surg* 2007, **246**(1):24–30.
21. Zhang Y, Shi J, Shi B, Song CY, Xie WF, Chen YX: **Self-expanding metallic stent as a bridge to surgery versus emergency surgery for obstructive colorectal cancer: a metaanalysis.** *Surg Endosc* 2012, **26**(1):110–119.
22. Zhao X, Liu B, Zhao E, Wang J, Cai M, Xia Z, Xia Q, Shuai X, Tao K, Wang G, Cai K: **The safety and efficiency of surgery with colonic stents in left-sided malignant colonic obstruction: a meta-analysis.** *Gastroenterol Res Pract* 2014, doi:10.1155/2014/407325.
23. Liu Z, Kang L, Li C, Huang M, Zhang X, Wang J: **Meta-analysis of complications of colonic stenting versus emergency surgery for acute left-sided malignant colonic obstruction.** *Surg Laparosc Endosc Percutan Tech* 2014, **24**(1):73–79. doi:10.1097/SLE.0000000000000030.

13

Spontaneous perforation of jejunal gastrintestinal stromal tumour (gist)

Somsubhra Datta Roy[1], Dawood Khan[1], Krishna K De[1] and Utpal De[1,2*]

Abstract

GIST is the commonest mesenchymal tumour of the gastrointestinal tract. Jejunal GIST is rare and spontaneous perforation of asymptomatic jejunal GIST is unique. A review of the English literature reveals only fifteen cases of perforated GIST till date. Pre-operative diagnosis is difficult. Diagnosis is confirmed on histopathology and immunohistochemistry. Complete removal with postoperative imatinib therapy entails optimal treatment. Perforated GIST is associated with high recurrence.

Keywords: Jejunum, GIST, Perforative peritonitis

Background

Gastro-intestinal stromal tumour (GIST) is most common mesenchymal tumour of gastrointestinal tract (G.I) tract (80%) [1]. The incidence of GIST is 10–20 million people per year with a malignant potential of 20-30% [1,2]. Presentations include abdominal mass (5-50%), obstruction (5%), haemorrhage and rarely perforation (0.8%) [1,2]. Spontaneous perforation of jejunal GIST is rare (Table 1) and unique. This article is an illustration of a similar case.

Case presentation

Forty six year old male presented to the emergency department with pain epigastrium, constipation, nausea, vomiting, fever and abdominal distension since two days. He had a past history of acid peptic disorder for which he was treated conservatively. On physical examination, patient was conscious and of normal built. Pallor, cyanosis, icterus and edema were absent. He was normotensive (124/70 mmHg), had tachycardia (110/min), fever (102.4°F) and hurried respiration (25/min). Abdominal examination revealed distension, board like rigidity, marked rebound tenderness, absent liver dullness and inaudible bowel sounds. Hernia sites were normal. Per-rectal examination did not reveal any significant abnormality. Examinations of other systems were within normal limits. A provisional diagnosis of peptic perforation was made.

Exploratory laparotomy was planned. Hematological examination revealed mild anemic with neutophilic leucocytosis [Hemoglobin – 9.8 g/dl, Total count-14,000/cu.mm (N85, L11, E10, B0, M0)]. Blood sugar (113 g/dl), liver function tests and serum electrolytes (Na-136 meq/lit, K- 4.2 meq/lit) were within normal limits. Viral markers were non-reactive. Abdominal roentgenogram showed free gas under both domes of diaphragm with diffuse ground glass opacity. Excessive gas in the abdomen with free fluid was noted in abdominal sonography.

The patient was resuscitated with intravenous fluids, ryles tube and antibiotics. Following adequate resuscitation, the patient was put up for operation. Midline laparotomy revealed purulent free fluid with flakes. On aspiration and removal of the flakes and fluid, a purplish coloured firm growth with everted margins, measuring 3×2 cm was found in the anti-mesenteric border of the jejunum, fifty cm from the duodeno-jejunal flexure. The growth had a central perforation with intestinal contents effusing through the rent (Figure 1). All other organs were normal. The growth was resected with five cm margin and an end to end, single layer, interrupted, anastomosis was performed using 2′0′ polyglycolic

* Correspondence: utpalde@vsnl.net
[1]Department of surgery, Medical College Hospital, 88, College Street, Kolkata 73, India
[2]Dankuni Housing Complex, L-4/9, Ph 3, Dankuni, Hooghly 713211, India

Table 1 Table showing published case reports on jejunal perforation

Serial number	Country	Journal	Patient paticulars	Date of publication
1	Greece	Journal of gastro-intetinal and liver diseases	66 yrs/ M	2006
2 *	China	Journal of Chinese oncology	69 yrs/ M	2008
3	Ankara	Turkish journal of gastroenterology	70 yrs/ M	2008
4	Turkey	Gastroenterology research	52 yrs / F	2009
5	Japan	Journal of abdominal emergency medicine	56 yrs/ M	2009
6 *	China	International journal of gastroentrology	69 yrs/ M	2009
7	Greece	World journal of surgical oncology	28 yrs/ F	2010
8	Istanbul	Turkish journal of gastroenterology	65 yrs/ M	2010
9	India	International journal of biomedical research	68 yrs / M	2010
10	India	Bombay hospital journal	55 yrs/ M	2011
11	China	Turkish journal of gastroenterology	45 yrs/ M	2011
12	Greece	journal of current surgery	56 yrs/ M	2011
13	Turkey	Journal of clinical and analytical medicne	61 yrs/ F	2012
14	India	The internet journal of surgery	35 yrs/ M	2012
15	India	Indian journal of surgery	22 yrs/ M	2012

* same case report published in different journal.

suture. Thorough peritoneal lavage was done with warm normal saline and abdomen was closed in layers. A tube drain was placed in the hepatorenal pouch of Morrison. The specimen was sent for histopathological examination.

Post operative period was uneventful and the patient was discharged on the tenth post-op day after stitch removal.

Histopathology (Figure 2) of the resected specimen showed, a submucosal nodular tumour composed of interlacing fascicles of spindle shaped cells with elongated, plump nuclei. There was mild nuclear pleomorphism and more than five mitotic figures per fifty high power fields.

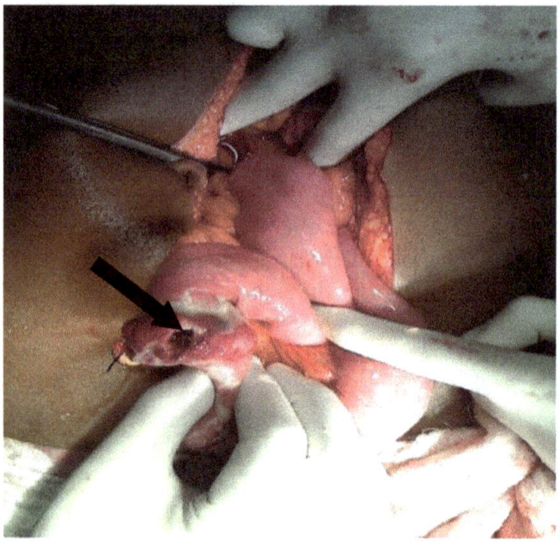

Figure 1 Peroperative photograph showing jejunal gist with perforation.

No tumour necrosis found. Pathologically it was jejunal GIST of intermediate risk. Surgical lines of resection were free. Immuno-histochemistry study revealed diffuse immunoreactivity for CD-117 (Figure 3), focal CD-34 positivity, negative for desmin, S-100 and SMA;Ki 67 less than 5%.

The patient is on six months follow-up receiving oral imatinib 300 mg twice a day.

Conclusion

GIST was first described by Mazor and Clark (1983) [1]. It originates from the interstitial cells of Cajal (ICC), located in the muscularis propria (myenteric plexus) responsible for triggering smooth muscle contraction [2,3]. The

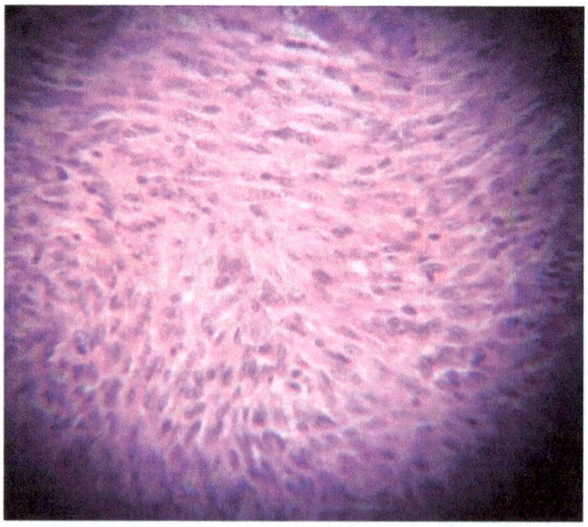

Figure 2 Histopathology of jejunal GIST.

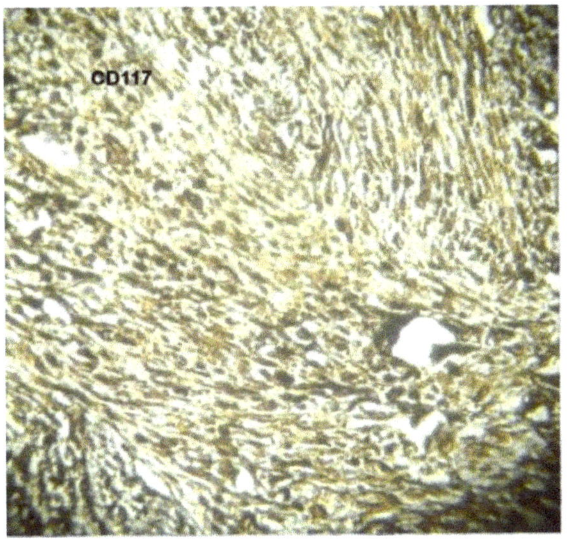

Figure 3 Immunohistochemistry for CD117 positivity.

basic pathology is an activating mutation (gain in function) of chromosome 4 which codes for c-Kit resulting in uncontrolled proliferation of stem cells that differentiate towards ICC. GIST is sporadic [3]. Familial forms with autosomal dominant inheritance have also been documented [3,4].

Isolated reports of GIST occurring concomitantly with paraganglioma, pulmonary chondroma, nerofibromatosis, pancreatic neuro-endocrine tumours, burkitt's lymphoma, osteosarcoma, neuroblastoma and melanoma have been documented [4].

90% of GIST occurs in adults more than 40 years of age (median age 63 years). There is slight male preponderance [4]. No documented elements indicating any association with geographic location, ethnicity, race or occupation has been elucidated [4,5].

The commonest site of GIST is stomach (60-70%) [2,3]. Jejunum accounts for 10% of all GI tract GIST's [1,3]. Sporadic reports of GISTs arising from the omentum, mesentery or retroperitoneum, have been documented but most of these are metastatic from gastric or intestinal primaries [4]. Extra-GIST has been reported in gall bladder, pancreas, liver and urinary bladder [4].

Presentation is erratic. Seventy percent are symptomatic at presentation, 20% are asymptomatic and 10% are detected at autopsy [5,6]. Common presentations include abdominal pain, palpable mass, gastro intestinal bleeding, fever, anorexia, weight loss and anaemia [7]. Isolated jejunal GIST associated with perforation and peritonitis is a rare and unique [1].

Perforation is usually attributed to replacement of bowel wall by tumour cells, tumour embolization leading to ischemia, necrosis together with raised intra-luminal pressure [4,5,7]. In view of the exophytic nature of the growth, intestinal obstruction occurs due to compression rather than luminal obstruction. As such intetstinal obstruction is a rare occurrence until the tumour attains enormous size.

Clinical diagnosis of GIST is based on index of suspicion [6,7]. Specific diagnostic signs and symptoms are absent. Chronicity is a rule. Acute atypical presentation includes hemorrhage and perforative peritonitis [1-10]. Preoperative imaging modalities like contrast enhanced abdominal computerized tomography (CT) aids in diagnosis [8]. The extent of the tumor, metastases and involvement of other organs can be assessed. A dedicated magnetic resonance imaging (MRI) provides better information than CT in the preoperative staging workup [7,8]. Endoscopy can diagnose gastric GISTs. Endoscopy demonstrates smooth, mucosa-lined protrusion of the bowel wall which may or may not show signs of bleeding or ulceration. Endoscopic ultrasound with guided fine-needle aspiration is diagnostic for primary lesions in 89% of the cases [8-10]. However, the relative usefulness of images depends on the site, duration and suspicion of GIST in patients presenting with undiagnosed abdominal lumps. The decisive diagnosis rests on the pathological and immunohistological tests [2,5-10]. Histopathologically GISTs are composed of spindle (70%), epithelioid and round cell or an admixture [6,8]. Similarities with histological picture of gastrointestinal leiomyosarcoma, leiomyoblastoma and poorly differentiated carcinomas may cause diagnostic dielemma, Immuno-histochemical assays for CD117 antigen (KIT) is the mainstay for diagnosis [9,10].

Diagnosis of asymptomatic GIST with acute presentation like perforation remains elusive. Accordingly, our provisional diagnosis was peptic perforation as free gas under diaphragm was noted in erect abdominal rhoentgenogram.

Optimal surgical treatment of GIST entails complete removal of the tumor with clear surgical margins including the adjacent involved organs [5-10]. Complete surgical resection entails 48-65% five-year survival [1]. Perforation of the tumor lowers the five-year survival to 24%, probably due to peritoneal dissemination [5]. Local and regional lymph node involvement is infrequent in GIST [6,8,10]. GIST's presenting with perforation, attention needs to be paid, in view of possible recurrence of the tumor. Abundant peritoneal lavage should be performed with distilled water to reduce the risk of peritoneal tumour spillage. Distilled water is used because of its cytolytic activity on suspended cells [7,9,10].

GIST response to conventional chemotherapy is very poor (<10%), while radiotherapy is only used in cases of intraperitoneal hemorrhage, when the precise location of the tumor is known, or for analgesic purposes [7,8].

STI571 (imatinib), acts as a powerful selective inhibitor of tyrosine-kinase, PDGFR (platelet derived growth factor receptor) and c-kit receptor [10]. Oral imatinib at doses >300 mg per day achieves curative results.

The prognostic factors of GIST include age at presentation, anatomic location, size (most important), histomorphology, immuno-histochemistry and molecular genetics [4,6-10].

Positron-emission tomography with 18F-fluoro-2-deoxy-D-glucose is a very useful tool for the postoperative follow-up of patients receiving imatinib [4,5,9,10].

The 5-year survival rate is 35%. It increases to 54% after complete surgical excision [1-10]. However 40% will recur within 18 – 24 months. Once recurrence has occurred median survival is 9–16 months [3,5,7,8,10].

Consent

"Written informed consent was obtained from the patient for publication of this Case report and any accompanying images. A copy of the written consent is available for review by the Editor-in-Chief of this journal".

Competing interests

The authors declare that they have no competing interests.

Authors' contributions

UD participated in the conception, design of the study, sequence alignment and drafted the manuscript. SD carried out the immunohistochemical studies. DK participated in the clinical and surgical management. KKD helped to draft the manuscript. All authors read and approved the final manuscript.

References

1. Efremidou EI, Liratzopoulos N, Papageorgiou MS, Romanidis K: **Perforated GIST of the small intestine as a rare cause of acute abdomen: surgical treatment and adjuvant therapy. Case report.** *J Gastrointestin Liver Dis* 2006, **15**:297–299.
2. Oida Y, Motojuku M, Morikawa G, Mukai M, Shimizu K, Imaizumi T, Makuuchi H: **Laparoscopic-assisted resection of gastrointestinal stromal tumor in small intestine.** *Hepatogastroenterology* 2008, **55**:146–149.
3. Miettinen M, Sobin LH, Lasota J: **Gastrointestinal stromal tumors presenting as omental masses–a clinicopathologic analysis of 95 cases.** *Am J Surg Pathol* 2009, **33**:1267–1275.
4. Sornmayura P: **Gastrointestinal stromal tumors (GISTs): a pathology view point.** *J Med Assoc Thai* 2009, **92**:124–135.
5. Steigen SE, Bjerkehagen B, Haugland HK, Nordrum IS, Løberg EM, Isaksen V, Eide TJ, Nielsen TO: **Diagnostic and prognostic markers for gastrointestinal stromal tumors in Norway.** *Mod Pathol* 2008, **21**:46–53.
6. Wilson SL, Wheeler WE: **Giant leiomyoma of the small intestine with free perforation into the peritoneal cavity.** *South Med J* 1992, **85**:667–668.
7. Shah SN: **Malignant gastrointestinal stromal tumor of intestine: a case report.** *Indian J Pathol Microbiol* 2007, **50**:357–359.
8. Huang CC, Yang CY, Lai IR, Chen CN, Lee PH, Lin MT: **Gastrointestinal stromal tumor of the small intestine: a clinicopathologic study of 70 cases in the postimatinib era.** *World J Surg* 2009, **33**:828–834.
9. Kingham TP, DeMatteo RP: **Multidisciplinary treatment of gastrointestinal stromal tumors.** *Surg Clin North Am* 2009, **89**:217–233.
10. Annaberdyev S, Gibbons J, Hardacre JM: **Dramatic response of a gastrointestinal stromal tumor to neoadjuvant imatinib therapy.** *World J Surg Oncol* 2009, **7**:30.

14

Typhoid intestinal perforations at a University teaching hospital in Northwestern Tanzania: A surgical experience of 104 cases in a resource-limited setting

Phillipo L Chalya[1*], Joseph B Mabula[1†], Mheta Koy[2†], Johannes B Kataraihya[2†], Hyasinta Jaka[2†], Stephen E Mshana[3†], Mariam Mirambo[3†], Mabula D Mchembe[4†], Geofrey Giiti[1†] and Japhet M Gilyoma[1†]

Abstract

Background: Typhoid intestinal perforation is still prevalent in many developing countries. Despite the advances in the management, the outcome in these patients in resource limited countries is still very poor. This study was to review our experiences on the surgical management of typhoid intestinal perforation and to determine the prognostic factors for mortality in our local setting.

Methods: This was a combined retrospective and prospective study of patients who were operated for typhoid intestinal perforation at Bugando Medical Centre between August 2006 and September 2011. Data collected were analyzed using SPSS computer software version 15.

Results: A total of 104 patients were studied representing 8.7% of typhoid fever cases. Males were affected twice more than the females (2.6:1). Their ages ranged from 8 to 76 years with a median age of 18.5 years. The peak age incidence was in the 11-20 years age group. Fever and abdominal pain were the most common presenting symptoms and majority of the patients (80.8%) perforated between within 14 days of illness. Chest and abdominal radiographs revealed pneumoperitonium in 74.7% of cases. Ultrasound showed free peritoneal collection in 85.7% of cases. Nine (10.2%) patients were HIV positive with a median CD4+ count of 261 cells/μl. The perforation-surgery interval was more than 72 hours in 90(86.5%) patients. The majority of patients (84.6%) had single perforations and ileum was the most common part of the bowel affected occurring in 86.2% of cases. Simple closure of the perforations was the most commonly performed procedure accounting for 78.8% of cases. Postoperative complication rate was 39.4% and surgical site infection was the most frequent complication in 55.5% of cases. Mortality rate was 23.1% and it was statistically significantly associated with delayed presentation, inadequate antibiotic treatment prior to admission, shock on admission, HIV positivity, low CD4 count (< 200 cells/μl), high ASA classes (III-V), delayed operation, multiple perforations, severe peritoneal contamination and presence of postoperative complications ($P < 0.001$). The median overall length of hospital stay was 28 days.

Conclusion: Typhoid intestinal perforation is still endemic in our setting and carries high morbidity and mortality. This study has attempted to determine the factors that statistically influence mortality in typhoid perforation in our environment. Appropriate measures focusing at these factors are vital in order to deliver optimal care for these patients in this region.

Keywords: Typhoid fever, Intestinal perforation, Surgical management, Prognostic factors, Tanzania

* Correspondence: drphillipoleo@yahoo.com
† Contributed equally
[1]Department of Surgery, Catholic University of Health and Allied Sciences-Bugando, Mwanza, Tanzania
Full list of author information is available at the end of the article

Background

Typhoid fever, a severe febrile illness caused primarily by a gram negative bacillus *Salmonella typhi*, has continued to be a public health problem in many developing countries [1,2]. Typhoid infection is generally transmitted by faeco-oral route and may occasionally lead to an epidemic, particularly in areas with poor sanitation and limited availability of clean, potable water [1-4]. It is a global health problem that can have a devastating impact on resource-poor countries like Tanzania and it is estimated that more than 33 million cases of typhoid fever occur annually causing more than 500,000 deaths [2,5,6]. While control of the infection has been achieved in developed countries by effective public health measures, developing countries continue to bear the burden of the disease, principally because many communities still fall short of standards for drinking water, hygiene and sanitation [2,7,8].

The surgical complications of typhoid fever are a cause of significant morbidity and mortality in many parts of Africa, particularly in sub-Saharan Africa where standard medical facilities are not yet readily available [4,6]. Intestinal perforation is a serious complication of typhoid fever and remains a significant surgical problem in developing countries, where it is associated with high mortality and morbidity, due to lack of clean drinking water, poor sanitation and lack of medical facilities in remote areas and delay in hospitalization [9]. The rates of perforation have been reported in literature to vary between 0.8% and 18% [10-13]. The high incidence of perforation in most developing countries has been attributed to late diagnosis and the emergence of multi-drug resistant and virulent strains of *Salmonella typhi* [14]. The disease affects mostly young adults who contribute enormously to the economy of third world countries [14-16]. It also affects children and it is most common in people in the low socio-economic strata [15].

The management of typhoid intestinal perforation poses diagnostic and therapeutic challenges to general surgeons practicing in resource-limited countries [6,15]. Surgery is considered the treatment of choice in order to improve the chances of survival of patients with this condition, who most often present late [17]. The management of these patients provides a number of unique challenges to the attending surgeon. Many of these patients present at and are managed in rural hospitals where resources are often very limited. The outcome of treatment of typhoid intestinal perforation may be poor especially in developing countries where late presentation of the disease coupled with lack of clean drinking water, poor sanitation, lack of diagnostic facilities and emergence of Multi-drug resistant (MDR) strains of *S. typhi* resulting from inappropriate and indiscriminate use of antibiotics are among the hallmarks of the disease [6,18]. Late presentation, inadequate preoperative resuscitation, delayed operation, number of perforations and the extent of fecal peritonitis have been found to have a significant effect on prognosis [19,20].

While mortality in the developed world has dropped to between 0% and 2% [21,22], mortality in the developing world remains high at between 9% and 22% [14,15,23]. The reasons for this state of affairs have not been evaluated in our setting. Despite the high mortality and morbidity of typhoid intestinal perforation in developing world like Tanzania, relatively a little is known about the pattern of this disease and its prognostic factors in our set up. The purpose of this study was to describe our experiences on the surgical management of typhoid intestinal perforation outlining the clinical profile and treatment outcome of this disease and to determine the prognostic factors for morbidity and mortality in our local setting. It is hoped that identification of these factors will help in policy decision making, prioritizing management and improving the quality of care in typhoid intestinal perforation.

Methods

This was a combined retrospective and prospective study of patients who were operated for typhoid intestinal perforation at Bugando Medical Centre between October 2006 and September 2011. Bugando Medical Centre (BMC) is a consultant, tertiary care and teaching hospital for the Catholic University of Health and Allied Sciences -Bugando (CUHAS-Bugando) with a bed capacity of 1000.

All patients who were operated for typhoid intestinal perforation during the study period were included in the study. Patients with incomplete data and those who failed to consent for HIV infection were excluded from the study. The details of patients who presented from October 2006 to September 2008 were retrieved retrospectively from patient registers kept in the Medical record departments, the surgical wards, and operating theatre. Patients who presented to the A & E department between October 2008 and September 2011 were prospectively enrolled in the study after signing an informed written consent for the study. The diagnosis of typhoid perforation was established by clinical features of typhoid fever and peritonitis which were supported by positive Widal test, detection of free air under the diaphragm on chest and abdominal radiographs and free intra peritoneal fluid on ultrasound abdomen and confirmed by intraoperative findings of oval perforation on the antimesenteric border of the intestine and an acutely inflamed and edematous intestine. Peritonitis was recorded as general when the whole abdomen was involved; it was recorded as local when peritonitis was limited to the lower abdomen. The patients who developed clinical features of peritonitis after typhoid fever and presented within 24 hours were labeled as *early* while those presented after 24 hours were marked as *late* cases. Inadequate prehospital therapy was defined as not being given a minimum of 3 days of effective antibiotic treatment for *S. Typhi* at the correct dose prior to admission. The time of typhoid intestinal perforation was subjectively determined as the time the patient felt an excruciating sharp pain with worsening of symptoms. In small children it was taken as the time the mother noticed abdominal distention, constipation and vomiting.

Preoperatively, all the patients had intravenous fluids to correct fluid and electrolyte deficits; nasogastric suction; urethral catheterization and broad-spectrum antibiotic coverage. Relevant preoperative investigations included packed cell volume, serum electrolytes, urea and creatinine, HIV testing (using Tanzania HIV Rapid Test Algorithm) and CD 4+ count (using FACS or FACSCALIBUR from BD Biosciences USA), Widal's test; chest and abdominal radiographs to detect air under the diaphragm. Abdominal ultrasound was also performed in some patients suspected to have abdominal collections. They had pre-operative anaesthetic assessment using the American Society of Anesthetists (ASA) classification [24] as shown in Table 1. To minimize variability in our study, the assignation of ASA class was performed by one consultant anesthetist adhering strictly to criteria above. After resuscitation all patients under general anaesthesia were subjected to exploratory laparotomy. Adequate hydration was indicated by an hourly urine output of 30 ml/hour. An initial systolic blood pressure (SBP) on each patient was also recorded on admission. Preoperative shock was defined as a preoperative systolic blood pressure of less than 90 mmHg.

Laparotomy was performed by a midline incision; all dirty yellow purulent material was aspirated from peritoneal cavity. General survey of peritoneal cavity was made. In patients with single perforation, the edge of the intestinal perforation was excised, and double-layer closure was done with chromic catgut or coated vicryl 2/0 and silk 2/0. Patients with multiple perforations had bowel resection and anastomosis. Ileostomy and damage control surgery was done in patients with ASA class VE. Copious peritoneal lavage was done with warm isotonic saline, 2 drains were placed, one in the pelvis, the other in the right paracolic gutter, and mass closure of the abdomen was done using nylon-1. The skin was closed with interrupted stitches of nylon-2/0. Post-operatively patients were kept nil orally till return of bowl sounds and at that time nasogastric tubes were removed. IV antibiotics were used for one week. Drains were removed on 6th post operative day. The postoperative outcome was monitored; patients in ASA classes IV and V were admitted into intensive care unit after surgery. Data on each patient were entered into a pro forma prepared for the study. The study variables included socio-demographic data (i.e. age and sex, level of education, occupation and area of residence), clinical presentation, HIV status, radiological findings, perforation-surgery interval, ASA classification, operative findings (such as type of peritonitis, degree of contamination and number of perforations), antibiotics used and surgical procedure performed. The variables studied in the postoperative period were postoperative complications, hospital stay and mortality.

Table 1 American Society of Anesthetists (ASA) classification

ASA class	Description
I	Healthy individual with no systemic disease
II	Mild systemic disease not limiting activity
III	Severe systemic disease that limits activity but is not incapacitating
IV	Incapacitating systemic disease which is constantly life threatening
V	Moribund, not expected to survive 24 hours with or without operation

Note: E is added to the class when the case is an emergency e.g. IIE refers to ASA class scheduled for emergency surgery

Statistical analysis

The statistical analysis was performed using statistical package for social sciences (SPSS) version 15.0 for Windows (SPSS, Chicago IL, U.S.A).The mean ± standard deviation (SD), median and ranges were calculated for continuous variables whereas proportions and frequency tables were used to summarize categorical variables. Continuous variables were categorized. Chi-square (χ^2) test were used to test for the significance of association between the independent (predictor) and dependent (outcome) variables in the categorical variables. The level of significance was considered as $P < 0.05$. Multivariate logistic regression analysis was used to determine predictor variables that predict the outcome.

Ethical consideration

Ethical approval to conduct the study was obtained from the CUHAS-Bugando/BMC joint institutional ethic review committee before the commencement of the study. Patients recruited prospectively were required to sign a written informed consent for the study and for HIV testing.

Results

Out of 1213 patients who presented to our centre with typhoid fever during the study period, 123 patients underwent emergency laparotomy for typhoid intestinal perforations. Of these, 19 patients were excluded from the study due to failure to meet the inclusion criteria and incomplete data. Thus, 104 patients were studied giving an average of 10 cases annually and represented 8.5% of cases. Of these, 21 (20.2%) patients were studied retrospectively and the remaining 83(79.8%) patients were studied prospectively.

Socio-demographic characteristics

Seventy- five (72.1%) patients were males and females were 29 (27.9%) with the male to female ratio of 2.6:1. Their ages ranged from 8 to 76 years with a median age of 18.5 years. The peak age incidence was in the 11-20 years age group accounting for 47.1% of cases (Table 2). Figure 1 shows distribution of age group by sex. Most of patients, 86 (82.7%) had either primary or no formal education and more than eighty percent of them were unemployed. The majority of patients, 78 (75.0%) came from the rural areas located a considerable distance from Mwanza City and more than three quarter of them had no identifiable health insurance.

Clinical presentation of patients with typhoid intestinal perforations

Fever and abdominal pain were common to all the patients (Table 3). The duration of illness (fever-perforation interval) was within 14 days in 84 (80.8%) patients and more than 14 days in 20(19.2%) patients. Most patients, 87 (83.7%) had perforation occurred prior to hospital admission, whereas in the remaining 17 (16.3%) patients perforation occurred during the course of hospitalization. Perforation- admission interval was within 24 hours (early presentation) in 16 (15.4%) patients and more than 24 hours (late presentation) in 88 (84.6%) patients. Adequate antibiotic treatment prior to admission was recorded in 26 (25.0%) patients whereas inadequate antibiotic treatment was recorded in 72 (69.2%) patients. Antibiotic treatment prior to admission was not documented in 6 (5.8%) patients. Inadequate treatment prior to admission was significant predictor of intestinal perforation (Odds ratio = 2.3, 95% Confidence interval = 1.4-4.6, $P = 0.002$).

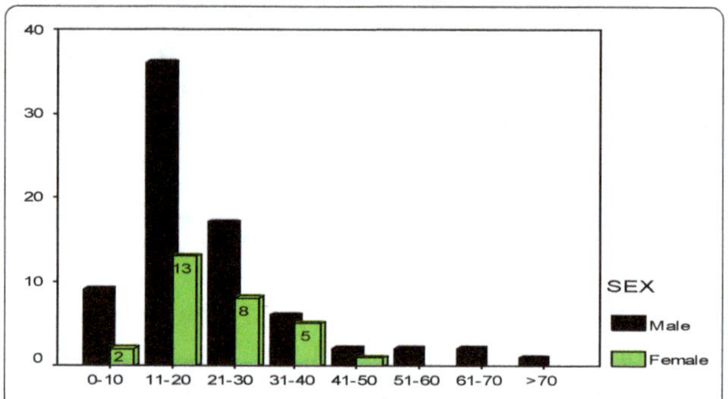

Figure 1 Age group distribution by sex.

Investigations

Ninety-nine (95.2%) of the patients had plain abdominal x-ray films available for review and demonstrated free gas under the diaphragm (pneumoperitonium) in 74 (74.7%) of them. Ultrasound done in 56 (53.8%) patients detected free peritoneal collections in 48 (85.7%) patients. Widal's test was positive (i.e. titre ≥ 1 in 160 dilutions) in 98(94.2%) patients. HIV status was known in 88 (84.6%) patients. Of these, 9 (10.2%) were HIV positive. Of the HIV positive patients, four (44.4%) patients were known cases on ant-retroviral therapy (ARV) and the remaining 5 (55.6%) patients were newly diagnosed patients. HIV status was not known in 16 (15.4%) patients. CD 4+ count among HIV positive patients was available in only 7 patients and ranged from 43 cells/μl to 720 cells/μl with the mean of 224 cells/μl and standard deviation of 78 cells/μl. The median and the mode were 261 cells/μl and 172 cells/μl respectively. A total of three HIV positive patients (42.9%) had CD4+ count below 200 cells/μl and the remaining 4 patients (57.1%) had CD4+ count of ≥200 cells/μl. Serum electrolytes revealed hypokalaemia and hyponatraemia in 34 and 21 patients respectively.

Table 2 Distribution of age group by sex

Age group (in years)	Males (N/%)	Females (N/%)	Total (N/%)
0-10	9 (8.7)	2 (1.9)	11 (10.6)
11-20	36 (34.6)	13 (12.5)	49 (47.1)
21-30	17 (16.3)	8 (7.7)	26 (24.0)
31-40	6 (5.8)	5 (4.8)	11 (10.6)
41-50	2 (1.9)	1 (1.0)	3 (2.9)
51-60	2 (1.9)	-	2 (1.9)
61-70	1 (1.0)	-	1 (1.0)
> 70	1 (1.0)	-	1 (1.0)
Total	75 (72.1)	29 (27.9)	104 (100)

Table 3 Clinical features of patients with typhoid

Clinical features	Frequency	Percentage
Fever	104	100
Abdominal pain	104	100
Vomiting	94	90.4
Diarrhea	88	84.6
Constipation	80	76.9
Abdominal distension	76	73.1
Dehydration	72	69.2
Shock	63	60.6
Feculent gastric aspirates	12	11.5
Jaundice	7	6.7

Histopathological examination of excised specimens from the edges of perforations was typical of chronic inflammation (infiltration by monocytes, lymphocytes, plasma cells) in the 97 (93.3%) patients. Blood and stool cultures were not done in any of the patients

Anesthetic assessment

All patients were assessed pre-operatively using the American Society of Anaesthetists (ASA) pre-operative grading as shown in Table 4.

Operative findings

All patients in this study underwent laparotomy. The perforation-surgery interval was within 24 hours in 14 (13.5%) patients and more than 24 hours in 90(86.5%) patients. The interval between presentations at the Accident and Emergency department and surgery (waiting time) ranged from 1-10 hours with a median of 6 hours. On operation the abdominal cavity was heavily contaminated (generalized peritonitis) in 96 (92.3%) patients while in 8 (7.7%) patients the peritoneal cavity was having minimal contamination (localized peritonitis). Eighty-eight (84.6%) had single perforation and the remaining 16 (15.4%) patients had multiple perforations. The median age of the patients with single perforation (45 years) was significantly higher than that of those with multiple perforations (14 years) ($P = 0.018$). A total of 109 perforations were identified and ileum was the most common part of the bowel affected and occurred in 86.2% of cases (Table 5). The median size of the perforations was 7.8 mm (2-28 mm). The median distance from ileocecal junction was 36 cm (range 8-98 cm). The amount of pus/faecal matter drained from the peritoneal cavity reflected the extent of contamination. The drainage was between 200 and 3000 mls with a mean of 628 mls. It was less than 1000 ml in15 (14.4%) patients and more than 1000 mls in 89 (85.6%) patients.

Surgical procedures

Perforations were surgically treated depending upon the number of perforations, general health status of patient and degree of faecal contamination. Simple closure of the perforations was the most commonly done procedure accounting for 78.8% of cases and this was generally done in two layers after excision the edges (Table 6). Eight (7.7%) patients had re-operation between 3 rd and 14th day post-operatively as follows: 4 (3.8%) patients for intra-abdominal abscess and 2 (1.9%) patients for burst abdomen and enterocutaneous fistula each respectively. Four (3.8%) patients were re-operated during the follow up period as follows: 3 (2.9%) patients underwent Mayo's repair for incisional hernia and 1 (1.9%) patient had laparotomy due to adhesive intestinal obstruction.

Table 4 Distribution of patients according to ASA classification

ASA classification	Number of patients	Percentage
I	8	7.7
II	20	19.2
III	40	38.5
IV	31	29.8
V	5	4.8
Total	104	100

Table 5 Distribution of patients according to anatomical site of perforations (N = 109)

Anatomical site	Frequency	Percentage
Jejunum	11	10.1
Ileum	94	86.2
Caecum	2	1.8
Appendix	1	0.9
Ascending colon	1	0.9
Total	109	100

Clinical outcome

Post-operative complications

Forty-one (39.4%) patients had 62 post-complications as shown in Table 7. Surgical site infection was the most common post-operative complication accounting for 55.5% of cases.

Length of hospital stay

The overall length of hospital stay (LOS) ranged from 7 to 64 days with a median of 28 days. The median LOS for non-survivors was 6 days (range 1-10 days). Patients who had post-complications stayed longer in the hospital and this was statistically significant ($P = 0.012$).

Mortality

In this study, twenty-four patients died giving a mortality rate of 23.1%. Table 8 shows predictors of mortality according to univariate and multivariate logistic regression analysis.

Follow up of patients

Of the survivors, seventy-six (95.0%) patients were discharged well and the remaining 4 (5.0%) were discharged

Table 6 Type of surgical procedures performed (N = 104)

Surgical procedure performed	Frequency	Percentage
Simple double layered closure	82	78.8
Bowel resection with anastomosis	10	9.6
Right hemicolectomy + ileo-transverse anastomosis	8	7.7
Exteriorization of perforation with ileostomy	2	1.9
Appendicectomy	2	1.9

Table 7 Post-operative complications (N = 62)

Post-operative complications	Response	Frequency	Percentage
Early postoperative complications	Surgical site infection	35	55.5
	Chest infections	16	25.8
	Septic shock	5	8.1
	Intra-abdominal abscess	4	6.5
	Enterocutaneous fistula	4	6.5
	Wound dehiscence/burst abdomen	2	3.2
	Post-operative paralytic ileus	2	3.2
	Renal failure	1	1.6
Late postoperative complications	Adhesive intestinal obstruction	4	6.5
	Incisional hernia	3	4.8
	Hypertrophic/Keloids	2	3.2

against medical advice. No patients were discharged with permanent disabilities. Out of 80 survivors, twenty-eight (35.0%) patients were available for follow up at three month after discharge and the remaining 52 (65.0%) patients were lost to follow up.

Discussion

Intestinal perforation is the most serious complication of typhoid fever in the developing world that presents a challenge to surgeons in that perforation leads to high morbidity and mortality, but development of perforation is also unpredictable [14,15,22-27]. The incidence of the disease varies considerably in different parts of the world [28]. The incidence of typhoid intestinal perforation had previously been reported as an indication of endemicity of typhoid fever in any locality [27,29-34].

In most parts of the world, perforation rate ranges from 0.6% to 4.9% of enteric fever cases [8,35], but in West Africa, higher rates of 10%-33% have been reported [28,29,31,36]. In this review, the rate of typhoid intestinal perforation represented 8.5% of cases which is significantly lower than that reported in Western Africa [29,31,36]. High rate of intestinal perforation in this region may be due to a more virulent strain of *Salmonella typhi* among West Africans, coupled with increased hypersensitivity reaction in the Peyer's patches in this sub-region, where the perforation rate is higher than other endemic areas. These differences in the incidence of the disease reflect differences in the rate of risk factors for typhoid intestinal perforation from one country to another. The figures for the rate of typhoid intestinal perforation in our study may actually be an underestimate and the magnitude of the problem may not be apparent because of high number of patients excluded from this study.

In the present study, the highest incidence of typhoid intestinal perforation occurred in the first and second decades of life which is in keeping with other studies done elsewhere [6,15,28]. The increasing occurrence of typhoid intestinal perforation in this age group in our setting can be explained by the fact that youths are generally more adventurous and mobile and are more likely to eat unhygienic food outside the home. There is also high risk of fecal contamination as they visit the toilets at school or public toilets. High incidence of the disease in this age group has a negative impact on the country's economy because this group represents the economically productive age group and portrays an economic lost both to the family and the nation. The fact that the economically productive age-group is mostly affected demands an urgent public policy response on preventive measures such as safe drinking water and appropriate sewage disposal, and typhoid vaccination.

In agreement with other studies [15,26,27,35,36], typhoid intestinal perforation in the present study was more common in males than in females. The exact reason for this male preponderance is not known although it is possible that men have an increased risk of exposure to typhoid fever resulting from spending longer time and consuming more food outdoors that may lead to more frequent contact with the causative bacteria.

Intestinal perforation resulting from typhoid fever has been reported to be more prevalent in people with low socio-economic status [15]. This observation is reflected in our study where most of patients had either primary or no formal education and more than eighty percent of them were unemployed. The majority of patients in the present study came from the rural areas located a considerable distance from Mwanza City and more than three quarter of them had no identifiable health insurance. Similar observation was reported by others [15,37]. This observation has an implication on accessibility to health care facilities and awareness of the disease.

The clinical presentation of typhoid intestinal perforation in our patients is not different from those in other geographical areas [6,15,26,27,38] with fever and

Table 8 Predictors of mortality according to univariate and multivariate logistic regression analysis

Independent (Predictor) Variable	Survivors (N/%)	Non-survivors (N/%)	Univariate analysis	Multivariate analysis				
			O.R.	95% C.I.	*P*-value	O.R.	95% C.I.	*P*-value
Age								
≤ 40	77(79.4)	22(22.6)						
> 40	5 (71.4)	2(28.6)	1.23	0.24-2.98	0.984	2.32	0.43-2.45	NS
Sex								
Male	58 (77.3)	17(22.7)						
Female	22 (75.9)	7 (24.1)	2.21	0.95-2.76	0.051	1.32	0.22-2.32	NS
Duration of illness								
Within 14 days	64 (76.2)	20 (23.8)						
After 14 days	16 (80.0)	4 (20.0)	1.11	0.57-1.98	0.454	1.67	0.78-2.11	NS
Perforation-admission interval								
Within 24 hours	15 (93.7)	1 (6.3)						
After 24 hours	65 (73.7)	23 (26.1)	2.43	1.34-3.54	0.024	1.67	1.12-3.43	**0.003**
Timing of operation								
Within 24 hours	12(85.7)	2(14.3)						
After 24 hours	68 (75.6)	22(24.4)	0.21	0.11-0.98	0.011	1.23	1.12-3.65	**0.034**
HIV status								
Positive	3 (33.3)	6(66.7)						
Negative	63 (79.7)	16 (20.3)						
Not known	14 (87.5)	2 (12.5)	3.54	2.46-4.98	0.031	0.23	0.11-0.98	**0.022**
CD4+ count (cells/μl)								
≤ 200	1(33.3)	2 (66.7)						
> 200	3(75.0)	1(25.0)	5.34	3.45-6.98	0.004	4.54	3.23-6.87	**0.000**
Prehospital antibiotic therapy								
Adequate	23 (88.5)	3 (11.5)						
Inadequate	52 (72.2)	20 (27.8)						
Not documented	7 (87.5)	1 (12.5)	2.87	2.11-4.50	0.021	3.11	1.45-7.86	**0.006**
ASA classes								
I-II (Low risk group)	26 (92.9)	2 (7.1)						
III-V (High risk group)	54 (71.1)	22 (28.9)	0.32	0.11-0.98	0.033	3.2	2.34-6.81	**0.012**
SBP on admission								
≤ 90 mmHg	22 (61.1)	14 (38.9)						
> 90 mmHg	58(85.3)	10 (14.7)	3.45	1.56-4.91	0.011	1.98	1.72-4.98	**0.000**
Type of peritonitis								
Generalized	74(77.1)	22 (22.9)						
Localized	6(75.0)	2(25.0)	1.95	0.98-2.75	0.967	0.32	0.11-1.63	NS
Amount of peritoneal fluid/pus								
≤ 1000 mls	13 (86.7)	2 (13.3)						
> 1000 ml	67(75.3)	22 (24.7)	1.52	1.18-2.22	0.023	1.22	1.09-1.76	**0.011**
Number of perforations								
Single	71 (80.7)	17 (19.3)						
Multiple	9 (56.2)	7(43.8)	1.54	1.11-4.87	0.012	2.89	2.33-5.98	**0.007**
Postoperative complications								
Present	25 (61.0)	16 (39.0)						
Absent	55 (87.3)	8 (12.7)	2.98	2.33-4.91	0.004	5.22	3.43-6.94	**0.000**

Keys: N = Number of patients, C.I. = Confidence interval, O.R. = Odds ratio, SBP = Systolic blood pressure abdominal pain being common to all the patients. In our study, perforation occurred early in the course of the disease and this has been recognized by others [28,29,31,36]. Patients who perforate during the first two weeks of the illness appear to have a better prognosis [36]. It has been observed that compromised nutritional status could possibly play a role in the poor prognosis of the patient who has been ill for more than 2 weeks and then develops a perforation [39], but this observation is yet to be proved. Typhoid intestinal perforation generally occurs in 2nd to 3 rd week of illness, this is because of mechanism of perforation in Peyer's patches of terminal ileum [12] but in developing countries cases are reported early within first week of illness [30], reason behind this observation is not clear but it is speculated to be due to low immune power, change in virulence of bacteria, hypersensitivity to Peyer's patches and ileal contents of bacteria. This observation is reflected in our study where more than fifty percent of patients developed perforation within 1-2 weeks of the illness. The mechanism of intestinal perforation in typhoid fever is hyperplasia and necrosis of Peyer's patches of the terminal ileum. The lymphoid aggregates of Peyer's patches extend from the lamina propria to the sub-mucosa, so that in the presence of hyperplasia the distance from the luminal epithelium to the serosa is bridged by lymphoid tissue. During the course of typhoid fever, *S. Typhi* is found within mononuclear phagocytes of Peyer's patches, and in cases with intestinal perforation, both this tissue and surrounding tissues show hemorrhagic areas, most often during the third week of the illness [3]. Tissue damage in Peyer's patches occurs, resulting in ulceration, bleeding, necrosis, and, in extreme cases, full-thickness perforation. The process leading to tissue damage is probably multifactorial, involving both bacterial factors and host inflammatory response [3,35].

Most patients with typhoid fever who were admitted to our centre, reported after they had perforated which is in keeping with other studies done elsewhere [15,23,28,40]. As reported by many authors [15,40], majority of patients in the present study presented late in poor general condition. This was found to be the most important factor influencing the outcome of surgical procedure as also emphasized by a number of authors [15,23,29,30,36,40]. In resource-poor countries, difficulties in diagnosis, patient transfer, and sub-therapeutic antibiotic treatment often result in delayed presentation to a hospital [3,15,28].

In agreement with other studies [15,23,28,40], the diagnosis of typhoid intestinal perforation in this study was made from clinical evaluation, laboratory investigation, identification of free air under the diaphragm on abdominal and chest radiographs and operative findings such as typical perforation on antimesenteric border, purulent collection and adhesion of bowel loops with friable pussy flecks. The value of the radiological investigation has been compared with other writers and with current radiological techniques; 80-90% of cases are correctly diagnosed. Findings from our study demonstrated free gas under the diaphragm on abdominal and chest radiographs in more than seventy percent of cases which is consistent with other studies [41,42]. A plain abdominal or chest radiograph with free air under the diaphragm is a fairly frequent but variable finding signifying perforated hollow viscus, but its absence does not exclude the diagnosis. Abdominal ultrasonography has also been found to be superior to plan radiographs in the diagnosis of free intra-peritoneal air as confirmed by the present study [43]. For the accurate diagnosis of typhoid intestinal perforation, blood for culture and sensitivity, urine for culture and sensitivity and stool for culture and sensitivity or bone marrow are required. None of these laboratory investigations was performed in our study mainly because of lack of facilities capable of performing these tests. It is very difficult to isolate *Salmonella typhi* from urine and stool specimens in most developing countries. This is often due to lack of culture media, expertise and sometimes previous exposure to inadequate doses of antibiotics. Another major problems relating to the laboratory is the abuse of the Widal's test. It is therefore recommended to carry out studies of baseline value of typhoid agglutinins in our setting as has been done in some areas to know the diagnostic utility of the Widal's test.

The clinical picture of typhoid intestinal perforation may be complex when typhoid fever occurs with HIV infected patients [44]. We could not find any study in the literature that shows the effect of HIV infection on outcome of patients with typhoid intestinal perforation. This observation provides room for research on this topic. The prevalence of HIV infection among patients with typhoid intestinal perforation in the present study, was 10.2% which is higher than 6.5% [45] in the general population in Tanzania. However, the overall HIV seroprevalence in this study may actually be an underestimate and the magnitude of the problem may not be apparent because many patients were excluded from the study due to failure to meet the inclusion criteria. We could not establish the reason for the high seroprevalence of HIV among these patients although it is possible that these patients have an increased risk of exposure to HIV infection. This calls for a need to research on this observation. HIV infection was found to be associated with poor postoperative outcome. This observation calls for routine HIV screening in patients suspected to have typhoid intestinal perforation.

Surgical intervention is considered to be the standard treatment of choice for patients with typhoid intestinal perforation [16,46]. In keeping with other studies

[4,6,12-15,25-28,33], all patients in the present study underwent surgical treatment. One of the many factors affecting the surgical outcome in patients with typhoid intestinal perforation is time interval between duration of illness and surgical intervention (perforation-surgery interval) [46,47]. Early surgery can minimize the complications while delayed surgery leads to severe peritonitis and septic shock. In the present study, the majority of patients were operated more than 24 hours after the onset of illness. Similar observation was reported by other studies done in developing countries [47]. Delayed definitive surgery in the present study may be attributed to late presentation due to lack of accessibility to health care facilities, lack of awareness of the disease as a result some patients with typhoid perforation may decide to take medications in the pre-hospital period with hope that the symptoms will abate. It is also possible that some clinicians managing the patients initially may not have considered perforation as a possible diagnosis. In resource-poor countries, difficulties in diagnosis, patient transfer, and inadequate antibiotic treatment often result in delayed presentation to a hospital [3,36].

The presence of single intestinal perforations in majority (84.6%) of our patients is consistent with other reports [6,15,29,30]. The median age of the patients with single perforations in the present study was significantly higher than that of those with multiple perforations which is line with other reporters [38,47]. We could not establish the reason for this observation. The number of intestinal perforation in patients with typhoid intestinal perforation has been reported to have an influence on prognosis. In the present study, patients with multiple perforations had significantly high mortality rates compared to those with single perforations. Beniwal *et al* [46] found that the number of perforation had effect on surgical outcome. Adesunkanmi *et al* [36] reported high incidence of residual abscess in patients with single perforation, Kaybal *et al* [48] reported better outcome in single perforation and worse prognosis in multiple perforations while Rehman [31] does not favor correlation of perforation to morbidity and mortality.

Although typhoid ulcers could occur anywhere from the stomach to the rectum [22], the terminal ileum is usually mostly involved due to the high concentration of Payer's patches. Whereas the ileum was the most common site of typhoid perforation in the present study, colonic involvement was very rare which is consistent with other studies [12,15,22,23,25,26,28,32,37]. It is postulated that colonic involvement is due to direct bacteria invasion while ileal lesions are due to enterotoxin produced from parasitizes macrophages that caused hyperplasia, necrosis and ulceration [49].

Early surgical interference is the optimal treatment option for perforation. However, the type of surgery to be applied is controversial. Many surgical techniques have been used, ranging from simple peritoneal drainage under local anaesthesia in moribund patients [15], excision of the edge of the ileal perforation, and simple transverse closure in two layers; as done for majority of our patients, segmental intestinal resection and primary anastomosis especially in multiple perforations or right hemicolectomy where the caecum is involved. Whereas, better results are reported with simple closure, in many series [15,25,26,38,39,41], others favour segmental ileal resection and anastomosis [50]. Those that favour simple closure argue, that in such very ill patients any prolonged procedure may jeopardize the outcome and that the ileum affected by typhoid fever, take sutures well without cutting through. Our practice in managing these patients is a simple closure in solitary perforations and segmental intestinal resection and primary anastomosis in multiple perforations, right hemicolectomy where the caecum is involved and ileostomy for severe peritoneal contamination. The role of ileostomy as a first line operation for typhoid perforation continues to be debated. It has been recommended for patients with severe peritoneal contamination; enhancing intestinal decompression with improved healing, early resolution of ileus and early start to enteral feeding [23,27]. The major drawback of ileostomy is the need for a second operation to restore intestinal continuity, the specialized care before closure and the attendant cost which reduces its popularity [27]. The challenge is even more conspicuous in a developing country like Tanzania where resources for caring of patients with ileostomy are limited. The management of stoma remains difficult in developing countries because of the shortage of suitable equipment in this respect and peristomal ulceration remains a major problem. Indeed, peristomal ulceration provokes skin pain, inducing the patient to self-limitation of food intake leading to severe malnutrition.

The use of antibiotics has been extensively discussed in the past. Chloramphenical with metranidazole used to be the antibiotic of choice [6,15] and is still used in some centers [23]. With increasing resistance of the organisms to Chloramphenical, Cephalosporins (e.g. Ceftriaxone) and Quinolones (e.g. ciprofloxacin) came into being with metranidazole added for the anaerobes and gentamicin for the gram-negative pathogens. This is the regimen commonly used in our centre. However, a recent study done in our centre has shown resistance of the organisms to this combination and highly sensitive to Imipenem and meropenem [51]. But unfortunately these drugs may not be readily available in many third world countries including Tanzania.

The overall complications rate in this series was 39.4% which is comparable to what was reported by others [13,23]. High complications rate was reported by

Kouame *et al* [27]. This difference in complication rates can be explained by differences in antibiotic coverage, meticulous preoperative care and proper resuscitation of the patients before operation, improved anesthesia and somewhat better hospital environment. In agreement with other studies [6,13,15,28,37], surgical site infection was the most common postoperative complications in the present study. High rate of surgical site infection in the present study may be attributed to contamination of the laparotomy wound during the surgical procedure.

The overall median duration of hospital stay in the present study was 28 days which is higher than that reported by other authors [15,22,23,25,31]. This can be explained by the presence of large number of patients with postoperative complications in our study.

In the developing world, mortality rates from typhoid perforation have been reported to range from 9-22%. The mortality rate of 23.1% in the present study is comparable to the rates reported from tropical countries such as 22.0% from Nigeria where chloramphenical is still the drug of first choice [14]. These figures are much higher than the rates reported from other tropical countries such as 6.8% from Nepal [52], and 10.5% from India [46]. A high mortality rate of 39.0% was also reported in Nigeria by Meier *et al* [53]. Exceptionally low mortality rates of 1.5-2% have been reported from some parts of the developed world, where socioeconomic infrastructures are well developed [21]. The reasons for the high mortality are multifactorial. In our experience in this study high mortality rate was attributed to delayed presentation, inadequate antibiotic treatment prior to admission, shock on admission, HIV positivity, low CD4 count (< 200 cells/μl), high ASA classes (III-V), delayed operation, multiple perforations, severe peritoneal contamination and presence of postoperative complications.

Self discharge by patient against medical advice is a recognized problem in our setting and this is rampant, especially amongst surgical patients. Similarly, poor follow up visits after discharge from hospitals remain a cause for concern. In the present study, only 35% of survivors were available for follow up which is in keeping with other studies done in developing countries [15]. These issues are often the results of poverty, long distance from the hospitals and ignorance.

The potential limitation of this study is the fact that information about some patients obtained retrospectively was incomplete and this might have introduced some bias in our findings. Also, data obtained retrospectively and failure to detect HIV infection during window period may have underestimated the prevalence of HIV infection in our study. However, despite these limitations, the study has highlighted our experiences with typhoid intestinal perforation and their outcome of surgical management in our limited-resource environment and has provided local data that can guide health care providers in the treatment of patients. The challenges identified in the management of these patients in our setting need to be addressed, in order to deliver optimal care for these patients and improve their treatment outcome.

Conclusion

Typhoid intestinal perforation is still endemic in our setting and carries high morbidity and mortality. Delayed presentation, inadequate antibiotic treatment prior to admission, shock on admission, HIV positivity, low CD4 count (< 200 cells/μl), high ASA classes (III-V), delayed operation, multiple perforations, severe peritoneal contamination and presence of postoperative complications were the main predictors of mortality in this study. Early and appropriate surgical intervention, effective perioperative resuscitation, postoperative intensive care procedures, safe anesthesia, and delivery of wide-spectrum antibiotics with low resistance are highly recommended in the management of typhoid intestinal perforation in this region. Emphasis should be on preventive measures such as safe drinking water and appropriate sewage disposal, and typhoid vaccination.

Acknowledgements

We would like to express our gratitude to all those who provided support in preparation of this manuscript. Special thanks go to the staff members of Medical records department of Bugando Medical Centre and our residents in surgical department for their support and cooperation rendered to us during data collection.

Author details

[1]Department of Surgery, Catholic University of Health and Allied Sciences-Bugando, Mwanza, Tanzania. [2]Department of Internal Medicine, Catholic University of Health and Allied Sciences-Bugando, Mwanza, Tanzania. [3]Department of Microbiology and Immunology, Catholic University of Health and Allied Sciences-Bugando, Mwanza, Tanzania. [4]Department of Surgery, Muhimbili University of Health and Allied Sciences, Dar Es Salaam, Tanzania.

Authors' contributions

PLC contributed in study design, literature search, data analysis, manuscript writing, editing and submission of the manuscript. JBM, MK, HJ, SEM, MM and GG participated in study design, data analysis, manuscript writing & editing. MDM participated in data analysis, literature search, manuscript writing & editing. JMG supervised the study and contributed in data analysis, manuscript writing & editing. All the authors read and approved the final manuscript.

Competing interests

The authors declare that they have no competing interests.

References

1. Crum NF: **Current trends in typhoid fever.** *Current Gastroenterol Rep* 2003, **5(4)**:279-86.
2. Ukwenya AY, Ahmed A, Garba ES: **Progress in management of typhoid perforation.** *Ann Afr Med* 2011, **10**:259-65.

3. Hosoglu S, Aldemir M, Akalin S, Geyik MF, Tacyildiz IH, Loeb M: **Risk factors for enteric perforation in patients with typhoid Fever.** *Am J Epidemiol* 2004, **160**:46-50.
4. Osifo OD, Ogiemwonyi SO: **Typhoid ileal perforation in children in Benin City.** *Afr J Paediatr Surg* 2010, **7**:96-100.
5. Perera N, Geary C, Wiselka M, Rajakumar K: **and Andrew Swann, R: Mixed Salmonella infection: case report and review of the literature.** *J Travel Med* 2007, **14(2)**:134-5.
6. Agbakwuru EA, Adesunkanmi AR, Fadiora SO, Olayinka OS, Aderonmu AO, Ogundoyin OO: **A review of typhoid perforation in rural African hospital.** *West Afr J Med* 2003, **22(1)**:22-5.
7. Crump JA, Luby SP, Mintz ED: **The global burden of typhoid fever.** *World Health Organ Bull* 2004, **82**:346-53.
8. Crump JA, Ram PK, Gupta SK, Miller MA, Mintz ED: **Part I Analysis of data gaps *Salmonella enterics*erotype *Typh*infection in low and medium human development index countries, 1984-2005.** *Epidemiol Infect* 2008, **136**:436-48.
9. Bhutta ZA: **Current concepts in the diagnosis and management of typhoid fever.** *Br Med J* 2006, **333**:78-82.
10. Kotan C, Kosem M, Tuncer I, Kisli E, Sönmez R, Çıkman Ö, Söylemez Ö, Arslantürk H: **Typhoid intestinal perforation: Review of 11 cases.** *Kolon Rektum Hast Derg* 2000, **11**:6-10.
11. Pegues DA, Miller SI: **Salmonella Species, Including Salmonella Typhi.** In *Mandell, Douglas, and Bennett's Principles and Practice of Infectious Diseases.* 7 edition. Edited by: Mandell GL, Bennett JE, Dolin R. Philadelphia: Elsevier Churchill Livingstone; 2009:2287-2903.
12. Atamanalp SS, Aydinli B, Ozturk G, Oren D, Basoglu M, Yildirgan MI: **Typhoid intestinal perforations: twenty-six year experience.** *World J Surg* 2007, **31**:1883-1888.
13. Sumer A, Kemik O, Dulger AC, Olmez A, Hasirci I, Kişli E, Vedat Bayrak V, Bulut G, Kotan C: **Outcome of surgical treatment of intestinal perforation in typhoid fever.** *World J Gastroenterol* 2010, **16**:4164-4168.
14. Otegbayo JA, Daramola OO, Onyegbatulem HC, Balogun WF, Oguntoye OO: **Retrospective analysis of typhoid fever in a tropical tertiary health facility.** *Trop Gastroenterol* 2002, **23**:9-12.
15. Ugwu BT, Yiltok SJ, Kidmas AT, Opalawa AS: **Typhoid intestinal perforation in North Central Nigeria.** *West Afr J Med* 2005, **24**:1-6.
16. Saxe JM, Crospey R: **Is operative management effective in the treatment of perforated typhoid?** *Am J Surg* 2005, **189**:342-4.
17. Talwarr S, Sharmad A, Mittala IND, Prasad P: **Typhoid enteric perforation.** *Aust N Z J Surg* 1997, **67**:351-3.
18. Rowe B, Ward LR, Threlfall EJ: **Multidrug-resistant *Salmonella typhi*a worldwide epidemic.** *Clin Infect Dis* 1997, **24**:S106-S109.
19. Parry EHO: **Typhoid Fever.** In *Principles of Medicine in Africa..* 2 edition. Edited by: Parry EHO. Oxford: Oxford University Press; 1984:268-76.
20. Ajao 0G: **Typhoid perforation: factors affecting mortality and morbidity.** *Int Surg* 1982, **67**:317-9.
21. Carmeli Y, Raz R, Scharpiro JAC: **Typhoid fever in Ethiopian immigrants to Israel and native - born Israelis: a comparative study.** *Clin Inf Dis* 1993, **16**:213-215.
22. Chang YT, Lin JY: **Typhoid colonic perforation in childhood: a ten year experience.** *World J Surg* 2006, **30**:242-7.
23. Edino ST, Yakubu AA, Mohammed AZ: **Abubakar.IS: Prognostic Factors in Typhoid ileal Perforation: A Prospective Study of 53 Cases.** *JAMA* 2007, **99**:1043-1045.
24. Wolters U, Wolf T, Stutzer H, Schroder T: **ASA classification and perioperative variables as predictors of postoperative outcome.** *British Journal of Anaesthesia* 1996, **77**:217-222.
25. Nuhu A, Dahwa S, Hamza A: **Operative management of typhoid ileal perforation in children.** *Afr J Paediatr Surg* 2010, **7**:9-13.
26. Edino ST, Mohammed AZ, Uba AF, Sheshe AA, Anumah M, Ochicha O, Yakubu AA, Alhassan SU, Mamman M: **Typhoid enteric perforation in North Western Nigeria.** *Nig J Med* 2004, **13**:345-9.
27. Koume J, Kouadio L, Turquin HT: **Typhoid ileal perforation: surgical experience of 64 cases.** *Acta Chir Belg* 2004, **104**:445-7.
28. Tade AO, Olateju SO, Osinupebi OA, Salami BA: **Typhoid Intestinal Perforations in a Tropical Tertiary Health Facility: A Prospective Study.** *East Cent Afr J Surg* 2011, **16(2)**:72.
29. Ameh EA: **Typhoid ileal perforation in children: A scourge in developing countries.** *Ann Trop Paediatr* 1999, **19**:267-72.
30. Uba AF, Chirdan LB, Ituen AM, Mohammed AM: **Typhoid intestinal perforation in children: A continuing scourge in a developing country.** *Pediatr Surg Int* 2007, **23**:33-9.
31. Rahman GA, Abubakar AM, Johnson AW, Adeniran JO: **Typhoid ileal perforation in Nigerian children: An analysis of 106 operative cases.** *Pediatr Surg Int* 2001, **17**:628-30.
32. Archibong AE, Ikpi EE, Enakirerhi G, Okoronkwo C: **Typhoid enteric perforation in children in Calabar, Nigeria.** *J Med Lab Sci* 2003, **12**:41-2.
33. Oheneh-Yeboah M: **Postoperative complications after surgery for typhoid ileal perforation in adults in Kumasi.** *West Afr J Med* 2007, **26**:32-6.
34. Abantanga FA: **Complications of typhoid perforation of the ileum in children after surgery.** *East Afr Med J* 1997, **74**:800-2.
35. van Basten JP, Stockenbrugger R: **Typhoid perforation: A review of literature since 1960.** *Trop Geogr Med* 1994, **46**:336-9.
36. Adesunkanmi ARK, Ajao OG: **Prognostic factors in typhoid ileal perforation: a prospective study in 50 patients.** *J R Coll Surg Edinb* 1997, **42**:395-399.
37. Ahmed HN, Niaz MP, Amin MA, Khan MH, Parhar AB: **Typhoid perforation still a common problem: situation in Pakistan in comparison to other countries of low human development.** *J Pak Med Assoc* 2006, **56(5)**:230-2.
38. Ekenze SO, Okoro PE, Amah CC, Ezike HA, Ikefuna AN: **Typhoid ileal perforation: Analysis of morbidity and mortality in 89 children.** *Niger J Clin Pract* 2008, **11**:58-62.
39. Ansari AG, Naqvi SQH, Ghumro AA, Jamali AH, Talpur AA: **Management of typhoid ileal perforation: A surgical experience of 44 cases.** *Gomal J Med Sci* 2009, **7(1)**:27-30.
40. Khan JA, Rehman S, Rasool AG, Qayyum A, Mehboob M: **A study of typhoid bowel perforation in Balochistan.** *Pak J Surg* 1998, **14(1&2)**:28-31.
41. Khan SH, Aziz SA, Ul-Haq MI: **Perforated peptic ulcers: A review of 36 cases.** *Professional Med J* 2011, **18(1)**:124-127.
42. Lee CW, Yip AW, Lam KH: **Pneumogastrogram in the diagnosis of perforated peptic ulcer.** *Aust N Z J-Surg* 1993, **63**:459-61.
43. Chen SC, Yen ZS, Wang HP, Lin FY, Hsu CY, Chen WJ: **Ultrasonography is superior to plain radiography in the diagnosis of pneumoperitonium.** *Br J Surg* 2002, **89**:351-354.
44. Wani RA, Parray FQ, Bhat NA, Wani MA, Bhat TH, Farzana F: **Non traumatic terminal ileal perforation.** *World J Emerg Surg* 2006, **1**:7.
45. Urassa M, Isingo R, Kumogola Y, Mwidunda P, Helelwa M, Changulucha J, Mngara J, Zaba B, Calleja T, Slaymaker E: **Effect of PMTCT availability on choice of ANC in Mwanza and Magu districts and its impact on HIV sentinel surveillanc.** *Tanzania: Report of ANC surveillance Mwanza and Magu Districts* 2007.
46. Beniwal US, Jindal D, Sharma J, Jain S, Shyman G: **Comparative study of operative procedures in typhoid perforation.** *Indian J Surg* 2003, **65**:172-7.
47. Kella N, Radhi PK, Shaikh AR, Leghari F: **Qureshi MA: Factors affecting the surgical outcome in typhoid intestinal perforation in children.** *Paed Surg* 2010, **16(4)**:567-570.
48. Kaybal I, Gokcora IH, Kaybal M: **A contemporary evaluation of enteric perforation in typhoid fever; analysis of 257 cases.** *Int Surg* 1990, **75**:96-100.
49. Elesha SO: **Pathology and pathogenesis of typhoid fever.** *Nig P Med J* 1994, **1**:38.
50. Shah AA, Wani KA, Wazir BS: **The ideal treatment of typhoid enteric perforation- resection anastomosis.** *Int Surg* 1999, **84**:35-8.
51. Mawalla B, Mshana SE, Chalya PL, Imirzalioglu C, Mahalu W: **Predictors of surgical site infections among patients undergoing major surgery at Bugando Medical Centre in Northwestern Tanzania.** *BMC Surgery* 2011, **11**:21.
52. Karmacharya B, Sharma VK: **Results of typhoid perforation management: our experience in Bir Hospital, Nepal.** *Kathmandu University Med J* 2006, **4**:22-24.
53. Meier DE, Tarpley JL: **Typhoid intestinal perforations in Nigerian children.** *World J Surg* 1998, **22**:319-323.

15

Pyogenic vertebral osteomyelitis complicating abdominal penetrating injury

Arianna Zefelippo[1,2*], Paola M Bertazzoni[1,2], Aldo M Marini[1], Paolo De Rai[1] and Ettore Contessini-Avesani[1,2]

Abstract

Pyogenic vertebral osteomyelitis is a rare condition usually associated with endocarditis or spinal surgery. However, it may also occur following abdominal penetrating trauma with associated gastrointestinal perforation. Diagnosis might be challenging and appropriate treatment is essential to ensure a positive outcome. In trans-abdominal trauma, 48 hours of broad-spectrum antibiotics is generally recommended for prophylaxis of secondary infections. A case report of vertebral osteomyelitis complicating trans-colonic injury to the retroperitoneum is presented and clinical management is discussed in the light of literature review.

Keywords: Vertebral osteomyelitis, Penetrating abdominal trauma, Post-traumatic infections

Background

Pyogenic vertebral osteomyelitis is a rare condition usually related to endocarditis or spinal procedures [1,2]. It may also develop as a complication of penetrating trauma of the spine [3] and it has been reported in literature in association with abdominal low-speed gunshot wounds [4-7] or stab wounds [8,9]. Trans-colonic injuries in particular appear to be at higher risk of developing secondary infections [3,10]. Diagnosis of vertebral osteomyelitis might be challenging due to subtle onset of symptoms and unspecific clinical features. Persistent back pain and fever, sometimes associated with neurological impairment, are the usual findings [1]. However, in trauma patients concurrent injuries may masquerade symptoms and delay diagnosis. Etiological diagnosis and correct clinical management are essential to ensure an appropriate therapy and to avoid complications. Treatment usually requires a long course of antibiotics and prolonged bed rest [2]. A case report of vertebral osteomyelitis complicating trans-colonic injury to the retroperitoneum is presented alongside a review of the literature.

* Correspondence: arianna.zefelippo@unimi.it
[1]General and Emergency Surgery Unit, Fondazione IRCCS Cà Granda Ospedale Maggiore Policlinico di Milano, via F. Sforza 35-20100, Milano, Italy
[2]General Surgery Post-graduation School, University of Milan, via F. Sforza 35-20100, Milano, Italy

Case presentation

A 21 year-old male was admitted to the emergency department for abdominal penetrating injury by a pointed metal stick (namely, a doner kebap spit). On primary survey, vital signs were normal and clinical examination demonstrated a single penetrating wound at the right inferior abdominal quadrant. No peritoneal free fluid was detected on ultrasound scan. Tetanus prophylaxis was administered. A thoraco-abdominal computed-tomography (CT) scan showed a retroperitoneal hematoma surrounding the sub-hepatic inferior vena cava with no intraperitoneal fluid or other abnormalities (Figure 1). A minimal tear of the vena cava was suspected to be the source of bleeding; due to hemodynamic stability, the patient was initially treated conservatively. After three hours of clinical observation, he developed peritonitis while vital signs remained normal and steady. Thoraco-abdominal CT scan was repeated in order to rule out any rebleeding in the retroperitoneum and to investigate possibility for endovascular treatment prior to surgery. The hematoma was unchanged compared to the first scan whereas free peritoneal air was demonstrated (Figure 2). At laparotomy, diffuse peritonitis secondary to perforation of the transverse colon was found. Perforation was repaired with direct suture and a sample of peritoneal fluid was collected for cultures. Retroperitoneum was left untouched. Postoperative recovery was uneventful. The patient received 5 days of intravenous

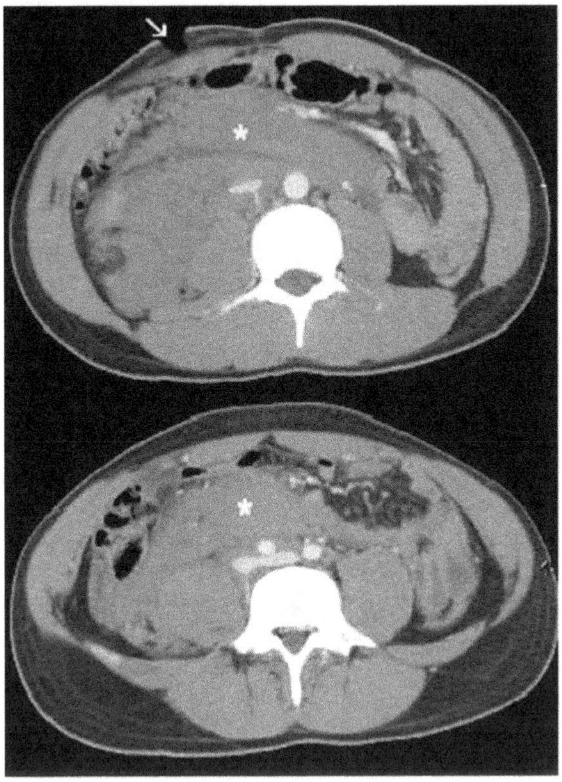

Figure 1 CT scan on admission. CT scan on admission showed a large retroperitoneal hematoma (*). Entrance site of penetrating wound is visible at right lower quadrant (arrow).

broad spectrum antibiotics (imipenem) and was discharged in 8 days.

Ten days later he was readmitted for fever and worsening lumbar pain radiating to the limbs bilaterally with minimal walking impairment. Blood exams revealed increased C-reactive protein (CRP) levels and leukocyte count. Abdominal CT scan showed no signs of intra or retroperitoneal abscess; the retroperitoneal hematoma appeared decreased in size. No evidence of chest or urinary tract infections was demonstrated. Eventually, magnetic resonance imaging (MRI) showed osteomyelitis at III and IV lumbar vertebrae with bone erosion and inflammation of disc space; a small collection in the paravertebral tissue at that level was also detected (Figure 3). No vertebral fractures or spinal involvement were demonstrated and clinical assessment was performed to confirm spinal stability. Given the results of cultures on peritoneal fluid collected at time of laparotomy, that showed polimicrobial contamination by Escherichia coli, Enterobacter cloacae, Candida albicans and Candida krusei, treatment was started with intravenous piperacillin/tazobactam and fluconazole. Ten sessions of hyperbaric oxygen therapy (HBOT) were administered in addition. Analgesia and bed rest were effective in alleviating symptoms. Clinical response to therapy was satisfactory and CRP levels were decreased after 2 weeks of treatment. Repeated sets of blood cultures were negative. The patient was discharged in 20 days on oral medications (ciprofloxacin, thrimethoprim and fluconazole) for 6 weeks and prescription for a back brace and physiotherapy. Clinical improvement was confirmed at 10 days follow-up. He made a full recovery in 2 months.

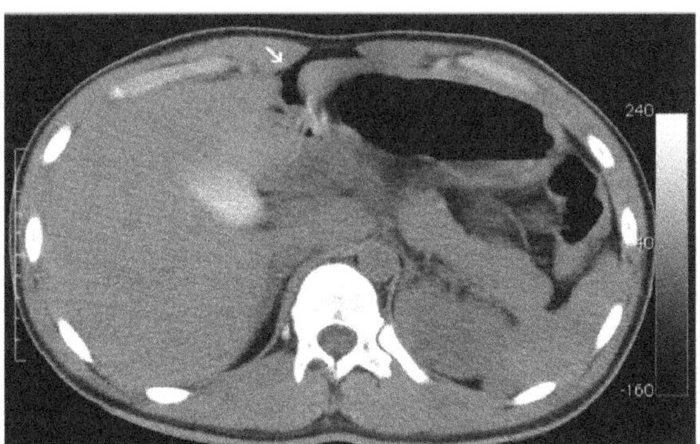

Figure 2 Repeated CT scan. A CT scan was repeated after the patient developed peritonitis. Peritoneal free air was detected (arrow).

Discussion

Pyogenic vertebral osteomyelitis is a rare disease that counts for 2-5% of all cases of osteomyelitis, with an annual incidence of 0.4 to 2.4/100′000 among European

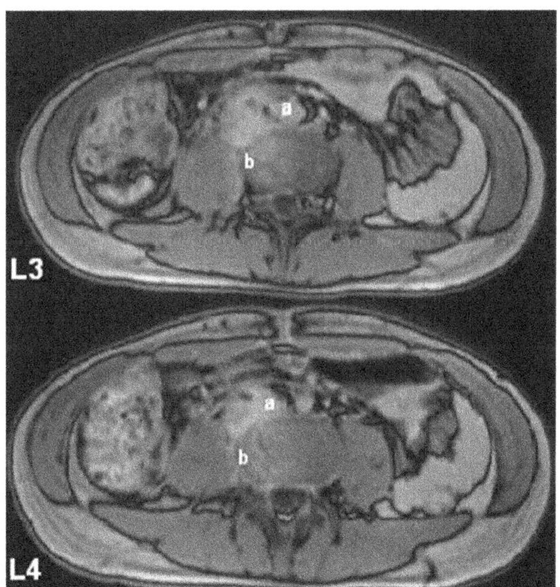

Figure 3 Diagnostic MRI. Contrast MRI demonstrated a small paravertebral collection **(a)** and osteomyelitis at L III – L IV with areas of bone erosion **(b)** (T1 weighted images are shown).

population [2]. Predisposing factors are intravenous drug use, immunosuppression, chronic illnesses and insulin-dependent diabetes mellitus. Typically, vertebral osteomyelitis is a complication of bacterial endocarditis and septicemia. Direct contamination associated with spinal surgery or epidural procedures appears to be of increasing importance among possible etiologies [1,2]. According to observational studies, Staphylococcus aureus (20-84%) and Enterobactericeae (33%) are the most common pathogens, with anaerobes (3%) and fungi (1-2%) rarely involved; less than 10% are polimicrobial infections [11]. In trauma setting, direct or trans-abdominal penetrating injuries to the spine are at risk of developing secondary infections, particularly when a hollow viscus is perforated [3,10]. In the presented case, a pointed metal stick caused a perforation of the transverse colon and a retroperitoneal injury. Bone infection was considered to be secondary to direct contamination from the peritoneum and treated accordingly. Diagnosis of pyogenic vertebral osteomyelitis is usually guided by clinical suspicion in the presence of persistent back pain and remitting fever. A wide range of neurological symptoms, including weakness, radiculopathy and sensory loss may also be shown by up to 30% of the patients [1]. It has to be noted that in trauma patients, concurrent injuries may mislead and delay diagnosis. In our case, fever, back pain and neurological impairment were at first attributed to superinfection of the retroperitoneal hematoma or possibly to an intra-abdominal abscess, before diagnosis of vertebral osteomyelitis was made. Adequate imaging should also support the clinical suspicion. In the presented case, CT scan of the abdomen failed to detect vertebral osteomyelitis that was subsequently diagnosed on MRI. Although plain X-ray and CT are frequently used as first step investigation for back pain, MRI is considered to be the gold standard for diagnosis of osteomyelitis. Moreover, MRI is superior to CT in defining involvement of neuronal and soft tissue and extension of the infective process [2]. Every effort should be taken to identify the pathogen, in order to ensure an appropriate antimicrobial therapy and prevent complications such as abscesses, extension of the infection to neuronal tissue, persistence or recurrence of infection, septicemia. Blood cultures have a high rate of positivity, reported to range between 30 and 75% [1]. If negative, percutaneous CT-guided biopsy to obtain material for cultures is generally recommended. Surgical biopsy in not recommended unless surgery has already been planned to drain an abscess or to treat spinal instability [2]. In our case, antimicrobial treatment was based on intraoperative cultures of peritoneal liquid whereas repeated sets of blood cultures remained negative. This therapy demonstrated to be effective and invasive diagnostic procedures were spared. 6 to 8 weeks of antibiotics is the recommended duration for treatment, which should be anyway adjusted according to clinical course. A positive

Table 1 Studies on spinal infections (including vertebral osteomyelitis) secondary to trans-abdominal injuries

Author	Study design	Mechanism of injury	Patients included	Incidence of spinal infections	Antibiotic coverage
Romanick 1985 [4]	Retrospective	Low speed gunshot wounds	20 →12 bowel perforations: → 4 upper GI tract → 8 colon	7/8 colon perforations	At least 2 days, broad spectrum
Roffi 1989 [5]	Retrospective	Low speed gunshot wounds	42 →14 colon perforations	3/14 colon perforations	Extended course (6 to 14 days)
Kihtir 1991 [15]	Retrospective	Gunshot wounds	21 → 5 colon perforations	0/21 patients	48 hours
Lin 1995 [13]	Retrospective	Low speed gunshot wounds	29 → 8 colon perforations	0/29 patients	2 to 5 days
Kumar 1998 [14]	Retrospective	Gunshot wounds	33 → 13 colon perforations	0/13 colon perforations	2 to 43 days
Quickgley 2006 [6]	Retrospective	Low speed gunshot wounds	114 → 27 bowel perforations: → 12 upper GI tract → 15 colon	4/27 bowel perforations (3/15 colon perforations)	5 days, broad spectrum
Rabinowitz 2012 [7]	Retrospective	Gunshot wounds	51 bowel perforations: → 25 upper GI tract → 26 colon	1/51 bowel perforations	24-48 hours broad spectrum for prophylaxis *vs* prolonged treatment for documented infections

response to therapy is defined by clinical improvement and decrease in CRP levels within 4 weeks [1]. Repeated MRI is usually unnecessary unless treatment failure or complications are suspected [2]. Treatment should be also focused towards alleviating symptoms, with extensive use of analgesia and bed rest. An appropriate rehabilitation plan is also advisable. HBOT has been increasingly used as adjuvant therapy for bone infections. Although lacking in high quality evidence, a number of studies have suggested HBOT to be effective in enhancing leukocyte bactericidal activity and antibiotic activity in hypoxic tissues, suppressing anaerobic pathogens, inducing angiogenesis and accelerating wound healing [12]. In our case, HBOT was administered in addition to standard treatment and proved to be beneficial.

Appropriate prophylaxis for infective complications in trauma patients has been largely investigated. Colon perforation is considered to be a risk factor for developing secondary infections and use of broad-spectrum antibiotic prophylaxis is generally recommended for at least 24–48 hours [3,10]. However, few published studies address the specific issue of spinal or paraspinal and vertebral infection following penetrating injuries associated with hollow viscus perforation. Results of a review of the literature focusing on this topic are summarized in Table 1. All case series included patients with trans-abdominal injuries to the spine caused by gunshot wounds. Reported incidence of osteomyelitis is very low, even in the presence of bowel perforation. As for prophylaxis, some authors recommend prolonged antibiotic coverage for at least 5 days [5,6,13,14] while a number of studies have showed no significant difference in the incidence of secondary infections when a short-term prophylaxis is administered [4,7,15]. It has to be noted that all these studies are characterized by the small number of patients included and by retrospective design. A recently published study included 51 patients with penetrating gunshot wounds to the spine following gastrointestinal perforation observed over 8 years of activity in a level 1 trauma center [7]. Patients received up to 48 hours perioperative antibiotic prophylaxis (35% of patients) unless damage control surgery was performed or a longer course of antibiotics was required for documented infections (65%). Only 1 patient developed a spinal infection, which occurred among the group that received prolonged antibiotic treatment. The author concluded questioning the necessity for extended prophylaxis for more than 48 hours. Although current evidence on this issue is poor, a 24–48 hours prophylaxis with large-spectrum antibiotics appears to be a reasonable approach in the event of penetrating abdominal wounds associated with hollow viscus perforation.

Conclusion

Pyogenic vertebral osteomyelitis is a rare complication that may occur following abdominal penetrating injury, especially when bowel is perforated. Diagnosis can be difficult and should be guided by high clinical suspicion. An accurate management and appropriate treatment are essential to ensure a positive outcome. 48 hours of broad-spectrum antibiotics is suggested for prophylaxis of secondary infections following trans-abdominal trauma.

Consent

Written informed consent was obtained from the patient for publication of this case report and accompanying images.

Competing interests

The authors declare that they have no competing interests.

Authors' contributions

AZ was involved in the clinical management of the patient and drafted the manuscript. PD and PB performed the operation and contributed in conceiving the manuscript. AM admitted the patient and reviewed the manuscript. All authors read and approved the final manuscript.

References

1. Zimmerli W: **Clinical practice. Vertebral osteomyelitis.** *N Engl J Med* 2010, **362:**1022–1029.
2. Pola E, Fantoni M: **Focus on spondylodiscitis.** *In Eur Rev Med Pharmacol Sci* 2012, **16**(Suppl 2):1–85.
3. Bono CM, Heary RF: **Gunshot wounds to the spine.** *Spine J* 2004, **4:**230–240.
4. Romanick PC, Smith TK, Kopaniky DR, Oldfield D: **Infection about the spine associated with low-velocity-missile injury to the abdomen.** *J Bone Joint Surg Am* 1985, **67:**1195–1201.
5. Roffi RP, Waters RL, Adkins RH: **Gunshot wounds to the spine associated with a perforated viscus.** *Spine* 1989, **14:**808–811.
6. Quickgley KJ, Place HM: **The role of debridement and antibiotics in gunshot wounds to the spine.** *J Trauma* 2006, **60:**814–820.
7. Rabinowitz RP, Tabatabai A, Stein DM, Scalea TM: **Infectious complications in GSW's through the gastrointestinal tract into the spine.** *Injury* 2012, **43:**1058–1060.
8. Harries TJ, Lichtman DM, Swafford AR: **Pyogenic vertebral osteomyelitis complicating abdominal stab wounds.** *J Trauma* 1981, **21:**75–79.
9. Myllynen P, Klossner O: **Pyogenic vertebral osteomyelitis as a complication of an abdominal stab wound.** *Ann Chir Gynaecol* 1982, **71:**344–346.
10. Luchette FA, Borzotta AP, Croce MA, O'Neill PA, Whittmann DH, Mullins CD, Palumbo F, Pasquale MD: **Practice management guidelines for prophylactic antibiotic use in penetrating abdominal trauma.** *J Trauma* 2000, **48:**508–515.
11. D'Agostino C, Scorzolini L, Massetti AP, Carnevalini M, D'Ettorre G, Venditti M, Vullo V, Orsi GB: **A seven-year prospective study on spondylodiscitis: epidemiological and microbiological features.** *Infection* 2010, **38:**102–107.
12. Fang RC, Galiano RD: **Adjunctive therapies in the treatment of osteomyelitis.** *Semin Plast Surg* 2009, **23:**141–147.
13. Lin SS, Vaccaro AR, Reisch S, Devine M, Cotler JM: **Low-velocity gunshot wounds to the spine with an associated transperitoneal injury.** *J Spinal Disord* 1995, **8:**136–144.
14. Kumar A, Wood GW, Whittle AP: **Low-velocity gunshot injuries of the spine with abdominal viscus trauma.** *J Orthop Trauma* 1998, **12:**514–517.
15. Kihtir T, Ivatury RR, Simon R, Stahl WM: **Management of transperitoneal gunshot wounds of the spine.** *J Trauma* 1991, **31:**1579–1583.

16

A rare cause of gastrointestinal phytobezoars: diospyros lotus

Gökhan Ertuğrul[1*], Murat Coşkun[1], Mahsuni Sevinç[1], Behzat Yelimlieş[1], Fisun Ertuğrul[2] and Toygar Toydemir[3]

Abstract

Aim: Diospyros Lotus ("Wild Date Palm of Trabzon or Persimmon"), which has been proven to cause phytobezoars, is a widely consumed fruit in the Black Sea and Northeast Anatolia regions of Turkey. The aim of the present study was to investigate the effects of Diospyros Lotus together with other predisposing factors, on the development of gastrointestinal phytobezoars and to discuss the treatment results in comparison to the literature.

Material and method: The records of 13 patients, who had been admitted to the General Surgery Clinic of Düzce Atatürk State Hospital between August 2008 and August 2011, were retrospectively reviewed. Demographic characteristics, predisposing factors, clinical and radiological findings, diagnostic and therapeutic methods, and the outcomes of the patients were recorded from the patient files. Written informed consent was obtained from each patient for publication of this research article and accompanying images.

Results: All the patients had a history of consuming Diospyros Lotus. Of the patients, 30,7% had a history of previous gastric surgery, 30,7% had diabetes mellitus and 23% had dental implants. None of the patients had hypothyroidism, which is another predisposing factor for phytobezoars.
The phytobezoars were located in the stomach alone in 23% of the patients, whereas 15,3% was detected in the jejunum and stomach, 15,3% was detected in the jejunum alone, and 46,1% was detected in the ileum alone.
All patients were treated with surgery, and there were no deaths.

Conclusion: Gastric phytobezoars are rare. Preventive measures have particular importance in the management of this condition, which is difficult to treat. For this purpose, excessive consumption of herbal nutrients containing a high amount of indigestible fibers such as Diospyros Lotus should be avoided in patients with a history of gastrointestinal surgery or poor oral and dental health.

Keywords: Gastrointestinal phytobezoars, Diospyros lotus (Persimmon)

Introduction

Gastrointestinal bezoar is a rarely encountered clinical condition difficult to diagnose and treat. They are classified according to their contents. Phytobezoar is the most common type of gastrointestinal system bezoars that occur due to excessive consumption of herbal nutrients including a high amount of indigestible fibers. Excessive consumption of Diospyros Lotus (Wild Date Palm of Trabzon, Persimmon), which is a traditional nutrient grown particularly in the Black Sea Region of Turkey and includes high amount of indigestible fibers, is thought to be responsible for the high prevalence of gastrointestinal phytobezoars in this region. (Figures 1 and 2: Diospyros Lotus)

Clinical picture, ranging from an asymptomatic condition to acute abdomen, depends on the amount of Diospyros Lotus consumed, as well as to the location of phytobezoar.

In addition to radiological imaging methods, upper gastrointestinal endoscopy is used in the diagnosis of phytobezoars.

Prevention is the primary goal in the management of phytobezoars, however when they occur, they have to be removed. Various endoscopic and surgical techniques, including gastric lavage, are used for treatment.

In the present study, the records of 13 patients who had undergone surgical intervention for gastrointestinal phytobezoars, considered to be caused by Diospyros

* Correspondence: mdgertugrul@gmail.com
[1]Department of General Surgery, Düzce Atatürk State Hospital, Muncurlu, Düzce, Turkey
Full list of author information is available at the end of the article

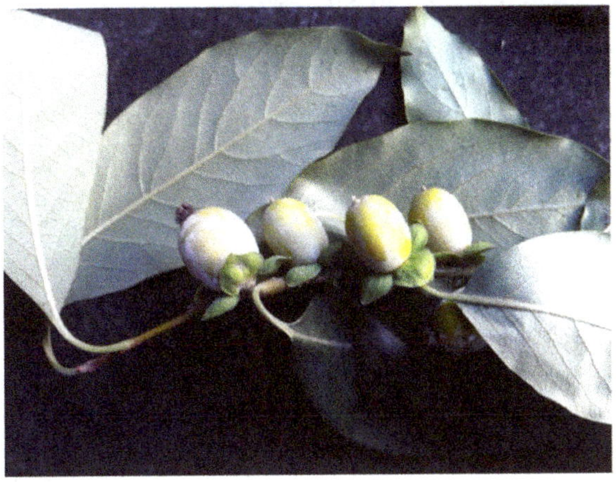

Figure 1 Diospyros Lotus.

Lotus consumption, were investigated. The aim of the study was to investigate the effects of Diospyros Lotus, which is a widely consumed fruit in our region, together with other predisposing factors on the development of gastrointestinal system phytobezoars, and to discuss the treatment results in comparison to the literature.

Material and method

The present study was designed as a retrospective study. The medical records of 13 patients, who had been admitted to the General Surgery Clinic of Düzce Atatürk State Hospital between August 2008 and August 2011, and had undergone surgical intervention with a diagnosis of gastric phytobezoar, were reviewed.

Demographic characteristics, predisposing factors, clinical and radiological findings, diagnostic and therapeutic methods were recorded from the patient records, and morbidity and mortality rates were estimated. Current information regarding the disease, such as recurrence, was obtained from the patients themselves, and recorded.

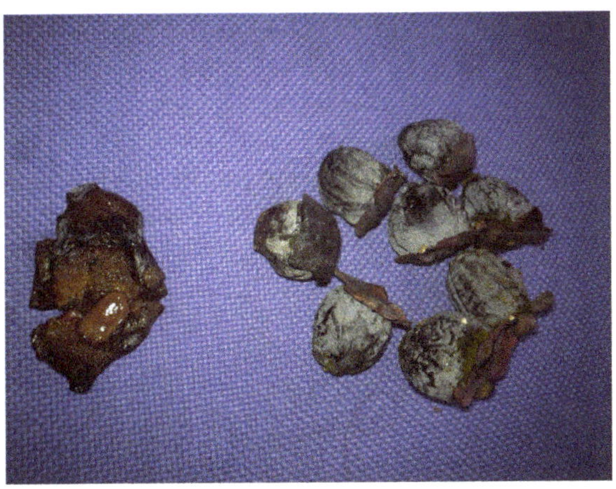

Figure 2 Diospyros Lotus.

Written informed consents were obtained from all patients for publication of this research article and accompanying images.

Results

Thirteen patients, (84,6% female) with a mean age of 54,4 years, were included in the study.

All the patients had a history of consuming Diospyros Lotus. Ten (76,9%) of these patients had been admitted to the hospital in November and December, harvesting time, when the fruit is highly consumed. The remaining three patients (23%) with a history of consumption dried Diospyros Lotus, had been admitted between March and June. Other predisposing factors included a history of gastric surgery in four (30,7%) patients [Antrectomy and Billroth II Surgery in one (7,6%) and Distal Subtotal Gastrectomy and Billroth II Anastomosis in three (23%) patients], diabetes mellitus, as a concomitant disease, in four (30,7%) patients and dental implants in three (23%) patients. Hypothyroidism, one of the predisposing factors, was identified in none of the patients (Table 1: Predisposing Factors).

All patients presented to the clinic with extensive abdominal pain, nausea and fecaloid vomiting. Physical examinations of the patients revealed abdominal distension, rigidity, and rebound tenderness, indicating an acute mechanical bowel obstruction.

Plain abdominal radiographs in the standing position showed nonspecific signs such as dilated loops of bowel and air-fluid levels. Diagnosis was based on the abdomen tomography in 11 patients (84,6%), and upper gastrointestinal endoscopy in two (15,3%) patients (Figure 3: Abdomen Tomography, Figure 4: Upper Gastrointestinal Endoscopy).

Phytobezoars were found in the stomach alone in three (23%), in the jejunum and stomach in two (15,3%), in the jejunum alone in two (15,3%), and in the ileum alone in six (46,1%) patients (Table 2: Location of Phytobezoars).

All patients underwent surgical intervention including gastrotomy in three (23%), gastrotomy together with manual fragmentation and milking into cecum in two (15,3%), enterotomy in five (38,4%), and manual fragmentation and milking into cecum in three (23%) patients. (Table 3: Surgical Treatment Methods) (Figure 5: Gastrotomy), (Figure 6: Manual Fragmentation and Milking into Cecum).

Table 1 Predisposing Factors

	n	%
Diospyros Lotus	13	100
History for Gastric Surgery	4	30,7
Diabetes Mellitus	4	30,7
Dental Prosthesis	3	23
Hypothyroidism	—	—

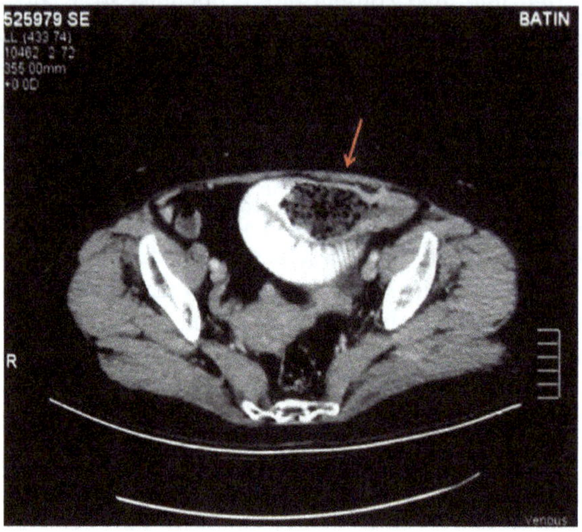

Figure 3 Abdomen Tomography.

Pathological examinations were performed. Macroscopically, the material was composed of plant fibers with the seed of Diospyros Lotus at the center. Microscopic examination revealed no cellular elements, but a material composed of plant fibers and food residue.

Only one (7,6%) patient developed wound site infection, which was treated with broad-spectrum antibiotics and daily dressings. None of the patients died.

The mean length of hospital stay was 10,5 days (range, 5–18 days).

The mean postoperative follow-up period was 21,3 months (range, 6–36 months), and no recurrence was observed.

Discussion

Gastrointestinal bezoars are classified according to their contents. Phytobezoars are the most common type of

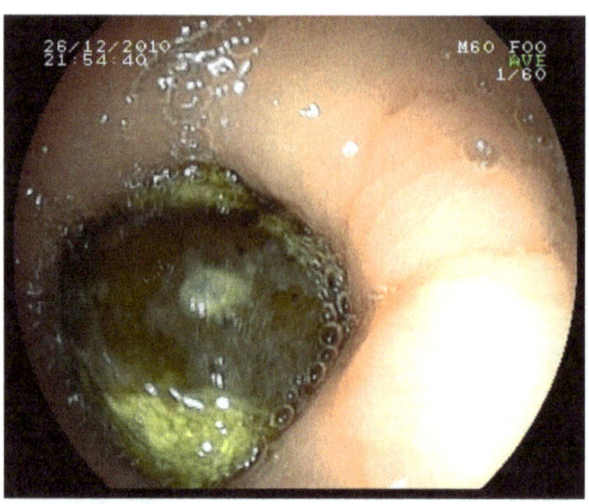

Figure 4 Upper Gastrointestinal Endoscopy.

Table 2 Location of Phytobezoars

	n	%
Stomach	3	23
Stomach + Jejunum	2	15,3
Jejunum	2	15,3
Ileum	6	46,1

bezoars, formed by excessive consumption of herbal nutrients. Celery, grape, prune, Diospyros Lotus and pineapple are the main nutrients responsible for phytobezoars. Such nutrients contain high amounts of indigestible fibers, such as cellulose, hemicellulose, lignin and fruit tannins. Trichobezoars, composed of hardened hair and hair-like fibers, are usually encountered in children with mental retardation and in adults with mental illness. Lactobezoar occurs in low birth weight infants fed with concentrated milk and formulas in the first week of life, pharmacobezoar occurs due the use of concentrated drug formulas (cholestyramine and kayexalate); and food bezoars occur due to the use of concentrated food formulas [1-5].

Various predisposing factors are responsible for gastrointestinal phytobezoars; the most important predisposing factors are loss of pyloric function, decreased gastric motility and acid secretion following gastric surgery, adhesions due to abdominal surgery, inadequate chewing, and excessive consumption of herbal nutrients including high amounts of indigestible fibers [3,5-9]. Furthermore, delayed gastric emptying, which results from diabetic neuropathy, hypothyroidism, and connective tissue diseases, forms a basis for the development of gastrointestinal phytobezoars[9-11]. Chisholm et al. retrospectively examined 13 patients with phytobezoars, and found that all the patients had a history of persimmon consumption, whereas 11 (84,6%) had a history of gastric surgery [12]. Krausz et al., in their retrospective study on 113 patients, showed that 106 (93,8%) patients had undergone gastric surgery, whereas 103 (91,1%) had a history of persimmon consumption [10]. In the present study, all 13 patients (100%) had a history of Diospyros Lotus consumption, whereas four (30,7%) had a history of previous gastric surgery. Furthermore, four (30,7%) patients had diabetes mellitus and three (23%) had a history of using dental implants.

Table 3 Surgical Therapy Methods

	n	%
Gastrotomy	3	23
Gastrotomy + Manuel Fragmentation and Milking to Cecum	2	15,3
Enterotomy	5	38,4
Manuel Fragmentation and Milking to Cecum	3	23

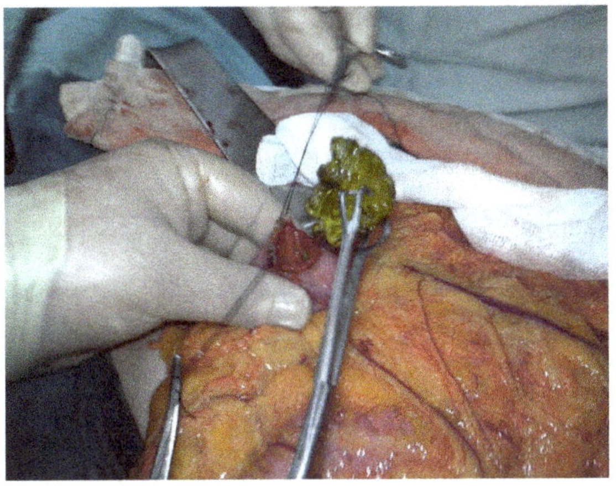

Figure 5 Gastrotomy.

The main clinical symptoms are abdominal pain, epigastric distress, nausea and vomiting. In addition, sensation of fullness, dyspepsia, dysphagia, anorexia, weight loss, and gastrointestinal bleeding may be seen [1,13-15]. Decreased bowel sounds, rebound tenderness, rigidity, distension, diarrhea, constipation, nausea and vomiting may be seen in complicated cases [10].

Small bowel obstruction is the most common major complication of phytobezoars. Moreover, gastritis, ulcer, and gastric perforation may be seen. Small bowel phytobezoars usually occur due to the extension of gastric phytobezoars [10,16]. However, small intestinal phytobezoars may also be seen in patients with underlying diseases, such as diverticulitis, stricture, and tumor [17-19]. Small bowel obstructions due to phytobezoars usually occur in the terminal ileum and jejunum, which are the narrowest parts of the small intestine [20]. Chisholm et al. identified phytobezoars in the stomach in two (12,5%), in the jejunum in four (25%), in the ileum in nine (56,2%), and in more than one region of the small intestine in two (12,5%) patients[12]. Krausz et al. detected phytobezoars in the stomach in 13 (11,5%), in the small intestine and stomach in 20 (17,6%), and in the small intestine in 80 (70,7%) patients[10]. In the present study, phytobezoars were located in the stomach alone in three (23%), in the jejunum and stomach in two (15,3%), in the jejunum alone in two (15,3%), and in the ileum alone in six (46,1%) patients.

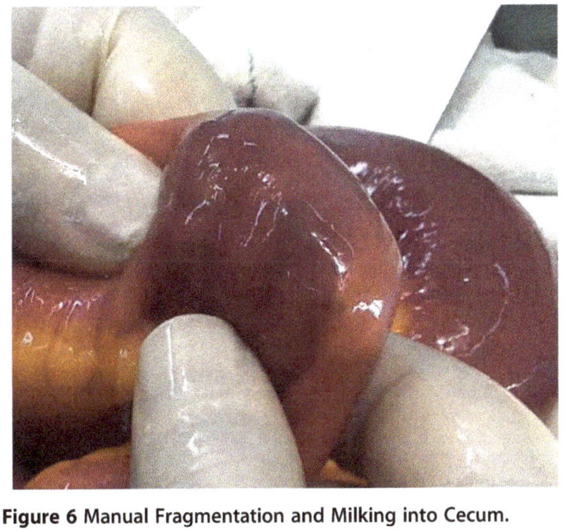

Figure 6 Manual Fragmentation and Milking into Cecum.

Upper gastrointestinal endoscopy and radiological imaging methods, such as plain abdominal radiography in the standing position, barium enema radiograph, abdominal ultrasound and abdominal computed tomography, are used for the diagnosis of gastrointestinal phytobezoars. Plain abdominal radiographs may show dilated intestinal loops, air-fluid levels and thickened intestinal wall [17]. Barium radiography is contraindicated in patients with suspected complete obstruction and perforation. Phytobezoars may appear as an echogenic intraluminal mass and a remarkable posterior acoustic shadowing on abdominal ultrasound [21-23]. A dilated small bowel loop with a well-defined, round-shaped, heterogeneous, intraluminal mass distally, is typical on abdominal computed tomography. It typically appears as an intraluminal soft tissue mass that contains air bubbles [9,17,24,25]. Upper gastrointestinal endoscopy can detect all of the gastric phytobezoars, but just 12% of the small bowel phytobezoars[26]. In the present study, diagnosis was made by abdominal tomography in 11 (84,6%), and upper gastrointestinal endoscopy in two patients.

Gastric lavage, and endoscopic or surgical techniques, can be used in the treatment of gastrointestinal phytobezoars.

L-cysteine, metoclopramide and cellulose, papain and cellulose, pineapple juice, normal saline solution, sodium bicarbonate, hydrochloric acid, pancrelipase, pancreatin, 1-2% zinc chloride, and coca cola are used for the disintegration of the bezoar during gastric lavage [3,19,27-29]. Hayashi et al. observed that there was a significant decrease in the size and a significant softening in the structure of the phytobezoar by giving 500–1000 ml coca cola before each meal for three weeks, and they removed the mass using endoscopic forceps [30].

The first successful outcomes concerning endoscopic removal of gastric phytobezoars were published in 1972 by McKechnie[31]. Endoscopic disintegration requires normal pyloric function and absence of duodenal obstruction [27]. If the phytobezoar is not large in size, it can be removed using a basket catheter or by direct aspiration [25].

Surgical therapy may be performed either by open or laparoscopic technique. Main surgical techniques include manual fragmentation and milking to cecum, gastrotomy, enterotomy, and resection and anastomosis in complicated cases. As the prevalence of concurrent gastric and small intestine phytobezoars is 17-21%, care should be given not to leave any residue during surgery [32,33]. Chisholm et al. performed endoscopic removal in one (6,2%), gastrotomy together with manual fragmentation and milking into cecum in one (6,2%), manual fragmentation and milking into cecum in nine (56,2%), enterotomy in four (25%), and small intestine resection and anastomosis in one (6,2%) patient [12]. In a study conducted by Krausz et al., 14 (12,3%) patients underwent gastrotomy, 62 patients (54,8%) underwent manual fragmentation and milking into cecum, 34 patients (30%) underwent enterotomy, and two patients (1,7%) underwent small intestine resection and anastomosis [10]. In the present study, three patients (23%) underwent gastrotomy, two patients (15,3%) underwent gastrotomy together with manual fragmentation and milking into cecum, five patients (38,4%) underwent enterotomy, and three patients (23%) underwent manual fragmentation and milking into cecum.

Krausz et al. reported early morbidity and mortality rates as 11,5% and 1,7%, respectively [10]; the morbidity rate was 7,6% in the present study, whereas no mortality was observed.

Conclusion

In conclusion, gastrointestinal phytobezoar is a rare clinical condition, difficult to treat and diagnose. Prevention is the best way to manage the disease. Therefore, excessive consumption of herbal nutrients, containing high amounts of indigestible fibers, such as Diospyros Lotus should be avoided by people with a history of gastric surgery or poor oral and dental health.

Consent

Written informed consents were obtained from all patients for publication of this research article and accompanying images. A copy of the written consent is available for review by the Editor-in-Chief of this journal.

Competing interests

I declare that I have no competing interests.

Authors' contributions

G E, M C, B Y and F E performed the surgeries. G E, M S and T T analyzed and interpreted the data. G E was the main author of the manuscript. All authors read and approved the final manuscript.

Author details

[1]Department of General Surgery, Düzce Atatürk State Hospital, Muncurlu, Düzce, Turkey. [2]Department of Anesthesiology and Reanimation, Düzce Atatürk State Hospital, Muncurlu, Düzce, Turkey. [3]Department of General Surgery, İstanbul Surgery Hospital, Nişantaşı, İstanbul, Turkey.

References

1. Andrus CH, Ponsky JL: **Bezoars: Classification, pathophysiology and treatment.** *Am J Gastroenterol* 1988, **83**:476–478.
2. Alsafwah S, Alzein M: **Small bowel obstruction due to trichobezoar: Role upper endoscopy in diagnosis.** *Gastrointes Endosc* 2000, **52**:784–786.
3. Saeed ZA, Rabassa AA, Anand BS: **An endoscopic method for removal of duodenal phytobezoars.** *Gastrointest Endosc* 1995, **41**(1):74–76.
4. Gurses N, Ozkan K, Ozkan A: **Bezoars-Analysis of seven cases.** *Kinder Chirurg* 1987, **42**:291–292.
5. Hayes PG, Rotstein OD: **Gastrointestinal phytobezoars: Presentation and management.** *Can J Surg* 1986, **29**:419–420.
6. Ko SF, Lee TY, Ng SH: **Small bowel obstruction due to phytobezoar: CT diagnosis.** *Abdom Imaging* 1997, **22**:471–473.
7. Minami A: **Gastric bezoars after gastrectomy.** *Am J Surg* 1973, **126**:421–424.
8. Buchholz RR, Hainsten AS: **Phytobezoars Following Gastric Surgery for Doudenal Ulcer.** *Surg Clin N Am* 1972, **52**:341–351.
9. Quiroga S, Alvarez-Castells A, Sebastiá MC, Pallisa E, Barluenga E: **Small bowel obstruction secondary to bezoar: CT diagnosis.** *Abdom Imaging* 1997, **22**:315–317.
10. Krausz MM, Moriel EZ, Ayalon A, Pode D, Durst AL: **Surgical aspects of gastrointestinal persimmon phytobezoar treatment.** *Am J Surg* 1986, **152**:526–530.
11. Norberg PB: **Intestinal obstruction due to food.** *Surgery Gynec Obstet* 1961, **113**:149–152.
12. Chisholm EM, Chung SCS, Leong HT: **Phytobezoar: an uncommon cause of small bowel obstruction.** *Ann R Coll Surg Engl* 1992, **74**:342–344.
13. Verstandig AG, Klin B, Blomm RA, Hadas I, Libson E: **Small Bowel Phytobezoars: Detection with Radiography.** *Radiology* 1989, **172**:705–707.
14. Mangold D, Woolam GL, Garcia-Rinaldi R: **Intestinal obstruction due to phytobezoars: observations in two patients hypothyroidism and previous gastric surgery.** *Arch Surg* 1978, **113**:1001–1003.
15. Rumley TO, Hocking MP, King CE: **Small bowel obstruction secondary to enzymatic digestion of gastric bezoars.** *Gastroenterology* 1983, **84**:627–629.
16. Escamilla C, Roblos-Campos R, Parrilla-Paricio P, Lujan-Mompean J, Liron-Ruiz R, Torralba-Martinez JA: **Intestinal obstruction and bezoars.** *J Am Coll Surg* 1994, **178**:285–288.
17. Kim JH, Ha HK, Sohn MJ, Kim AY, Kim TK, Kim PN, Lee MG, Myung SJ, Yang SK, Jung HY: **CT findings of phytobezoar associated with small bowel obstruction.** *Eur Radiol* 2003, **13**:299–304.
18. Frazzini VI, English WJ, Bashist B, Moore E: **Small bowel obstruction due to phytobezoar formation within Meckel diverticulum: CT findings.** *J Comput Asit Tomogr* 1996, **20**:390–392.
19. Lorimer JW, Allen MW, Toa H, Burns B: **Small-bowel carcinoid presenting in association with a phytobezoar.** *Can J Surg* 1991, **34**:331–333.
20. Teo M, Wong CH, Chui CH: **Food bolus - an uncommon cause of small intestinal obstruction.** *Aust N Z J Surg* 2003, **73**(Suppl 1):A47.
21. Ko YT, Lim JH, Lee DH, Yoon Y: **Small intestinal phytobezoar Sonographic detection.** *Abdom Imaging* 1993, **18**:271–273.
22. McCracken S, Jongeward R, Silver TM, Jafri SZ: **Gastric trichobezoar: Sonographic findings.** *Radiology* 1986, **161**:123–124.
23. Frager DH, Baer JW, Mollinelli B, Friedman M: **Role of CT in evaluating patients with small-bowel obstruction.** *Semin US CT MR* 1995, **16**:127–140.
24. Frager D, Medwid SW, Baer JW, Mollinelli B, Friedman M: **CT of small-bowel obstruction: Value in establishing the diagnosis and determining the degree and cause.** *Am J Roentgenol* 1994, **162**:37–41.
25. Fukuya T, Hawes DR, Lu CC, Chang PJ, Barloon TJ: **CT diagnosis of small-bowel obstruction: Efficacy in 60 patients.** *Am J Roentgenol* 1992, **158**:765–769.
26. Naveau S, Poynard T, Zourabichvili O, Poitrine A, Chaput JC: **Gastric phytobezoar destruction by Nd: YAG laser therapy (letter).** *Gastrointest Endosc* 1986, **32**:430–431.
27. Gáyá J, Barranco L, Llompart A, Reyes J, Obrador A: **Persimmon bezoars: A successful combined therapy.** *Gastrointest Endosc* 2002, **55**:581–583.
28. Ladas SD, Triantafyllou K, Tzathas C, Tassios P, Rokkas T, Raptis SA: **Gastric phytobezoars may be treated by nasogastric Coca-Cola lavage.** *European J Gastroenterol Hepatol* 2002, **14**:801–803.
29. Stanten A, Peters HE: **Enzymatic dissolution of phytobezoars.** *Am J Surg* 1975, **130**:259–261.
30. Kazuki Hayashi, Hirotaka Ohara, Itaru Naitoh: **Persimmon Bezoar Successfully Treated by Oral Intake of Coca- Cola: A case report.** *Cases Journal* 2008, **1**:385.

Cholecystectomy for acute cholecystitis: How time-critical are the so called "golden 72 hours"? Or better "golden 24 hours" and "silver 25–72 hour"?

Peter Ambe[1,4*], Sebastian A Weber[2], Hildegard Christ[3] and Dirk Wassenberg[4]

Abstract

Introduction: Early cholecystectomy within 72 hours has been shown to be superior to late or delayed cholecystectomy with regard to outcome and cost of treatment. Recently, immediate cholecystectomy within 24 hours of onset of symptom was proposed as standard procedure for the management of fit patients presenting with acute cholecystitis. We sort to find out if there are any differences in surgical outcomes between patients managed within 24 h and those managed 25-72 h following symptom begin for acute cholecystitis.

Patients and methods: A retrospective analysis was performed. The outcomes of patients undergoing laparoscopic cholecystectomy within 24 h were compared to those of patients managed 25-72 h following symptom onset for acute cholecystitis.

Results: 35 patients managed 25-72 h following begin of symptoms were matched with 35 patients with similar baseline features, medical comorbidities and disease severity managed within 24 hours of symptom onset. There were no significant differences in the duration of surgery, postoperative complications, rate of conversion and length of hospital stay.

Conclusion: Immediate laparoscopic cholecystectomy for acute cholecystitis within 24 hour of symptom onset is not superior to surgery 25–72 hour after symptoms begin. Laparoscopic cholecystectomy for acute cholecystitis therefore can be safely performed anytime within the golden 72 h.

Keywords: Acute cholecystitis, Laparoscopic cholecystectomy, Early cholecystectomy, Immediate cholecystectomy, Gallbladder inflammation, Tokyo guidelines, Timing of cholecystectomy

Introduction

Acute cholecystitis (AC) is a common diagnosis in the surgical practice with a clear indication for surgery. Although widely discussed in the past, unequivocal evidence exists supporting the superiority of early laparoscopic cholecystectomy within 72 hours over delayed LC with respect to outcome and cost of treatment [1-8]. This trend was confirmed in a recently published randomized study in patients managed within 24 hours of admission [9]. Cholecystectomy however, may not always be possible within 24 hours of admission for many different reasons. In such cases, surgery should be performed within 72 hours as recommended in several guidelines [10-12]. The aim of this study was to compare the outcomes of patients undergoing LC within 24 h of symptom begin on one hand to those of patients managed 25 to 72 h after symptom begin for AC on the other hand.

Patients and methods

A retrospective review of the charts of patients undergoing cholecystectomy for AC from January 2009 to December 2013 in the department of surgery of a

* Correspondence: peter.ambe@helios-kliniken.de
[1]Helios Klinikum Wuppertal, Department of Surgery II, Witten/Herdecke University, Heusner Strasse 40, 42283 Wuppertal, Germany
[4]Department of General, visceral and thoracic surgery, St. Remigius Hospital Opladen, An St. Remigius 26, 51379 Leverkusen, Germany
Full list of author information is available at the end of the article

primary care hospital in Germany was performed. Baseline characteristics including age, sex, body mass index (BMI) and medical comorbidities as defined by the American Society of Anesthesiology (ASA) were retrieved for each patient.

Acute cholecystitis was diagnosed as outlined in the Tokyo guidelines [13,14]. The diagnosis was confirmed during surgery and following histopathology. Only patients managed within 72 hours of symptom begin were included for analysis. All patients were placed on intravenous antibiotics upon admission which was continued after surgery. Perioperative data including the duration of anesthesia, the duration of surgery, conversion to open surgery, postoperative complications and the length of postoperative hospital stay were retrieved from surgical documentation sheets, surgeon's notes and discharge records.

All surgeries in this study were performed by experienced attending surgeons. Laparoscopic cholecystectomy [15] was carried out using four incisions with pneumoperitoneum installed via a sub-umbilical mini-laparotomy with the maximum intraabdominal pressure kept at 12 mmHg.

The data collected was analyzed using the Statistical Package for Social Science (SPSS®), IBM, version 22. The study population was statistically described using absolute case numbers, percentages, medians and interquartile ranges. Significances were calculated using the Fisher' s exact test with levels of significance set at $p < 0.05$.

Patients operated upon 25 to 72 h after symptom begin (study group) were matched with regard to baseline and clinical features (same gender, similar ages, disease severity, BMI, ASA and APACHE II Scores) as well as disease severity grade (as outlined in the Tokyo guidelines) with patients operated upon within 24 h following symptom begin (control group). Both groups were comparable with regard to demographic and clinical characteristics.

Primary endpoints included the duration of anesthesia, the duration of surgery and postoperative complications. Secondary endpoints included the length postoperative of hospital stay and hospital mortality.

Results

Within the period of investigation 152 cases of AC were managed surgically. The distribution of study population is represented in Figure 1. Thirty-five patients were managed within 25-72 h following symptom begin (study group). Thirty-five patients with similar characteristics to those of the study group were selected from the 105 patients managed within 24 h of symptom begin, Table 1. The demographic characteristics of the study population are summarized in Table 2. Both groups were comparable in all cases.

There was no significant difference in the duration of anesthesia, the duration of surgery and the length of postoperative hospital stay amongst both groups. Five cases (14.2%) were converted to open cholecystectomy in the group managed within 24 h, while 3 cases (8.6%) were converted in the group operated upon within 25-72 h of symptom onset. This difference was not statistically significant, $p = 0.23$.

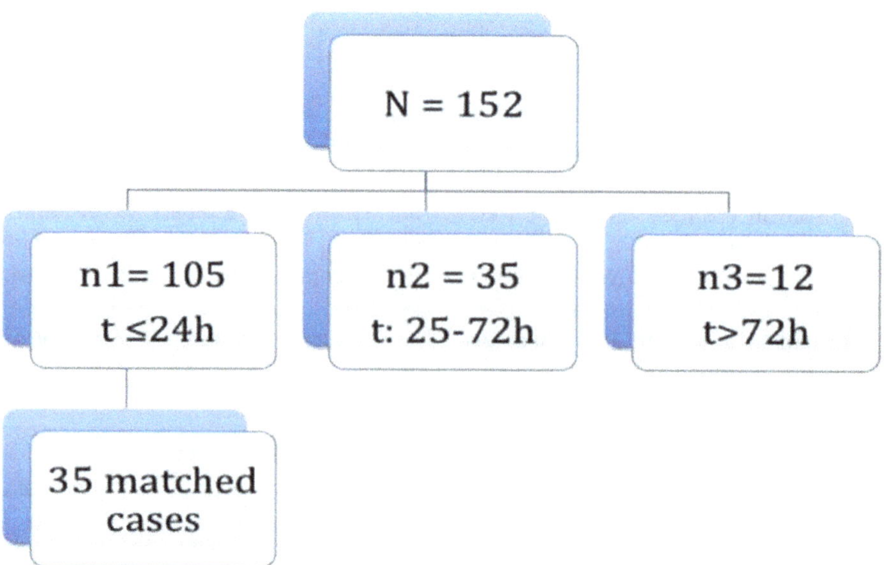

Figure 1 Distribution of the study population. 35 Patients undergoing surgery 25-72 h following symptom begin were compared to 35 selected patients with similar demographic and clinical parameter from the groups managed within 24 h of symptom onset.

Table 1 Patients with similar baseline and clinical characteristics were selected from the group managed within 24 h and matched with those managed 25-72 h

Case number	Gender		Age/yrs		ASA		BMI		Severity grade		APACHE II score	
	≤24 h	25- 72 h	≤24 h	25- 72 h	≤24 h	25- 72 h	≤24 h	25- 72 h	≤24 h	25- 72 h	≤24 h	25- 72 h
1	M	M	69	68	2	2	32.4	23.8	1	1	5	7
2	M	M	74	74	3	3	35.2	26.1	2	3	9	7
3	F	F	69	70	3	3	32.4	35.8	2	2	8	6
4	M	M	82	84	4	3	28.7	27.4	3	3	18	17
5	F	F	30	22	2	2	25.5	25.4	2	2	1	1
6	F	F	68	61	1	2	26.2	41.5	2	2	6	5
7	F	F	39	39	2	2	32.3	24.8	1	1	2	1
8	M	M	76	74	4	4	34.9	33.1	3	3	18	19
9	M	M	74	74	3	4	25.1	26.8	2	3	17	18
10	M	M	80	76	2	2	28.4	23.6	2	1	14	13
11	F	F	46	45	2	1	38.6	28.7	1	1	3	2
12	M	M	42	43	2	2	28.1	27.0	1	1	2	2
13	F	F	37	37	2	1	26.3	29.7	1	1	1	1
14	F	F	60	55	2	2	32.8	31.0	1	1	4	4
15	F	F	84	81	2	1	25.4	20.8	2	1	11	14
16	M	M	76	71	3	3	31.6	25.6	1	1	11	11
17	M	M	57	60	2	2	29.6	29.0	1	1	5	8
18	F	F	45	47	2	2	31.3	33.2	1	1	3	2
19	M	M	34	31	1	1	26.2	17.0	1	1	1	1
20	F	F	43	42	3	3	29.4	26.6	1	1	2	3
21	F	F	76	71	3	3	27.2	31.6	2	1	9	6
22	M	M	56	56	2	1	24.2	24.7	1	1	6	6
23	M	M	43	45	1	2	24.2	22.0	1	1	1	2
24	M	M	80	79	3	3	16.2	19.4	1	2	9	9
25	F	F	51	54	2	2	24.8	24.4	1	1	4	3
26	M	M	52	59	2	2	28.7	26.2	1	1	4	4
27	M	M	73	74	2	2	30.8	29.2	2	1	8	5
28	F	F	61	65	3	3	26.0	33.5	3	3	15	13
29	F	F	82	83	3	3	31.2	21.5	1	1	7	5
30	M	M	65	61	2	1	25.7	26.5	1	1	8	5
31	M	M	64	63	2	2	25.1	21.6	1	2	9	7
32	M	M	79	77	3	3	33.9	31.2	3	3	13	11
33	M	M	82	87	3	3	29.9	27.6	2	3	19	18
34	M	M	71	76	2	2	30.2	33.8	1	1	11	11
35	F	F	68	63	2	1	30.2	34.1	1	1	11	11

Both groups were comparable in terms of demographic and clinical parameters.

Two complications, including one patient with pneumonia and one with wound infection, were recorded in the group operated upon within 24 hours (5.7%). Five complications, including three patients with bile leak, one patient with wound infection and one patient with acute renal failure, were recorded in the group managed between 25-72 h of symptom begin (14.2%). This difference was not statistically significant ($p = 0.42$), Table 3. There was no mortality in both groups.

Discussion

The optimal timing of surgery for patients with AC has been a topic of controversy in the past. Initially, patients were managed conservatively with the aim of "cooling

Table 2 Summary of the baseline characteristics of the cohort

Feature		≤24 h	25 - 72 h	P-value
Gender (F/M)		15/20	15/20	/
Median age (interquartil range)		68.0 (30.0)	63.0 (27.0)	0.32
Median BMI (interquartil range)		28.7 (5.9)	26.8 (6.8)	0. 19
ASA	1-2	22	22	/
	3-4	13	13	

Both groups were comparable with regard to demographic characteristics.

down" the inflammation, and then perform cholecystectomy weeks later. The heterogeneity of patients suffering from AC and their medical co-morbidities it difficult to standardize treatment [16]. Acute cholecystitis was once considered a relative contraindication for LC at the beginning of the laparoscopic era, mainly due to high rates of complications and conversion. This trend however changed following growing expertise in laparoscopy. Nowadays, laparoscopic cholecystectomy is the gold standard for the management of benign gallbladder disorders and belongs to one of the most commonly performed procedures in surgery [17,18]. Current data suggest that early LC for acute cholecystitis is superior to late or delayed LC with regard to outcome and cost of treatment [2,19].

The term „early“ is rather vaguely defined in the literature [20,21]. In some series, „early“ defines the begin of symptoms while the same term is used with regard to the time of admission in other series. In this study, "early" was defined with respect to symptom begin. Generally speaking, early cholecystectomy is performed within a time interval of 72 h, the so called golden 72 h [22].

In a recently published multi-center randomized study by Gutt et. al., laparoscopic cholecystectomy performed within 24 h of admission was shown to be superior to delayed LC with regard to outcome. The authors concluded that immediate LC should become the treatment of choice for operable patients with AC [9]. This conclusion however, cannot be generally applied at all levels of patient care. Furthermore, immediate LC may not always be possible for different reasons. A number of patients presenting with AC may require special consultations and correction of co-morbidities (e.g. those on oral anticoagulation treatment) before undergoing surgery. Besides, experienced laparoscopic surgeons may not be available within 24 h, as may be the case in quiet a number of primary care hospitals. In such cases, LC should be performed within 72 h.

The aim of this study was to compare the outcomes of patients with AC managed within 24 h of symptom begin to those of patients managed 25-72 h following symptom onset. Data of patients undergoing LC in a primary care hospital in Germany was retrospectively analyzed. Thirty-five patients with AC managed within 24 h were matched (similar baseline characteristics, comorbidities and disease severity) with 35 patients managed 25 - 72 h after symptom onset. All surgeries were performed laparoscopically by surgical attendings with expertise in laparoscopy.

Surgery for acute cholecystitis could be time critical. According to Zhu et. al., gallbladder inflammation during the first 72 h of onset of symptoms may not involve structures within the triangle of Calot [23]. Surgical dissection within this critical period therefore appears easiest due to lack of organized adhesions. Cholecystectomy within this time frame reduces the risk of injury to the structures within the triangle of Calot. This is reflected in the low rates of complication and conversation.

There was no significant difference amongst both groups with respect to the duration of anesthesia and the duration of surgery. Equally, there was no significant difference in the rates of conversion and morbidity between both groups. All cases of conversion were due to the inability to clearly identify the structures within the space of calot.

Interestingly, three cases of bile leak were recorded in the study group. These complications occurred in patients with severity grade III and histopathologic evidence of necrotizing cholecystitis.

We could not prove any difference in outcome between the group managed within 24 h and that managed 25 - 72 h of onset of symptoms. Our results therefore suggest that it is not necessary to perform LC for AC within 24 h following symptom onset.

Taken together, a division of the critical time frame, i.e. the so called "golden 72 h" for the surgical management of acute cholecystitis into a more favorable "golden 24 h" and a less favorable "silver 25-72 h" could not be justified in this series.

Table 3 Summary of the perioperative data

Parameters	≤24 h	25-72 h	P-value
Median duration of anaesthesiology (interquartile range)	120.0 (45.0) min	115.0 (35.0) min	0.82
Median duration of surgery (interquartile range)	70.0 (35.0) min	65.0 (30.0) min	0.23
Rate of complication	5.7%	14.2%	0.42
Median duration of postoperative stay (interquartile range)	7.0 (3.0) min	6.0 (2.0)	0.65

Min: minutes.

This study is limited by the relatively small size of the cohorts and the retrospective study design. Since the study did not include consecutive patients, there might have been some degree of bias in the selection of the patients for the matching group. Therefore the trend shown in this study must be validated in prospective studies with larger case numbers.

Conclusion

Laparoscopic cholecystectomy for acute cholecystitis must not be performed within 24 h of admission. The golden 72 h time frame however should be maintained where possible.

Competing interests

The authors declare that they have no competing interests.

Authors' contribution

Study concept and design: PA, SW. Data collection: PA, DW. Statistical analysis: PA, HD. Interpretation: PA;SW;CH;DW. Drafting the manuscript: PA. Critical review and approval: PA; SW; HC; DW. All authors read and approved the final manuscript.

Author details

[1]Helios Klinikum Wuppertal, Department of Surgery II, Witten/Herdecke University, Heusner Strasse 40, 42283 Wuppertal, Germany. [2]Department of Internal Medicine, St. Elisabeth Hospital Hohenlind, 50377 Köln, Germany. [3]Department of medical statistics and epidemiology, University of Cologne, Cologne, Germany. [4]Department of General, visceral and thoracic surgery, St. Remigius Hospital Opladen, An St. Remigius 26, 51379 Leverkusen, Germany.

References

1. Gurusamy K, Samraj K, Gluud C, Wilson E, Davidson BR: **Meta-analysis of randomized controlled trials on the safety and effectiveness of early versus delayed laparoscopic cholecystectomy for acute cholecystitis.** *Br J Surg* 2010, **97**(2):141–150.
2. Gurusamy KS, Koti R, Fusai G, Davidson BR: **Early versus delayed laparoscopic cholecystectomy for uncomplicated biliary colic.** *Cochrane Database Syst Rev* 2013, **6**, CD007196.
3. Lau B, DiFronzo LA: **An acute care surgery model improves timeliness of care and reduces hospital stay for patients with acute cholecystitis.** *Am Surg* 2011, **77**(10):1318–1321.
4. Lau H, Lo CY, Patil NG, Yuen WK: **Early versus delayed-interval laparoscopic cholecystectomy for acute cholecystitis: a metaanalysis.** *Surg Endosc* 2006, **20**(1):82–87.
5. Lee AY, Carter JJ, Hochberg MS, Stone AM, Cohen SL, Pachter HL: **The timing of surgery for cholecystitis: a review of 202 consecutive patients at a large municipal hospital.** *Am J Surg* 2008, **195**(4):467–470.
6. Overby DW, Apelgren KN, Richardson W, Fanelli R: **Society of American G, Endoscopic S: SAGES guidelines for the clinical application of laparoscopic biliary tract surgery.** *Surg Endosc* 2010, **24**(10):2368–2386.
7. Papi C, Catarci M, D'Ambrosio L, Gili L, Koch M, Grassi GB, Capurso L: **Timing of cholecystectomy for acute calculous cholecystitis: a meta-analysis.** *Am J Gastroenterol* 2004, **99**(1):147–155.
8. Wilson E, Gurusamy K, Gluud C, Davidson BR: **Cost-utility and value-of-information analysis of early versus delayed laparoscopic cholecystectomy for acute cholecystitis.** *Br J Surg* 2010, **97**(2):210–219.
9. Gutt CN, Encke J, Köninger J, Harnoss JC, Weigand K, Kipfmüller K, Schunter O, Götze T, Golling MT, Menges M, Klar E, Feilhauer K, Zoller WG, Ridwelski K, Ackmann S, Baron A, Schön MR, Seitz HK, Daniel D, Stremmel W, Büchler MW: **Acute cholecystitis: Early versus delayed cholecystectomy, a multicenter randomized trial (ACDC Study, NCT00447304).** *Ann Surg* 2013, **258**(3):385–393.
10. Mayumi T, Takada T, Kawarada Y, Nimura Y, Yoshida M, Sekimoto M, Miura F, Wada K, Hirota M, Yamashita Y, Nagino M, Tsuyuguchi T, Tanaka A, Gomi H, Pitt HA: **Results of the Tokyo Consensus Meeting Tokyo Guidelines.** *J Hepato-Biliary-Pancreat Surg* 2007, **14**(1):114–121.
11. Miura F, Takada T, Strasberg SM, Solomkin JS, Pitt HA, Gouma DJ, Garden OJ, Buchler MW, Yoshida M, Mayumi T, Okamoto K, Gomi H, Kusachi S, Kiriyama S, Yokoe M, Kimura Y, Higuchi R, Yamashita Y, Windsor JA, Tsuyuguchi T, Gabata T, Itoi T, Hata J, Liau KH; Tokyo Guidelines Revision Comittee: **TG13 flowchart for the management of acute cholangitis and cholecystitis.** *J Hepato-Biliary-Pancreat Sci* 2013, **20**(1):47–54.
12. Takada T, Strasberg SM, Solomkin JS, Pitt HA, Gomi H, Yoshida M, Mayumi T, Miura F, Gouma DJ, Garden OJ, Büchler MW, Kiriyama S, Yokoe M, Kimura Y, Tsuyuguchi T, Itoi T, Gabata T, Higuchi R, Okamoto K, Hata J, Murata A, Kusachi S, Windsor JA, Supe AN, Lee S, Chen XP, Yamashita Y, Hirata K, Inui K, Sumiyama Y, *et al*: **TG13: Updated Tokyo Guidelines for the management of acute cholangitis and cholecystitis.** *J Hepato-Biliary-Pancreat Sci* 2013, **20**(1):1–7.
13. Sekimoto M, Takada T, Kawarada Y, Nimura Y, Yoshida M, Mayumi T, Miura F, Wada K, Hirota M, Yamashita Y, Strasberg S, Pitt HA, Belghiti J, de Santibanes E, Gadacz TR, Hilvano SC, Kim SW, Liau KH, Fan ST, Belli G, Sachakul V: **Need for criteria for the diagnosis and severity assessment of acute cholangitis and cholecystitis: Tokyo Guidelines.** *J Hepato-Biliary-Pancreat Surg* 2007, **14**(1):11–14.
14. Yokoe M, Takada T, Strasberg SM, Solomkin JS, Mayumi T, Gomi H, Pitt HA, Garden OJ, Kiriyama S, Hata J, Gabata T, Yoshida M, Miura F, Okamoto K, Tsuyuguchi T, Itoi T, Yamashita Y, Dervenis C, Chan AC, Lau WY, Supe AN, Belli G, Hilvano SC, Liau KH, Kim MH, Kim SW, Ker CG; Tokyo Guidelines Revision Committee: **TG13 diagnostic criteria and severity grading of acute cholecystitis (with videos).** *J Hepato-Biliary-Pancreat Sci* 2013, **20**(1):35–46.
15. Ferrarese AG, Solej M, Enrico S, Falcone A, Catalano S, Pozzi G, Marola S, Martino V: **Elective and emergency laparoscopic cholecystectomy in the elderly: our experience.** *BMC Surg* 2013, **13**(Suppl 2):S21.
16. Campanile FC, Catena F, Coccolini F, Lotti M, Piazzalunga D, Pisano M, Ansaloni L: **The need for new "patient-related" guidelines for the treatment of acute cholecystitis.** *World J Emerg Surg : WJES* 2011, **6**(1):44.
17. Agresta F, Ansaloni L, Baiocchi GL, Bergamini C, Campanile FC, Carlucci M, Cocorullo G, Corradi A, Franzato B, Lupo M, Mandalà V, Mirabella A, Pernazza G, Piccoli M, Staudacher C, Vettoretto N, Zago M, Lettieri E, Levati A, Pietrini D, Scaglione M, De Masi S, De Placido G, Francucci M, Rasi M, Fingerhut A, Uranüs S, Garattini S: **Laparoscopic approach to acute abdomen from the Consensus Development Conference of the Societa Italiana di Chirurgia Endoscopica e nuove tecnologie (SICE), Associazione Chirurghi Ospedalieri Italiani (ACOI), Societa Italiana di Chirurgia (SIC), Societa Italiana di Chirurgia d'Urgenza e del Trauma (SICUT), Societa Italiana di Chirurgia nell'Ospedalita Privata (SICOP), and the European Association for Endoscopic Surgery (EAES).** *Surg Endosc* 2012, **26**(8):2134–2164.
18. Campanile F, Carrara A, Motter M, Ansaloni L, Agresta F: **Laparoscopy and Acute Cholecystitis: The Evidence.** In *Laparoscopic Cholecystectomy.* Edited by Agresta F, Campanile FC, Vettoretto N. Springer International Publishing; 2014:59–72.
19. Johner A, Raymakers A, Wiseman SM: **Cost utility of early versus delayed laparoscopic cholecystectomy for acute cholecystitis.** *Surg Endosc* 2013, **27**(1):256–262.
20. Degrate L, Ciravegna AL, Luperto M, Guaglio M, Garancini M, Maternini M, Giordano L, Romano F, Gianotti L, Uggeri F: **Acute cholecystitis: The golden 72-h period is not a strict limit to perform early cholecystectomy. Results from 316 consecutive patients.** *Langenbeck's Arch Surg* 2013, **398**(8):1129–1136.
21. Gomes RM, Mehta NT, Varik V, Doctor NH: **No 72-hour pathological boundary for safe early laparoscopic cholecystectomy in acute cholecystitis: A clinicopathological study.** *Ann Gastroenterol* 2013, **26**(4):340–345.
22. Ambe P, Esfahani BJ, Tasci I, Christ H, Köhler L: **Is laparoscopic cholecystectomy more challenging in male patients?** *Surg Endosc Interv Tech* 2011, **25**(7):2236–2240.
23. Zhu B, Zhang Z, Wang Y, Gong K, Lu Y, Zhang N: **Comparison of laparoscopic cholecystectomy for acute cholecystitis within and beyond 72 h of symptom onset during emergency admissions.** *World J Surg* 2012, **36**(11):2654–2658.

18

The role of open abdomen in non-trauma patient: WSES Consensus Paper

Federico Coccolini[1*], Giulia Montori[1], Marco Ceresoli[1], Fausto Catena[2], Ernest E. Moore[3], Rao Ivatury[4], Walter Biffl[5], Andrew Peitzman[6], Raul Coimbra[7], Sandro Rizoli[8], Yoram Kluger[9], Fikri M. Abu-Zidan[10], Massimo Sartelli[11], Marc De Moya[12], George Velmahos[12], Gustavo Pereira Fraga[13], Bruno M. Pereira[13], Ari Leppaniemi[14], Marja A. Boermeester[15], Andrew W. Kirkpatrick[16], Ron Maier[17], Miklosh Bala[18], Boris Sakakushev[19], Vladimir Khokha[20], Manu Malbrain[21], Vanni Agnoletti[22], Ignacio Martin-Loeches[23], Michael Sugrue[24], Salomone Di Saverio[25], Ewen Griffiths[26], Kjetil Soreide[27,28], John E. Mazuski[29], Addison K. May[30], Philippe Montravers[31], Rita Maria Melotti[32], Michele Pisano[1], Francesco Salvetti[1], Gianmariano Marchesi[33], Tino M. Valetti[33], Thomas Scalea[34], Osvaldo Chiara[35], Jeffry L. Kashuk[36] and Luca Ansaloni[1]

Abstract

The open abdomen (OA) is defined as intentional decision to leave the fascial edges of the abdomen un-approximated after laparotomy (laparostomy). The abdominal contents are potentially exposed and therefore must be protected with a temporary coverage, which is referred to as temporal abdominal closure (TAC). OA use remains widely debated with many specific details deserving detailed assessment and clarification. To date, in patients with intra-abdominal emergencies, the OA has not been formally endorsed for routine utilization; although, utilization is seemingly increasing. Therefore, the World Society of Emergency Surgery (WSES), Abdominal Compartment Society (WSACS) and the Donegal Research Academy united a worldwide group of experts in an international consensus conference to review and thereafter propose the basis for evidence-directed utilization of OA management in non-trauma emergency surgery and critically ill patients. In addition to utilization recommendations, questions with insufficient evidence urgently requiring future study were identified.

Keywords: Open abdomen, Laparostomy, Non-trauma, Peritonitis, Pancreatitis, Vascular emergencies, Fistula, Nutrition, Re-exploration, Re-intervention, Closure, Biological, Synthetic, Mesh, Technique, Timing

Background

The decision by a surgeon to utilize the open abdomen (OA) technique is a dramatically non-anatomic situation that dramatically increases resource utilization and has potential severe side effects. It is, however, often dramatically effective at countering the drastically impaired physiology of critical illness when no other perceived options exist. There are both mandatory and relative indications for OA use, which are heavily influenced by the primary pathophysiologic insults and responses to intra-abdominal sepsis and inflammation, both inherent to the patient and induced through medical treatments.

* Correspondence: federico.coccolini@gmail.com
[1]General, Emergency and Trauma Surgery dept., Papa Giovanni XXIII Hospital, Piazza OMS 1, 24127 Bergamo, Italy
Full list of author information is available at the end of the article

The abdominal compartment is dramatically affected in both its contents and the characteristics of the abdominal wall. Several factors as systemic inflammatory response syndrome, increased vascular permeability, and aggressive crystalloid resuscitation predispose to fluid sequestration leading to peritoneal fluid formation. Patients with severe sepsis and septic shock commonly receive large amounts of resuscitation fluids and may develop excessive gut edema and diminished contractility and motility. These changes in combination with sequestration of second and third space fluids and forced closure of an abdominal wall with altered compliance may result in increased intra-abdominal pressure (IAP) ultimately leading to intra-abdominal hypertension (IAH) or even abdominal compartment syndrome (ACS) [1, 2].

The pathophysiologic implications of elevated IAP have been restarted to be studied in deep during the last 20 years [2–4]. In 2013, The Abdominal Compartment Society (WSACS) updated the previously published definition and guidelines for the management of intra-abdominal hypertension [5]. Elevated IAP constitutes IAH and was classified into four grades: (1) grade I IAP 12–15 mmHg, (2) grade II IAP 16–20 mmHg, (3) grade III IAP 21–25 mmHg, and (4) grade IV IAP >25 mmHg. Elevated IAP commonly causes marked deficits in loco-regional and whole body perfusion that may result in organ failure [5]. An uncontrolled IAH, with an IAP exceeding 20 mmHg and new onset organ failure, is defined as an abdominal compartment syndrome (ACS) [2, 5]. ACS is a syndrome and not a disease, as such, it can have many causes and it can occur in many disease processes, it is an all or nothing phenomenon, while IAH is a more graded continuum. ACS in turn has further effects on intra-abdominal organs, as well as indirect effects on the other organ(s) and system(s). The ACS is a potentially and frequently lethal complication characterized by effects on splanchnic, cardiovascular, pulmonary, renal, and central nervous systems [2, 5]. While medical therapies should be attempted, the ACS is rapidly lethal and opening of the abdominal cavity conducted promptly if medical interventions do not quickly alleviate or temporize the situation. If surgery has been undertaken for the index disease, leaving the abdomen temporarily open is often required to prevent inducing ACS in a critically ill pro-inflammatory patient with visceral edema and ongoing resuscitation. Whether leaving the abdomen open will primarily influence the septic response is also intriguing but unproven at the present time.

The OA procedure is defined as intentionally leaving the fascial edges of the abdomen un-approximated (laparostomy). The abdominal contents are exposed and thus must be protected with a temporary coverage, which is itself termed a temporary abdominal coverage (TAC) [2, 6]. The OA technique, when used appropriately, may be useful in the management of surgical patients with compromised general conditions due to any critical illness/injury but most frequently cases of intra-abdominal sepsis and severe pancreatitis are seen recently [7]. Despite many serious potential complications, the OA is perceived to be a life-saving intervention in catastrophically injured patients [2]. Compared to trauma patients, however, patients undergoing OA management for intra-abdominal non-trauma emergencies have greater risks subsequent to OA utilization, including entero-atmospheric fistula (EAF) and a "frozen abdomen", intra-abdominal abscesses, and lower rates of definitive fascial closure [8, 9] with resultant large ventral hernia defects. This discrepancy in risks and benefits, along with economic considerations [10], was the primary reason the WSACS suggested not routinely using the OA for septic cases versus traumatic cases [5]. Thus, every effort should be exerted to attempt abdominal closure as soon as the patient can physiologically tolerate it.

Methods

The recommendations are formulated and graded according to the *modified Grading of Recommendations Assessment, Development and Evaluation* (GRADE) hierarchy of evidence from the GRADE Group, summarized in the Table 1 [11].

The WSES and Abdominal Compartment Society together with the Donegal Research Academy united a group of subject-matter experts coordinated by a central coordinator to review and summarize the evidence and thereafter to express their evidence-based opinion on important issues concerning OA utilization in non-trauma patients:

Which non-trauma patients can benefit from OA techniques and for which specific critical conditions is indicated (example, peritonitis, vascular emergencies, and severe pancreatitis)?

What is the optimum TAC technique for use in non-trauma patients?

Is there a role for fluid instillation?

What is the optimum timing of re-exploration before definitive closure in non-trauma patients?

What is the optimum timing to definitively close an OA in non-trauma patients?

What are the optimum adjunctive techniques to definitively close an OA in non-trauma patients considering both non-mesh-mediated techniques and mesh-mediated techniques?

What is the optimum treatment to treat frozen abdomen and enteral fistulas?

What nutritional support is indicated in OA?

A central project coordinator compiled the answers and statements derived from the first round of presentations and discussions. The statements were discussed during the Consensus Conference held in Dublin (Ireland) in July 2016. Once an agreement was reached within the experts groups, a final round of discussion among a larger group of experts led to the final version of recommendations reflecting the final expert-consensus document (Table 2).

Open abdomen in peritonitis

The open abdomen is an option for emergency surgery patients with severe peritonitis and septic shock under the following circumstances: abbreviated laparotomy due to the severe physiological derangement, or the need for a deferred intestinal anastomosis or a planned second look

Table 1 "Modified Grading of Recommendations Assessment, Development and Evaluation (GRADE)" hierarchy of evidence from the American College of Chest Physicians task force by Guyatt and colleagues [11]

Grade of recommendation	Clarity of risk/benefit	Quality of supporting evidence	Implications
1A			
Strong recommendation, highquality evidence	Benefits clearly outweigh risk and burdens, or vice versa	RCTs without important limitations or overwhelming evidence from observational studies	Strong recommendation, applies to most patients in most circumstances without reservation
1B			
Strong recommendation, moderate-quality evidence	Benefits clearly outweigh risk and burdens, or vice versa	RCTs with important limitations (inconsistent results, methodological flaws, indirect analyses or imprecise conclusions) or exceptionally strong evidence from observational studies	Strong recommendation, applies to most patients in most circumstances without reservation
1C			
Strong recommendation, lowquality or very lowquality evidence	Benefits clearly outweigh risk and burdens, or vice versa	Observational studies or case series	Strong recommendation but subject to change when higher quality evidence becomes available
2A			
Weak recommendation, high-quality evidence	Benefits closely balanced with risks and burden	RCTs without important limitations or overwhelming evidence from observational studies	Weak recommendation, best action may differ depending on the patient, treatment circumstances, or social values
2B			
Weak recommendation, moderate-quality evidence	Benefits closely balanced with risks and burden	RCTs with important limitations (inconsistent results, methodological flaws, indirect or imprecise) or exceptionally strong evidence from observational studies	Weak recommendation, best action may differ depending on the patient, treatment circumstances, or social values
2C			
Weak recommendation, Low-quality or very lowquality evidence	Uncertainty in the estimates of benefits, risks, and burden; benefits, risk, and burden may be closely balanced	Observational studies or case series	Very weak recommendation; alternative treatments may be equally reasonable and merit consideration

for intestinal ischemia, or persistent source of peritonitis (failure of source control), or extensive visceral edema with the concern for development of abdominal compartment syndrome (grade 2C).

In severe secondary peritonitis, some patients may experience a disease progression to severe sepsis and septic shock experiencing progressive organ dysfunction, hypotension, myocardial depression, and coagulopathy and a staged approach may be required [12]. These are often hemodynamically unstable and unfit for immediate complex surgical interventions [12]. If the patient is not in a condition to be undergone to a definitive repair and/or abdominal wall closure, the intervention should be abbreviated due to suboptimal local conditions for healing and global susceptibility to spiraling organ failure. For instance, intestinal continuity restoration can be deferred to a subsequent surgical intervention, which is particularly important in hypotensive patients who are receiving inotropes [13]. In facing the impossibility to completely obtain a source control of the contamination in a single operation or if extensive visceral edema and decreased abdominal wall compliance increases the risk of ACS development, primary fascial closure should not be attempted and the abdomen should be left open [14]. The rationale for using the OA is to leave the abdomen open and to treat the infected peritoneal cavity like an "open abscess" with subsequent re-operations involving generous irrigations and potentially active TAC techniques [15] to definitively control the contamination while also preventing IAH progression to ACS. No definitive data exist about the management of severe peritonitis with the open abdomen. Robledo et al. compared open versus closed abdomen procedures in 40 patients with severe secondary peritonitis; no significant differences in mortality rates were found (55% open vs. 30% closed). The study was interrupted at the first interim analysis for high relative risk and odds ratios for death in the open group (1.83 and 2.85, respectively) [16]. However, the TAC technique that was selected as the "intervention" would be relatively contraindicated in current OA management. Some other

Table 2 Statement Grid

	Statements
Open Abdomen indication:	
➢ Peritonitis	The open abdomen is an option for emergency surgery patients with severe peritonitis and septic shock under the following circumstances: abbreviated laparotomy due to the severe physiological derangement, or the need for a deferred intestinal anastomosis or a planned second look for intestinal ischemia, or persistent source of peritonitis (failure of source control), or extensive visceral edema with the concern for development of abdominal compartment syndrome (Grade 2C).
➢ Vascular Emergencies	The open abdomen should be strongly considered following management of hemorrhagic vascular catastrophes such as ruptured abdominal aortic aneurysm (Grade 1C) The open abdomen should be considered following surgical management of acute mesenteric ischemic insults (Grade 2C).
➢ Pancreatitis	In patients with severe acute pancreatitis unresponsive to step-up conservative management surgical decompression and leaving the abdomen open is effective in treating abdominal compartment syndrome (Grade 2C) Leaving the abdomen open after surgical necrosectomy for infected pancreatic necrosis is not recommended excepted in those situation at high risk of abdominal compartment syndrome (Grade 1C)
Optimal technique for temporary abdominal closure	Negative pressure wound therapy with continuous fascial traction is suggested as the preferred technique for temporary abdominal closure (Grade 1B). Temporary Abdominal Closure without Negative pressure wound therapy (e.g., mesh alone, Bogota bag) whenever possible should NOT be applied for the purpose of temporary abdominal closure, because of low delayed fascial closure rate and being accompanied by a significant intestinal fistula rate (Grade 1B).
Is there a role for NPWT with Fluid Instillation?	There is inadequate evidence to make a recommendation regarding use of negative pressure wound therapy in combination with fluid instillation in patients with temporary abdominal closure (NOT GRADED).
Planning re-exploration before definitive closure	- In critically ill non-trauma patients with open abdomen, once any requirements for on-going resuscitation have ameliorated, early re-operation with the intention of closing the abdomen should be given a high priority (Grade 1C). - In critically ill patients with open abdomen, re-laparotomy with concern for ongoing ischemia/ contamination reoperation should be conducted no later than 24–48 h after the index operation, with the duration from the index operation shortening with increasing degrees of patient non-improvement and hemodynamic instability (Grade 1C).
Best timing to definitively close an open abdomen	- Fascia should be closed as soon as possible (Grade 1C). - Acidosis (pH <7.25), hypothermia (temperature < 34 °C) and coagulopathy (TEG, INR) are not predictive of the need for maintaining the open abdomen in non-trauma patients (Grade 2A). - The abdomen should be maintained open in non-trauma patients if the source of contamination persists, if a condition of haemodynamic instability persists meaning in presence of on-going fluid resuscitation or vasopressor support necessity, if a deferred intestinal anastomosis is needed, if there is the necessity for a planned second look for ischemic intestine and lastly if there are concerns about abdominal compartment syndrome development (Grade 2C). - Early fascia closure (within 7 days) should be the strategy for management of the open abdomen once the source control has been reached, the severe sepsis has been controlled meaning that the patient is haemodynamically stable and the hypoperfusion has been definitively corrected, no further surgical re-exploration is needed and there are no concerns for abdominal compartment syndrome (Grade 2C).
Best solution to definitively close an open abdomen	
➢ *Non-mesh mediated techniques*	- Primary fascia closure is the ideal solution to restore the abdominal closure (2A). - Component separation is an effective technique; however, it's early use is NOT recommended in fascial temporary closure. It should be considered only for definitive closure or reconstructive interventions (Grade 2C) - Planned ventral hernia (skin graft or skin closure only) remains an option for complicated open abdomen (i.e. in the presence of entero-atmospheric fistula or in cases with a protracted open abdomen due to underlying diseases) or in those low resource setting where no other facilities are present (Grade 2C)
➢ *Mesh mediated techniques*	- A fascial bridge using prosthetic mesh (polypropylene, polytetrafluoruroethylene (PTFE) and polyester products) should NOTt be recommended to achieve definitive fascial closure in patients with open abdomen and should be placed only in patients without other alternatives (Grade 1B). - Biologic meshes are reliable for definitive abdominal wall reconstruction in the presence of a large wall defect, bacterial contamination, comorbidities and difficult wound healing. NPWT can be used combined with biologic mesh to facilitate granulation and skin closure (Grade 2B). - Non–cross-linked biologic meshes seem to be preferred in sublay position when the linea alba can be reconstructed. Non–cross-linked biologic mesh is easily integrated, with reduced fibrotic reaction and lesser infection and removal rate (Grade 2B).

Table 2 Statement Grid *(Continued)*

	- The long-term outcome of a bridging non–cross-linked biologic mesh is laxity of the abdominal wall and a high rate of recurrent ventral hernia. In the bridge position (no linea alba closure), cross-linked biologic meshes maybe associated with less ventral hernia recurrence (Grade 2B).
Best treatment for open abdomen and entero-atmospheric fistulas	- Several clinical circumstances may contribute to the development of entero-atmospheric fistula and few risk factors may predict its development. Awareness of this complication and avoidance of contributing conditions for its development are mandatory; moreover preemptive measures are imperative (Grade 1C). - The management of entero-atmospheric fistula should be personalized according to standard classification and grading system. Current different classification schemes echo the problematic and challenging issues related to their management (Grade 1C) - The caloric intake and protein demands of patients with entero-atmospheric fistula increase; the Nitrogen balance should be corrected and protein supplemented. Nutrition should be started immediately upon recognition of entero-atmospheric fistula (Grade 1C) - Entero-atmospheric fistula effluent isolation is essential for proper wound healing. Separating the wound into different compartments in order to facilitate the collection of fistula output is of paramount importance (Grade 2A). - Many methods for wound care exist; however in the presence of entero-atmospheric fistula in open abdomen, negative pressure wound therapy makes effluent isolation feasible and wound healing conceivable (Grade 2A). Definitive management of entero-atmospheric fistula should be delayed to after the patient has recovered and the wound completely healed (Grade 1C).
Nutritional support	- Open abdomen patients are in a hyper-metabolic condition; an immediate and adequate nutritional support is mandatory (Grade 1C). - Open abdomen techniques result in a significant nitrogen loss that must be replaced with a balanced nutrition regimen (Grade 1C). - Early enteral nutrition should be started as soon as possible if the gastrointestinal tract allows (Grade 1C). - Enteral nutrition should be delayed in patients with high output fistula with no possibility to obtain feeding access distal to the fistula (Grade 2C) - Oral feeding is not contraindicated; whenever it's possible it could be started as soon as the patient is able to eat (Grade 2C).
Patient Mobilization	- To date, no recommendations can be made about early mobilization of patients with open abdomen.

cohort studies showed the effectiveness of OA technique in treating severe peritonitis. At present, however, no definitive data from randomized trials exist.

Open abdomen in vascular emergencies

The open abdomen should be strongly considered following management of hemorrhagic vascular catastrophes such as ruptured abdominal aortic aneurysm (grade 1C).

The open abdomen should be considered following surgical management of acute mesenteric ischemic insults (grade 2C).

The ACS has been well described in the setting of ruptured abdominal aortic aneurysm (rAAA) [17]. Rupture of aortic as well as iliac or visceral aneurysm often results in life-threatening hemorrhagic shock. The combination of severe shock and massive resuscitation contributes to retroperitoneal, mesenteric, and bowel wall edema and production of ascites that can increase abdominal pressure and lead to ACS. Intra-abdominal hypertension occurs in up to 50% of patients following AAA repair, and ACS occurs in 8–20%. Mortality after rAAA is as high as 30–50%; of note, mortality is generally twice as high among patients who develop ACS compared with those who do not [18].

Consequently, prevention of ACS, if possible, would be of tremendous benefit to the patient.

In prospective non-randomized studies, the incidence of ACS is reduced when prophylactic OA is employed [19]. Unfortunately, selection criteria for employing OA are not well defined; the surgeon might consider inability to close the fascia without tension; use of aortic balloon occlusion catheter; and preoperative blood loss >5 L [19, 20]. Such criteria should prompt the surgeon to consider temporary OA utilization. When the abdomen is closed primarily, postoperative monitoring of IAP is recommended, with vigilance for ACS as reflected by elevated airway pressures, reduced cardiac output, or oliguria. Concerns for infection of aortic grafts with OA are allayed by existing data, indicating a relatively low rate [21]. Patients are often selected for endovascular repair (EVAR) of rAAA if they have less hemodynamic compromise. Although it is less common, ACS still occurs after EVAR [17]. The major risk factor appears to be massive resuscitation. These patients should have vigilant monitoring for elevated IAP and the onset of ACS.

Mesenteric ischemia may result from arterial (thrombotic, embolic, or low perfusion) or venous (venous thrombosis) insults. Fundamental principles of management include making the diagnosis, restoration of intestinal perfusion, and assessment of bowel viability with resection as necessary. The bowel ischemia leads to bowel wall and mesenteric edema, as well as ascites production; reperfusion of the bowel can exacerbate bowel edema and ascites and thus increase risk of ACS. For this reason, OA use should be considered following restoration of perfusion in a patient with acute mesenteric ischemia. As there are no reliable independent predictors of ACS in this setting, the surgeon should assess bowel swelling and the patient's physiology to make this decision [22, 23]. Another reason to consider temporary OA following mesenteric ischemia is to facilitate second-look laparotomy to assess bowel viability and perform bowel anastomosis as needed [24]. Bowel resection is much less common in the setting of venous thrombosis than arterial occlusion, so the patients with mesenteric venous thrombosis probably do not require OA as often as those with acute arterial occlusion [25]; although, IAP should be followed.

Open abdomen in pancreatitis

In patients with severe acute pancreatitis unresponsive to step-up conservative management, surgical decompression and leaving the abdomen open is effective in treating abdominal compartment syndrome (grade 2C).

Leaving the abdomen open after surgical necrosectomy for infected pancreatic necrosis is not recommended except in those situations at high risk of abdominal compartment syndrome (grade 1C).

Acute pancreatitis (AP) is a mild self-limiting disease in the majority of cases, even though the 15% of patients with AP progress to severe disease identified by development of persistent organ failure [26]. Multiple organ failure (MOF) is the factor mainly associated to mortality in AP, as a counterpart in absence of organ dysfunction or if it transient the risk of dying is very low [27–29]. However, in those with severe AP, MOF develops generally early, with over half of the patients exhibiting organ dysfunction's signs at hospital admission and in any case, most part of them develops within the first 4 days after admission [28, 30]. More than half of the deaths happen within the first week from onset of AP and generally within a week after MOF first symptoms [31]. Principal treatments of MOF are support therapies: vasopressors, fluid replacement, and renal replacement therapy and mechanical ventilation if indicated. During AP, IAH/ACS may aggravate MOF, and therefore, constant IAP measurements are crucial to identify patients with high risk of developing ACS [32]. ACS should be prevented and treated, whenever possible, with non-operative management. Surgical decompression is the last but the most effective tool to decrease the IAP, and it should not be postponed if the patient presents ACS manifestation [5, 33].

In the event of AP, the risk to develop subsequent infections (i.e., bacteremia, pneumonia and infection of pancreatic or peripancreatic necrosis) is increased. The first week of illness is crucial for the extra-pancreatic infection occurrence, whereas pancreatic necrosis usually becomes infected later [34]. Some factors are associated to an increased risk of infected necrosis: the presence of organ failure, early bacteremia, and the extent of pancreatic necrosis [34]. Surgical necrosectomy is the last resort if more conservative management including percutaneous drainage failure [35]. Patients with persistent organ failure complicated with infected pancreatic necrosis face a very high mortality risk [36].

Optimal technique for temporary abdominal closure

Negative pressure wound therapy with continuous fascial traction is suggested as the preferred technique for temporary abdominal closure (grade 1B).

Temporary abdominal closure without negative pressure wound therapy (e.g., *mesh alone, Bogota bag) whenever possible should NOT be applied for the purpose of temporary abdominal closure, because of low delayed fascial closure rate and being accompanied by a significant intestinal fistula rate (grade 1B).*

There is inadequate evidence to make a recommendation regarding use of negative pressure wound therapy in combination with fluid instillation in patients with temporary abdominal closure (NOT GRADED).

The perceived indications and subsequent treatment choices in managing OA differ among surgeons. The existing techniques result in different risk of entero-atmospheric fistula (EAF) and the different rate of delayed fascial closure. Overall, 74 relevant studies exist for a total of 4358 patients: 3461 (79%) with peritonitis. The described OA indications are considerably different. Thirty-eight out of 78 series described negative pressure wound therapy (NPWT) TAC systems. NPWT with a dynamic component (mesh-mediated fascial traction or dynamic sutures) gives the best results in terms of delayed fascial closure, but dynamic sutures result more often in fistula. NPWT without a dynamic component (Barker's VAC or commercial products) for the use of temporary fascial closure has a moderate delayed fascial closure rate and a fistula rate similar to mesh closure without NPWT.

Several TAC techniques exist that could be used alone or combined together. Six-eight series reported about one TAC technique. Ten series described patients managed with combined TAC systems. NPWT was used alone in 32 studies [37–68], and in 6 studies, NWPT is combined with fascial traction (mesh or sutures) [69–74] and eight series described the use of meshes (non-absorbable and/or absorbable) [75–81]. Six series reported about the Bogota-bag use [75, 82–86]; five, about Zipper [87–91]; and other five, about dynamic retention sutures [92–96]. Two more series described loose packing [97, 98]. Lastly, the Wittmann patch was used in one series [99]. The remnant three series applied different TAC systems [82, 100, 101]. The delayed fascial closure rate ranged from 3.2 to 100%.

Twenty-two series were prospective, and ten out of them described NPWT (608 patients) showing a weighted fascial closure rate of 53.9% and an EAF rate of 9.8%. The four prospective series on NPWT with fascial traction (411 patients) showed a weighted fascial closure rate of 77.8% and an EAF rate of 4.3%. Including retrospective studies data per closure type are in line with the aforementioned results. With the highest weighted fascial closure rate for NPWT with fascial traction (73.1%) and dynamic retention sutures (73.6%). TAC using a mesh or zipper showed the lowest delayed closure rates (34.2 and 34.0% respectively). Nine series were not exhaustive in describing eventual fascial closure attempts [16, 45, 75, 81, 87, 89, 98, 102, 103].

Is there a role for NPWT with fluid instillation?

There are no series published on the use of NPWT with instillation in situations of TAC in non-trauma patients or in trauma patients. Recently, a systematic review performed by an expert consensus group has been published underlining the need of more evidence to support the fluid instillation and giving no recommendation of its use in abdominal wound [104].

Planning re-exploration before definitive closure

In critically ill non-trauma patients with open abdomen, once any requirements for on-going resuscitation have ameliorated, early re-operation with the intention of closing the abdomen should be given a high priority (grade 1C).

In critically ill patients with open abdomen, re-laparotomy with concern for ongoing ischemia/contamination re-operation should be conducted no later than 24–48 h after the index operation, with the duration from the index operation shortening with increasing degrees of patient non-improvement and hemodynamic instability (grade 1C).

A related question for clinicians is when to re-operate (if ever) for the sole purpose of "revise" when there is recognition that closing an abdomen will not be possible. This question may be further conceptually complicated in an attempt to distinguish indications to re-operate because the patient is not improving or deteriorating and there is fear that contamination or ischemia is ongoing and those cases of non-improvement or only modest improvement in whom there is operation intention to "wash" the peritoneal cavity and to "change" the TAC dressing or device. No RCTs or meta-analyses examining the timing of re-operation in OA patients exist. Guidelines and review papers did not generally discuss timing of re-operation [8, 105]. In the position paper of the WSES, it is recommended that as a general principle, patients should be taken back to the operating room at 24–48 h after the initial surgery [2]. Other expert opinions come from the survey of Trauma Association of Canada in 2006, and the majority of responders indicated the best timing included between 24 and 72 h [106, 107]. Pommerening et al. utilized the American Association for the Surgery of Trauma (AAST) Open Abdomen Registry to evaluate time to the first re-operation on trauma OA patients as a predictor of primary fascial closure using a hierarchical multivariate logistic regression analysis [108]. Adjusting for other factors, including resuscitation volumes, increasing delay to the first re-operation was associated with a decreased likelihood of primary fascial closure (PFC), with a 1.1% decrease in PFC rates for every hour after 24 h from the index operation [108]. Further, there was a trend (95% CI 1.0–3.25 OR) of increased complications in patients having the first re-operation after 48 h [108].

It should be clearly understood however that extrapolation of these findings regarding the timing of re-operation in trauma patients might not be directly applicable to non-trauma patients with OA. It is becoming apparent that infected and non-infected patients with auto-activation of the immune responses leading to multi-organ dysfunction syndrome (MODS) and MOF have more fundamental differences than previously appreciated [109]. Fundamental evidences from basic science are emerging justifying the OA in critically ill/injured patents in order to manipulate the systemic immune response and ameliorate the bio mediator burdens of catastrophic illness [110–113]. There are also newly described populations of fully mature indwelling peritoneal macrophages that migrate locally within the peritoneal cavity within an hour of injury [114]. Whether mechanically removing such cell populations through scheduled "wash-outs" is beneficial or harmful is a completely unstudied question. Thus, the timing of re-operation is more complex in non-trauma patients and urgently requires further study. Lastly, in critically ill patients with an OA, re-laparotomy with the intention of cleaning or "washing-out" the abdomen has an unknown priority and should be subjected to future randomized study.

Best timing to definitively close an open abdomen

Fascia should be closed as soon as possible (grade 1C).

Acidosis (pH <7.25), hypothermia (temperature <34 °C), and coagulopathy (TEG, INR) are not predictive of the need for maintaining the open abdomen in non-trauma patients (grade 2A).

The abdomen should be maintained open in non-trauma patients if the source of contamination persists, if a condition of hemodynamic instability persists meaning in the presence of an on-going fluid resuscitation or vasopressor support necessity, if a deferred intestinal anastomosis is needed, if there is the necessity for a planned second look for ischemic intestine, and lastly if there are concerns about abdominal compartment syndrome development (grade 2C).

Early fascia closure (within 7 days) should be the strategy for management of the open abdomen once the source control has been reached, the severe sepsis has been controlled meaning that the patient is hemodynamically stable and the hypoperfusion has been definitively corrected, no further surgical re-exploration is needed, and there are no concerns for abdominal compartment syndrome (grade 2C).

The early definitive abdominal closure is the first goal to achieve in order to reduce the OA complications rate [115], (i.e., EAF, fascial retraction with loss of abdominal wall domain, and incisional hernias) [115, 116]. The primary closure rates have a bimodal distribution, with early closure depending on postoperative intensive care management and delayed closure depending on the choice of the TAC technique [117]. Mortality, complications, and length of stay were compared between early and delayed fascial closure in a meta-analysis [118]. 3125 patients were included and 1942 (62%) successfully achieved early fascial closure. Early fascial closure is a factor significantly associated with a reduced mortality (12.3 versus 24.8%, RR 0.53, $P < 0.0001$) and complication rate (RR, 0.68, $P < 0.0001$). Early fascial closure is commonly performed within 4–7 days of the initial laparostomy [13]. No major technical difficulties are described to obtain primary fascial closure within few days from the index operation. Patients having abdominal sepsis are less likely to achieve an early fascial closure [119] and therefore should have closure attempts performed as soon as possible after severe abdominal sepsis is controlled [120].

Best solution to definitively close an open abdomen

Often the OA, particularly if prolonged, results in fascia retraction and consequently in large abdominal wall defects that require complex abdominal wall reconstruction. Moreover, the situation is often complicated by a contaminated field [121] with high risk of infections and wound complications, such as wound infections, seromas, fistula formation, recurrence of the defect, and mortality [122–124].

Non-mesh-mediated techniques

Primary fascia closure is the ideal solution to restore the abdominal closure (grade 2A).

Component separation is an effective technique; however, its early use is NOT recommended in fascial temporary closure. It should be considered only for definitive closure or reconstructive interventions (grade 2C).

Planned ventral hernia (skin graft or skin closure only) remains an option for complicated open abdomen (i.e., in the presence of entero-atmospheric fistula or in cases with a protracted open abdomen due to underlying diseases) or in those low-resource setting where no other facilities are present (grade 2C).

Abdominal component separation is most commonly considered an elective procedure for ventral hernia repair [118]. One important technique described for the reconstruction of the abdominal wall is the component separation. The technique of anterior component separation consists in a relaxing incision made in the aponeurosis of the external oblique muscle, a separation of the external and internal oblique muscle and the incision of the rectus fascia to achieve the advancement of the abdominal wall to cover the defect. This technique has been well studied and described in elective giant ventral hernia repair, and it provides an effective technique with a recurrence rate of 16% [125, 126] but a very relevant complication rate of 50%. Other surgical techniques that have been described include the posterior component separation: the rectus sheath is opened and the posterior rectus fascia and rectus muscle are separated. At the lateral margin of the rectus muscle, the aponeurosis of the transverse abdominis muscle is incised with the separation of the internal oblique muscle from the transverse abdominis muscle.

However, the use of abdominal component separation technique was recently described in acute fascia closure after open abdomen in a small case series by Rasilainen et al. [127] with 75% of primary fascia closure. At present, there is not enough evidence to support component separation in the acute setting due to the related high morbidity and the fact that these techniques can only be performed on a patient once, so that if ill timed, future options are not available. Therefore, a valuable alternative option for closure of the open abdomen remains the planned ventral hernia: its main goal is to cover abdominal viscera to prevent complications such as EAF. The abdominal wall defect could be closed only with skin suture and or a skin graft put on the underlying granulating tissue creating a planned laxity. After physiologic recovery and a significant period of scar and adhesion maturation, the complete restoration of the patient's abdominal wall through reconstructive techniques can be undertaken as an elective procedure.

Mesh-mediated techniques

A fascial bridge using prosthetic mesh (polypropylene, polytetrafluoruroethylene (PTFE) and polyester products) should not be recommended to achieve definitive fascial closure in patients with open abdomen and should be placed only in patients without other alternatives (grade 1B).

Biologic meshes are reliable for definitive abdominal wall reconstruction in the presence of a large wall defect, bacterial contamination, comorbidities, and difficult wound healing. NPWT can be used combined with biologic mesh to facilitate granulation and skin closure (grade 2B).

Non-cross-linked biologic meshes seem to be preferred in sublay position when the linea alba can be reconstructed. Non-cross-linked biologic mesh is easily integrated, with reduced fibrotic reaction and lesser infection and removal rate (grade 2B).

The long-term outcome of a bridging non-cross-linked biologic mesh is laxity of the abdominal wall and a high rate of recurrent ventral hernia. In the bridge position (no linea alba closure), cross-linked biologic meshes maybe associated with less ventral hernia recurrence (grade 2B).

Two meta-analyses exist on BP in abdominal wall defect. The first, by Sharrock et al. investigated the management and closure of OA in trauma patients [128]. Among the included studies, the point estimate recurrence rate of ventral hernia after 1 year of BP positioning was 51%. However, the authors highlighted the small number of included studies and their poor quality; moreover, as above mentioned, great differences exist between trauma and septic patients and great caution should be addressed in interpretation of this result. A systematic review and meta-analysis by Atema et al. [129] investigated the utilization of BP in abdominal wall reconstruction. They clearly stated that the poor quantity and quality of available data strongly limits taking a clear message from the results. Biological material in infected fields had a recurrence rate of 30% compared with 7% of synthetic material, but data were derived from a single study and does not justify the use of synthetic materials, especially as a bridge position after OA.

The "bridging" technique refers to using some mesh (either prosthetic or biologic) to physically interpose between native abdominal wall fascia that either cannot or should not be primarily opposed. Thus, such fascial defects can be closed with a mesh in a bridging position. In general, non-absorbable synthetic materials (i.e., polypropylene mesh) reinforce any fascial repair through a combination of mechanical tension and intense inflammatory reaction, resulting in the entrapment of the mesh into scar tissue. However, in a bridging position, there is no native tissue to protect viscera from the mesh and thus, the persistent inflammatory response combined with the contaminated field may induce local side effects such as adhesions, erosions, and fistula formation [130–135]. International guidelines on emergency repair of abdominal wall hernia therefore do *not* recommend the use of synthetic meshes in contaminated fields [136].

Biological prosthesis (BP) has been designed to perform as permanent surgical prosthesis in the abdominal wall repair, minimizing mesh-related complications [137]. The rationale of their usage in OA is based on the premise that the implantation of a biologic material triggers a cascade of events leading to new healthy tissue deposition and prosthesis remodeling. The presence of vital tissue therefore allows for perfusion and a native immune response preventing mesh infection and abscess formations. The ideal BP will also maintain mechanical characteristics of a synthetic mesh with a sufficient mechanical strength to withstand the physiological and anatomic stresses of the human abdominal wall. Such an ideal BP should also tolerate adjunctive NPWT to facilitate wound healing, granulation, and skin closure [100, 138].

Discordant data have been published about the use of BP to bridge a wide defect of the abdominal wall. The evidence is limited with few studies, all non-randomized, and with an overall small number of cases. Further among heterogeneous patients reported, recurrence rates have ranged between 0 and 100% [139–152]. When used as a bridge to close the fascia defect, the reported recurrence rate in a large retrospective series was >80% [153]. Another study by Booth and colleagues compared primary fascia closure with mesh reinforcement with the use of the mesh as a bridge and demonstrated a higher recurrence rate in the mesh in a bridge position (8 vs. 56%, $p < 0.001$) [154].

Several studies investigated the best anatomical position in terms of BP function, but were not specifically focused on OA reconstruction. Nonetheless, evidence, including that from randomized trials, suggest that implanting the BP in the sublay position results in a lower recurrence and complication rate [155–157]. However, it should be stressed that the data included was not specific for the OA situation and the heterogeneity among patients and indications was very high, resulting in a poor level of evidence.

Two meta-analyses exist on BP in abdominal wall defect. The first, by Sharrock et al. investigated the management and closure of OA in trauma patients [128]. Among the included studies, the point estimate recurrence rate of ventral hernia after 1 year of BP positioning was 51%. However, the authors highlighted the small number of included studies and their poor quality; moreover, as above mentioned, great differences exists between trauma and septic patients and great caution should be addressed in interpretation of this result.

A systematic review and meta-analysis by Atema et al. [129] investigated the utilization of BP in abdominal wall reconstruction; the poor quantity and quality of available data strongly limits the results. Biological material in infected fields had a recurrence rate of 30% compared with 7% of synthetic material, but data were derived from a single study and does not justify the use of synthetic materials, especially as a bridge position after OA.

In conclusion, no definitive evidence-based conclusions could be obtained currently from the literature. The

BJORK CLSSIFICATION 2009		BJORK CLASSIFICATION 2016	
GRADE	DESCRIPTION	GRADE	DESCRIPTION
1 A	Clean OA without adherence between bowel and abdominal wall or fixity	1 A	Clean OA without adherence between bowel and abdominal wall or fixity
B	Contaminated OA without adherence/fixity	B	Contaminated OA without adherence/fixity
		C	Enteric leak, no fixation
2 A	Clean OA developing adherence/fixity	2 A	Clean OA developing adherence/fixity
B	Contaminated OA developing adherence/fixity	B	Contaminated OA developing adherence/fixity
		C	Enteric leak, developing fixation
3 A	OA complicated by fistula formation	3 A	Clean, frozen abdomen
		B	Contaminated, frozen abdomen
4	Frozen OA with adherent/fixed bowel; unable to close surgically; with or without fistula	4	Established enteroatmospheric fistula, frozen abdomen

Fig. 1 Open Abdomen classification according to Bjork et al. [168]

available evidence is really weak: most of the cited meta-analysis included rather poor quality retrospective case series. There is also great heterogeneity among the indications for mesh implantation, the anatomic positioning of the mesh, and the type of mesh. This further weakens the quality of the evidences. Thus, well-performed randomized trials comparing different type of meshes and the techniques of mesh positioning are urgently required.

Best treatment for open abdomen and entero-atmospheric fistulas

Several clinical circumstances may contribute to the development of entero-atmospheric fistula and few risk factors may predict its development. Awareness of this complication and avoidance of contributing conditions for its development are mandatory; moreover, preemptive measures are imperative (grade 1C).

The management of entero-atmospheric fistula should be personalized according to standard classification and grading system. Current different classification schemes echo the problematic and challenging issues related to their management (grade 1C).

The caloric intake and protein demands of patients with entero-atmospheric fistula increase; the nitrogen balance should be corrected and protein supplemented. Nutrition should be started immediately upon recognition of entero-atmospheric fistula (grade 1C).

Entero-atmospheric fistula effluent isolation is essential for proper wound healing. Separating the wound into different compartments in order to facilitate the collection of fistula output is of paramount importance (grade 2A).

Many methods for wound care exist; however, in the presence of entero-atmospheric fistula in an open abdomen, negative pressure wound therapy makes effluent isolation feasible and wound healing conceivable (grade 2A).

Definitive management of entero-atmospheric fistula should be delayed to after the patient has recovered and the wound completely healed (grade 1C).

Enteric fistula is a severe complication following abdominal surgery. The opening of a fistula onto dehisced wound therefore exposing and communicating the bowel and its effluent to the atmosphere is defined as EAF. The incidence of EAF varies from 4.5 to 25% in the trauma setting [158] and from 5.7 and 17.2% in non-trauma patients [105]. The presence of this complication dramatically increases considerably mortality, length of stays, and costs [159].

Many factors may contribute to the development of EAF. All linked as a "vicious cycle": the lack of overlying soft tissue, with its blood supply, precludes spontaneous healing and the exposed viscera predispose to additional disruptions in the gastrointestinal tract. EAFs may result from various etiologies: anastomotic dehiscence or disruption, iatrogenic injury during dissection or inappropriate handling, and presence of synthetic prosthetic material (i.e., mesh) and from the prolonged exposure of bowel [160–163]. ACS and severe IAH may result in reduced bowel blood supply and therefore contribute to EAF development [68]. A prospective analysis of 517 trauma emergency laparotomies showed that large bowel resections, large volume fluid resuscitation (>5 L/24 h), and increased number of re-explorations were significantly associated with an increased incidence of EAF

[158]. Preemptive measures could be undertaken in order to prevent this complication: early abdominal wall closure, bowel coverage with omentum or skin, and no direct application of NPWT on the viscera are some of these measures [112, 164, 165].

Several classifications and grading systems of EAF exist. Schein and Decker proposed in 1991 a grading system based on the fistula location. Grade IV indicates a fistula related to large abdominal wall defects with grades IVa and IVb indicating the site of the fistula in regards to its location [166]. EAF can be classified based on the fistula effluent output: low (<200 ml/day), moderate (200-500 ml/day), and high (>500 ml/day) [167]. Bjork et al. proposed a classification based on the presence of adhesions of the bowel in the setup of the open abdomen as well as the association to the fistula formation (Fig. 1), and this was later adapted by WSACS [168]. Di Saverio et al. proposed a comprehensive classification based on the combination of different criteria as anatomical location, output, exposure, and number of fistulas [169]. As a general principle, a single, superficial fistula located in the lower GI tract with a low output has a higher probability of spontaneous closure rather than multiple fistulas deep in the wound with high output [169, 170]. According to this principle, the management should be tailored to each clinical situation and individualized accordingly. In conclusion, the presence of several different classifications represents the true difficulties in the management of EAF in OA. Level of evidence is poor and many recommendations are based on expert opinion suggestions.

EAF is a poorly predictable and, above all, avoidable complication. When patients develop EAF, an accurate and tailored management scheme should be adopted. Nutrition plays a key role in the management of these patients and should be always kept in mind as a fundamental part of the treatment. The open abdomen strategy may result in fluid and electrolytes loss resulting in acid-base derangements [8]. The anatomy and the characteristics of the EAF(s) should be defined in order to plan the best treatment option [171]. Parenteral nutrition (TPN) should be started immediately after the patient resuscitation. Enteral nutrition in OA patients has been well studied demonstrating a reduction in infectious complications preserving the intestinal mucosal barrier and its immunological function [172–174]. Enteral nutrition in patients with an EAF is has but may increase fistula output. Only small series of patients with EAF treated with EN exists; therefore, no strong evidence can support these treatments and further studies are needed [175, 176]. The use of octreotide analogs is controversial. No evidence exists about the use of somatostatin and octreotide in managing of EAF. Few studies suggest that octreotide may reduce fistula output by diminishing GI secretions [177] while others argue their benefit due to this agents' reduction in splanchnic blood flow and reduction in immune function [178, 179].

The main goal in the management of EAF should be the closure of the fistula. Differently from common GI fistulas, the EAF is not a true fistula since a fistula tract does not exist. The lack of surrounding tissues prevents the spontaneous closure. The goal of the treatment should be focused on trying to isolate the fistula effluent and enhancing the formation of granulation tissues surrounding it. Several different techniques were described and proposed in the literature to control and treat EAF, and some attempts to standardize its management exist [169, 170]. A patient diagnosed with EAF in the setup of OA should be treated by medical personnel familiar with this complication and its consequences.

Accurate fistula definition and anatomy should be made. Sepsis control and management is important. Diversion of the fistula output in order to maintain clean the peritoneal cavity is mandatory. Fistula effluent should be measured in order to facilitate fluid balance and to ensure skin protection from its digestive nature on the skin. This will enhance and allow better patient care and mobility.

Several different dressing and techniques were described for the management of EAF, each one with relatively small case series and discordant results with a consequent poor level of evidence [162, 170, 180–183]. Proposed treatments vary from primary suture and fibrin glue for small exposed distal fistula to a fistula suspension fixating the fistula edges to the skin. Several variants of NPWT with devices for fistula isolation and diversion were described with promising outcomes.

The several techniques are described in detail elsewhere and are not in the scope of the current position paper [170]. The described method to manage NPWT in patients with EAF in the setup of OA should be applied depending on surgeon preference, skills, and expertise and according to hospital facilities and material availability. Generally, negative pressure wound therapy, with specifically described variants, is the most accepted technique. EAF isolation and proper wound management will enable skin grafting and converting EAF to a more controllable one with ease of applying effluent collection bag. The definitive treatment, i.e., closure of the fistula and repairing the abdominal wall defect should be postponed at least 6 months and only after the patient and the wound healed completely.

Nutritional support

Open abdomen patients are in a hyper-metabolic condition; an immediate and adequate nutritional support is mandatory (grade 1C).

Open abdomen techniques result in a significant nitrogen loss that must be replaced with a balanced nutrition regimen (grade 1C).

Early enteral nutrition should be started as soon as possible if the gastrointestinal tract allows (grade 1C).

Enteral nutrition should be delayed in patients with high output fistula with no possibility to obtain feeding access distal to the fistula (grade 2C).

Oral feeding is not contraindicated; whenever its possible, it could be started as soon as the patient is able to eat (grade 2C).

The hyper-catabolic state of critically ill patients is associated with muscle proteolysis, acute protein malnutrition, immune function impairment, and subclinical development of MOF. Several studies clearly demonstrated malnutrition as a fundamental risk factor associated to poor outcomes during hospital stay [184]. Furthermore, in a critically ill patient, OA leads to significant nitrogen loss estimated to be 2 g per liter of abdominal fluid output. This issue requires adequate consideration and an adjusted integration [185]. For this reason, the measurement of the abdominal fluid loss is mandatory [185]. This loss in nitrogen and protein is ulterior greatly increased in the presence of EAF. A particular attention must be given to this critical aspect because patients with OA are the sickest, most inflamed, and subsequently most hypermetabolic among surgical patients. During the OA patient management, once the resuscitation is almost completed and the GI tract allows it, EN should be started as soon as possible. Thus, it will bring beneficial effects for the patient as faster fascia closure and lower pneumonia and fistula rate [173, 186, 187]. If malnutrition occurs, mucosal atrophy and malabsorption are among the earliest consequences. Gut-associated lymphoid tissue seems to be diminished, and as a consequence, it can increase the risk for disseminated infection due to bacterial translocation through the intestinal wall [188]. EN helps in maintaining gut mucosal barrier in good shape and function; as a consequence, it has been demonstrated to enhance immunity and IgA secretion, to prevent muscle atrophy, and lastly to decreases systemic inflammation and oxidative injury [188, 189]. Early EN within the first 24–48 h is demonstrated to improve wound healing, decrease catabolism, preserve GI tract integrity, and finally, it reduces complications, length of hospital stay, and costs. Compared to TPN early EN decreases septic complications especially in abdominal trauma and traumatic brain injuries. A retrospective, single-institution study comparing DCS interventions with open abdomen performed to treat ACS, 43 patients underwent early (<4 days) and 35 late (>4 days) EN. Early EN significantly increased primary closure (74% vs. 49%), reduced the fistula rate (9% vs. 26%) with no difference in infections and but with a significant reductions in hospitalization costs [186].

Patient mobilization

To date, no recommendations can be made about early mobilization of patients with open abdomen.

Patients with an open abdomen generally should not be mobilized out of bed until their abdomens are definitively closed, for risk of evisceration [190]. This statement was extrapolated from trauma literature [191]. However, prolonged bed rest is associated with significant increase in complication rate. More recent attention has been focused on intensive care unit (ICU)-acquired weakness and the long-term adverse functional sequelae for ICU survivors, particularly in the physical domain and this has led to an increased interest in early mobilization in the ICU as a potential means of prevention [192–196]. The optimal timing for initiation of mobilization of patients with OA has yet to be defined. Early mobilization is currently defined as occurring within the first 2 to 5 days of ICU admission [197].

Patients with open abdomen managed with NPWT however, may be mobilized by active or passive transfer. Further research must occur to provide the rationale to early mobilization prior to definitive abdominal closure.

Conclusions

Management of the open abdomen remains a very controversial domain, in which many techniques are still debated. Many important issues remain to be addressed through carefully designed and rigorously conducted studies. Until better data is available, the use of the OA should be carefully tailored to each single patient taking care to not overuse this effective tool. Every effort should be exerted to attempt abdominal closure as soon as the patient can physiologically tolerate it. Finally, all the precautions should be considered to minimize the complication rate.

Abbreviations

AAST: American Association for the Surgery of Trauma; ACS: Abdominal compartment syndrome; AP: Acute pancreatitis; BP: Biological prosthesis; EAF: Entero-atmospheric fistula; EN: Enteral nutrition; EVAR: Endovascular repair; GRADE: Grading of Recommendations Assessment, Development and Evaluation; IAH: Intra-abdominal hypertension; IAP: Intra-abdominal pressure; INR: International Normalized Ratio; MODS: Multi-organ dysfunction syndrome; MOF: Multiple organ failure; NPWT: Negative pressure wound therapy; OA: Open abdomen procedure; PTFE: Polytetrafluoruroethylene; rAAA: Ruptured abdominal aortic aneurysm; RCT: Randomized controlled trial; TAC: Temporal abdominal closure; TEG: Thromboelastography; TPN: Parenteral nutrition; WSACS: The Abdominal Compartment Syndrome; WSES: World Society of Emergency Surgery

Acknowledgements

Special thanks to Ms. Franca Boschini (Bibliographer, Medical Library, Papa Giovanni XXIII Hospital, Bergamo, Italy) for the precious bibliographical work.

Funding

None.

Authors' contributions

FCo, GMo, MC, FCa, EEM, RI, WB, AP, RC, SR, YK, FMA-Z, MSa, MDM, GV, GPF, BMP, AL, MAB, AK, RM, MB, BS, VK, MM, VA, MIL, MSu, SDS, EG, KS, JEM, AKM, PM, RMM, MP, FS, GMa, TMV, TS, OC, JLK, and LA did the manuscript conception and draft, critically revised the manuscript, and contributed with important scientific knowledge giving the final approval. All authors read and approved the final manuscript.

Competing interest

Manu LNG Malbrain is Founding President and current Treasurer of the Abdominal Compartment Society (WSACS, www.wsacs.org). He is also a member of the executive committee of the International Fluid Academy (IFA). The IFA is integrated within the not-for-profit charitable organization iMERiT (International Medical Education and Research Initiative) under Belgian Law. The IFA website (http://www.fluidacademy.org) is now an official SMACC (Social Media and Critical Care) affiliated site, and its content is based on the philosophy of FOAM (Free Open Access Medical Education—#-FOAMed). He is a member of the medical advisory board of Pulsion Medical Systems (Maquet Getinge group) and consults for Acelity, ConvaTec, Spiegelberg and Holtech Medical.

Andrew Kirkpatrick has consulted for the Innovative Trauma Corporative, Acelity Corp., and Cook Medical Corp. The authors declare that they have no competing interests.

Author details

[1]General, Emergency and Trauma Surgery dept., Papa Giovanni XXIII Hospital, Piazza OMS 1, 24127 Bergamo, Italy. [2]Emergency and Trauma Surgery, Parma Maggiore hospital, Parma, Italy. [3]Denver Health, Denver, CO 80204, USA. [4]Trauma Surgery, Virginia Commonwealth University, Richmond, VA 23284, USA. [5]Acute Care Surgery, The Queen's Medical Center, Honolulu, HI 96813, USA. [6]Department of Surgery, Trauma and Surgical Services, University of Pittsburgh School of Medicine, Pittsburgh 15213, USA. [7]Department of Surgery, UC San Diego Health System, San Diego 92103, USA. [8]Trauma & Acute Care Service, St Michael's Hospital, Toronto, ON, Canada. [9]Division of General Surgery Rambam Health Care Campus, Haifa, Israel. [10]Department of Surgery, College of Medicine and Health Sciences, UAE University, Al-Ain, United Arab Emirates. [11]Department of Surgery, Macerata Hospital, Macerata, Italy. [12]Department of Trauma, Emergency Surgery and Surgical Critical Care, Massachusetts General Hospital, Boston, MA 02114, USA. [13]Faculdade de Ciências Médicas (FCM) – Unicamp Campinas, São Paulo, Brazil. [14]Second Department of Surgery, Meilahti Hospital, Helsinki, Finland. [15]Academic Medical Center Amsterdam, Amsterdam, The Netherlands. [16]Department of Surgery, Foothills Medical Centre, Calgary, Canada. [17]Department of Surgery, Harborview Medical Centre, Seattle 98104, USA. [18]General Surgery Department, Hadassah Medical Centre, Jerusalem, Israel. [19]First Clinic of General Surgery, University Hospital/UMBAL/St George Plovdiv, Plovdiv, Bulgaria. [20]General Surgery, Mozir Hospital, Mozir City, Belarus. [21]ICU and High Care Burn Unit, Ziekenhius Netwerk Antwerpen, Antwerpen, Belgium. [22]ICU Department, Bufalini Hospital, Cesena, Italy. [23]Critical Care Centre, Corporasiò Sanitaria Park Tauli, Sabdel, Spain. [24]General Surgery Department, Letterkenny Hospital, Letterkenny, Ireland. [25]General and Trauma Surgery Department, Maggiore Hospital, Bologna, Italy. [26]Upper Gatrointestinal Surgery, Birmigham Hospital, Birmigham, UK. [27]Department of Gastrointestinal Surgery, Stavanger University Hospital, Stavanger, Norway. [28]Department of Clinical Medicine, University of Bergen, Bergen, Norway. [29]Department of Surgery, School of Medicine, Washington University, Saint Louis, MO 63130, USA. [30]Departments of Surgery and Anesthesiology, Division of Trauma and Surgical Critical Care, Vanderbilt University Medical Center, Nashville, TN 37232, USA. [31]Département d'Anesthésie-Réanimation, CHU Bichat Claude-Bernard-HUPNVS, Assistance Publique-Hôpitaux de Paris, University Denis Diderot, Paris, France. [32]ICU department Sant'Orsola-Malpighi University Hospital, Bologna, Italy. [33]ICU Department, Papa Giovanni XXIII Hospital, Bergamo, Italy. [34]Trauma Surgery department, University of Maryland School of Medicine, Baltimore, MD 21201, USA. [35]Emergency and Trauma Surgery department, Niguarda Hospital, Milan, Italy. [36]General Surgery department, Assuta Medical Centers, Tel Aviv, Israel.

References

1. Bailey J, Shapiro MJ. Abdominal compartment syndrome. Crit Care. 2000;4:23–9.
2. Sartelli M, Abu-Zidan FM, Ansaloni L, Bala M, Beltrán MA, Biffl WL, et al. The role of the open abdomen procedure in managing severe abdominal sepsis: WSES position paper. World J Emerg Surg. 2015;10:35.
3. Van Hee R. Historical highlights in concept and treatment of abdominal compartment syndrome. Acta Clin Belg. 2007;62:9–15.
4. Demetriades D. Total management of the open abdomen. Int Wound J. 2012;9:17–24.
5. Kirkpatrick AW, Roberts DJ, De Waele J, Jaeschke R, Malbrain MLNG, De Keulenaer B, et al. Intra-abdominal hypertension and the abdominal compartment syndrome: updated consensus definitions and clinical practice guidelines from the World Society of the Abdominal Compartment Syndrome. Intensive Care Med. 2013;39:1190–206.
6. Leppäniemi AK. Laparostomy: why and when? Crit Care. 2010;14:216.
7. Ivatury RR. Update on open abdomen management: achievements and challenges. World J Surg. 2009;33:1150–3.
8. Coccolini F, Biffl W, Catena F, Ceresoli M, Chiara O, Cimbanassi S, et al. The open abdomen, indications, management and definitive closure. World J Emerg Surg. 2015;10:32.
9. Sartelli M, Catena F, Ansaloni L, Coccolini F, Corbella D, Moore EE, et al. Complicated intra-abdominal infections worldwide: the definitive data of the CIAOW Study. World J Emerg Surg. 2014;9:37.
10. van Ruler O, Mahler CW, Boer KR, Reuland EA, Gooszen HG, Opmeer BC, et al. Comparison of on-demand vs planned relaparotomy strategy in patients with severe peritonitis: a randomized trial. JAMA. 2007;298:865–72.
11. Guyatt G, Gutterman D, Baumann MH, Addrizzo-Harris D, Hylek EM, Phillips B, et al. Grading strength of recommendations and quality of evidence in clinical guidelines: report from an american college of chest physicians task force. Chest. 2006;129:174–81.
12. Moore LJ, Moore FA. Epidemiology of sepsis in surgical patients. Surg Clin North Am. 2012;92:1425–43.
13. Ordóñez CA, Sánchez ÁI, Pineda JA, Badiel M, Mesa R, Cardona U, et al. Deferred primary anastomosis versus diversion in patients with severe secondary peritonitis managed with staged laparotomies. World J Surg. 2010;34:169–76.
14. Plantefeve G, Hellmann R, Pajot O, Thirion M, Bleichner G, Mentec H. Abdominal compartment syndrome and intraabdominal sepsis: two of the same kind? Acta Clin Belg. 2007;62:162–7.
15. Schein M. Surgical management of intra-abdominal infection: is there any evidence? Langenbeck's Arch Surg. 2002;387:1–7.
16. Robledo FA, Luque-de-León E, Suárez R, Sánchez P, De-la-Fuente M, Vargas A, et al. Open versus closed management of the abdomen in the surgical treatment of severe secondary peritonitis: a randomized clinical trial. Surg Infect. 2007;8:63–72.
17. Rubenstein C, Bietz G, Davenport DL, Winkler M, Endean ED. Abdominal compartment syndrome associated with endovascular and open repair of ruptured abdominal aortic aneurysms. J Vasc Surg. 2015;61:648–54.
18. Reite A, Soreide K, Ellingsen CL, Kvaløy JT, Vetrhus M. Epidemiology of ruptured abdominal aortic aneurysms in a well-defined Norwegian population with trends in incidence, intervention rate, and mortality. J Vasc Surg. 2015;61:1168–74.
19. Ersryd S, Djavani-Gidlund K, Wanhainen A, Björck M. Abdominal compartment syndrome after surgery for abdominal aortic aneurysm: a Nationwide Population Based Study. Eur J Vasc Endovasc Surg. 2016;52:158–65.
20. Björck M. Management of the tense abdomen or difficult abdominal closure after operation for ruptured abdominal aortic aneurysms. Semin Vasc Surg. 2012;25:35–8.
21. Acosta S, Wanhainen A, Bjorck M. Temporary abdominal closure after abdominal aortic aneurysm repair: a systematic review of contemporary observational studies. Eur J Vasc Endovasc Surg. 2016;51:371–8.

22. Kougias P, Lau D, El Sayed HF, Zhou W, Huynh TT, Lin PH. Determinants of mortality and treatment outcome following surgical interventions for acute mesenteric ischemia. J Vasc Surg Off Publ Soc Vasc Surg [and] Int Soc Cardiovasc Surgery, North Am Chapter 2007;46:467–474.
23. Tilsed JVT, Casamassima A, Kurihara H, Mariani D, Martinez I, Pereira J, et al. ESTES guidelines: acute mesenteric ischaemia. Eur J Trauma Emerg Surg. 2016;42:253–70.
24. Bruns BR, Ahmad SA, O'Meara L, Tesoriero R, Lauerman M, Klyushnenkova E, et al. Nontrauma open abdomens: a prospective observational study. J Trauma Acute Care Surg. 2016;80:631–6.
25. Schermerhorn ML, Giles KA, Hamdan AD, Wyers MC, Pomposelli FB. Mesenteric revascularization: management and outcomes in the United States, 1988–2006. J Vasc Surg. NIH Public Access; 2009;50:341–348.e1.
26. Banks PA, Bollen TL, Dervenis C, Gooszen HG, Johnson CD, Sarr MG, et al. Classification of acute pancreatitis—2012: revision of the Atlanta classification and definitions by international consensus. Gut. 2013;62:102–11.
27. Halonen KI, Pettilä V, Leppäniemi AK, Kemppainen EA, Puolakkainen PA, Haapiainen RK. Multiple organ dysfunction associated with severe acute pancreatitis. Crit Care Med. 2002;30:1274–9.
28. Buter A, Imrie CW, Carter CR, Evans S, McKay CJ. Dynamic nature of early organ dysfunction determines outcome in acute pancreatitis. Br J Surg. 2002;89:298–302.
29. Mofidi R, Duff MD, Wigmore SJ, Madhavan KK, Garden OJ, Parks RW. Association between early systemic inflammatory response, severity of multiorgan dysfunction and death in acute pancreatitis. Br J Surg. 2006;93: 738–44.
30. Mentula P, Kylänpää-Bäck M-L, Kemppainen E, Takala A, Jansson S, Kautiainen H, et al. Decreased HLA (human leucocyte antigen)-DR expression on peripheral blood monocytes predicts the development of organ failure in patients with acute pancreatitis. Clin Sci (Lond). 2003;105:409–17.
31. Mole DJ, Olabi B, Robinson V, Garden OJ, Parks RW. Incidence of individual organ dysfunction in fatal acute pancreatitis: analysis of 1024 death records. HPB. 2009;11:166–70.
32. De Waele JJ, Leppäniemi AK. Intra-abdominal hypertension in acute pancreatitis. World J Surg. 2009;33:1128–33.
33. Mentula P, Hienonen P, Kemppainen E, Puolakkainen P, Leppäniemi A. Surgical decompression for abdominal compartment syndrome in severe acute pancreatitis. Arch Surg. 2010;145:764–9.
34. Besselink MG, Van Santvoort HC, Boermeester MA, Nieuweohuijs VB, Van Goor H, Dejong CHC, et al. Timing and impact of infections in acute pancreatitis. Br J Surg. 2009;96:267–73.
35. van Santvoort HC, Besselink MG, Bakker OJ, Hofker HS, Boermeester MA, Dejong CH, et al. A step-up approach or open necrosectomy for necrotizing pancreatitis. N Engl J Med. 2010;362:1491–502.
36. Petrov MS, Shanbhag S, Chakraborty M, Phillips ARJ, Windsor JA. Organ failure and infection of pancreatic necrosis as determinants of mortality in patients with acute pancreatitis. Gastroenterology. 2010;139:813–20.
37. Tsuei BJ, Skinner JC, Bernard AC, Kearney PA, Boulanger BR. The open peritoneal cavity: etiology correlates with the likelihood of fascial closure. Am Surg. 2004;70:652–6.
38. Rao M, Burke D, Finan PJ, Sagar PM. The use of vacuum-assisted closure of abdominal wounds: a word of caution. Color Dis. 2007;9:266–8.
39. Carlson GL, Patrick H, Amin AI, McPherson G, MacLennan G, Afolabi E, et al. Management of the open abdomen: a national study of clinical outcome and safety of negative pressure wound therapy. Ann Surg. 2013;257:1154–9.
40. Pliakos I, Papavramidis TS, Michalopoulos N, Deligiannidis N, Kesisoglou I, Sapalidis K, et al. The value of vacuum-assisted closure in septic patients treated with laparostomy. Am Surg. 2012;78:957–61.
41. Barker DE, Green JM, Maxwell RA, Smith PW, Mejia VA, Dart BW, et al. Experience with vacuum-pack temporary abdominal wound closure in 258 trauma and general and vascular surgical patients. J Am Coll Surg. 2007;204:784–92.
42. Oetting P, Rau B, Schlag PM. Abdominal vacuum device with open abdomen. Chirurg. 2006;77(586):588–93.
43. Kritayakirana K, Maggio PM, Brundage S, Purtill MA, Staudenmayer K, Spain DA. Outcomes and complications of open abdomen technique for managing non-trauma patients. J Emerg Trauma Shock. 2010;3:118–22.
44. Prichayudh S, Sriussadaporn S, Samorn P, Pak-Art R, Sriussadaporn S, Kritayakirana K, et al. Management of open abdomen with an absorbable mesh closure. Surg Today. 2011;41:72–8.
45. Adkins AL, Robbins J, Villalba M, Bendick P, Shanley CJ. Open abdomen management of intra-abdominal sepsis. Am Surg. 2004;70:137–40.
46. Amin AI, Shaikh IA. Topical negative pressure in managing severe peritonitis: a positive contribution? World J Gastroenterol. 2009;15:3394–7.
47. Bosscha K, Hulstaert PF, Visser MR, van Vroonhoven TJ, van der Werken C. Open management of the abdomen and planned reoperations in severe bacterial peritonitis. Eur J Surg. 2000;166:44–9.
48. Cipolla J, Stawicki SP, Hoff WS, McQuay N, Hoey BA, Wainwright G, et al. A proposed algorithm for managing the open abdomen. Am Surg. 2005;71:202–7.
49. López-Quintero L, Evaristo-Méndez G, Fuentes-Flores F, Ventura-González F, Sepúlveda-Castro R. Treatment of open abdomen in patients with abdominal sepsis using the vacuum pack system. Cir Cir. 2010;78:317–21.
50. Padalino P, Dionigi G, Minoja G, Carcano G, Rovera F, Boni LDR. Fascia-to-fascia closure with abdominal topical negative pressure for severe abdominal infections: preliminary results in a department of general surgery and intensive care unit. Surg Infect. 2010;11:523–52.
51. Schmelzle M, Alldinger I, Matthaei H, Aydin F, Wallert I, Eisenberger CF, et al. Long-term vacuum-assisted closure in open abdomen due to secondary peritonitis: a retrospective evaluation of a selected group of patients. Dig Surg. 2010:329–35.
52. Pliakos I, Michalopoulos N, Papavramidis TS, Arampatzi S, Diza-Mataftsi E, Papavramidis S. The effect of vacuum-assisted closure in bacterial clearance of the infected abdomen. Surg Infect. 2014;15:18–23.
53. Wondberg D, Larusson HJ, Metzger U, Platz A, Zingg U. Treatment of the open abdomen with the commercially available vacuum-assisted closure system in patients with abdominal sepsis: low primary closure rate. World J Surg. 2008;32:2724–9.
54. Khan A, Hsee L, Mathur S, Civil I. Damage-control laparotomy in nontrauma patients: review of indications and outcomes. J Trauma Acute Care Surg. 2013;75:365–8.
55. Brock WB, Barker DE, Burns RP. Temporary closure of open abdominal wounds: the vacuum pack. Am Surg. 1995;61:30–5.
56. Caro A, Olona C, Jimenez A, Vadillo J, Feliu F, Vicente V. Treatment of the open abdomen with topical negative pressure therapy: a retrospective study of 46 cases. Int Wound J. 2011;8:274–9.
57. Fieger AJ, Schwatlo F, Mündel DF-X, Schenk M, Hemminger F, Kirchdorfer B, et al. Abdominal vacuum therapy for the open abdomen—a retrospective analysis of 82 consecutive patients. Zentralbl Chir. 2011;136:56–60.
58. Horwood J, Akbar F, Maw A. Initial experience of laparostomy with immediate vacuum therapy in patients with severe peritonitis. Ann R Coll Surg Engl. 2009;91:681–7.
59. Ozguc H, Paksoy E, Ozturk E. Temporary abdominal closure with the vacuum pack technique: a 5-year experience. Acta Chir Belg. 2008;108:414–9.
60. Perez D, Wildi S, Demartines N, Bramkamp M, Koehler C, Clavien PA. Prospective evaluation of vacuum-assisted closure in abdominal compartment syndrome and severe abdominal sepsis. J Am Coll Surg. 2007;205:586–92.
61. Pérez Domínguez L, Pardellas Rivera H, Cáceres Alvarado N, López Saco Á, Rivo Vázquez Á, Casal NE. Vacuum assisted closure: utilidad en el abdomen abierto y cierre diferido. Experiencia en 23 pacientes. Cir Esp. 2012;90:506–12.
62. Plaudis H, Rudzats A, Melberga L, Kazaka I, Suba O, Pupelis G. Abdominal negative-pressure therapy: a new method in countering abdominal compartment and peritonitis—prospective study and critical review of literature. Ann Intensive Care. 2012;2(Suppl 1):S23.
63. Shaikh IA, Ballard-Wilson A, Yalamarthi S, Amin AI. Use of topical negative pressure in assisted abdominal closure does not lead to high incidence of enteric fistulae. Color Dis. 2010;12:931–4.
64. Smith LA, Barker DE, Chase CW, Somberg LB, Bradford Brock W, Phillip BR. Vacuum pack technique of temporary abdominal closure: a four-year experience. Am Surg. 1997;63:1102–8.
65. Wilde JW, Loudon MA. Modified opsite® sandwich for temporary abdominal closure: a non-traumatic experience. Ann R Coll Surg Engl. 2007;89:57–61.
66. Zielinski MD, Goussous N, Schiller HJ, Jenkins D. Chemical components separation with botulinum toxin A: a novel technique to improve primary fascial closure rates of the open abdomen. Hernia. 2013;17:101–7.
67. Bertelsen CA, Fabricius R, Kleif J, Kristensen B, Gögenur I. Outcome of negative-pressure wound therapy for open abdomen treatment after nontraumatic lower gastrointestinal surgery: analysis of factors affecting delayed fascial closure in 101 patients. World J Surg. 2014;38:774–81.
68. Richter S, Dold S, Doberauer JP, Mai P, Schuld J. Negative pressure wound therapy for the treatment of the open abdomen and incidence

of enteral fistulas: a retrospective bicentre analysis. Gastroenterol Res Pract. 2013;2013:6–11.

69. Fortelny RH, Hofmann A, Gruber-Blum S, Petter-Puchner AH, Glaser KS. Delayed closure of open abdomen in septic patients is facilitated by combined negative pressure wound therapy and dynamic fascial suture. Surg Endosc Other Interv Tech. 2014;28:735–40.
70. Kafka-Ritsch R, Birkfellner F, Perathoner A, Raab H, Nehoda H, Pratschke J, et al. Damage control surgery with abdominal vacuum and delayed bowel reconstruction in patients with perforated diverticulitis Hinchey III/IV. J Gastrointest Surg. 2012;16:1915–22.
71. Kleif J, Fabricius R, Bertelsen CA, Bruun J, Gögenur I. Promising results after vacuum-assisted wound closure and mesh-mediated fascial traction. Dan Med J. 2012;59
72. Kafka-Ritsch R, Zitt M, Schorn N, Stroemmer S, Schneeberger S, Pratschke J, et al. Open abdomen treatment with dynamic sutures and topical negative pressure resulting in a high primary fascia closure rate. World J Surg. 2012;36:1765–71.
73. Acosta S, Bjarnason T, Petersson U, Pålsson B, Wanhainen A, Svensson M, et al. Multicentre prospective study of fascial closure rate after open abdomen with vacuum and mesh-mediated fascial traction. Br J Surg. 2011;98:735–43.
74. Huang Q, Zhao R, Yue C, Wang W, Zhao Y, Ren J, et al. Fluid volume overload negatively influences delayed primary facial closure in open abdomen management. J Surg Res. 2014;187:122–7.
75. García Iñiguez JA, Orozco CF, Muciño Hernández MI, Ortega AL, Trabaldo SS, Cortés Flores AO, Hermosillo Sandoval JMOA. Complications of the management of secondary peritonitis with contained-open abdomen. Comparison of the Bogota's bag vs polypropylene mesh. Rev Gastroenterol Mex. 2004;69:147–55.
76. Schein M. Planned reoperations and open management in critical intra-abdominal infections: prospective experience in 52 cases. World J Surg. 1991;15:537–45.
77. Gentile AT, Feliciano PD, Mullins RJ, Crass RA, Eidemiller LR, Sheppard BC. The utility of polyglycolic acid mesh for abdominal access in patients with necrotizing pancreatitis. J Am Coll Surg. 1998;186:313–8.
78. Losanoff JE, Kjossev KT. Mesh-foil laparostomy. J Am Coll Surg. 1997;185:89–92.
79. Töns C, Schachtrupp A, Rau M, Mumme T, Schumpelick V. Abdominal compartment syndrome: prevention and treatment. Chirurg. 2000;71:918–26.
80. Schachtrupp A, Höer J, Töns C, Klinge U, Reckord U, Schumpelick V. Intra-abdominal pressure: a reliable criterion for laparostomy closure? Hernia. 2002;6:102–7.
81. Sökmen S, Atila K, Bora S, Astarcloğlu H, Çoker A, Füzün M. Evaluation of prosthetic mesh closure in semiopen-abdomen patients. Hernia. 2002;6:124–9.
82. Martinez-Ordaz JL, Cruz-Olivo PA, Chacon-Moya E, de la Fuente-Lira M, Chavelas-Lluck M, Blanco-Benavides R. Management of the abdominal wall in sepsis. Comparison of two techniques. Rev Gastroenterol Mex. 2004;69:88–93.
83. Gönüllü D, Köksoy FN, Demiray O, Özkan SG, Yücel T, Yücel O. Laparostomy in patients with severe secondary peritonitis. Ulus Travma ve Acil Cerrahi Derg. 2009;15:52–7.
84. Kirshtein B, Roy-Shapira A, Lantsberg L, Mizrahi S. Use of the "Bogota bag" for temporary abdominal closure in patients with secondary peritonitis. Am Surg. 2007;73:249–52.
85. Manterola C, Moraga J, Urrutia S. Contained laparostomy with a Bogota bag. Results of case series. Cir Esp. 2011;89:379–85.
86. Doyon A, Devroede G, Viens D, Saito S, Rioux A, Echavé V, et al. A simple, inexpensive, life-saving way to perform iterative laparotomy in patients with severe intra-abdominal sepsis. Color Dis. 2001;3:115–21.
87. Hakkiluoto A, Hannukainen J. Open management with mesh and zipper of patients with intra-abdominal abscesses or diffuse peritonitis. Eur J Surg. 1992;158:403–5.
88. Hubens G, Lafaire C, De Praeter M, Ysebaert D, Vaneerdeweg W, Heytens L, et al. Staged peritoneal lavages with the aid of a Zipper system in the treatment of diffuse peritonitis. Acta Chir Belg. 1994;94:176–9.
89. Hedderich GS, Wexler MJ, McLean AP, Meakins JL. The septic abdomen: open management with Marlex mesh with a zipper. Surgery. 1986;99:399–408.
90. Zingales F, Moschino P, Carniato S, Fabris G, Vittadello F, Corsini A. Laparostomy in the treatment of severe peritonitis: a review of 60 cases. Chir Ital. 2001;53:821–6.
91. Ercan F, Korkmaz A, Aras N. The zipper-mesh method for treating delayed generalized peritonitis. Surg Today. 1993;23:205–14.
92. Koniaris LG, Hendrickson RJ, Drugas G, Abt P, Schoeniger LO. Dynamic retention: a technique for closure of the complex abdomen in critically ill patients. Arch Surg. 2001;136:1359–62. discussion 1363
93. Reimer MW, Yelle JD, Reitsma B, Doumit G, Allen MA, Bell MS. Management of open abdominal wounds with a dynamic fascial closure system. Can J Surg. 2008;51:209–14.
94. Salman AE, Yetisir F, Aksoy M, Tokac M, Yildirim MB, Kilic M. Use of dynamic wound closure system in conjunction with vacuum-assisted closure therapy in delayed closure of open abdomen. Hernia. 2014;18:99–104.
95. Verdam FJ, Dolmans DEJGJ, Loos MJ, Raber MH, De Wit RJ, Charbon JA, et al. Delayed primary closure of the septic open abdomen with a dynamic closure system. World J Surg. 2011;35:2348–55.
96. Haddock C, Konkin DE, Blair NP. Management of the open abdomen with the abdominal reapproximation anchor dynamic fascial closure system. Am J Surg. 2013;205:528–33.
97. Anderson ED, Mandelbaum DM, Ellison EC, Carey LC, Cooperman M. Open packing of the peritoneal cavity in generalized bacterial peritonitis. Am J Surg. 1983;145:131–5.
98. Hollender LF, Bur F, Schwenck D, Pigache P. The "left-open abdomen". Technic, indication and results. Chirurg. 1983;54:316–9.
99. Wittmann DH. Staged abdominal repair: development and current practice of an advanced operative technique for diffuse suppurative peritonitis. Acta Chir Austriaca. 2000;32:171–8.
100. Dietz UA, Wichelmann C, Wunder C, Kauczok J, Spor L, Strauß A, et al. Early repair of open abdomen with a tailored two-component mesh and conditioning vacuum packing: a safe alternative to the planned giant ventral hernia. Hernia. 2012;16:451–60.
101. Losanoff J, Kjossev K. Palisade dorsoventral lavage for neglected peritonitis. Am J Surg. 1997;173:134–5.
102. Ivatury RR, Nallathambi M, Rao PM, Rohman M, Stahl WM. Open management of the septic abdomen: therapeutic and prognostic considerations based on APACHE II. Crit Care Med. 1989;17:511–7.
103. Wittmann DH, Aprahamian C, Bergstein JM. Etappenlavage: advanced diffuse peritonitis managed by planned multiple laparotomies utilizing zippers, slide fastener, and Velcro analogue for temporary abdominal closure. World J Surg. 1990;14:218–26.
104. Kim PJ, Attinger CE, Olawoye O, Crist BD, Gabriel A, Galiano RD, et al. Negative pressure wound therapy with instillation: review of evidence and recommendations. Wounds a Compend Clin Res Pract. 2015;27:S2–19.
105. Atema JJ, Gans SL, Boermeester MA. Systematic review and meta-analysis of the open abdomen and temporary abdominal closure techniques in non-trauma patients. World J Surg. 2015;39:912–25.
106. Karmali S, Evans D, Laupland KB, Findlay C, Ball CG, Bergeron E, et al. To close or not to close, that is one of the questions? Perceptions of Trauma Association of Canada surgical members on the management of the open abdomen. J Trauma. 2006;60:287–93.
107. Kirkpatrick AW, Laupland KB, Karmali S, Bergeron E, Stewart TC, Findlay C, et al. Spill your guts! Perceptions of Trauma Association of Canada member surgeons regarding the open abdomen and the abdominal compartment syndrome. J Trauma. 2006;60:279–86.
108. Pommerening MJ, Dubose JJ, Zielinski MD, Phelan HA, Scalea TM, Inaba K, et al. Time to first take-back operation predicts successful primary fascial closure in patients undergoing damage control laparotomy. Surg (United States). 2014;156:431–8.
109. Singer M, Deutschman CS, Seymour CW, Shankar-Hari M, Annane D, Bauer M, et al. The Third International Consensus Definitions for Sepsis and Septic Shock (Sepsis-3). JAMA. 2016;315:801–10.
110. Emr B, Sadowsky D, Azhar N, Gatto LA, An G, Nieman GF, et al. Removal of inflammatory ascites is associated with dynamic modification of local and systemic inflammation along with prevention of acute lung injury: in vivo and in silico studies. Shock. 2014;41:317–23.
111. Kubiak BD, Albert SP, Gatto LA, Snyder KP, Maier KG, Vieau CJ, et al. Peritoneal negative pressure therapy prevents multiple organ injury in a chronic porcine sepsis and ischemia/reperfusion model. Shock. 2010;34:525–34.
112. Cheatham ML, Demetriades D, Fabian TC, Kaplan MJ, Miles WS, Schreiber MA, et al. Prospective study examining clinical outcomes associated with a negative pressure wound therapy system and Barker's vacuum packing technique. World J Surg. 2013;37:2018–30.
113. Kirkpatrick AW, Roberts DJ, Faris PD, Ball CG, Kubes P, Tiruta C, et al. Active negative pressure peritoneal therapy after abbreviated laparotomy: the intraperitoneal vacuum randomized controlled trial. Ann Surg. 2015;262:38–46.
114. Wang J, Kubes P. A reservoir of mature cavity macrophages that can rapidly invade visceral organs to affect tissue repair. Cell. 2016;165:668–78.

115. Demetriades D, Salim A. Management of the open abdomen. Surg Clin North Am. 2014;94:131–53.
116. Regner JL, Kobayashi L, Coimbra R. Surgical strategies for management of the open abdomen. World J Surg. 2012;36:497–510.
117. Godat L, Kobayashi L, Costantini T, Coimbra R. Abdominal damage control surgery and reconstruction: world society of emergency surgery position paper. World J Emerg Surg. 2013;8
118. Ramirez OM, Ruas E, Dellon AL. "Components separation" method for closure of abdominal-wall defects: an anatomic and clinical study. Plast Reconstr Surg. 1990;86:519–26.
119. Paul JS, Ridolfi TJ. A case study in intra-abdominal sepsis. Surg Clin North Am. 2012;92:1661–77.
120. Lambertz A, Mihatsch C, Röth A, Kalverkamp S, Eickhoff R, Neumann UP, et al. Fascial closure after open abdomen: initial indication and early revisions are decisive factors—a retrospective cohort study. Int J Surg. 2015;13:12–6.
121. Rasilainen SK, Juhani MP, Kalevi LA. Microbial colonization of open abdomen in critically ill surgical patients. World J Emerg Surg. 2015;10:25.
122. Leber GE, Garb JL, Alexander AI, Reed WP. Long-term complications associated with prosthetic repair of incisional hernias. Arch Surg. 1998;133:378–82.
123. Mathes SJ, Steinwald PM, Foster RD, Hoffman WY, Anthony JP. Complex abdominal wall reconstruction: a comparison of flap and mesh closure. Ann Surg. 2000;232:586–96.
124. Choi JJ, Palaniappa NC, Dallas KB, Rudich TB, Colon MJ, Divino CM. Use of mesh during ventral hernia repair in clean-contaminated and contaminated cases: outcomes of 33,832 cases. Ann Surg. 2012;255:176–80.
125. de Vries Reilingh TS, van Goor H, Charbon JA, Rosman C, Hesselink EJ, van der Wilt GJ, et al. Repair of giant midline abdominal wall hernias: "components separation technique" versus prosthetic repair : interim analysis of a randomized controlled trial. World J Surg Springer. 2007;31: 756–63.
126. Yegiyants S, Tam M, Lee DJ, Abbas MA. Outcome of components separation for contaminated complex abdominal wall defects. Hernia. 2012;16:41–5.
127. Rasilainen SK, Mentula PJ, Leppäniemi AK. Components separation technique is feasible for assisting delayed primary fascial closure of open abdomen. Scand J Surg. 2016;105:17–21.
128. Sharrock AE, Barker T, Yuen HM, Rickard R, Tai N. Management and closure of the open abdomen after damage control laparotomy for trauma. A systematic review and meta-analysis. Injury. Elsevier Ltd. 2015; 47:296–306.
129. Atema JJ, de Vries FEE, Boermeester MA. Systematic review and meta-analysis of the repair of potentially contaminated and contaminated abdominal wall defects. Am J Surg Elsevier Inc. 2016;212:982–95.
130. Dinsmore RC, Calton WC, Harvey SB, Blaney MW. Prevention of adhesions to polypropylene mesh in a traumatized bowel model. J Am Coll Surg. 2000;191:131–6.
131. van 't Riet M, de Vos van Steenwijk PJ, Bonthuis F, Marquet RL, Steyerberg EW, Jeekel J, et al. Prevention of adhesion to prosthetic mesh: comparison of different barriers using an incisional hernia model. Ann Surg. 2003;237:123–8.
132. Konstantinovic ML, Lagae P, Zheng F, Verbeken EK, De Ridder D, Deprest JA. Comparison of host response to polypropylene and non-cross-linked porcine small intestine serosal-derived collagen implants in a rat model. BJOG An Int J Obstet Gynaecol. 2005;112:1554–60.
133. Fansler RF, Taheri P, Cullinane C, Sabates B, Flint LM. Polypropylene mesh closure of the complicated abdominal wound. Am J Surg. 1995;170:15–8.
134. Voyles CR, Richardson JD, Bland KI, Tobin GR, Flint LM, Polk HC. Emergency abdominal wall reconstruction with polypropylene mesh: short-term benefits versus long-term complications. Ann Surg. 1981;194:219–23.
135. Brown GL, Richardson JD, Malangoni MA, Tobin GR, Ackerman D, Polk HC. Comparison of prosthetic materials for abdominal wall reconstruction in the presence of contamination and infection. Ann Surg. 1985;201:705–11.
136. Sartelli M, Coccolini F, van Ramshorst GH, Campanelli G, Mandalà V, Ansaloni L, et al. WSES guidelines for emergency repair of complicated abdominal wall hernias. World J Emerg Surg. 2013;8:50.
137. Cornwell KG, Landsman A, James KS. Extracellular matrix biomaterials for soft tissue repair. Clin Podiatr Med Surg. 2009;26:507–23.
138. Caviggioli F, Klinger FM, Lisa A, Maione L, Forcellini D, Vinci V, et al. Matching biological mesh and negative pressure wound therapy in reconstructing an open abdomen defect. Case Rep Med. Hindawi Publishing Corporation; 2014;2014:235930.
139. Badylak SF. Xenogeneic extracellular matrix as a scaffold for tissue reconstruction. Transpl Immunol. 2004;12:367–77.
140. Winters JC. InteXen tissue processing and laboratory study. Int Urogynecol J Pelvic Floor Dysfunct. 2006;17
141. Petter-Puchner AH, Dietz UA. Biological implants in abdominal wall repair. Br J Surg. 2013;100:987–8.
142. Montori G, Coccolini F, Manfredi R, Ceresoli M, Campanati L, Magnone S, et al. One year experience of swine dermal non-crosslinked collagen prostheses for abdominal wall repairs in elective and emergency surgery. World J Emerg Surg. 2015;10:28–35.
143. Primus FE, Harris HW. A critical review of biologic mesh use in ventral hernia repairs under contaminated conditions. Hernia. 2013;17:21–30.
144. Gurrado A, Franco IF, Lissidini G, Greco G, De Fazio M, Pasculli A, et al. Impact of pericardium bovine patch (Tutomesh®) on incisional hernia treatment in contaminated or potentially contaminated fields: retrospective comparative study. Hernia. 2015;19:259–66.
145. de Moya MA, Dunham M, Inaba K, Bahouth H, Alam HB, Sultan B, et al. Long-term outcome of acellular dermal matrix when used for large traumatic open abdomen. J Trauma Inj Infect Crit Care. 2008;65:349–53.
146. Ginting N, Tremblay L, Kortbeek JB. Surgisis® in the management of the complex abdominal wall in trauma: a case series and review of the literature. Injury. 2010;41:970–3.
147. Patton JH, Berry S, Kralovich KA. Use of human acellular dermal matrix in complex and contaminated abdominal wall reconstructions. Am J Surg. 2007;193:360–3.
148. Maurice SM, Skeete DA. Use of human acellular dermal matrix for abdominal wall reconstructions. Am J Surg. 2009;197:35–42.
149. Lin HJ, Spoerke N, Deveney C, Martindale R. Reconstruction of complex abdominal wall hernias using acellular human dermal matrix: a single institution experience. Am J Surg. 2009;197:599–603.
150. Diaz JJ, Conquest AM, Ferzoco SJ, Vargo D, Miller P, Wu Y-C, et al. Multi-institutional experience using human acellular dermal matrix for ventral hernia repair in a compromised surgical field. Arch Surg. 2009; 144:209–15.
151. Lee EI, Chike-Obi CJ, Gonzalez P, Garza R, Leong M, Subramanian A, et al. Abdominal wall repair using human acellular dermal matrix: a follow-up study. Am J Surg. 2009;198:650–7.
152. Pomahac B, Aflaki P. Use of a non-cross-linked porcine dermal scaffold in abdominal wall reconstruction. Am J Surg. Elsevier Inc; 2010;199:22–7.
153. Abdelfatah MM, Rostambeigi N, Podgaetz E, Sarr MG. Long-term outcomes (>5-year follow-up) with porcine acellular dermal matrix (Permacol) in incisional hernias at risk for infection. Hernia. 2015;19:135–40.
154. Booth JH, Garvey PB, Baumann DP, Selber JC, Nguyen AT, Clemens MW, et al. Primary fascial closure with mesh reinforcement is superior to bridged mesh repair for abdominal wall reconstruction. J Am Coll Surg. 2013;217:999–1009.
155. Chand B, Indeck M, Needleman B, Finnegan M, Van Sickle KR, Ystgaard B, et al. A retrospective study evaluating the use of Permacol™ surgical implant in incisional and ventral hernia repair. Int J Surg Elsevier Ltd. 2014;12:296–303.
156. Holihan JL, Nguyen DH, Nguyen MT, Mo J, Kao LS, Liang MK. Mesh location in open ventral hernia repair: a systematic review and network meta-analysis. World J Surg. 2016;40:89–99
157. Eriksson A, Rosenberg J, Bisgaard T. Surgical treatment for giant incisional hernia: a qualitative systematic review. Hernia. 2014;18:31–8.
158. Bradley MJ, Dubose JJ, Scalea TM, Holcomb JB, Shrestha B, Okoye O, et al. Independent predictors of enteric fistula and abdominal sepsis after damage control laparotomy: results from the prospective AAST Open Abdomen registry. JAMA Surg. 2013;148:947–54.
159. Teixeira PGR, Inaba K, Dubose J, Salim A, Brown C, Rhee P, et al. Enterocutaneous fistula complicating trauma laparotomy: a major resource burden. Am Surg. 2009;75:30–2.
160. Martinez JL, Luque-De-Leon E, Mier J, Blanco-Benavides R, Robledo F. Systematic management of postoperative enterocutaneous fistulas: factors related to outcomes. World J Surg. 2008;32:436–43.
161. Tavusbay C, Genc H, Cin N, Kar H, Kamer E, Atahan K, et al. Use of a vacuum-assisted closure system for the management of enteroatmospheric fistulae. Surg Today. Springer Japan; 2015;45:1102–1111.
162. D'Hondt M, Devriendt D, Van Rooy F, Vansteenkiste F, D'Hoore A, Penninckx F, et al. Treatment of small-bowel fistulae in the open abdomen with topical negative-pressure therapy. Am J Surg. Elsevier Inc; 2011;202:e20–4.

163. Marinis A, Gkiokas G, Argyra E, Fragulidis G, Polymeneas G, Voros D. "Enteroatmospheric fistulae"-gastrointestinal openings in the open abdomen: a review and recent proposal of a surgical technique. Scand J Surg. 2013;102:61–8.
164. Schecter WP, Ivatury RR, Rotondo MF, Hirshberg A. Open abdomen after trauma and abdominal sepsis: a strategy for management. J Am Coll Surg. 2006;203:390–6.
165. Carlson GL, Patrick H, Amin AI, McPherson G, MacLennan G, Afolabi E, et al. Management of the open abdomen. Ann Surg. 2013;257:1154–9.
166. Schein M, Decker GAG. Postoperative external alimentary tract fistulas. Am J Surg. Elsevier; 1991;161:435–438.
167. Schecter WP, Hirshberg A, Chang DS, Harris HW, Napolitano LM, Wexner SD, et al. Enteric fistulas: principles of management. J Am Coll Surg. Elsevier Inc; 2009;209:484–91.
168. Björck M, Kirkpatrick AW, Cheatham M, Kaplan M, Leppäniemi A, de Waele JJ. Amended classification of the open abdomen. Scand J Surg. 2016;105:5–10.
169. Di Saverio S, Tarasconi A, Inaba K, Navsaria P, Coccolini F, Costa Navarro D, et al. Open abdomen with concomitant enteroatmospheric fistula: attempt to rationalize the approach to a surgical nightmare and proposal of a clinical algorithm. J Am Coll Surg. 2015;220:e23–33.
170. Di Saverio S, Tarasconi A, Walczak DA, Cirocchi R, Mandrioli M, Birindelli A, et al. Classification, prevention and management of entero-atmospheric fistula: a state-of-the-art review. Langenbeck's Arch Surg. 2016;401:1–13.
171. Polk TM, Schwab CW. Metabolic and nutritional support of the enterocutaneous fistula patient: a three-phase approach. World J Surg. 2012;36:524–33.
172. Moore FA, Feliciano D V, Andrassy RJ, McArdle AH, Booth F V, Morgenstein-Wagner TB, et al. Early enteral feeding, compared with parenteral, reduces postoperative septic complications. The results of a meta-analysis. Ann Surg. Lippincott, Williams, and Wilkins; 1992;216:172–83.
173. Dissanaike S, Pham T, Shalhub S, Warner K, Hennessy L, Moore EE, et al. Effect of immediate enteral feeding on trauma patients with an open abdomen: protection from nosocomial infections. J Am Coll Surg. 2008;207:690–7.
174. Byrnes MC, Reicks P, Irwin E. Early enteral nutrition can be successfully implemented in trauma patients with an "open abdomen.". Am J Surg. 2010;199:359–63.
175. Reinisch A, Liese J, Woeste G, Bechstein W, Habbe N. A retrospective, observational study of enteral nutrition in patients with enteroatmospheric fistulas. Ostomy Wound Manage. 2016;62:36–47.
176. Yin J, Wang J, Yao D, Zhang S, Mao Q, Kong W, et al. Is it feasible to implement enteral nutrition in patients with enteroatmospheric fistulae? A single-center experience. Nutr Clin Pract. 2014;29:656–661.
177. Nubiola P, Badia JM, Martinez-Rodenas F, Gil MJ, Segura M, Sancho J, et al. Treatment of 27 postoperative enterocutaneous fistulas with the long half-life somatostatin analogue SMS 201-995. Ann Surg. 1989;210:56–8.
178. Lattuada D, Casnici C, Crotta K, Mastrotto C, Franco P, Schmid HA, et al. Inhibitory effect of pasireotide and octreotide on lymphocyte activation. J Neuroimmunol. 2007;182:153–9.
179. Cooper AM, Braatvedt GD, Qamar MI, Brown H, Thomas DM, Halliwell M, et al. Fasting and post-prandial splanchnic blood flow is reduced by a somatostatin analogue (octreotide) in man. Clin Sci. 1991;81:169–75.
180. Navsaria PH, Bunting M, Omoshoro-Jones J, Nicol AJ, Kahn D. Temporary closure of open abdominal wounds by the modified sandwich-vacuum pack technique. Br J Surg. 2003;90:718–22.
181. Al-Khoury G, Kaufman D, Hirshberg A. Improved control of exposed fistula in the open abdomen. J Am Coll Surg. 2008;206:397–8.
182. Layton B, DuBose J, Nichols S, Connaughton J, Jones T, Pratt J. Pacifying the open abdomen with concomitant intestinal fistula: a novel approach. Am J Surg. Elsevier Inc; 2010;199:e48–50.
183. Rekstad LC, Wasmuth HH, Ystgaard B, Stornes T, Seternes A. Topical negative-pressure therapy for small bowel leakage in a frozen abdomen: a technical report. J Trauma Acute Care Surg. 2013;75:487–91.
184. Giner M, Laviano A, Meguid MM, Gleason JR. In 1995 a correlation between malnutrition and poor outcome in critically ill patients still exists. Nutrition. 1996;12:23–9.
185. Cheatham ML, Safcsak K, Brzezinski SJ, Lube MW. Nitrogen balance, protein loss, and the open abdomen. Crit Care Med. 2007;35:127–31.
186. Collier B, Guillamondegui O, Cotton B, Donahue R, Conrad A, Groh K, et al. Feeding the open abdomen. JPEN J Parenter Enteral Nutr. 2007;31:410–5.
187. Cothren CC, Moore EE, Ciesla DJ, Johnson JL, Moore JB, Haenel JB, et al. Postinjury abdominal compartment syndrome does not preclude early enteral feeding after definitive closure. Am J Surg. 2004;188:653–8.
188. Marik PE, Zaloga GP. Meta-analysis of parenteral nutrition versus enteral nutrition in patients with acute pancreatitis. BMJ. 2004;328:1407–10.
189. McClave SA, Heyland DK. The physiologic response and associated clinical benefits from provision of early enteral nutrition. Nutr Clin Pract. 2009;24:305–15.
190. Panel OAA, Campbell A, Chang M, Fabian T, Franz M, Kaplan M, et al. Management of the open abdomen: from initial operation to definitive closure. Am Surg. 2009;75:S1–22.
191. Engels PT, Beckett AN, Rubenfeld GD, Kreder H, Finkelstein JA, da Costa L, et al. Physical rehabilitation of the critically ill trauma patient in the ICU. Crit Care Med. 2013;41:1790–801.
192. Truong A, Fan E, Brower R, Needham D. Bench-to-bedside review: mobilizing patients in the intensive care unit—from pathophysiology to clinical trials. Crit Care. 2009;13:216.
193. Pavy-Le Traon A, Heer M, Narici MV, Rittweger J, Vernikos J. From space to Earth: advances in human physiology from 20 years of bed rest studies (1986-2006). Eur J Appl Physiol. 2007;101:143–94.
194. Herridge MS. Building consensus on ICU-acquired weakness. Intensive Care Med. 2009;35:1–3.
195. Cuthbertson BH, Roughton S, Jenkinson D, Maclennan G, Vale L. Quality of life in the five years after intensive care: a cohort study. Crit Care. 2010;14:R6.
196. Burtin C, Clerckx B, Robbeets C, Ferdinande P, Langer D, Troosters T, et al. Early exercise in critically ill patients enhances short-term functional recovery. Crit Care Med. 2009;37:2499–505.
197. Hodgson CL, Berney S, Harrold M, Saxena M. Clinical review: early patient mobilization in the ICU. Crit Care. 2013;17:207.

19

Antibiotics alone versus appendectomy to treat uncomplicated acute appendicitis in adults

Leonardo Lima Rocha[1,2], Felipe Martin Bianco Rossi[3], Camila Menezes Souza Pessoa[1], Flavia Nunes Dias Campos[1], Carlos Eduardo Fonseca Pires[3] and Milton Steinman[2,3*]

Abstract

Background: Primary appendectomy is the current standard of care for treating uncomplicated acute appendicitis, but interest in conservative treatment with antibiotics alone has been increasing in recent years. Clinical trials so far have shown controversial results.

Methods: A series of meta-analyses were reviewed. Studies comparing surgery versus antibiotics alone for treating uncomplicated acute appendicitis in adults were included. Descriptive statistics and data on treatment effects were retrieved and summarized.

Results: The conservative approach has a success rate of around 60 % and is associated with shorter pain duration, reduced analgesic medication, faster resolution of the inflammation process, lower expenses and quicker return to work. On the other hand, medical treatment leads to high (up to 20 %) readmission rates and more often requires surgery. An operative approach is associated with higher treatment success rates (>90 %) and very a low mortality rate.

Conclusion: Based on the current body of evidence, the use of antibiotics for primary treatment of uncomplicated acute appendicitis cannot be routinely recommended. Appendectomy remains the gold-standard treatment.

Keywords: Appendicitis, Appendectomy, Antibiotics, Conservative, Surgery, Meta-analysis

Introduction

Acute appendicitis is the most common cause of inflammatory acute abdomen [1]. The incidence of acute appendicitis varies from 250,000 to 280,000 cases per year in the United States, which accounts for more than 1 million hospital days per year [2] and a cost of more than 3 billion dollars [3]. For more than a century, acute appendicitis has been treated by surgery, i.e., appendectomy [4, 5], with mortality rates as low as 0.07 to 0.7 % [6, 7]. Nevertheless, surgical intervention is associated with greater pain, adherence and hernia development, ileus, venous thromboembolic events, cardiopulmonary complications and increased costs.

During the 1950s, an initial non-operative approach for acute appendicitis was attempted, but it was not generally accepted at the time [8]. Appendicitis complicated by appendicular abscess/phlegmon may be managed with antibiotics and non-operative strategies with reduced complication rates compared to surgery [9], like other acute inflammatory intestinal conditions – i.e. diverticulitis and enterocolitis [10]. In this sense, antibiotic therapy may be associated with reduced costs of treatment, avoiding operation and its consequent complications. However, the use of antibiotics alone as primary therapy for uncomplicated acute appendicitis is still being assessed, and studies have shown conflicting results so far [11, 12].

The aim of this study is to review available meta-analyses comparing antibiotics alone versus appendectomy for uncomplicated acute appendicitis in adults.

* Correspondence: milton.steinman@einstein.br
[2]Telemedicine Service, Hospital Israelita Albert Einstein, Av. Albert Einstein, 2 andar, bloco D, São Paulo CEP: 05651-901, Brazil
[3]Surgery Department, Hospital Israelita Albert Einstein, São Paulo, Brazil
Full list of author information is available at the end of the article

Materials and methods

Study selection

We included all meta-analyses with retrospective or prospective observational and/or experimental studies and compared clinical (antibiotics alone) versus surgical (open or laparoscopic appendectomy) treatment for suspected uncomplicated acute appendicitis in adults (>18 years-old). Uncomplicated acute appendicitis was defined as acute inflammation of the appendix in the absence of an abscess, phlegmon, free perforation or peritonitis. We excluded meta-analyses enrolling patients with complicated appendicitis, without quality evaluation of individual studies, and children.

Search strategy

We searched MEDLINE, Embase, and The Cochrane Library databases up to June 2015 for meta-analysis in adults without language restrictions. The following MeSH (Medical Subject Headings) terms were used: "appendicitis", "meta-analysis", "appendectomy", and "anti-bacterial agents" with Boolean terms. The "related article" function and article references were searched to add other eligible meta-analyses. Experts in the field were also consulted for suggestions on further studies.

Data extraction

Two different authors (L.L.R. and F.M.B.R.) independently performed the search and retrieved eligible meta-analyses based on previously set inclusion and exclusion criteria. In case of no two authors consensus, a third one (M.S.) was contacted. The data extracted from each study included: first author, year of publication, geographic region, number and design of studies included, inclusion and exclusion criteria, studied population characteristics, statistical analysis (e.g. data on treatment effect, random and/or fixed models; heterogeneity), primary and secondary outcomes and study limitations.

Statistical analysis

Descriptive statistics summarizing the included studies were calculated. The mean ± standard deviation was used for normally distributed continuous variables. The median and interquartile range was used for non-normally distributed continuous variables. Odds ratio and 95 % confidence interval were calculated for specific outcomes from data available in the individual studies whenever not directly calculated by the meta-analysis authors. The meta-analysis pooled results, including the measures of central tendency and measures of treatment effect plus their associated 95 % confidence interval (CI) and p-value when available, were extracted and summarized. Ratios were calculated between appendectomy and antibiotics alone groups whenever applicable.

Results

A total of eight meta-analyses were retrieved [11, 13–19] and their general characteristics are shown in Table 1. The mean number of pooled patients included in each meta-analysis was 862 ± 211, which accounts for a mean of 403 ± 74 patients in the primary antibiotic therapy group and a mean of 458 ± 163 patients in the primary appendectomy group. The mean number of studies included was 4.38 ± 1.07. Generally, the quality of the individual studies was deemed low to moderate by different scales. From all the meta-analyses included, there were eight different individual studies, in different combinations

Table 1 Characteristics of included meta-analyses comparing antibiotics alone versus appendectomy in patients with acute uncomplicated appendicitis

Author (year)	Patients included			Study included	Study design	Quality evaluation
	Total	A	S			
Varadhan et al. (2010) [13]	661	350	311	3 [24–26]	RCT	2.7[a]
Liu et al. (2011) [14]	1201	433	768	6 [24–29]	RCT Observational	≥5[b]
Ansaloni et al. (2011) [15]	741	390	351	4 [24–26, 28]	RCT	Poor
Wilms et al. (2011) [16]	901	415	486	5 [25, 26, 28–30]	RCT	Low-moderate
Mason et al. (2012) [17]	980	510	470	5 [24–26, 28, 30]	RCT	1.8[a]
Varadhan et al. (2012) [18]	900	470	430	4 [24–26, 30]	RCT	Moderate[c]
Liu et al. (2014) [19]	983	391	592	5 [24–26, 29, 31]	RCT	3.2[a]
Kirby et al. (2015) [11]	531	268	263	3 [25, 26, 30]	RCT	N/A

[a]Mean Jadad score
[b]NOQAS
[c]GRADE system
Abbreviations: *A* antibiotics therapy group, *S* surgery group, *RCT* randomized controlled trial, *NOQAS* Newcastle-Ottawa Quality Assessment Scale, *GRADE* Grading of Recommendations Assessment, Development and Evaluation, *N/A* data not available

[20–27], with the majority being prospective studies (87.5 %). Only one meta-analysis included a retrospective study [23].

The main outcome metrics of each meta-analysis are illustrated in Table 2. Conservative therapy with antibiotic therapy was associated with significantly reduced minor (i.e. superficial wound infection, prolonged postoperative course, diarrhea, *Clostridium difficile* infection, fungal infection, etc.) and major (i.e. abscess formation, peritonitis, deep wound infection, reoperation, small bowel obstruction, postoperative cardiac events and venous thromboembolism) complication rates in most meta-analyses. The exception was the study by Kirby et al. [11], which reported a risk ratio of 7.71 (95%CI 2.33, 25.53) for major complications (i.e. peritonitis or abscess after the primary intervention) in patients assigned to antibiotic groups.

The conservative treatment was associated with faster recovery from inflammatory response, as evaluated by a better temperature curve, neutrophils count and C-reactive protein levels. Also, patients treated with antibiotics alone experienced significantly less pain duration and analgesic medication consumption. Regarding the return to daily activities, patients treated with antibiotics alone had a faster return to work (WMD, −5.20 95%CI −6.99, −3.40 days; $p < 0.001$) and less sick leave duration (MD, −0.19 95%CI −0.33, −0.06; $p = 0.005$). At the 1-year follow-up, there was no significant difference between groups in terms of perforation rates (10.6 % versus 9.3 %; p = NS) [11].

Table 2 Measured outcomes from different meta-analyses comparing appendectomy versus antibiotics alone for acute uncomplicated appendicitis

Outcome	Measure of Effect (95 % CI)	*p*-value	Heterogeneity	Authors' conclusion
Complications	0.43 (0.15, 1.21) [13]	0.11	Moderate	
	0.31 (0.19, 0.49) [14]	<0.05	Not present	
	1.92 (1.30, 2.85) [15]	N/A	Not present	
	0.83 (0.72, 0.91) [16]	N/A	Low	Favors antibiotics
	0.54 (0.37, 0.78) [17]	0.001	Moderate	
	0.69 (0.54, 0.89) [18]	0.004	Not present	
	0.86 (0.59, 1.26) [19]	0.44	Not present	
Treatment efficacy	4.54 (3.02, 6.82) [13]	<0.001	N/A	
	6.01 (4.27, 8.47) [15]	N/A	Not present	Favors surgery
	Crosses NI margin [16]	N/A	N/A	
	8.89 (5.94, 13.32) [18]	<0.001	N/A	
Treatment failure	6.9 % ± 4.4 % [14]	N/A	N/A	Favors surgery
	6.72 (3.48, 12.99) [17]	<0.001	Moderate	
Readmissions	15 % [13]			
	14.2 ± 10.6 % [14]			Favors surgery
	20 % [18]			
Complicated appendicitis	0.46 (0.19, 1.12) [18]	0.09	High	
	0.58 (0.18, 1.90) [18]	0.37	Moderate	Inconclusive
	0.73 (0.29, 1.84) [15]	N/A	Not present	
Pain/Analgesia	ATB less pain [15]	<0.001	N/A	
	−1.55 (−1.96, −1.14) [17]	<0.001	Not present	Favors antibiotics
	−0.13 (−0.28, 0.03) [17]	0.11	Low	
Length of hospital stay	0.11 (−0.22, 0.43) [13]	0.53	Moderate	
	0.66 (0.44, 0.87) [15]	<0.001	Low	
	0.34 (−0.06, 0.73) [17]	0.09	Low	Inconclusive
	0.34 (−0.19, 0.87) [18]	0.20	Low	
	0.01 (−0.01, 0.03) [19]	0.26	High	
Time to return to work	−0.19 (−0.33, −0.06) [17]	0.005	Not present	Favor antibiotics
	−5.20 (−6.99, −3.40) [19]	<0.001	High	

Abbreviations: *ACI* confidence interval, *ATB* antibiotics, *NI* non-inferiority, *N/A*, data not available

Comparing treatment efficacy, appendectomy was significantly more efficient than antibiotics alone (OR, 6.01 95%CI 4.37, 8.46) when overall treatment was analyzed. Comparing cure up to 1 year, the comparison was inconclusive according to a 20 % non-inferiority margin set by Wilms et al. [16] For the first 24 to 48 h (6.9 % versus 7.3 %) and initial hospitalization (OR, 2.43 95%CI 0.94, 6.33; $p = 0.07$), both treatments were equivalent in terms of treatment failures. On the other hand, exclusive antibiotic therapy was associated with a higher rate of readmission, which varied between 14.2 and 20 %. And from these readmissions, the absolute majority of patients were treated by the surgical approach, with a second course of antibiotics used in only a few cases (data not shown).

In the majority of meta-analyses, the length of hospital stay was not significantly different between the two groups (Table 2). The exception was the meta-analysis by Wilms et al. [16], which concluded that patients submitted to appendectomy had a reduction of 34 % in their length of hospital stay compared to conservative therapy (OR, 0.66 95%CI 0.44, 0.87).

The meta-analysis by Ansaloni et al. [15] was the only one that addressed costs. In this study, conservative therapy was associated with a mean cost reduction of USD 1257 per patient treated (USD 2893 versus USD 4150).

Discussion

To the best of our knowledge, this is the first study to assess a series of meta-analyses comparing appendectomy to antibiotics for uncomplicated acute appendicitis. The results of our review of this series of meta-analyses showed that conservative treatment with antibiotics for uncomplicated acute appendicitis is associated with less complications, faster recovery from an inflammatory state, shorter pain duration and reduced consumption of analgesic medication, faster return to work and reduced costs. Conversely, conservative treatment is associated with significantly higher treatment failure and readmission rates compared to primary appendectomy.

Treating appendicitis implies understanding acute appendicitis as a spectrum of disease, ranging from mild spontaneous resolution cases (up to 20 %) [28] through perforation and generalized peritonitis. In this sense, the actual challenge is to distinguish those patients who will spontaneously resolve the inflammatory state from those who will develop complications (gangrene, abscess, perforation and peritonitis). Some studies attempted to determine the risk factors for complicated appendicitis [29–31]. The main risk factors associated with complicated appendicitis are clinical (i.e. male sex, age ≥60 years of age and onset of symptoms) and laboratorial (i.e. leukocytosis, elevated C-reactive protein and bilirubin). Imaging investigations may improve diagnosis, avoiding conservative treatment of patients with complicated appendicitis [32].

CT scan, US and clinical exam, or a combination of these were used to diagnosis uncomplicated acute appendicitis. The CT scan in acute appendicitis has the highest diagnostic sensitivity and specificity, [28] increasing the appendectomy rate, especially in patients with lower Alvarado score [33, 34]. On the other hand, it is related to radiation exposure. The use of combined clinical scores (i.e. Alvarado score and Appendicitis Inflammatory Response score) allied with rational use of imaging methods (i.e. no routine use of CT scan, US in most cases) showed to be nearly as reliable as CT scan for diagnosis of acute appendicitis [35].

Antibiotics success rates as primary therapy for uncomplicated acute appendicitis varied from 58.3 to 73.4 %. As much as 42 % of patients primarily treated with antibiotics will require appendectomy later on in the disease's course [13]. Treating patients with uncomplicated appendicitis initially with antibiotics is safe even if an appendectomy is required later [36]. The use of prophylactic antibiotics during appendectomy is associated with a 3-fold reduction in the incidence of wound infection after appendectomy [37]. In the included studies, the surgical wound infection rate in patients undergoing primary appendectomy was 2.8 % when antibiotic prophylaxis was employed and 11.8 % when it was not [20, 26]. This may have introduced a bias in the meta-analyses that used wound infection as a primary outcome [18], since studies that did not use prophylactic antibiotics may be prone to favor the conservative treatment group [21]. Another issue is the use of heterogeneous antibiotic schemes, which includes oral, intravenous or mixed courses and mono/multi drug therapy. Some antibiotic schemes, such as amoxicillin plus clavulanic acid for Escherichia coli, may be ineffective for treating common gastrointestinal tract bacteria.

Open appendectomy, albeit largely performed worldwide, is associated with longer pain duration and analgesic consumption, longer time to return to work and sick leave, and higher rates of wound infection compared to laparoscopic appendectomy [38]. Patients were submitted to open appendectomy in the majority of studies included. This may have contributed to the significant differences in pain and analgesic consumption, time to work and wound infection rates observed between antibiotics and surgery groups.

All the studies suffered from several methodological limitations and the majority of the outcomes studied in individual meta-analyses presented some degree of heterogeneity, making it challenging to draw definitive conclusions. The study by Hansson et al. [20] showed a very high crossover rate (47.5 %) mainly from antibiotics to the appendectomy group, this might have introduced bias to meta-analyses, which includes this study. Due to the reduced number of enrolled patients, no subgroup analyses were performed to account for possible confounders such as sex, age, diagnostic assessment, surgical procedure (open versus laparoscopic), and use of prophylactic antibiotics to cite a few. Additionally, unblinded outcome assessment may overestimate the effects of treatment and lack of allocation concealment may have introduced selection bias to the analysis.

The recently published APPAC randomized clinical trial [36] was a well-designed adequately powered non-inferiority study comparing antibiotics (ertapenem for 3 days plus levofloxacin and metronidazole for 7 days) to appendectomy. It included in the primary analysis 272 patients in the appendectomy group and 256 in the antibiotic therapy group. The primary endpoint for surgery (successful completion of appendectomy) occurred in 99.6 % (95 %CI 98 %, 100 %) and the primary endpoint for antibiotic therapy group (discharge from hospital without need for appendectomy and no recurrent appendicitis within 1-year follow-up) occurred in 72.7 % (95 %CI 66.8 %, 78 %). The difference between treatments was −27 % (95%CI −31.6 %, ∞; $p = 0.89$), which crossed the non-inferiority margin of 24 %. The rate of complicated appendicitis did not differ between groups, and the antibiotics group presented lower complication rates. The length of stay was significantly higher in the antibiotics group, though not clinically significant. The ASAA (www.clinicaltrials.gov, NCT01421901) is another well-designed study whose findings will be published soon. The inclusion of these studies in future meta-analyses will help improve the methodological quality and robustness of the results.

Conclusion

Appendectomy is considered the gold standard for treating uncomplicated acute appendicitis. Nevertheless, for a selected subgroup of patients with no risk factors for complicated appendicitis and/or high surgical risk, conservative therapy with antimicrobials may be safe and effective. The decision to treat patients with acute uncomplicated appendicitis must be made on an individual basis and these patients may be followed closely.

Abbreviations

CI: Confidence interval; CT: Computed tomography; GRADE: Grading of Recommendations Assessment, Development and Evaluation; LOS: Length of stay; MD: Mean difference; N/A: Data not available; NI: Non-inferiority; NS: Not statistically significant; NOQAS: Newcastle-Ottawa Quality Assessment Scale; OR: Odds ratio; RCT: Randomized controlled trial; RR: Risk ratio; US: Ultrasonography; WMD: Weighted mean difference.

Competing interests

All authors declare no conflicts of interest related to this manuscript.

Authors' contributions

L.L.R. and M.S. were responsible for the study concept and design. L.L.R. and F.M.B.R. carried out the literature search. All authors were involved in acquisition of data from the individual meta-analyses included. L.L.R. and M.S. were responsible for analysis and interpretation of data. L.L.R. drafted the manuscript and performed the statistical analysis. All authors critically reviewed the manuscript for important intellectual content. M.S. was the study supervisor. All authors read and approved the final version of the manuscript.

Acknowledgements

We are indebted to Mario de Almeida Correia for critically reviewing this manuscript and James Joseph Hesson for English review.

Author details

[1]Intensive Care Unit, Hospital Israelita Albert Einstein, São Paulo, Brazil. [2]Telemedicine Service, Hospital Israelita Albert Einstein, Av. Albert Einstein, 2 andar, bloco D, São Paulo CEP: 05651-901, Brazil. [3]Surgery Department, Hospital Israelita Albert Einstein, São Paulo, Brazil.

References

1. Humes DJ, Simpson J. Acute appendicitis. BMJ. 2006;333:530–4.
2. Addiss DG, Shaffer N, Fowler BS, Tauxe RV. The epidemiology of appendicitis and appendectomy in the United States. Am J Epidemiol. 1990;132:910–25.
3. Davies GM, Dasbach EJ, Teutsch S. The burden of appendicitis-related hospitalizations in the United States in 1997. Surg Infect (Larchmt). 2004;5:160–5.
4. Fitz RH. Perforating inflammation of the vermiform appendix. Am J Med Sci. 1886;92:321–46.
5. McBurney C. Experiences with early operative interference in cases of disease of the vermiform appendix. N Y Med J. 1889;50:1676–84.
6. Blomqvist P, Ljung H, Nyren O, Ekbom A. Appendectomy in Sweden 1989–1993 assessed by the Inpatient Registry. J Clin Epidemiol. 1998;51:859–65.
7. Margenthaler JA, Longo WE, Virgo KS, Johnson FE, Oprian CA, Henderson WG, et al. Risk factors for adverse outcomes after the surgical treatment of appendicitis in adults. Ann Surg. 2003;238:59–66.
8. Coldrey E. Five years convervative treatment of acute appendicitis. J Int Coll Surg. 1959;32:255–61.
9. Simillis C, Symeonides P, Shorthouse AJ, Tekkis PP. A meta-analysis comparing conservative treatment versus acute appendectomy for complicated appendicitis (abscess or phlegmon). Surgery. 2010;147:818–29.
10. Wong WD, Wexner SD, Lowry A, Vernava 3rd A, Burnstein M, Denstman F, et al. Practice parameters for the treatment of sigmoid diverticulitis–supporting documentation. The Standards Task Force. The American Society of Colon and Rectal Surgeons. Dis Colon Rectum. 2000;43:290–7.
11. Kirby A, Hobson RP, Burke D, Cleveland V, Ford G, West RM. Appendicectomy for suspected uncomplicated appendicitis is associated with fewer complications than conservative antibiotic management: a meta-analysis of post-intervention complications. J Infect. 2015;70:105–10.
12. Mason RJ. Surgery for appendicitis: is it necessary? Surg Infect (Larchmt). 2008;9:481–8.
13. Varadhan KK, Humes DJ, Neal KR, Lobo DN. Antibiotic therapy versus appendectomy for acute appendicitis: a meta-analysis. World J Surg. 2010;34:199–209.
14. Liu K, Fogg L. Use of antibiotics alone for treatment of uncomplicated acute appendicitis: a systematic review and meta-analysis. Surgery. 2011;150:673–83.
15. Ansaloni L, Catena F, Coccolini F, Ercolani G, Gazzotti F, Pasqualini E, et al. Surgery versus conservative antibiotic treatment in acute appendicitis: a systematic review and meta-analysis of randomized controlled trials. Dig Surg. 2011;28:210–21.
16. Wilms IM, de Hoog DE, de Visser DC, Janzing HM. Appendectomy versus antibiotic treatment for acute appendicitis. Cochrane Database Syst Rev. 2011;11:CD008359.

17. Mason RJ, Moazzez A, Sohn H, Katkhouda N. Meta-analysis of randomized trials comparing antibiotic therapy with appendectomy for acute uncomplicated (no abscess or phlegmon) appendicitis. Surg Infect (Larchmt). 2012;13:74–84.
18. Varadhan KK, Neal KR, Lobo DN. Safety and efficacy of antibiotics compared with appendicectomy for treatment of uncomplicated acute appendicitis: meta-analysis of randomised controlled trials. BMJ. 2012;344:e2156.
19. Liu ZH, Li C, Zhang XW, Kang L, Wang JP. Meta-analysis of the therapeutic effects of antibiotic versus appendicectomy for the treatment of acute appendicitis. Exp Ther Med. 2014;7:1181–6.
20. Hansson J, Korner U, Khorram-Manesh A, Solberg A, Lundholm K. Randomized clinical trial of antibiotic therapy versus appendicectomy as primary treatment of acute appendicitis in unselected patients. Br J Surg. 2009;96:473–81.
21. Styrud J, Eriksson S, Nilsson I, Ahlberg G, Haapaniemi S, Neovius G, et al. Appendectomy versus antibiotic treatment in acute appendicitis. a prospective multicenter randomized controlled trial. World J Surg. 2006;30:1033–7.
22. Eriksson S, Granstrom L. Randomized controlled trial of appendicectomy versus antibiotic therapy for acute appendicitis. Br J Surg. 1995;82:166–9.
23. Liu K, Ahanchi S, Pisaneschi M, Lin I, Walter R. Can acute appendicitis be treated by antibiotics alone? Am Surg. 2007;73:1161–5.
24. Malik AA, Bari SU. Conservative management of acute appendicitis. J Gastrointest Surg. 2009;13:966–70.
25. Turhan AN, Kapan S, Kutukcu E, Yigitbas H, Hatipoglu S, Aygun E. Comparison of operative and non operative management of acute appendicitis. Ulus Travma Acil Cerrahi Derg. 2009;15:459–62.
26. Vons C, Barry C, Maitre S, Pautrat K, Leconte M, Costaglioli B, et al. Amoxicillin plus clavulanic acid versus appendicectomy for treatment of acute uncomplicated appendicitis: an open-label, non-inferiority, randomised controlled trial. Lancet. 2011;377:1573–9.
27. Gibeily GJ, Ross MN, Manning DB, Wherry DC, Kao TC. Late-presenting appendicitis: a laparoscopic approach to a complicated problem. Surg Endosc. 2003;17:725–9.
28. Cobben LP, de Van Otterloo AM, Puylaert JB. Spontaneously resolving appendicitis: frequency and natural history in 60 patients. Radiology. 2000;215:349–52. 28. Paulson EK, Kalady MF, Pappas TN (2003) Clinical practice. Suspected appendicitis. N Engl J Med 348: 236–242.
29. Barreto SG, Travers E, Thomas T, Mackillop C, Tiong L, Lorimer M, et al. Acute perforated appendicitis: an analysis of risk factors to guide surgical decision making. Indian J Med Sci. 2010;64:58–65.
30. Sheu BF, Chiu TF, Chen JC, Tung MS, Chang MW, Young WR. Risk factors associated with perforated appendicitis in elderly patients presenting with signs and symptoms of acute appendicitis. ANZ J Surg. 2007;77:662–6.
31. McGowan DR, Sims HM, Zia K, Uheba M, Shaikh IA. The value of biochemical markers in predicting a perforation in acute appendicitis. ANZ J Surg. 2013;83:79–83.
32. Nomura O, Ishiguro A, Meakawa T, Nagai A, Kuroda T, Sakai H. Antibiotic administration can be an independent risk factor for therapeutic delay of pediatric acute appendicitis. Pediatr Emerg Care. 2012;28:792–5.
33. Petrosyan M, Estrada J, Chan S, Somers S, Yacoub WN, Kelso RL, et al. CT scan in patients with suspected appendicitis: clinical implications for the acute care surgeon. Eur Surg Res. 2008;40:211–9.
34. Alvarado A. A practical score for the early diagnosis of acute appendicitis. Ann Emerg Med. 1986;15:557–64.
35. Saverio D, Sibilio A, Giorgini E, Biscardi A, Villani S, Coccolini F, et al. The NOTA Study (Non Operative Treatment for Acute Appendicitis): prospective study on the efficacy and safety of antibiotics (amoxicillin and clavulanic acid) for treating patients with right lower quadrant abdominal pain and long-term follow-up of conservatively treated suspected appendicitis. Ann Surg. 2014;260:109–17.
36. Salminen P, Paajanen H, Rautio T, Nordström P, Aarnio M, Rantanen T, et al. Antibiotic therapy vs appendectomy for treatment of uncomplicated acute appendicitis: the APPAC randomized clinical trial. JAMA. 2015;313:2340–8.
37. Andersen BR, Kallehave FL, Andersen HK. Antibiotics versus placebo for prevention of postoperative infection after appendicectomy. Cochrane Database Syst Rev. 2005;20:CD001439.
38. Sauerland S, Jaschinski T, Neugebauer EA. Laparoscopic versus open surgery for suspected appendicitis. Cochrane Database Syst Rev. 2010;10:CD001546.

20

Global validation of the WSES Sepsis Severity Score for patients with complicated intra-abdominal infections

Massimo Sartelli[1*], Fikri M. Abu-Zidan[2], Fausto Catena[3], Ewen A. Griffiths[4], Salomone Di Saverio[5], Raul Coimbra[6], Carlos A. Ordoñez[7], Ari Leppaniemi[8], Gustavo P. Fraga[9], Federico Coccolini[10], Ferdinando Agresta[11], Asrhaf Abbas[12], Saleh Abdel Kader[13], John Agboola[14], Adamu Amhed[15], Adesina Ajibade[16], Seckin Akkucuk[17], Bandar Alharthi[18], Dimitrios Anyfantakis[19], Goran Augustin[20], Gianluca Baiocchi[21], Miklosh Bala[22], Oussama Baraket[23], Savas Bayrak[24], Giovanni Bellanova[25], Marcelo A. Beltràn[26], Roberto Bini[27], Matthew Boal[4], Andrey V. Borodach[28], Konstantinos Bouliaris[29], Frederic Branger[30], Daniele Brunelli[31], Marco Catani[32], Asri Che Jusoh[33], Alain Chichom-Mefire[34], Gianfranco Cocorullo[35], Elif Colak[36], David Costa[37], Silvia Costa[38], Yunfeng Cui[39], Geanina Loredana Curca[40], Terry Curry[6], Koray Das[41], Samir Delibegovic[42], Zaza Demetrashvili[43], Isidoro Di Carlo[44], Nadezda Drozdova[45], Tamer El Zalabany[46], Mushira Abdulaziz Enani[47], Mario Faro[48], Mahir Gachabayov[49], Teresa Giménez Maurel[50], Georgios Gkiokas[51], Carlos Augusto Gomes[52], Ricardo Alessandro Teixeira Gonsaga[53], Gianluca Guercioni[54], Ali Guner[55], Sanjay Gupta[56], Sandra Gutierrez[57], Martin Hutan[58], Orestis Ioannidis[59], Arda Isik[60], Yoshimitsu Izawa[61], Sumita A. Jain[62], Mantas Jokubauskas[63], Aleksandar Karamarkovic[64], Saila Kauhanen[65], Robin Kaushik[56], Jakub Kenig[66], Vladimir Khokha[67], Jae Il Kim[68], Victor Kong[69], Renol Koshy[44], Avidyl Krasniqi[70], Ashok Kshirsagar[71], Zygimantas Kuliesius[72], Konstantinos Lasithiotakis[73], Pedro Leão[74], Jae Gil Lee[75], Miguel Leon[76], Aintzane Lizarazu Pérez[77], Varut Lohsiriwat[78], Eudaldo López-Tomassetti Fernandez[79], Eftychios Lostoridis[80], Raghuveer Mn[81], Piotr Major[82], Athanasios Marinis[83], Daniele Marrelli[84], Aleix Martinez-Perez[85], Sanjay Marwah[86], Michael McFarlane[87], Renato Bessa Melo[88], Cristian Mesina[89], Nick Michalopoulos[90], Radu Moldovanu[91], Ouadii Mouaqit[92], Akutu Munyika[93], Ionut Negoi[94], Ioannis Nikolopoulos[95], Gabriela Elisa Nita[10], Iyiade Olaoye[96], Abdelkarim Omari[97], Paola Rodríguez Ossa[7], Zeynep Ozkan[98], Ramakrishnapillai Padmakumar[99], Francesco Pata[100], Gerson Alves Pereira Junior[101], Jorge Pereira[102], Tadeja Pintar[103], Konstantinos Pouggouras[80], Vinod Prabhu[104], Stefano Rausei[105], Miran Rems[106], Daniel Rios-Cruz[107], Boris Sakakushev[108], Maria Luisa Sánchez de Molina[109], Charampolos Seretis[110], Vishal Shelat[111], Romeo Lages Simões[9], Giovanni Sinibaldi[112], Matej Skrovina[113], Dmitry Smirnov[114], Charalampos Spyropoulos[115], Jaan Tepp[116], Tugan Tezcaner[117], Matti Tolonen[8], Myftar Torba[118], Jan Ulrych[119], Mustafa Yener Uzunoglu[120], David van Dellen[121], Gabrielle H. van Ramshorst[122], Giorgio Vasquez[123], Aurélien Venara[30], Andras Vereczkei[124], Nereo Vettoretto[125], Nutu Vlad[126], Sanjay Kumar Yadav[127], Tonguç Utku Yilmaz[128], Kuo-Ching Yuan[129], Sanoop Koshy Zachariah[130], Maurice Zida[131], Justas Zilinskas[63] and Luca Ansaloni[10]

* Correspondence: massimosartelli@gmail.com
[1]Department of Surgery, Macerata Hospital, Macerata, Italy
Full list of author information is available at the end of the article

Abstract

Background: To validate a new practical Sepsis Severity Score for patients with complicated intra-abdominal infections (cIAIs) including the clinical conditions at the admission (severe sepsis/septic shock), the origin of the cIAIs, the delay in source control, the setting of acquisition and any risk factors such as age and immunosuppression.

Methods: The WISS study (WSES cIAIs Score Study) is a multicenter observational study underwent in 132 medical institutions worldwide during a four-month study period (October 2014-February 2015). Four thousand five hundred thirty-three patients with a mean age of 51.2 years (range 18–99) were enrolled in the WISS study.

Results: Univariate analysis has shown that all factors that were previously included in the WSES Sepsis Severity Score were highly statistically significant between those who died and those who survived ($p < 0.0001$). The multivariate logistic regression model was highly significant ($p < 0.0001$, $R2 = 0.54$) and showed that all these factors were independent in predicting mortality of sepsis. Receiver Operator Curve has shown that the WSES Severity Sepsis Score had an excellent prediction for mortality. A score above 5.5 was the best predictor of mortality having a sensitivity of 89.2 %, a specificity of 83.5 % and a positive likelihood ratio of 5.4.

Conclusions: WSES Sepsis Severity Score for patients with complicated Intra-abdominal infections can be used on global level. It has shown high sensitivity, specificity, and likelihood ratio that may help us in making clinical decisions.

Keywords: Intra-abdominal, Infections, Sepsis, Septic shock

Background

Intra-abdominal infections (IAIs) include several different pathological conditions [1] and are usually classified into uncomplicated and complicated. In complicated IAIs (cIAIs), the infectious process extends beyond the organ, and causes either localized peritonitis or diffuse peritonitis. The treatment of patients with complicated intra-abdominal infections involves both source control and antibiotic therapy. Complicated IAIs are an important cause of morbidity and may be associated with poor prognosis. However the term "complicated intra-abdominal infections" describes a wide heterogeneity of patient populations, making it difficult to suggest a general treatment regimen and stressing the need of an individualized approach to decision making.

Early prognostic evaluation of complicated intra-abdominal infections is crucial to assess the severity and decide the aggressiveness of treatment. Many factors influencing the prognosis of patients with cIAIs have been described, including advanced age, poor nutrition, pre-existing diseases, immunosuppression, extended peritonitis, occurrence of septic shock, poor source control, organ failures, prolonged hospitalization before therapy, and infection with nosocomial pathogens [2–10].

Recently the World Society of Emergency Surgery (WSES) designed a global prospective observational study (CIAOW Study) [11, 12]. All the risk factors for occurrence of death during hospitalization were evaluated and then discussed with an international panel of experts. The most significant variables, adjusted to clinical criteria, were used to create a severity score for patients with cIAIs including the clinical conditions at admission (severe sepsis/septic shock), the origin of the cIAIs, the delay in source control, the setting of acquisition and any risk factors such as age and immunosuppression (Appendix).

There may be different causes of sepsis, health care standards, and differences in underlying health status, economical differences that make prediction of sepsis on global level difficult. The WSES addressed this issue in the present study which aims to validate a previous score on a global level.

Methods

Ethical statement

The study met the standards outlined in the Declaration of Helsinki and Good Epidemiological Practices. This study did not change or modify the laboratory or clinical practices of each centre and differences of practices were kept as they are. The data collection was anonymous and identifiable patient information was not submitted.

Individual researchers were responsible for complying with local ethical standards and hospital registration of the study.

Study population

This multicenter observational study was run in 132 medical institutions from 54 countries worldwide during a four-month period (October 2014-February 2015). Inclusion criteria were patients older than 18 years with complicated intra-abdominal sepsis (cIAIs) who had surgical management or interventional radiological drainage. cIAIs was defined as an infectious process that proceeded beyond the organ, and caused either localized peritonitis/abscess or diffuse peritonitis [13]. Patients who were younger than 18 years, or those who had pancreatitis, or primary peritonitis were excluded from the study. Severe sepsis was defined as sepsis-induced tissue hypoperfusion or organ dysfunction (any of the following thought to be due to the infection): hypotension (<90/60 or MAP < 65), lactate above upper limits laboratory normal, Urine output < 0.5 mL/kg/h for more than 2 h despite adequate fluid resuscitation, Creatinine > 2.0 mg/dL (176.8 μmol/L), Bilirubin > 2 mg/dL (34.2 μmol/L), Platelet count < 100,000 μL, Coagulopathy (international normalized ratio > 1.5), Acute lung injury with Pao2/Fio2 < 250 in the absence of pneumonia as infection source. Septic shock was defined as severe sepsis associated with refractory hypotension (BP < 90/60) despite adequate fluid resuscitation [14].

WSES Sepsis Severity Score for patients with complicated Intra-abdominal infections is shown in Appendix.

Data monitoring and collection

The study was monitored by the coordination center, which investigated and verified missing or unclear data submitted to the central database. This study was performed under the direct supervision of the Board of Directors of WSES. In each centre, the coordinator collected and compiled data in an online case report system. Data were entered directly through a web-based computerized database. Data were entered either by a drop menu for categorical data like the source of infection or numbers for continuous variables such as age. Data collected included demographic data of the patient and disease characteristics, demographical data, type of infection (community- or healthcare-acquired), severity criteria and origin of infection and surgical procedures performed.

Statistical analysis

Sepsis status was coded as ordinal data for testing the logistic regression (not for scoring) as follows: no sepsis = 0, sepsis = 2, severe sepsis = 3, septic shock = 4). The source of sepsis was analysed as categorical data in the logistic regression, and the age as continuous data, while healthcare associated infection, delay in management, and immunosuppression as binomial data. The variables used in this scoring system in the patients who survived and those who died were compared using univariate analysis. This included Fisher's exact test or Pearson Chi-Square as appropriate for categorical data and Mann–Whitney U-test for continuous or ordinal data. Significant factors were then entered into a direct logistic regression model. A p value of ≤ 0.05 was considered significant. Data were analyzed with PASW Statistics 21, SPSS Inc, USA.

Results

Four thousand six hundred fifty-two cases were collected in the online case report system. One hundred twenty-nine cases did not meet the inclusion criteria. Four thousand five hundred thirty-three patients with a mean age of 51.2 years (range 18–99) were enrolled in the WISS study. One thousand nine hundred thirty-five patients (42.7 %) were women and 2598 (57.3 %) were men.

Among these patients, 3966 (87.5 %) were affected by community-acquired IAIs while the remaining 567 (12.5 %) suffered from healthcare-associated infections. One thousand six hundred twenty-seven patients (35.9 %) were affected by generalized peritonitis while 2906 (64.1 %) suffered from localized peritonitis or abscesses. Seven hundred ninety-one patients (17.4 %) were admitted in critical condition (severe sepsis/septic shock). The various sources of infection are outlined in Table 1. The most frequent source of infection was acute appendicitis; 1553 cases (34.2 %) involved complicated appendicitis.

The overall mortality rate was 9.2 % (416/4533).

Table 2 shows the univariate analysis comparing patients with complicated intra-abdominal infection who survived and those who died. The analysis shows that all factors included in the Sepsis Severity Score were highly significantly different between those who died and those who survived ($p < 0.0001$ in all variables). Accordingly all factors were entered into a direct logistic regression model (Table 3). The direct logistic regression model was highly significant ($p < 0.0001$, $R2 = 0.54$) and showed that all factors included in the Sepsis Severity Score were significant independent

Table 1 Source of infection in 4553 patients from 132 hospitals worldwide (15 October 2014–15 February 2015)

Source of infection	Number (%)
Appendicitis	1553 (34.2 %)
Cholecystitis	837 (18.5 %)
Post-operative	387 (8.5 %)
Colonic non diverticular perforation	269 (5.9 %)
Gastro-duodenal perforations	498 (11 %)
Diverticulitis	234 (5.2 %)
Small bowel perforation	243 (5.4 %)
Others	348 (7.7 %)
PID	50 (1.1 %)
Post traumatic perforation	114 (2.5 %)
Missing	
Total	4553 (100 %)

PID pelvic inflammatory disease

Table 2 Univariate analysis of patients with complicated intra-abdominal infection comparing patients who survived ($n = 4117$) and patient who died ($n = 416$)

Variable	Survided (%) $n = 4117$	Died (%) $n = 416$	p value
Sepsis status			<0.0001
No sepsis	1914 (46.5 %)	23 (5.5 %)	
Sepsis	1725 (41.9 %)	80 (19.2 %)	
Severe sepsis	404 (9.8 %)	157 (37.7 %)	
Septic shock	74 (1.8 %)	156 (37.5 %)	
Healthcare associated infection	433 (10.5 %)	134 (32.2 %)	<0.0001
Source of infection			<0.0001
Appendicitis	1536 (37.3 %)	17 (4.1 %)	
Cholecystitis	809 (19.7 %)	28 (6.7 %)	
Colonic non diverticular perforation	204 (5 %)	65 (15.6 %)	
Diverticulitis	203 (4.9 %)	31 (7.5 %)	
Gastro-duodenal perforation	431 (10.5 %)	67 (16.2 %)	
PID	50 (1.2 %)	0 (0)	
Postoperative	415 (10.1 %)	86 (20.7 %)	
Small bowel perforation	174 (4.2 %)	69 (16.6 %)	
Post-traumatic	104 (2.5 %)	10 (2.4 %)	
Others	259 (6.3 %)	53 (12.7 %)	
Delay in source control	2015 (48.9 %)	341 (82 %)	<0.0001
Median age years (range)	48 (18–97)	79 (18–99)	<0.0001
Immunosuppresion	292 (7.1)	120 (28.8 %)	<0.0001
Sepsis severity score	3 (0–17)	10 (0–17)	<0.0001

Data presented as median range or number percentage as appropriate
PID pelvic inflammatory disease
p value = Fisher's exact test, Pearson Chi-Square, or Mann Whitney U test as appropriate

Table 3 Direct logistic regression model with factors affecting mortality of patients complicated intra-abdominal infection, global study of 132 centres, ($n = 4553$)

Score variable	B	S.E.	Wald test	*P* value	OR	OR 95 % C.I.	
						Lower	Upper
Sepsis status	1.57	0.08	365.59	<0.0001	4.81	4.09	5.65
Setting of infection acquisition	0.6	0.18	10.49	0.001	1.81	1.27	2.6
Source of infection[a]			59.38	<0.0001			
Colonic non-diverticulical perforation	−0.26	0.27	0.97	0.33	0.77	0.46	1.3
Diverticulitis diffuse peritonitis	−0.26	0.34	0.51	0.48	0.78	0.40	1.54
Postoperative diffuse peritonitis	−0.005	0.29	0	0.99	1.00	0.56	1.76
Remaining sources	−1.2	0.21	32.47	<0.0001	0.30	0.20	0.46
Delay in management	1.47	0.17	78.53	<0.0001	4.33	3.13	5.99
Age	0.04	0.004	103.58	<0.0001	1.04	1.04	1.05
Immunosuppression	1.24	0.17	55.79	<0.0001	3.46	2.5	4.79
Constant	−7.52	0.41	342.24	<0.0001	0.001		

OR odds ratio
[a]Compared with small bowel perforation

Table 4 Direct logistic regression model showing the ability of WSES Sepsis Severity Score in predicting mortality of patients complicated intra-abdominal infection, global study of 132 centres, ($n = 4553$)

Variable	B	S.E.	Wald	*P* value	OR	OR 95 % C.I.	
						Lower	Upper
WSESSCORE	0.58	0.02	639.59	<0.0001	1.784	1.706	1.866
Constant	−5.79	0.19	958.74	<0.0001	.003		

OR odds ratio

predictors of mortality. Accordingly the ability of the score to predict mortality was tested by a direct logistic regression which is shown in Table 4. Again, this model using only the sepsis severity score was highly significant ($p < 0.0001$, R2 = 0.5). The odds of death increased by 0.78 by an increase on one score which is remarkable.

Figure 1 shows that WSES Sepsis Severity Score had a very good ability of distinguishing those who survived from those who died. The overall mortality rate was 9.2 % (416/4533). This was 0.63 % for those who had a score of 0–3, 6.3 % for those who had a score of 4–6, and 41.7 % for those who had a score of ≥ 7. The receiver operating characteristic curve showed that the best cutoff point for predicting mortality was a Sepsis Severity Score. 5.5 was the best predictor of mortality having a sensitivity of 89.2 %, a specificity of 83.5 % and a positive likelihood ratio of 5.4 (Fig. 2).

Discussion

Complicated intra-abdominal infections remain an important source of patient morbidity and may be frequently associated with poor clinical prognosis. Treatment of patients with cIAIs, has been usually described to achieve satisfactory results if adequate management is established [15]. However, results from published clinical trials may not be representative of the true morbidity and mortality rates of such severe infections. First of all, patients who have perforated appendicitis are usually over-represented in clinical trials. Furthermore patients with intra-abdominal infection enrolled in clinical trials have often an increased likelihood of cure and survival. In fact the trial eligibility criteria usually restrict the inclusion of patients with co-morbid diseases that would increase the death rate of patients with intra-abdominal infections [16]. In the WISS study we enrolled all the patients older than 18 years old with complicated intra-abdominal infections in the study-period and the overall mortality rate was 9.2 % (416/4533). Stratification of the patient's risk is essential in order to optimize the treatment plan. Patients with intra-abdominal infections are generally classified into low risk and high risk. "High risk" is generally intended to describe patients with a high risk for treatment failure and mortality. In high risk patients the increased mortality associated with inappropriate management cannot be reversed by subsequent modifications. Therefore early prognostic

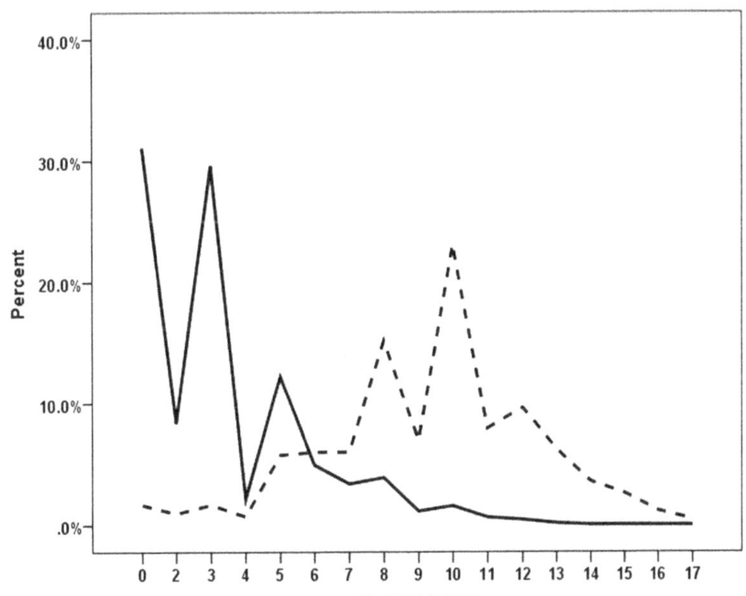

Fig. 1 Distribution of the percentile WSES Sepsis Severity Score of complicated intra-abdominal infection patients for those who survived (*solid line*) ($n = 4117$) and those who died (*interrupted line*) ($n = 416$)

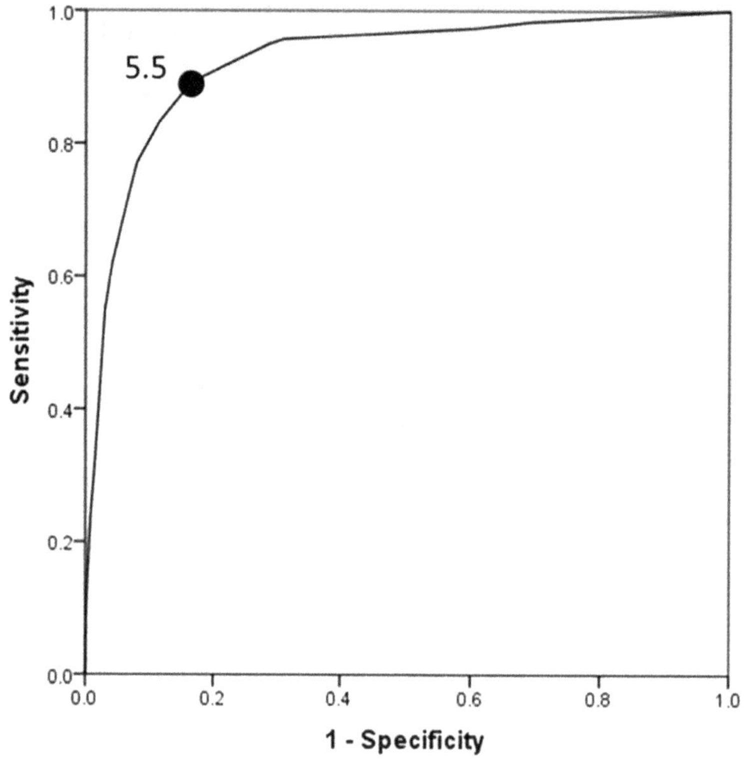

Fig. 2 Receiver operating characteristic curve for the best WSES Sepsis Severity Score that predicted mortality in patients having complicated intra-abdominal infection, global study of 132 centres, ($n = 4553$)

evaluation of complicated intra-abdominal infections is important to assess the severity and decide the aggressiveness of treatment.

Scoring systems can be roughly divided into two groups: disease-independent scores for evaluation of serious patients requiring care in the intensive care unit (ICU) such as APACHE II and Simplified Acute Physiology Score (SAPS II) and peritonitis-specific scores such as Mannheim Peritonitis Index (MPI) [17].

Although considered a good marker, APACHE II value in peritonitis has been questioned because of the difficulty of the APACHE II to evaluate interventions despite the fact that interventions might significantly alter many of the physiological variables. Moreover it requires appropriate software to be calculated [18].

The MPI is specific for peritonitis and easy to calculate. MPI was designed by Wacha and Linder in 1983 [19]. It was based on a retrospective analysis of data from 1253 patients with peritonitis. Among 20 possible risk factors, only 8 proved to be of prognostic relevance and were entered into the Mannheim Peritonitis Index, classified according to their predictive power. After 30 years, identifying a new clinical score to assess the severity the cIAIS would be clinically relevant in order to modulate the aggressiveness of treatment according the type of infection and the clinical characteristics of the patients.

WSES Sepsis Severity Score is a new practical clinical severity score for patients with complicated intra-abdominal infections. It is specific for cIAIs and easy to calculate, even during surgery. It may be relevant in order to modulate the aggressiveness of treatment particularly in higher risk patients.

The score is illustrated in Appendix. The statistical analysis shows that the sepsis severity score has a very good ability of distinguishing those who survived from those who died. The overall mortality was 0.63 % for those who had a score of 0–3, 6.3 % for those who had a score of 4–6, 41.7 % for those who had a score of ≥ 7. In patients who had a score of ≥ 9 the mortality rate was 55.5 %, those who had a score of ≥ 11 the mortality rate was 68.2 % and those who had a score ≥ 13 the mortality rate was 80.9 %.

Conclusions

Given the sweeping geographical distribution of the participating medical centers, WSES Sepsis Severity Score for patients with complicated Intra-abdominal infections can be used on global level. It has shown high sensitivity, specificity, and likelihood ratio that may help us in making clinical decisions.

Appendix

Table 5 WSES sepsis severity score for patients with complicated Intra-abdominal infections (Range: 0–18)

Clinical condition at the admission	
• Severe sepsis (acute organ dysfunction) at the admission	3 score
• Septic shock (acute circulatory failure characterized by persistent arterial hypotension. It always requires vasopressor agents) at the admission	5 score
Setting of acquisition	
• Healthcare associated infection	2 score
Origin of the IAIs	
• Colonic non-diverticular perforation peritonitis	2 score
• Small bowel perforation peritonitis	3 score
• Diverticular diffuse peritonitis	2 score
• Post-operative diffuse peritonitis	2 score
Delay in source control	
• Delayed initial intervention [Preoperative duration of peritonitis (localized or diffuse) > 24 h)]	3 score
Risk factors	
• Age>70	2 score
• Immunosuppression (chronic glucocorticoids, immunosuppresant agents, chemotherapy, lymphatic diseases, virus)	3 score

Competing interests
The authors declare that they have no competing interests.

Authors' contributions
MS designed the study and wrote the manuscript. FMA-Z performed statistical analysis. All authors participated in the study. All authors read and approved the final manuscript.

Author details
[1]Department of Surgery, Macerata Hospital, Macerata, Italy. [2]Department of Surgery, College of Medicine and Health Sciences, UAE University, Al-Ain, United Arab Emirates. [3]Department of Emergency Surgery, Maggiore Hospital, Parma, Italy. [4]General and Upper GI Surgery, Queen Elizabeth Hospital, Birmingham, UK. [5]Department of Surgery, Maggiore Hospital, Bologna, Italy. [6]Department of Surgery, UC San Diego Medical Center, San Diego, USA. [7]Fundación Valle del Lili, Universidad del Valle, Cali, Colombia. [8]Abdominal Center, University Hospital Meilahti, Helsinki, Finland. [9]Division of Trauma Surgery, Hospital de Clinicas, School of Medical Sciences, University of Campinas, Campinas, Brazil. [10]General and Emergency Surgery, Papa Giovanni XXIII Hospital, Bergamo, Italy. [11]General Surgery, ULSS19 del Veneto, Adria, RO, Italy. [12]Department of Surgery, Mansoura University Hospital, Mansoura, Egypt. [13]Department of General Surgery, Al Ain Hospital, Al-Ain City, United Arab Emirates. [14]Department of Surgery, Kwara State General Hospital, Ilorin, Nigeria. [15]Department of Surgery, Ahmadu Bello University Teaching Hospital Zaria, Kaduna, Nigeria. [16]Department of Surgery, LAUTECH Teaching Hospital, Osogbo, Nigeria. [17]Department of General Surgery, Training and Research Hospital of Mustafa Kemal University, Hatay, Turkey. [18]Depatment of Surgery, King Fahad Medical City, Riyadh, Saudi Arabia. [19]Primary Health Care Centre of Kissamos, Chania, Greece. [20]Department of Surgery, University Hospital Center, Zagreb, Croatia. [21]Clinical and Experimental Surgery, Brescia Civil Hospital, Brescia, Italy. [22]Trauma and Acute Care Surgery Unit, Hadassah Hebrew University Medical Center, Jerusalem, Israel. [23]Department of Surgery, Bizerte Hospital, Bizerte, Tunisia. [24]Department of General Surgery, Istanbul Training and Research Hospital, Istanbul, Turkey. [25]Surgical II Division, S. Chiara Hospital, Trento, Italy. [26]Department of General Surgery, Hospital San Juan de Dios de La Serena, La Serena, Chile. [27]Department of General and Emergency Surgery, SG Bosco Hospital, Turin, Italy. [28]Emergency Surgery Department, 1st Municipal Hospital, Novosibirsk State Medical University, Novosibirsk, Russian Federation. [29]Department of Surgery, University Hospital of Larissa, Larissa, Greece. [30]Visceral Surgery, CHU, Angers, France. [31]Chirurgia Generale, Ospedale di Città di Castello, Città di Castello, Italy. [32]Department of Emergency Surgery, Umberto I Hospital, "La Sapienza" University, Rome, Italy. [33]Department of Surgery, Kuala Krai Hospital, Kelantan, Malaysia. [34]Department of Surgery, Regional Hospital, Limbe, Cameroon. [35]General and Emergency Surgery, Policlinico Paolo Giaccone, Palermo, Italy. [36]Department of General Surgery, Samsun Education and Research Hospital, Samsun, Turkey. [37]Department of General and Digestive Tract Surgery, Alicante University General Hospital, Alicante, Spain. [38]Department of Surgery, CHVNG/E, EPE, Vila Nova de Gaia, Portugal. [39]Department of Surgery, Tianjin Nankai Hospital, Tianjin, China. [40]Department of General Surgery, Emergency Municipal Hospital Pascani, Pascani, Iasi, Romania. [41]Department of Surgery, Numune Training and Research Hospital, Adana, Turkey. [42]Department of Surgery, University Clinical Center, Tuzla, Bosnia and Herzegovina. [43]Department General Surgery, Kipshidze Central University Hospital, Tbilisi, Georgia. [44]Department of Surgery, Hamad General Hospital, Doha, Qatar. [45]Department of Surgery, Riga East Clinical University Hospital, Riga, Latvia. [46]Department of Surgery, Bahrain Defence Force Hospital, Manama, Bahrain. [47]King Fahad Medical City, Riyadh, Saudi Arabia. [48]Division of General and Emergency Surgery, Hospital Estadual Mario Covas, ABC School of Medicine, Santo André, Brazil. [49]Department of Surgery 1, Vladimir City Clinical Hospital of Emergency Medicine, Vladimir, Russian Federation. [50]Cirugía General y Digestiva, Hospital Universitario Miguel Servet, Zaragoza, Spain. [51]2nd Department of Surgery, Aretaieio University Hospital, Athens, Greece. [52]Department of Surgery, Hospital Universitário Terezinha de Jesus, Faculdade de Ciências Médicas e da Saúde de Juiz de Fora, Juiz de Fora, Brazil. [53]Department of Surgery, Hospital Escola Padre Albino, Catanduva, Brazil. [54]Department of Surgery, Ascoli Piceno Hospital, Ascoli Piceno, Italy. [55]Department of General Surgery, Trabzon Kanuni Training and Research Hospital, Trabzon, Turkey. [56]Department of Surgery, Government Medical College and Hospital, Chandigarh, India. [57]Hospital Universitario del Valle, Universidad del Valle, Cali, Colombia. [58]2nd Surgical Department of Medical Faculty Comenius University, University Hospital Bratislava, Bratislava, Slovakia. [59]2nd Surgical Department, General Hospital of Kavala, Kavala, Greece. [60]Department of Surgery, Mengucek Gazi Training Research Hospital, Erzincan, Turkey. [61]Department of Emergency and Critical Care Medicine, Jichi Medical University, Shimotsuke, Japan. [62]Department of Surgery, S M S Hospital, Jaipur, India. [63]Department of Surgery, Hospital of Lithuanian University of Health Sciences, Kaunas, Lithuania. [64]Clinic for Emergency Surgery, Medical Faculty University of Belgrade, Belgrade, Serbia. [65]Division Digestive Surgery and Urology, Turku University Hospital, Turku, Finland. [66]3rd Department of General Surgery, Jagiellonian Univeristy Collegium Medium, Kraków, Poland. [67]Department of Emergency Surgery, City Hospital, Mozyr, Belarus. [68]Department of Surgery, Ilsan Paik Hospital, Inje University College of Medicine, Goyang, Republic of Korea. [69]Department of Surgery, Edendale Hospital, Pietermaritzburg, South Africa. [70]Department of Surgery, University Clinical Center of Kosovo, Pristina, Kosovo. [71]Department of General Surgery, Krishna Hospital, Karad, India. [72]Department of General Surgery, Republican Vilnius University Hospital, Vilnius, Lithuania. [73]Department of Surgery, York Teaching Hospital NHS Foundation Trust, York, UK. [74]General Surgery/Coloretal Unit, Braga Hospital, Life and Health Sciences Research Institute (ICVS), School of Health Sciences, University of Minho, Braga, Portugal. [75]Department of Surgery, Yonsei University College of Medicine, Seoul, South Korea. [76]Department of Surgery, Hospital La Paz, Madrid, Spain. [77]Cirugía de Urgencias, Hospital Universitario Donostia, Donostia, Spain. [78]Department of Surgery, Faculty of Medicine Siriraj Hospital, Mahidol University, Bangkok, Thailand. [79]Department of Surgery, Insular University Hospital of Gran Canaria, Las Palmas, Spain. [80]1st Department of Surgery, Kavala General Hospital, Kavala, Greece. [81]Department of General Surgery, Mysore Medical College and Research Institute, Government Medical College Hospital Mysore, Mysore, India. [82]2nd Department of Surgery, Jagiellonian University Medical College, Krakow, Poland. [83]First Department of Surgery, Tzaneio Hospital, Piraeus, Greece. [84]Department of General Surgery and Surgical Oncology, Le Scotte Hospital, Siena, Italy. [85]Department of Surgery, University Hospital, Valencia, Spain. [86]Department of Surgery,

Post-Graduate Institute of Medical Sciences, Rohtak, India. [87]Department of Surgery, Radiology, University Hospital of the West Indies, Kingston, Jamaica. [88]General Surgery Department, Centro Hospitalar de São João, Porto, Portugal. [89]Second Surgical Clinic, Emergency Hospital of Craiova, Craiova, Romania. [90]3rd Department of Surgery, Haepa University Hospital, Thessaloniki, Greece. [91]Department of Surgery, CH Armentieres, Arras, France. [92]Surgery Department, University Hospital Hassan II, Fez, Morocco. [93]Department of Surgery, Onandjokwe Hospital, Ondangwa, Namibia. [94]Department of Surgery, Emergency Hospital of Bucharest, Bucharest, Romania. [95]Department of General Surgery, Lewisham & Greenwich NHS Trust, London, UK. [96]Department of Surgery, University of Ilorin Teaching Hospital, Ilorin, Nigeria. [97]Department of Surgery, King Abdalla University Hospital, Irbid, Jordan. [98]Department of Surgery, Elazig Training and Research Hospital, Elazig, Turkey. [99]Department of Laparoscopic and Metabolic Surgery, Sunrise Hospital, Kochi, India. [100]Department of Surgery, Sant'Antonio Abate Hospital, Gallarate, Italy. [101]Division of Emergency and Trauma Surgery, Ribeirão Preto Medical School, Ribeirão Preto, Brazil. [102]Surgery 1 Unit, Centro Hospitalar Tondela Viseu, Viseu, Portugal. [103]Department of Surgery, UMC Ljubljana, Ljubljana, Slovenia. [104]Department of Surgery, Bharati Medical College and Hospital, Sangli, India. [105]Department of Surgery, Insubria University Hospital, Varese, Italy. [106]Abdominal and General Surgery Department, General Hospital Jesenice, Jesenice, Slovenia. [107]Department of Surgery, Hospital de Alta Especialidad de Veracruz, Veracruz, Mexico. [108]General Surgery Department, Medical University, University Hospital St George, Plovdiv, Bulgaria. [109]Department of Surgery, Fundación Jimenez Díaz, Madrid, Spain. [110]Department of Surgery, Good Hope Hospital, Heart of England NHS Foundation Trust, Birmingham, UK. [111]Department of General Surgery, Tan Tock Seng Hospital, Novena, Singapore. [112]Departement of Surgery, Fatabenefratelli Isola Tiberina Hspital, Rome, Italy. [113]Department of Surgery, Hospital and Comprehensive Cancer Centre Novy Jicin, Novy Jicin, Czech Republic. [114]Department of General Surgery, Clinical Hospital at Chelyabinsk Station of OJSC "Russian Railroads", Chelyabinsk, Russian Federation. [115]3th Department of Surgery, Iaso General Hospital, Athens, Greece. [116]Department of Surgery, North Estonia Medical Center, Tallin, Estonia. [117]Department of Surgery, Baskent University Ankara Hospital, Ankara, Turkey. [118]General Surgery Service, Trauma University Hospital, Tirana, Albania. [119]1st Department of Surgery - Department of Abdominal, Thoracic Surgery and Traumatology, General University Hospital, Prague, Czech Republic. [120]Department of General Surgery, Sakarya Teaching and Research Hospital, Sakarya, Turkey. [121]Department of Renal and Pancreas Transplantation, Manchester Royal Infirmary, Manchester, UK. [122]Department of Surgery, Red Cross Hospital, Beverwijk, Netherlands. [123]Emergency Surgery, Arcispedale S.Anna Azienda Ospedaliero-Universitaria di Ferrara, Ferrara, Italy. [124]Department of Surgery, Medical School University Pecs, Pecs, Hungary. [125]Department of Surgery, Montichiari Hospital, Ospedali Civili Brescia, Brescia, Italy. [126]1st Surgical Clinic, St. Spiridon Hospital, Iasi, Romania. [127]Department of Surgery, Rajendra Institute of Medical Sciences, Ranchi, India. [128]Department of Surgery, Kocaeli University Training and Research Hospital, Kocaeli, Turkey. [129]Trauma and Emergency Surgery Department, Chang Gung Memorial Hospital, Taoyuan City, Taiwan. [130]Department of Surgery, MOSC Medical College Kolenchery, Cochin, India. [131]General and Digestive Surgery Department, Teaching Hospital Yalgado Ouedraogo, Ouagadougou, Burkina Faso.

References

1. Sartelli M, Viale P, Catena F, Ansaloni L, Moore E, Malangoni M, et al. 2013 WSES guidelines for management of intra-abdominal infections. World J Emerg Surg. 2013;8(1):3.
2. Mulari K, Leppäniemi A. Severe secondary peritonitis following gastrointestinal tract perforation. Scand J Surg. 2004;93(3):204–8.
3. Horiuchi A, Watanabe Y, Doi T, Sato K, Yukumi S, Yoshida M, et al. Evaluation of prognostic factors and scoring system in colonic perforation. World J Gastroenterol. 2007;13(23):3228–31.
4. Evans HL, Raymond DP, Pelletier SJ, Crabtree TD, Pruett TL, Sawyer KG. Tertiary peritonitis (recurrent diffuse or localized disease) is not an independent predictor of mortality in surgical patients with intra-abdominal infection. Surg Infect. 2001;2:255–65.
5. McLauchlan GJ, Anderson ID, Grant IS, Fearon KCH. Outcome of patients with abdominal sepsis treated in an intensive care unit. Br J Surg. 1995;82:524–9.
6. Koperna T, Schulz F. Prognosis and treatment of peritonitis: Do we need new scoring systems? Arch Surg. 1996;131:180–6.
7. Pacelli F, Doglietto GB, Alfieri S, Piccioni E, Sgadari A, Gui D, et al. Prognosis in intra-abdominal infections. Multivariate analysis on 604 patients. Arch Surg. 1996;131:641–5.
8. Ohmann C, Yang Q, Hau T, Wacha H, the Peritonitis Study Group of the Surgical Infection Society Europe. Prognostic modelling in peritonitis. Eur J Surg. 1997;163:53–60.
9. Montravers P, Gauzit R, Muller C, Marmuse JP, Fichelle A, Desmonts JM. Emergence of antibiotic-resistant bacteria in cases of peritonitis after intra-abdominal surgery affects the efficacy of empirical antimicrobial therapy. Clin Infect Dis. 1996;23:486–94.
10. Prabhu V, Shivani A. An overview of history, pathogenesis and treatment of perforated peptic ulcer disease with evaluation of prognostic scoring in adults. Ann Med Health Sci Res. 2014;4(1):22–9.
11. Sartelli M, Catena F, Ansaloni L, Leppaniemi A, Taviloglu K, van Goor H, et al. Complicated intra-abdominal infections in Europe: a comprehensive review of the CIAO study. World J Emerg Surg. 2012;7(1):36.
12. Sartelli M, Catena F, Ansaloni L, Coccolini F, Corbella D, Moore EE, et al. Complicated intra-abdominal infections worldwide: the definitive data of the CIAOW Study. World J Emerg Surg. 2014;9:37.
13. Sartelli M. A focus on intra-abdominal infections. World J Emerg Surg. 2010;5:9.
14. Dellinger RP, Levy MM, Rhodes A, Annane D, Gerlach H, Opal SM, et al. Surviving Sepsis Campaign Guidelines Committee including The Pediatric Subgroup. Surviving Sepsis Campaign: international guidelines for management of severe sepsis and septic shock, 2012. Intensive Care Med. 2013;39(2):165–228.
15. Mazuski JE, Solomkin JS. Intra-abdominal infections. Surg Clin North Am. 2009;89(2):421–37.
16. Merlino JI, Malangoni MA, Smith CM, Lange RL. Prospective randomized trials affect the outcomes of intraabdominal infection. Ann Surg. 2001;233(6):859–66.
17. Komatsu S, Shimomatsuya T, Nakajima M, Amaya H, Kobuchi T, Shiraishi S, et al. Prognostic factors and scoring system for survival in colonic perforation. Hepatogastroenterology. 2005;52:761–64.
18. Koperna T, Semmler D, Marian F. Risk stratification in emergency surgical patients: is the APACHE II score a reliable marker of physiological impairment? Arch Surg. 2001;136(1):55–9.
19. Wacha H, Linder MM, Feldman U, Wesch G, Gundlach E, Steifensand RA. Mannheim peritonitis index – prediction of risk of death from peritonitis: construction of a statistical and validation of an empirically based index. Theor Surg. 1987;1:169–77.

21

A historical review of surgery for peritonitis secondary to acute colonic diverticulitis: from Lockhart-Mummery to evidence-based medicine

Roberto Cirocchi[1], Sorena Afshar[2], Salomone Di Saverio[3*], Georgi Popivanov[4], Angelo De Sol[5], Francesca Gubbiotti[6], Gregorio Tugnoli[3], Massimo Sartelli[7], Fausto Catena[8], David Cavaliere[9], Renata Taboła[10], Abe Fingerhut[11,12] and Gian Andrea Binda[13]

Abstract

The management of patients with colonic diverticular perforation is still evolving. Initial lavage with or without simple suture and drainage was suggested in the late 19th century, replaced progressively by the three-stage Mayo Clinic or the two-stage Mickulicz procedures. Fears of inadequate source control prompted the implementation of the resection of the affected segment of colon with formation of a colostomy (Hartman procedure) in the 1970's. Ensuing development of the treatment strategies was driven by the recognition of the high morbidity and mortality and low reversal rates associated with the Hartman procedure. This led to the wider use of resection and primary anastomosis during the 1990's.

The technique of lavage and drainage regained popularity during the 1990's. This procedure can also be performed laparoscopically with the advantage of faster recovery and shorter hospital stay. This strategy allows resectional surgery to be postponed or avoided altogether in many patients; and higher rates of primary resection and anastomosis can be achieved avoiding the need for a stoma. The three recent randomized controlled trials comparing laparoscopic peritoneal lavage alone to resectional surgery reported inconsistent outcomes.

The aim of this review is to review the historical evolution and future reflections of surgical treatment modalities for diffuse purulent and feculent peritonitis. In this review we classified the various surgical strategies according to Krukowski et al. and Vermeulen et al. and reviewed the literature related to surgical treatment separately for each period.

Keywords: Acute diverticulitis, Emergency surgery, Perforated diverticulitis, Laparoscopic lavage, Colorectal surgery, Acute care surgery, Hartmann resection

Background

Colonic diverticulosis is an increasingly common clinical condition in Western Europe and North America [1]. Most people with colonic diverticula will remain completely asymptomatic. However, 10–20% of patients with diverticulosis will manifest symptoms and signs of illness. Symptomatic diverticular disease (DD) can be separated into DD without inflammation (75%) and with inflammation or diverticulitis [2]. The former can also be painful in spite of the lack of inflammation [2]. Acute diverticulitis is defined as acute inflammation of a colonic diverticulum [3]. Peridiverticular and pericolic infections are a result of microscopic or macroscopic perforation of a diverticulum. The spectrum of acute diverticulitis varies between mild diverticulitis and diffuse feculent peritonitis [4]. Starting in 1978, Hinchey's classification has been used for the staging of complicated diverticulitis [5]. Several modifications of Hinchey's traditional classification have been proposed [6, 7] (Table 1).

The European Association for Endoscopic Surgeons (EAES) classification system divides the severity of

* Correspondence: salo75@inwind.it; salomone.disaverio@gmail.com
[3]General (Colorectal) Emergency and Trauma Surgery Service, Maggiore Hospital Regional Emergency Surgery and Trauma Center – Bologna Local Health District, Bologna, Italy
Full list of author information is available at the end of the article

Table 1 Hinchey classification of perforated diverticulitis

Hinchey stage	Features of disease
Stage I[a]	Diverticulitis with a pericolic abscess
Stage II[b]	Diverticulitis with a distant abscess (this may be retroperitoneal or pelvic)
Stage III	Purulent peritonitis
Stage IV	Fecal peritonitis

[a]Stage I has been divided into Ia (phlegmon) and Ib (confined pericolic abscess)
[b]Stage II has been divided into distant abscesses amendable for percutaneous drainage (stage IIa) and complex abscesses associated with a possible fistula (stage IIb)

diverticulitis into three different grades of disease [8] (Table 2). In-hospital mortality after emergency surgery for acute perforated diverticulitis is high (29%) and the Hinchey stage has been found to be a significant predictive factor for mortality [9].

The main cause for the high mortality rate is due to sepsis and prognosis is associated with severity of peritonitis as measured by scoring systems such as the Acute Physiology and Chronic Health Evaluation (APACHE), Mannheim peritonitis index (MPI) and Sequential Organ Failure Assessment (SOFA) [10, 11]. SOFA score was developed to assess organ dysfunction and morbidity and in contrast to APACHE II it allows serial follow-up [11]. The predictive value for death at admission and after 72 h is 75% and 84% respectively [12].

According to current practice guidelines, patients with generalized peritonitis should undergo emergency surgery, as suggested by Mikulicz in 1889 [13]. However, despite intensive research carried out during the last century, the best treatment algorithm is yet to be determined.

The aim of this review is to expose the historical evolution and future reflections of surgical treatment modalities for purulent and feculent peritonitis.

Methods

Surgical strategies were stratified according to the classifications proposed by Krukowski et al. and Vermeulen et al. [14, 15] (Table 3). We reported the essential literature relating to surgical treatment separately for each decade from 1900 to 2016. Only the highest grade of evidence published for each topic was noted for each period. The hierarchy of evidence grading system proposed by the Centre for Evidence-Based Medicine of Oxford was used [16].

Table 2 European Association for Endoscopic Surgeons classification system for colonic diverticulitis (1999)

Grade of disease	Description	Clinical state of the patient
I	Symptomatic uncomplicated disease	Pyrexia, abdominal pain, CT findings consistent with diverticulitis
II	Recurrent symptomatic disease	Recurrence of Grade I
III	Complicated disease	Bleeding, abscess formation, phlegmon, colonic perforation, purulent and fecal peritonitis, stricture, fistula and obstruction

Table 3 Operative Procedures

Conservative: perforated colon retained in peritoneal cavity

1. Suture of perforation
2. Drainage
3. Transverse colostomy
4. Caecostomy
5. Any combination of 1–4

Radical: perforated colon eliminated from peritoneal cavity

1. No resection
   - Exteriorization
2. Resection
   a. Without anastomosis
      - Hartmann's procedure
      - Sigmoid resection with mucous fistula
      - Paul-Mickulicz procedure
   b. With anastomosis
      - Without defunctioning stoma
      - With defunctioning stoma

This systematic review was performed in accordance with the Preferred Reporting Items for Systematic Reviews and Meta-analyses (PRISMA) standards (Fig. 1) [17]. We conducted a systematic literature search using PubMed employing the terms perforated OR peritonitis AND diverticulitis; we search in the published papers from January 1st 1990 to May 2016 [18]. The PubMed function "related articles" was used to broaden each search, and the reference list of all potentially eligible studies was analysed. In addition, a manual search method including the Science Citation Index Expanded, Scopus and Google Scholar databases was performed. After this initial screening process, two authors (RT, RC) independently assessed eligibility of full-text papers. The final decision on eligibility was reached by consensus between the two authors. When multiple articles were published from a single study group and where overlapping study periods were reported, only the most recent article was considered to avoid duplication of data. Data were extracted based on an intention-to-treat principle. Any disagreement was resolved through discussion with a reassessment of the data and/or by involving a senior author.

Results

The PRISMA flow diagram for systematic reviews is presented in Fig. 1. We identified 2,403 publications using

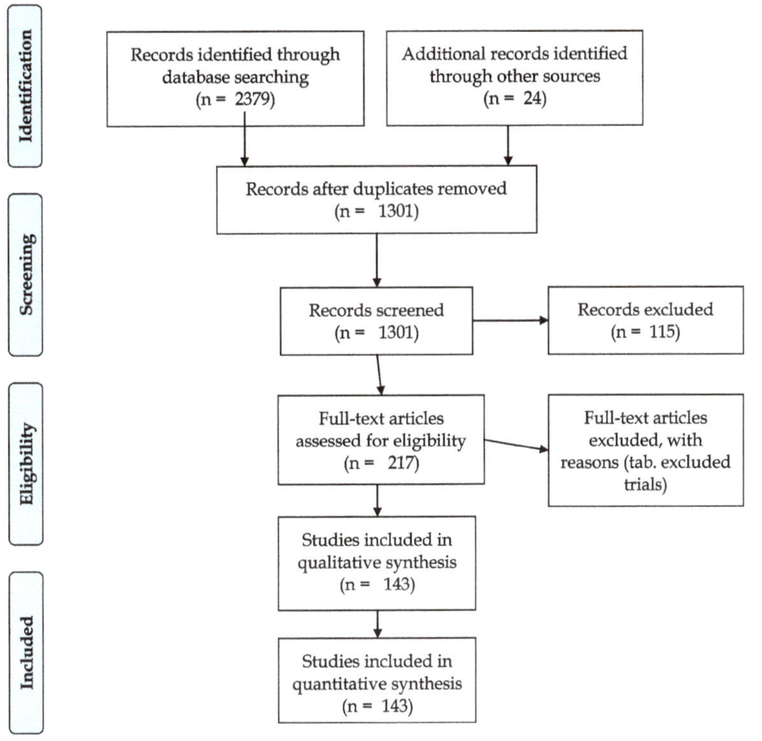

Fig. 1 Prisma flow diagram of the study

the literature search strategy described above and additional searches through other sources. After excluding 2,186 records following the duplicate removed and the review of the titles and abstracts, 217 abstracts eligible for full-text evaluation remained. After full-text assessment we identified 143 publications that fulfilled the inclusion criteria.

Surgical treatment of acute generalized peritonitis from diverticulitis was described as early as 1910 by Lockhart-Mummery [19] who advocated washing the peritoneum and abdominal drainage, combined, if possible, with suture of the colonic perforation (Tables 4 and 5) [19–113].

In the same decade Mikulicz described his two-stage technique of intestinal resection and anastomosis in a well-known article entitled "Surgical Experiences with Intestinal Carcinoma" presented for the first time to the Thirty-First Congress of the German Society of Surgery in 1903 [114]. Along with the description of details of his technique for intestinal resection, he also reported his personal experience in 106 patients, 16 of whom underwent a two-stage technique because he considered performing the initial anastomosis to be too hazardous for the treatment of intestinal cancer and so advocating to limiting the procedure in some cases to the resection and a double-barreled colostomy. Mikulicz strongly recommended this two-stage technique for all resections and anastomoses of the large and small bowel when the bowel was obstructed. This technique was then subsequently adopted for the treatment of diverticulitis.

In 1924 an observational study from the Mayo Clinic advocated drainage and suture of the colonic perforation as well as selective use of a diverting colostomy [115]. However, in some cases, fecal fistulas developed and some became chronic. In cases of substantial infection in or close to the colon, or in the presence of a colovesical fistula or fistula with other structures, the mortality decreased substantially with use of a diverting colostomy. However, in some cases the local suture of the perforation had been unsatisfactory because of difficulties visualizing the perforation, as well as difficulty in suturing edematous bowel wall. During the same decade Henri Hartmann proposed his surgical technique consisting of sigmoid resection, burying the rectal stump and performing terminal colostomy for the treatment of rectal cancer, as an alternative to abdomino-perineal resection, commonly called Hartmann's procedure (HP) [116]. Hartmann had not originally advocated subsequent restoration of intestinal continuity.

In 1930 Rankin and Brown standardized the three-stage procedure developed by Mayo in 1907 [21, 115]. The first stage of the procedure consisted of peritoneal lavage, drainage of any abscess and creation of a proximal colostomy. The second stage was performed after a period of 2 to 4 months and involved resection of the sigmoid colon with end-to-end anastomosis. The third

Table 4 Included studies published up to 1980

Author Year	Center Nation	Years of study	Level of evidence	Patients	Treatment
Lockart-Mummery 1910	St Mark Hospital (London) England	1910	5	Peritonitis from perforated diverticulitis	Toilette of the peritoneum and abdominal drainage ± suture
Judd and Pollock 1924	Mayo Clinic (Rochester, Minn.) USA	1907–24	4	Perforated diverticulitis	Toilette of the peritoneum and abdominal drainage ± suture
Wheeler 1930	Dublin Ireland	1930	5	Peritonitis from perforated diverticulitis	Caecostomy associated at Mikulicz' procedure
Rankin 1930	Mayo Clinic (Rochester, Minn.) USA	1916–28	4	Perforated diverticulitis	Resection of diverticulun and suture Three-stage procedure: proximal colostomy. resection of the sigmoid colon, closure of the colostomy after a few weeks
Eggers 1931	Lenox Hill Hospital (New York) USA	1931	4	Peritonitis from perforated diverticulitis	Toilette of the peritoneum and abdominal drainage
Conway 1931	New York Hospital (New York) USA	NR	4	Peritonitis from perforated diverticulitis	Mikulicz' procedure
Lockart-Mummery 1934	St Mark Hospital (London) England	1934	5	Peritonitis from perforated diverticulitis	Toilette of the peritoneum and abdominal drainage ± suture
Hunt 1934	Los Angeles USA	NR	5	Perforated diverticulitis	Drainage and colostomy - Mikulicz' procedure
Eggers 1941	Lenox Hill Hospital (New York) USA	1938–39	4	Peritonitis from perforated diverticulitis	Toilette of the peritoneum and abdominal drainage – Drainage and colostomy –Mikulicz' procedure
Smithwick 1942	Massachusetts General Hospital (Boston) USA	1925–42	4	Peritonitis from perforated diverticulitis	Toilette of the peritoneum and abdominal drainage ± suture - Drainage and colostomy - Mikulicz' procedure
Pemberton 1947	Mayo Clinic (Rochester, Minn.) USA	1908–45	4	Perforated diverticulitis	Drainage and colostomy - Mikulicz' procedure
Arnheim 1950	Mount Sinai Hospital (New York) USA	1927–37	4	Peritonitis from perforated diverticulitis	Drainage and colostomy - Mikulicz' procedure
Boyden 1950	Portland, USA	NR	4	Peritonitis from perforated diverticulitis	Drainage and colostomy - Mikulicz' procedure - Hartman procedure
Hughes 1952	Monash University (Melburne) Australia	1941–51	4	Peritonitis from perforated diverticulitis	Drainage – Drainage and colostomy – Exteriorization of the affected loop
Lloyd-Davies 1953	Kent and Canterbury Hospital (Canterbury) England	NR	5	Peritonitis from perforated diverticulitis	Drainage and colostomy
Welch 1953	Massachusetts General Hospital (Boston) USA	1942–53	4	Perforated diverticulitis	Drainage and colostomy
Lewis 1953	Yale Medical School (New Haven) USA	NR	4	Perforated diverticulitis	Drainage and colostomy
Edwards 1954	Surgeon to King's College Hospital, (London) England	NR	5	Peritonitis from perforated diverticulitis	Drainage – Drainage and colostomy – Exteriorization of the affected loop
Scarborough 1954	Stanford University (San Francisco) USA	1954	5	Peritonitis from diverticulitis	Drainage and colostomy
Welch 1955	Massachusetts General Hospital (Boston) USA	1942–55	4	Perforated diverticulitis	Drainage and colostomy

Table 4 Included studies published up to 1980 *(Continued)*

Gregg 1955	State University of New York (New York) USA	NR	4	Perforated diverticulitis	Resection with anastomosis and covering stoma
Ransom 1956	University of Michigan (Ann Harbor) USA	1934–51	4	Peritonitis from perforated diverticulitis	Drainage and colostomy
Bacon 1956	University of Pennsylvania (Philadelphia) USA	1940–1955	4	Perforated diverticulitis	Drainage – Drainage and colostomy –Mikulicz' procedure - Exteriorization of the affected loop
Belding 1957	Medical Clinic (Riverside) USA	1951–52	4	Peritonitis from perforated diverticulitis	Resection with anastomosis
MacLaren 1957	Royal Infirmary, (Edinburgh) United Kingdom	NR	4	Perforated diverticulitis	Resection with anastomosis
Ryan 1958	St Vincent's (Melbourne) Australia	1954–56	4	Peritonitis from perforated diverticulitis	Drainage - Drainage and colostomy - Resection with anastomosis
McGregor 1958	Temple University, (Philadelphia) USA	1940–57	4	Peritonitis from perforated diverticulitis	Drainage and colostomy
O'Brein 1959	Hamilton General Hospital (Ontario) Canada	1952–59	4	Perforated diverticulitis	Drainage and colostomy
Brown 1960	Western Infirmary, (Glasgow) England	1945–56	4	Peritonitis from perforated diverticulitis	Drainage – Drainage and colostomy –Mikulicz' procedure
Greig 1960	South Down Group of Hospitals Northern Ireland	1952–59	4	Peritonitis from perforated diverticulitis	Drainage – Drainage and colostomy
Boyden 1961	The Portland Clinic, (Portland) USA	NR	5	Peritonitis from diverticulitis	Hartmann' procedure
Donald 1961	(Birmingham) USA	NR	4	Peritonitis from diverticulitis	Drainage and colostomy
Beard 1961	St. George Hospital (London) England	NR	4	Peritonitis from diverticulitis	Drainage and colostomy
Stauton 1962	Morriston Hospital (Swansea) England	1955–59	4	Peritonitis from diverticulitis	Exteriorization of the affected loop
Estrada 1962	Vancouver General Hospital (Vancouver) Canada	NR	4	Peritonitis from diverticulitis	Drainage – Drainage and colostomy
Hughes 1963	Monash University (Melburne) Australia	1951–61	4	Peritonitis from diverticulitis	Drainage – Drainage and colostomy – Exteriorization of the affected loop
Linder 1962	Brooklyn Women's Hospital (New York) USA	NR	5	Perforated diverticulitis	Exteriorization of the affected loop
Hartley 1964	Addenbrooke's Hospital Cambridge (London) England	1950–60	4	Perforated diverticulitis	Drainage – Drainage and colostomy
Large 1964	Royal Berkshire Hospital (Reading) England	NR	4	Perforated diverticulitis	Resection with anastomosis
Madden 1965	St Clare Hospital (New York) USA	1949–65	4	Perforated diverticulitis	Drainage and colostomy - Resection with anastomosis and covering stoma
Cochrane 1965	Fulham Hospital (London) England	1965	5	Perforated diverticulitis	Drainage and colostomy - Exteriorization of the affected loop
Dawson 1965	King's College Hospital (London) England	1953–58	4	Peritonitis from diverticulitis	Drainage and colostomy –Mikulicz' procedure - Exteriorization of the affected loop
Bacon 1966	University of Pennsylvania (Philadelphia) USA	NR	4	Peritonitis from diverticulitis	Drainage and colostomy

Table 4 Included studies published up to 1980 *(Continued)*

Smiley 1966	University of South California (Los Angeles) USA	1961–65	4	Peritonitis from diverticulitis	Drainage and colostomy - Mikulicz' procedure – Hartmann' procedure
Bolt 1966	West Middlesex Hospital, (London) England	1948–57	4	Peritonitis from diverticulitis	Drainage and colostomy - Exteriorization of the affected loop
Byrne 1966	St. Vincent Hospital, (Los Angeles) USA	1962–66	4	Perforated diverticulitis	Hartmann' procedure
Watkins 1966	Washington University USA	1960–66	4	Peritonitis from diverticulitis	Exteriorization of the affected loop
Moseley 1966	Peter Bent Brigham Hospital (Boston), USA	1945–63	4	Peritonitis from diverticulitis	Drainage and colostomy - Hartmann' procedure
Giffin 1967	Barnes Hospital (St. Louis) USA	1956–66	4	Peritonitis from diverticulitis	Drainage and colostomy - Exteriorization of the affected loop - Hartmann' procedure - Resection with anastomosis
Levy 1967	University of Pennsylvania (Philadelphia) USA	1953–64	4	Peritonitis from diverticulitis	Drainage and colostomy - Exteriorization of the affected loop - Hartmann' procedure
Localio 1967	New York Medical Center (New York) USA	NR	4	Peritonitis from diverticulitis	Drainage and colostomy - Mikulicz' procedure
Colcock 1968	Lahey Clinic (Boston) USA	1947–67	4	Perforated diverticulitis	Drainage and colostomy - Mikulicz' procedure – Hartmann' procedure
Roxburgh 1968	Middlesex Hospital, (London) England	1964–67	4	Peritonitis from diverticulitis	Mikulicz' procedure – Hartmann' procedure - Resection with anastomosis and covering stoma
Rodkey 1969	Massachusetts General Hospital (Boston) USA	NR	4	Perforated diverticulitis	Drainage and colostomy - Mikulicz' procedure
Moore 1969	Exter Hospital (Exeter) England	1960–67	4	Perforated diverticulitis	Hartmann' procedure
Dandekar 1969	New Rochelel Hospital (New York) England	1960–66	4	Peritonitis from diverticulitis	Drainage and colostomy - Exteriorization of the affected loop - Hartmann' procedure - Resection with anastomosis
Fenger 1969	Kommunehospitalet (Copenhagen) Denmark	1950–67	4	Perforated diverticulitis	Drainage and colostomy - Hartmann' procedure
Reiss 1969	Meir Hospital (Kfar Saba) Israel	NR	4	Perforated diverticulitis	Drainage, colostomy and suture
Tagart 1969	Newmarket Community Hospital (Newmarket) England	1962–65	4	Peritonitis from diverticulitis	Drainage - Drainage and colostomy - Exteriorization of the affected loop - Hartmann' procedure - Resection with anastomosis - Resection with anastomosis and covering stoma
Botsford 1969	Harvad Medical School (Boston) USA	1950–67	4	Peritonitis from diverticulitis	Drainage and colostomy - Hartmann' procedure - Mikulicz' procedure
Mitty 1969	St Vincent Hospital (New York) USA	1958–67	4	Perforated diverticulitis	Drainage and colostomy
Killingkack 1970	Audit Australia	1967–69	4	Peritonitis from diverticulitis	Drainage - Drainage and colostomy - Exteriorization of the affected loop - Hartmann' procedure - Mikulicz' procedure
Garnjobst 1970	Department of Surgery Providence Hospital (Portland) Oregon	1954–1969		diverticulitis	

Table 4 Included studies published up to 1980 *(Continued)*

Reilly 1970	Plymouth General Hospital, (Plymouth) England	NR	5	Peritonitis from diverticulitis	Drainage – Drainage and colostomy- Hartmann' procedure
Ponka 1970	Henry Ford Hospital Detroit USA	1963–67	4	Peritonitis from diverticulitis	Drainage and colostomy- Hartmann' procedure
Barabas 1971	Royal Postgraduate Medical School (London) England	NR	4	Peritonitis from perforated diverticulitis	Drainage - Drainage and colostomy - Exteriorization of the affected loop - Hartmann' procedure - Resection with anastomosis
Botsford 1971	Harvad Medical School Massachusetts (Boston) USA	1950–70	4	Perforated diverticulitis	Drainage and colostomy - Mikulicz' procedure – Hartmann' procedure
Byrne 1971	Boston City Hospital (Boston) USA	NR	4	Peritonitis from perforated diverticulitis	Drainage and colostomy – Hartmann' procedure
Miller 1971	Roosvelt Hospital (New York) USA	1957–69	4	Peritonitis from perforated diverticulitis	Drainage and colostomy – Hartmann' procedure
Watkins 1971	Washington Medical School, (Washington) USA	NR	4	Peritonitis from perforated diverticulitis	Exteriorization of the affected loop
Whelan 1971	Saint Vincent Hospita, Worchester. USA	1956–70	4	Peritonitis from perforated diverticulitis	Drainage and colostomy – Hartmann' procedure
Endrey-Walder 1973	Mayo Clinic (Rochester)	1961–70	4	Peritonitis from perforated diverticulitis	Drainage and colostomy – Resection and anastomosis with or without covering stoma
Labow 1973	Muhlemberg Hospital, (Painfield) USA	NR	4	Peritonitis from perforated diverticulitis	Drainage and colostomy - Hartmann' procedure
Graves 1973	Vanderbilt University, (Nashville) USA	NR	4	Peritonitis from perforated diverticulitis	Drainage and colostomy - Hartmann' procedure - Resection and anastomosis
Laimon 1974	University of British Columbia, (Vancouver) Canada	NR	5	Peritonitis from perforated diverticulitis	Hartmann' procedure
Tagart 1974	Newmarket Community Hospital (Newmarket) England	NR	5	Peritonitis from perforated diverticulitis	Mikulicz' procedure - Hartmann' procedure
Rodkey 1974	Massachusetts General Hospital (Boston)	1964–73	4	Peritonitis from perforated diverticulitis	Drainage and colostomy - Hartmann' procedure
Ryan 1974	St Vincent Hospital (Melburne) Australia	NR	4	Peritonitis from perforated diverticulitis	Drainage - Drainage and colostomy - Mikulicz' procedure - Hartmann' procedure - Resection with anastomosis
Tolins 1975	Albert Einstein College of Medicine, New York	196873	4	Perforated diverticulitis	Drainage and colostomy - Hartmann' procedure
Nilsson 1976	Centralsarettet, (Halmastated) Sweden	1963–72	4	Peritonitis from perforated diverticulitis	Drainage - Drainage and colostomy - Mikulicz' procedure - Hartmann' procedure - Resection with anastomosis
Berardi 1976	Veerans Administration Hospital (Des Moines) USA	1969–73	5	Peritonitis from perforated diverticulitis	Drainage and colostomy

Table 4 Included studies published up to 1980 *(Continued)*

Saegesser 1975	Bern Switzerland	NR	5	Peritonitis from perforated diverticulitis	Mikulicz' procedure
Classen 1976	Union Memorial Hospital (Baltimore) USA	1965–75	4	Perforated diverticulitis	Drainage and colostomy - Exteriorization of the affected loop
Himal 1977	McGill University (Montreal), Canada	NR	4	Perforated diverticulitis	Drainage and colostomy - Exteriorization of the affected loop - Hartmann' procedure
Eng 1977	New York School of Medicine (New York), USA	1971–75	4	Peritonitis from perforated diverticulitis	Hartmann' procedure
Nahrwold 1977	Milton S. Hershey Medical Center, (Hershey), USA	NR	4	Perforated diverticulitis	Hartmann' procedure
Sweatman 1977	Birmingham (USA)	1962–72	4	Peritonitis from perforated diverticulitis	Drainage and colostomy - Hartmann' procedure - Resection with anastomosis
Hinckey 1978	Montreal General Hospital (Montreal) Canada	NR	4	Peritonitis from perforated diverticulitis	Drainage and colostomy - Hartmann' procedure
Malafosee 1978	Hopital Saint-Antomine (Paris) France	1964–74	4	Peritonitis from diverticulitis	Drainage and colostomy - Hartmann' procedure - Exteriorization of the affected loop - Resection with anastomosis
Morgenstern 1979	Cedars-Sinai Medical Centers (Los Angeles) USA	1965–78	4	Perforated diverticulitis	Drainage and colostomy
Howe 1979	University of Arkansas (Little Rock) USA	1967–77	4	Perforated diverticulitis	Drainage and colostomy - Hartmann' procedure
Nunes 1979	Spokane (USA)	1971–78	4	Peritonitis from perforated diverticulitis	Hartmann' procedure
Haglund 1979	University of Gotheborg, Gotheborg, Sweden	1962–73	4	Peritonitis from perforated diverticulitis	Drainage and colostomy - Hartmann' procedure - Exteriorization of the affected loop - Resection and anastomosis with a covering stoma
Thow 1980	Cale Clinic (Urbana) USA	1971–76	4	Peritonitis from perforated diverticulitis	Resection with anastomosis
Theile 1980	Princess Alexandra Hospital (Brisbane) Australia	NR	4	Peritonitis from perforated diverticulitis	Drainage - Drainage and colostomy - Hartmann' procedure
Greif 1980	Beth Israel Medical Center (Boston) USA	NR	5	Peritonitis from perforated diverticulitis	Mikulicz' procedure

Table 5 Conclusion of studies reported the use of peritoneal lavage and drainage, published up to 1980

Author	Technique	Quote from publication
Lockart-Mummery 1910	The toilette of the peritoneum and abdominal drainage was the only technique performed. The visible colonic perforation, if possible to find, can be closed by suture	"Perforation and general peritonitis. In these cases, though a careful toilet of the peritoneum and the establishment of adequate drainage may suffice, it is advisable, if possible to find, and close by suture, the perforation of colon"
Judd and Pollock 1924	The toilette of the peritoneum and abdominal drainage was the only technique performed. The visible colonic perforation, if possible to find, can be closed by suture	"We have operated on a number of patients who had abscesses, either just draining the abscess, or draining and suturing the opening left in the colon at the point of perforation of the diverticulum"
Eggers 1931	A taylor surgery. In the arsenal of the surgeon there is also the toilette of the peritoneum and abdominal drainage.	"In four patients an acute perforation took place into the- free-peritoneal cavity. One of them was drained early and recovered, another was treated expectantly for peritonitis without knowledge at that time of the underlying cause, and finally recovered, while the other two died"
Eggers 1941	A taylor surgery. In the arsenal of the surgeon there is also the toilette of the peritoneum and abdominal drainage	"Drainage only"
Smithwick 1942	A taylor surgery. In the arsenal of the surgeon there is also the toilette of the peritoneum and abdominal drainage. The visible colonic perforation, if possible to find, can be closed by suture	"Acute perforation. Principally ± drainage suture"
Hughes 1952	A taylor surgery. In the arsenal of the surgeon there is also the toilette of the peritoneum and abdominal drainage	"Laparotomy and simple drainage of the abdomen"
Edwards 1954	A taylor surgery. In the arsenal of the surgeon there is also the toilette of the peritoneum and abdominal drainage. The visible colonic perforation, if possible to find, can be closed by suture	"The prognosis after early operation in patients with no previous history, or a history of short duration, is excellent, for the bowel wall is still flexible and the perforation can readily be found and easily closed. The closure is reinforced by omentum and the pelvis drained. The real problem is in the surgical management of those cases in which there has been a long history of recurrent attacks of diverticulitis and in which at exploration the bowel is found to be immensely thickened and congested, and particularly in those in whom the actual point of perforation cannot be identified. In such an event the safest procedure is to exteriorize the bowel, if this is practicable. An alternative is to attempt to seal off the inflamed area with pericolic fat and omentum; in the old and the very ill patient the operation may need to be restricted to this procedure".
Bacon 1956	A taylor surgery. In the arsenal of the surgeon there is also the toilette of the peritoneum and abdominal drainage. The visible colonic perforation, if possible to find, can be closed by suture	"Once the diverticulum rupture is discovered and the surround bowel wall is to be fairly normal it can be quickly repaired"
Ryan 1958	A taylor surgery. In the arsenal of the surgeon there is also the toilette of the peritoneum and abdominal drainage.	"Drainage alone was carried out"
Brown 1960	A taylor surgery. In the arsenal of the surgeon there is also the toilette of the peritoneum and abdominal drainage. The visible colonic perforation, if possible to find, can be closed by suture	"Laparotomy and peritoneal drainage was the operation most commonly performed as palliative measure. Identification and suture of a ruptured diverticulum in the distal colon is usually impossible owing to the friable state of tissues involved, but on occasion it can be achieved"
Greig 1960	A taylor surgery. In the arsenal of the surgeon there is also the toilette of the peritoneum and the abdominal drainage.	"Laparatomy and drainage only"

stage consisted of closure of the colostomy a few weeks after the second stage to ensure healing of the anastomosis.

In 1934 Lockhart-Mummery changed his original surgical technique, based only on peritoneal toilette and abdominal drainage by adding the use of a proximal diverting colostomy [23]. The right half of the transverse colon was used to create the colostomy. This approach was subsequently shown to leave the left colon and splenic flexure free from adhesions and favor the ensuing sigmoidectomy [117]. However, drainage and colostomy were associated with a higher mortality and morbidity because further leakage occurred from the site of perforation in spite of the proximal colostomy in some cases. Moreover, the inflamed colon could represent a source of sepsis and leaving this *in situ* was not seen as an attractive option. For these reasons, many surgeons, including Arhneim and Egger, favored the Mikulicz procedure [24, 118]. However, while most surgeons approved the theoretical advantages of Mikulicz' exteriorization, they believed that this technique could be performed in very limited cases, because of the surrounding adhesions and edematous bowel [25, 119].

The three-stage procedure was the standard treatment of acute diverticulitis until the late 1940's. "Palliative" treatment, consisting of formation of a colostomy alone, without subsequent resection, was almost partially abandoned during this period. Interval closure of the colostomy without colon resection led to a high proportion of aggravation of symptoms– over 45 and 70% of patients, in Smithwick's and Pemberton*et al.*'s experiences, respectively [27, 28]. During this period, the use of the HP for the treatment of recto-sigmoid cancer decreased in favor of resection and primary anastomosis (PRA). At the same time, HP gained in popularity as a treatment of complications of DD and other emergency conditions while antibiotics were introduced into clinical practice. In 1950 Boyden articulated this approach and proposed a technical variation: a long distal bowel stump was exteriorized through the hypogastrium [29].

During this period, drainage of pus and formation of a proximal colostomy with the aim of controlling severe sepsis was not longer popular: fecal diversion was thought to limit peritonitis and surgeons avoided source control in fear of spreading infection. In the 50's such 'palliative' operations were increasingly considered as unsatisfactory. The resection of the inflamed colonic segment followed by an anastomosis was suggested as a more 'bold' alternative. The improvement of anesthetic techniques and antibiotic therapy supported this approach of "eliminating the source of sepsis", as stated by Crile in 1954 or "source control" as later coined by Marshall [120, 121]. It seems that a direct approach to the source of contamination, with diversion or resection of diseased segments, drainage of abscess, and suction of most of the pus and feces from abdominal cavity, gave the patient the best chance of survival [120]. Also during this period PRA with or without proximal protective colostomy was increasingly reported [32–35]. The results were good in the presence of a minimum peri-diverticular contamination or intra-mesenteric abscess [34].

The gold standard surgical treatment of complicated diverticulitis was the three-stage procedure with the drainage and colostomy as first stage. Stauton and Smiley supported the diversion of the perforated loop with sigmoid colostomy in the left iliac fossa plus drainage and colostomy [49, 50, 59–61]. Transverse colostomy was discouraged for fecal peritonitis as it might leave fecal residue proximal to the perforation [122]. Certainly the septic focus was removed from the peritoneal cavity, but the toxins were not removed from the circulation and still exerted their systemic effect [123, 124].

During the 1970s HP gained renewed popularity, because eradicating the source of sepsis had proved its superiority to mere diversion in terms of mortality and complications. Subsequent colostomy closure became an increasingly routine procedure, well standardized and progressively feasible [5, 84–113].

In the 1980s a landmark systematic review by Krukowski and Matheson was published [125]. The two authors examined the mortality in 36 case series (821 cases of diverticulitis associated with purulent or fecal peritonitis) published between 1957 and 1984 that compared resection versus colostomy without resection. All patients underwent emergency surgery: mortality was 12% in the 316 who underwent resection versus 29% in the 505 who underwent colostomy without resection. Although there was a high risk of selection bias (patients in better health were more likely to undergo resection while patients with poor health status were more likely to receive a colostomy), this report found that, with antibiotics and better fluid resuscitation therapy, a substantial number of patients could undergo resection as an emergency procedure with an acceptable mortality rate. In addition, advocates of resection argued that emergency colectomy avoided the risk of missing colonic cancer (which was estimated to occur in 2–7% of the cases) and decreased morbidity [125].

The 1990s saw the emergence of two-stage resection and HP supported by two RCTs published in Denmark and France [126, 127]. Kronborg, in a single-center study published in 1993, examined 62 patients operated on for diverticulitis complicated with peritonitis, 46 of whom were classified as Hinchey III (purulent peritonitis). Twenty-one were randomized to transverse colostomy, suture and omentoplasty without resection with 100% survival. Six of the 25 patients (24%) randomized to acute resection without primary anastomosis died postoperatively [126]. Kronborg concluded that simple suture of the perforation and omentoplasty with proximal diversion was safer and more effective than acute resection in purulent peritonitis and comparable in effectiveness [126]. Hospital stay was shorter and there were fewer inflammatory relapses after acute resection. Twenty-seven different surgeons operated on the 62 enrolled patients during 14 years. This RCT was suspended early due to slow recruitment (an average of four patients each year) and used subgroup analysis without statistical adjustment, and consequently lacked statistical power [126]. In contrast, the French multicenter prospective RCT included 103 patients with either purulent (Hinchey III) or fecal peritonitis (Hinchey IV) [127]. The primary endpoint was post-operative peritonitis. For the 48 patients who were randomized to colostomy (with perforation closure by suture in the Hinchey IV cases), the postoperative peritonitis rate was high, up to 20%. In contrast, for the other 55 patients randomized to HP emergency resection, the postoperative peritonitis rate was significantly lower, less than 2%. Three studies were published from 1985 to 2000 where the HP was compared to the three-stage technique (Table 6) [126, 128, 129]. Our recent meta-analysis of these three studies analyzed the overall mortality as the primary outcome [130]. A total of 159 patients had colonic resection versus 105 who maintained perforated diseased segment of colon after proximal diversion or suture of the colon perforation. Overall, mortality was 13.6% (20/147) in the colonic resection group versus 24.6% (18/73) after proximal diversion or suture of the colon perforation (with perforated diseased segment of colon maintained). Statistical analysis failed to show a statistically significant lower overall perioperative mortality rate in the colonic resection group compared to the other group (OR 0.53, 95% CI 0.16 to 0.73, $P = 0.31$) and heterogeneity among the included studies was high ($Tau^2 = 0.71$, $Chi^2 = 5.31$, $I^2 = 62\%$) [130]. In 2000, the American Society of Colon and Rectal Surgeons based on expert review of the evidence concluded that segmental colonic resection followed by an end colostomy (i.e., HP) was the most suitable procedure for perforated diverticulitis with peritonitis [131].

During this period a number of systematic reviews and meta-analysis were published comparing PRA versus HP (Table 7) [130, 132–135].

The first published was Salem's review in 2004 [132]. This review identified 98 studies (published between 1957 and 2003) on the surgical management of perforated diverticulitis complicated with peritonitis. Perioperative mortality data from patients with diverticular peritonitis undergoing HP ($n = 1{,}051$) was calculated for 54 studies. Overall cumulative mortality rate was 19.6% (18.8% for HP and 0.8% for subsequent procedures to restore intestinal continuity). The surgical site infection rate was 29.1% (24.2% for HP and 4.9% for reversal). Stoma complications and anastomotic leaks (after restoring intestinal continuity) occurred in 10.3% and 4.3%, respectively. Of 569 reported cases of PRA from 50 studies, the associated mortality rate was 9.9% (range 0–75%) with an anastomotic leak rate of 13.9% (range, 0–60%) and a surgical site infection rate of 9.6% (range, 0–26). In patients with diverticular peritonitis who underwent PRA the reported mortality and morbidity rates were not higher than those in patients undergoing HP, suggesting that PRA was a safe operative option in this specific population.

However, in 2006, Constantinides et al. published a systematic review of 15 observational studies (13 retrospectives and 2 prospective nonrandomized studies published from 1984 to 2004) comparing PRA with HP for acute diverticulitis in emergency surgery [133]. They found that peri-operative mortality was lower in those patients who underwent PRA compared with those who underwent HP. In addition, there was a trend favoring PRA for surgical complications (surgical site infections, abscesses, and peritonitis). However, it has to be borne in mind that this review was at high risk of selection bias because of the primarily retrospective character of case series Notwithstanding, these data showed that: 1)

Table 6 Hartman procedure vs to three stages technique

	Study type	Cases		Age (yr)	Pathology	Hinchey stage			
						Hinchey </= 2		Hinchey > 2	
		Resection	Trasverse colostomy and drainage			resection	colostomy and drainage	resection	colostomy and drainage
Nagorney et al. (1985)	R	90	31	CR 61 vs TCD 65	P	–	–	90	31
Finlay et al. (1987)	R	38	40	D	P, A	12	29	26	11
Kronborg et al. (1993)	RCT	31	31	CR 73 vs TCD 71	P	–	–	31	31

RCT randomized controlled trial, *R* retrospective observational trial
CR colon resection, *TDC* transverse colostomy and drainage
Pathology: *P* peritonitis, *A* abscess; *O* obstruction, *DD* diverticular disease

Table 7 Systematic review: primary resection with anastomosis vs Hartmann's procedure

Authors	Type of review	Number of studies included	Number of patients included	Conclusion
Salem 2004	systematic review	98	1.051	"Reported mortality and morbidity in patients with diverticular peritonitis who underwent primary anastomosis were not higher than those in patients undergoing Hartmann's procedure were. This suggests that primary anastomosis is a safe operative alternative in certain patients with peritonitis. Despite inclusion of only patients with peritonitis in this analysis, selection bias may have been a limitation and a prospective, randomized trial is recommended."
Constantinides 2006	systematic review and metanalysis	15	963	"Patients selected for primary resection and anastomosis have a lower mortality than those treated by Hartmann's procedure in the emergency setting and comparable mortality under conditions of generalized peritonitis (Hinchey > 2). The retrospective nature of the included studies allows for a considerable degree of selection bias that limits robust and clinically sound conclusions. This analysis highlights the need for high-quality randomized trials comparing the two techniques
Abbas 2007	systematic review	18	884	"This review suggests that surgical resection and primary anastomosis in acute diverticulitis with peritonitis compares favourably with Hartmann's procedure in terms of peri-operative complications. The need for revision of Hartmann's procedure could be subsequently avoided. Some articles showed that patients with severe peritonitis, who had a diverting stoma, in the setting of resection and primary anastomosis, had the lowest complication rate. However, the quality of these studies was poor with the presence of selection bias."
Cirocchi 2013	systematic review and metanalysis	14	1041	*"Despite numerous published articles on operative treatments for patients with generalized peritonitis from perforated diverticulitis, we found a marked heterogeneity between included studies limiting the possibility to summarize in a meta-analytical method the data provided and make difficult to synthesize data in a quantitative fashion. The advantages in the group of colon resection with primary anastomosis in terms of lower mortality rate and postoperative stay should be interpreted with caution because of several limitations. Future randomized controlled trials are needed to further evaluate different surgical treatments for patients with generalized peritonitis from perforated diverticulitis."*
Lorusso 2016	systematic review and metanalysis	24	4.062	*"Our meta-analysis shows that the PRA technique is better than HP for all considered outcomes. Due to the high variability of the included studies, further randomized controlled trials would be required to confirm these results".*

emergency PRA could be performed in selected cases with a low incidence of anastomotic leak (roughly 6%); 2) PRA and HP had similar operative times; and 3) for the most severe cases (Hinchey IV), PRA and the HP had similar mortality (14.1 vs. 14.4%).

In 2006, the American Society of Colon and Rectal Surgeons updated their guidelines for the treatment of sigmoid diverticulitis dating from 2000 [136]. Emergency sigmoid resection was deemed mandatory for diverticulitis with peritonitis, and the alternatives to the HP consisted of PRA with or without a de-functioning stoma. The role of the PRA (particularly without the use of a de-functioning stoma) remained unclear.

In 2007, Abbas published a systematic review of trials conducted between 1966 and 2003 [134]. Eighteen non-randomized studies reporting on 884 matched patients with complicated diverticulitis were included. There were no significant differences found between PRA and HP in terms of mortality, morbidity, sepsis, surgical site complications, duration of operation or antibiotic therapy. However, again the risk of selection bias was high.

Successively a RCT comparing PRA and HP was published [137]. The study protocol called for a de-functioning ileostomy within the PRA procedure. Ninety patients were randomized to PRA or HP in 14 centres in eight countries during a 9-year period [137]. Thirty-four PRA patients were compared to 56 HP patients. There were no statistically significant differences found in terms of age ($P = 0.481$), gender ($P = 0.190$), Hinchey stage III and IV ($P = 0.394$) and Mannheim Peritonitis Index ($P = 0.145$). There were no statistically significant differences found in mortality (2.9 vs. 10.7%; $P = 0.247$) or morbidity (35.3 vs. 46.4%; $P = 0.38$) after PRA or HP. The rate of restoration of intestinal continuity was similar in both groups (64.7% after PRA and 60% after HP, $P = 0.659$) after a similar lag time between emergency operation and elective stoma reversal ($P = 0.43$). The main difference between the two groups was the post-operative complication rate after restoration of intestinal continuity that differed statistically significantly (4.5 vs. 23.5% after PRA and HP, respectively; $P = 0.05$). However, it is impossible to draw firm conclusions from this RCT because of early termination and enrolment of only 15% of its calculated sample size (600 patients to achieve 90% power to detect 10% difference in mortality).

Another systematic review and meta-analysis on the same topic, published in 2013, compared PRA and HP [130] for the treatment of diverticulitis complicated by peritonitis, including the above mentioned RCT [137]. The overall morbidity rate was 17% (40/235) and 28.37% (84/296) in the PRA and HP groups, respectively (OR 0.46, 95% CI 0.23 to 0.90, $P = 0.02$). The re-intervention rate after PRA did not differ significantly between the two groups (15.2% versus 24.1% in the PRA and HP, respectively; OR 1.06, 95% CI 0.24 to 4.73, $P =$ 0.94). Successively another RCT was published on this topic; Oberkofler and colleagues randomized 62 patients in four centres with acute perforation of left colon (Hinchey III and IV) to HP ($n = 30$) or PRA (with de functioning ileostomy, $n = 32$) with a planned procedure to restore intestinal continuity after 3 months in both groups [138]. Both groups were similar at baseline (Hinchey III: 76% vs. 75% and Hinchey IV: 24% vs. 25%, for HP vs. PRA respectively). The primary outcome was the overall complication rate that was similar in both groups (80% vs. 84%, $P = 0.813$). The outcomes after the primary colon resection were also similar (mortality 13% vs. 9% and morbidity 67% vs. 75% in HP vs. PRA). This is the first RCT that seems to favour PRA in patients with complicated diverticulitis with peritonitis. However, there is evidence of bias, as highlighted by Panis in his comments, therefore no firm conclusions can be drawn [139]. Succesively Lorusso published a systematic review including 24 studies, in [135] which reported the same our results (Table 8) [137, 138, 140–162].

Recently laparoscopic peritoneal lavage (LPL) with drainage and antibiotics has been recently introduced into the surgical practice with aim to decrease the rate of HP [163, 164]. In 2009, Toorenvliet's systematic review identified 231 patients with acute diverticulitis who underwent LPL, drainage and antibiotics therapy [165]. In 95.7% of patients this minimally invasive procedure permitted adequate control of the abdominal and systemic sepsis, with low rates of mortality (1.7%), morbidity (10.4%) and stoma (1.7%). Most patients subsequently had a delayed elective laparoscopic PRA. Patients who did not undergo subsequent resection had a long recurrence free period. The authors concluded that LPL was an effective and safe treatment of peritonitis secondary to perforated diverticulitis [165].

However, the use of peritoneal lavage without primary resection in generalized peritonitis originating from perforated diverticulitis remains controversial. Recently three RCT (DILALA-trial, SCANDIV-trial, LADIES trial) including a total of 343 participants (178 in the lavage group versus 175 in the resection group) have been published on this topic (Table 9) [166–168].

The DILALA trial included patients with only Hinchey III peritonitis diagnosed by laparoscopy and with 1-year re-operation rate as primary outcome. The preliminary analysis of the short-term results (12 weeks) in 76 patients reported no statistically significant difference regarding morbidity and mortality, statistically significant longer period of abdominal drainage but shorter hospital stay in the LPL group compared to HP group [167].

LADIES was a two-arm trial with 1-year morbidity and mortality as the primary outcome. The LOLA arm compared laparoscopic lavage with sigmoidectomy in 90 patients with Hinchey III diverticulitis [166]. The trial could not prove the superiority of LPL and was terminated due to increased adverse events in this group despite the lack of statistical significance.

In contrast, the SCANDIV trial was able to report on the totality of 199 patients randomized to laparoscopic lavage or to laparoscopic/open resection with or without anastomosis [168]. The primary outcome was 90-day major complications rate according to the Clavien-Dindo classification. The authors reported a non-statistically significant higher incidence of the primary outcome in the LPL group and comparable mortality. However, there were statistically significantly higher rate of abscesses, secondary peritonitis and re-operations and in the LPL group along with missed malignancy in four cases. Despite the shorter operative time in the LPL group (72 vs 149 min), the hospital stay was similar in both groups. However, the study has several limitations such as inclusion of patients with Hinchey I and II and participation of more experienced surgeons in the resection group, which might be a source of significant bias [169].

Slim recently published a letter in which the three RCTs were examined and none showed laparoscopic lavage to be superior. In relation to three meta-analysis of these studies could respond to the question raised by this editorial, but "... came to opposite conclusions....." [170].

We published the fourth meta-analysis, that failed to demonstrate significant benefits (Table 10) [171–174]. Overall the quality of evidence was low because of serious concern regarding the risk of bias and imprecisions. A significantly increased rate of intra-abdominal abscess formation (RR = 2.54, 95% CI 1.34 to 4.83) (moderate

Table 8 Evidence about primary resection with anastomosis vs Hartmann's procedure

	Study type	Cases		Pathology	Hinchey stage			
					Hinchey </= 2		Hinchey > 2	
		PRA	HP		PRA	HP	PRA	HP
Hold et al. (1990)	R	99	76	DD, P, A	83	45	16	31
Gooszen et al. (2001)	R	32	28	DD, P, A	11	9	21	19
Schilling et al. (2001)	PNR	13	42	DD, P	0	0	13	42
Regenet et al. (2003)	PNR	27	33	DD, P	0	0	27	33
Richter et. Al (2006)	PNR	36	5	DD, P	0	0	36	5
Trenti et al. (2011)	R	27	60	P	0	0	58	69
Oberkofler et al. (2012)	RCT	32	30	(DD) P	0	0	32	30
Alanis et al. (1989)	R	34	26	DD,P,A	31	19	3	7
Alizai (2013)	R	26	72	DD,P,A	16	24	10	48
Blair (2002)	R	33	634	DD,P,A	24	31	9	32
Berry (1989)	R	27	47	DD,P,A,O,F,B	NR	NR	NR	NR
Gawlick (2012)	R	340	1678	DD,P,A	NR	NR	NR	NR
Herzog (2011)	R	21	19	DD,P,A,O,B	NR	NR	NR	NR
Kourtesis (1988)	R	23	10	DD,P,A, F	NR	6	0	4
Mäkelä (2005)	R	64	93	DD,P	62	19	2	0
Mueller (2011)	R	47	26	DD,P,A	45	14	2	12
Pastenak (2010)	R	46	65	DD,P,A	34	17	12	48
Saccomani (1993)	R	26	8	DD,P,A,F	NR	NR	NR	NR
Smirniotis (1992)	R	6	18	DD,P,A	6	10	0	8
Stumpf (2007)	R	36	30	DD,P,A,O	NR	NR	NR	NR
Tabbara (2010)	R	18	176	DD,P,A,S	16	69	2	107
Zingg et al. (2009)	PNR	46	65	DD, P	34	17	12	48
Binda et al. (2012)	RCT	34	56	P	0	0	34	56
Tudor (1994)	PNR	76	77	DD,P,A,B,O,F	29	20	8	44
Vermeulen (2007)	R	61	139	DD,P,A	35	44	26	95

RCT randomized controlled trial, *PNR* prospective, nonrandomized, *R* retrospective
PRA primary resection and anastomosis, *HP* Hartmann's operation
Pathology: *P* peritonitis, *A* abscess, *O* obstruction, *DD* diverticular disease
F fistula, *B* bleeding (dc chronic diverticulitis)

quality of evidence), was seen with this approach. However, LPL does not appear inferior to traditional surgical resection and may achieve reasonable outcomes (lower rate of post-operative wound infections, R = 0.10, 95% CI 0.02 to 0.51) and less hospital resources (shorter duration of post-operative hospital stay during index admission, WMD =−2.03, 95% CI −2.59 to −1.47).

Discussion

This review analyzes the best scientific evidence for over a century of surgery for complicated DD stratifying the technical solutions over time.

It is difficult to draw firm conclusions based on the available evidence. The studies were principally retrospective and prone to bias, irrespective of the decade in question. Also the few currently available RCTs have limitations and therefore have not been able to provide clear recommendations.

Since the publication of Graser in 1899, DD has been a subject of increasing interest for clinicians and surgeons [175]. DD is more frequent in Western countries (especially left-sided) and a trend toward increased frequency has been noted with estimated prevalence of 20–60% [176].

Despite the intensive research since the beginning of the last century, decisions regarding if and when to operate on patients with diverticulitis remains a topic of substantial debate. The debate between supporters of non-operative and traditional techniques has existed over this time and persists to this day. However, no

Table 9 RCTs about abdominal laparoscopic lavage: characteristics

Name of trial Trial registry entries	Type of trial	Country	Participants	Inclusion criteria	Exclusion criteria	Study number	Time of study
LADIES ClinicalTrials.gov Identifier: NCT01317485	Multicentre two-armed randomised trial: 34 teaching hospitals and eight academic hospitals in Belgium, Italy, and the Netherlands	The Netherlands	Patients with generalised purulent and faecal peritonitis from sigmoid diverticulitis	Clinical signs of peritonitis. Free gas on and/or diffuse fluid on CT LOLA arm: Only patients with purulent perforated diverticulitis without overt perforation	Dementia Previous sigmoidectomy Prior pelvic irradiation, Chronic treatment with high-dose steroids (>20 mg daily) Being aged younger than 18 years or older than 85 years Preoperative shock needing inotropic support Patients with Hinchey I and II Patients with Hinchey IV peritonitis or overt perforation were excluded from the DIVA group	LOLA arm: 264 DIVA arm: 212	LOLA arm: between July 2010, and the early termination of the trial February 2013
DILALA trial ISRCTN for clinical trials ISRCTN82208287	Multicentre randomised trial	Sweden-Denmark	Perforated non-faeculent diverticulitis	Hinchey grade III at diagnostic laparoscopy, i.e. free fluid	Hinchey grade I - II at laparoscopy i.e. no free fluid Hinchey grade IV at laparoscopy, i.e. gross faecal contamination. Other pathology than diverticulitis diagnosed as explanation of peritonitis	80	Between February 2010 until February 2014
SCANDIV ClinicalTrials.gov Identifier: NCT01047462	Multicentre randomised trial	Sweden-Norvey	Perforated non-faeculent diverticulitis	Patients with generalised peritonitis	Pregnancy Bowel obstruction	199	Between February 2010 until June 2014

Table 10 Meta-analysis about laparoscopic abdominal lavage

	Cirocchi		Ceresoli	Angenete	Marshall
	All Hinchey	Hinchey III	Hinchey III	Hinchey III	Hinchey III
Post-operative mortality at index admission or within 30 days from index intervention	RR 1.33, 95% CI 0.37 to 4.74	RR 3.01, 95% CI 0.48 to 18.93	OR 0.93; 95% C.I. 0.23–3.82; $P = 0.92$	RR 1.34, 95% CI 0.59–3.04	RR 1.34, 95% CI 0.37 to 4.79
Mortality at 90 days	RR 1.27, 95% CI 0.60 to 2.69	Not performed[j]	OR 0.83; 95% C.I. 0.32–2.11; $P = 0.69$	RR 0.86, 95% CI 0.40–1.83	RR 0.86, 95% CI 0.40 to 1.84
Mortality at 12 months	RR 0.84, 95% CI 0.38 to 1.88	Not performed[j]	OR 0.74 $P = 0.51$	RR 0.54, 95% CI 0.38–0.76	
Reoperation at index admission or within 30 days from index intervention	RR 1.93, 95% CI 0.71 to 5.22	RR = 1.40, 95% CI 0.71 to 4.90	OR 3.75, $P = 0.006$	RR 1.34, 95% CI 0.59–3.04	RR 3.03, 95% CI 1.16 to 7.89
At 90 days follow reoperations	Not analyzed[a]	Not performed[j]	NR	RR 1.71, 95% CI 0.85–3.43	NR
At 12 months follow reoperations	RR 0.57, 95% CI 0.39 to 0.86	Not performed[j]	OR 0.32, $P = 0.0004$	RR 0.54, 95% CI 0.38–0.76	NR
Intra-abdominal abscesses at index admission or within 30 days from index intervention	Not analyzed[b]	Not performed[j]	OR 3.50; 95% C.I. 1.79–6.86; $P = 0.0003$	NR	NR
Intra-abdominal abscesses at 90 days	RR = 2.54, 95% CI 1.34 to 4.83	Not performed[j]	NR	NR	NR
Wound infections	RR = 0.10, 95% CI 0.02 to 0.51	Not performed[j]	OR 0.14; 95% C.I. 0.04–0.45; $P = 0.0009$	NR	NR
Morbidity at 90 days	Not performed[j]	Not performed[j]	OR 1.70; 95% C.I. 1.00–2.87; $P = 0.05$	NR	NR
Presence of stoma at 12 months	RR = 0.50, 95% CI 0.14 to 1.75	Not performed[j]	OR 0.44 $P = 0.27$	NR	RR 0.50, 95% CI 0.14 to 1.76
Operating time	Not analyzed[c]	Not performed[j]	NR	NR	NR
Post-operative persistent peritonitis	Not analyzed[d]	Not performed[j]	NR	NR	NR
Post-operative secondary peritonitis	Not analyzed[e]	Not performed[j]	NR	NR	NR
Length of post-operative hospital stay during index admission.	WMD −2.03, 95% CI−2.59 to−1.47	Not performed[j]	NR	NR	NR
Adverse events within 90 days by Dindo-Clavien grade I-II	Not analyzed[f]	Not performed[j]	NR	NR	NR
Adverse events within 90 days by Dindo-Clavien grade IIIa	Not analyzed[g]	Not performed[j]	NR	NR	NR
Adverse events within 90 days by Dindo-Clavien grade IIIb	RR 1.40, 95% CI 0.47 to 4.17	Not performed[j]	NR	RR 1.46, 95% CI 0.99–2.20	NR
Adverse events within 90 days by Dindo-Clavien grade IVa	RR 0.59, 95% CI 0.20 to 1.75	Not performed[j]	NR	NR	NR
Adverse events within 90 days by Dindo-Clavien grade IVb	RR 0.62, 95% CI 0.10 to 3.75	Not performed[j]	NR	NR	NR
Total length of hospital stays within 12 months.	Not analyzed[h]	Not performed[j]	NR	NR	NR
Quality of Life	Not analyzed[i]	Not performed[j]	NR	NR	NR
	NR	NR	NR	NR	

Table 10 Meta-analysis about laparoscopic abdominal lavage *(Continued)*

Post-operative ICU admission	RR 0.85, 95% CI 0.40 to 1.78

NR not reported
[a]Two trials (LADIES and DILALA) reported this outcome, but the LADIES reported only the abscesses needing percutaneous drainage, differently the DILALA reported only the abscess underwent surgical reintervention
[b]Only one trial (SCANDIV) reported this outcome
[c]This outcome was reported in the SCANDIV although a definition of operating time was not provided. In the DILALA trial, the duration of surgery, and time between end of surgery and the end of anesthesia was reported. In the LADIES trial, the results of a comparative analysis were provided in the absence of the primary data. Because of the incongruous reports of operating time, for these reasons the analysis of this outcome was not performed
[d]Only the DILALA trial analyzed this outcome as persistent peritonitis
[e]Only the SCANDIV trial analyzed this outcome of persistent peritonitis
[f]Only the DILALA trial reported this outcome
[g]Only the DILALA trial reported this outcome
[h]Only the DILALA trial reported this outcome
[i]All the included trials reported this outcome; however, the data of quality of life questionnaires were not comparable
[j]Lack of data

single treatment strategy has dominated in terms of efficacy or safety.

Diverticulitis is complicated in approximately 10–25% of all cases. Operations are traditionally reserved for complicated diverticulitis (colon perforation and peritonitis, abscess, fistula, or stenosis). After a first acute attack of diverticulitis, approximately 20–30% of patients undergo surgery, around a half of these cases being performed as an emergency. Of these, 15–40% tend to be young patients (less than 50 years old). The mortality of emergency operations is between 10 and 20% while in elective surgery it is less than 2% [177] The condition has a great social and financial impact. In USA about 313.000 hospitalizations are due to diverticular disease with more 50.000 bowel resections annually [178, 179].

A retrospective cost analysis from USA found that treatment of DD for 1 financial year was 5.3% of the total annual budget of General Surgery [180]. At present, diverticulitis is the associated diagnosis for one third of all colostomies and/or colon resections [132].

Recent literature has reported an increase in the incidence of DD among younger patients. In a large review of the Nationwide Inpatient Sample (NIS) of 267,000 admissions for AD between 1998 and 2005, incidence rates increased dramatically in 18 to 44 year-olds and 45 to 64 year-olds, while they remained stable in 65 to 74 year-olds and actually decreased in persons 75 years of age or older [181].

Generally, more aggressive treatments have been used in patients in better health with less aggressive options reserved for patients in a poor state of health. Therefore, direct comparisons between such treatments in an observational study setting could lead to the erroneous conclusion that the more aggressive interventions are associated with lower morbidity and mortality than the conservative options.

It is interesting to note that some of the oldest described therapeutic options, such as the peritoneal lavage and drainage or surgery in several stages, are still very relevant today. This is particularly true on the background of the new potent antimicrobial agents, improved ICU management, the wider use of percutaneous drainage and last, but not least due to the growing experience with laparoscopic surgery.

Antimicrobial therapy plays an important role in the management peritonitis from complicated acute diverticulitis. Judicious use of antibiotics should be considered an integral part of good clinical practice. It can maximize the utility and therapeutic efficacy of treatment, and minimize the risks associated with emerging infections and the selection of resistant pathogens. Antimicrobial therapy is typically empiric because critically-ill patients need immediate treatment and microbiological data usually requires more than 24/36 h for the identification of pathogens and antibiotic susceptibility pattern.

In the last years several guidelines have been published in literature in the setting of intra-abdominal infections [182–186]. However, consideration of local epidemiological data and regional resistance profiles should be essential for antibiotic selection.

Considering the intestinal micro biota, patients with acute diverticulitis requires antibiotics toward gram-positive and gram-negative bacteria, as well as for anaerobes. Most of the complicated acute diverticulitis is community acquired infection. In these condition the main resistance threat in intra-abdominal infections may posed by Extended-Spectrum Beta-Lactamase (ESBL)-producing Enterobacteriaceae, which are becoming common in community-acquired infections worldwide [182]. The most significant risk factors for ESBL producing infection include prior exposure to antibiotics and co morbidities requiring concurrent antibiotic therapy [182].

The duration of therapy should be shortened as much as possible if there no signs of ongoing infections. Patients who have signs of sepsis beyond 5 to 7 days of treatment need diagnostic investigation to determine an ongoing uncontrolled source of infection [187].

In the management of critically ill patients with sepsis and septic shock clinical signs and symptoms as well as inflammatory response markers such as pro calcitonin, although debatable, may assist in guiding antibiotic treatment [187].

However, the variety of available treatments and the paucity of good quality evidence make clinical decision making difficult for surgeons especially in emergency setting.

Tracking the development of current surgical practice is very important due to several reasons. Firstly, we pay tribute to our teachers who paved the way to our current achievements. Secondly, analyzing historical procedures allows us to understand that these are still very relevant despite the technological advancements; we can still learn from them and further develop such techniques.

The treatment of complicated DD in the early decades was dominated either by only lavage with/without suture or different stage-procedures. In the 70's HP gradually became increasingly popular and a routine procedure with acceptable mortality and morbidity, probably due to higher rate of successful colostomy closure at the second stage. The period 1991–2000 is characterized by increased frequency of the re-sectional surgery but the first two RCTs reported controversial results. From 2001 until now there has been a marked shift in surgical practice toward PRA and wider use of the laparoscopic approach with or without resection. This is probably due to the growing recognition that Hartmann's reversal is not a benign procedure with 49-55% morbidity and 20% mortality rates [188–190]. Moreover, a large number of patients never undergo restoration (48–74%), albeit that patients with diverticular disease have significantly higher reversal rate (83%) [190, 191].

The studies published in 2001–2016 can be divided into two categories – comparing HP versus resection with PRA and those investigating the effectiveness of LPL, drainage and antibiotic therapy as an initial approach versus resection.

Several comparative studies published in this period reported improved outcome after resection with primary anastomosis in contrast to Hartmann's procedure such as those of Salem et al., Constantinides et al., whereas the work of Abbas et al. showed similar results with respect to morbidity and mortality rates, duration of the operation and antibiotic therapy [132–134]. Two RCTs directly compared PRA and HP. Binda et al. reported no significant difference in mortality and morbidity rates, but significantly lower complication rate after intestinal continuity restoration in PRA versus HP [137]. However, it was stopped due to insufficient recruitment rate. A other trial found similar complication rate [138]. A recent systematic review [130] found that despite the growing body of the literature there is a marked heterogeneity between studies, which precludes the possibility to draw valid conclusions. PRA was associated with lower, but insignificant mortality rate and significantly shortened hospital stay. Generally, the benefit of PRA seems to be of lower mortality rate and shorter postoperative stay. The studies failed to write a definitive word on this issue, because their premature conclusion and bias, and, for many reasons (the laparoscopic lavage procedure's widespread included), nowadays a study like this seems impractical.

The second group of studies has been dealing with the still controversial role of LPL with drainage and antibiotic therapy. Recently there has been a steady trend toward this approach as a definitive treatment or as bridge procedure to subsequent delayed resection due to the well-known advantages of the laparoscopic surgery and in order to reduce the rate of HP.

The systematic review of Toorenviliet et al. reported adequate control of the infection and successful delayed laparoscopic resection in most of the cases [165].

The more recent systematic review analyzed 19 studies on LPL with follow-up between 1.5 and 96 months. In 24% of the cases it was sufficient treatment with reintervention rate 5% and 30-day mortality 4.8%. Readmission rate was 7% with redo surgery in 69% of the cases of which 92% underwent PRA. In 36% two-stage laparoscopic management was performed [192].

None recent RCT trials [166–168] did show any significant advantage of LPL with respect to post-operative mortality and surgical re-interventions. The overall picture seems to be mostly of equivalence, except for higher reoperation rates in the LPL group, as seen in two out of the three trials. It is noteworthy that re-operation after LPL in the prematurely terminated LADIES trial did not result in excess mortality. The SCANDIV study was strongly criticized by some due to several limitations such as inclusion of patients with Hinchey I and II and participation of more experienced surgeons in the resection group which may be sources of significant bias [169, 193].

Furthermore in early 1980 some authors reported the routine use of ureteral catheters to minimize the incidence of ureteral injury during colorectal surgery (from 0.2 to 4.5%) [194–197]. In the following decades, with introduction of laparoscopic colectomy the prophylactic placement of ureteral catheters during colorectal surgery has been recommended for prevention of ureteral injuries [198, 199]; so some surgeons reported the use of lighted ureteral stents during colectomy [200]. In complicated diverticulitis the sigmoidectomy is a surgical challenge for the fibrotic adherences with the ureter. Moshe Schein reported that *"Severely" plastered diverticulitis has been referred to by some as "malignant diverticulitis" and claimed to be a contra-indication to resection. Using an appropriate technique and staying "near the bowel" an experienced surgeon should be able to resect any sigmoid"* [107, 201, 202]. It follow that in these complicated diverticulitis the prophylactic placement of ureteral catheters can reduce the ureteral injuries. The use of prophylactic ureteral catheters was reported in the surgical treatment of complicated diverticulitis, but the use of these catheters was performed only in election surgery and often during laparoscopic colectomy.

The last problem are the localized peritonitis, that not properly treated can evolve into an abdominal abscess, that are associated with an acute mortality of 5–10%. Treatment of these abscess depends on size, localization and patient's general condition. Though solid supporting evidence is lacking, most abscess ≤ 3 cm in diameter are treated safely with antibiotics. For larger abscesses there is much evidence supporting the advantages of percutaneous drainage combined with antibiotics [203–205]. There is no evidence supporting a specific drainage or the aspiration technique. If an abscess cannot be drained percutaneously, an urgent surgical procedure is advised. Resection with primary anastomosis is the intervention of choice: there is increasing evidence that a drainage through a laparoscopic approach can be successful avoiding a further resection or deferiing it to an elective setting. After a successful percutaneous drainage of an abscess there is no agreement or evidence supporting a conservative or surgical policy [206].

Despite limitations due to the lack of strong evidence for the reasons discussed above, we summarize and propose a treatment for various clinical scenarios below:

- Patient in a good general condition with Hinchey I or II – Initially stabilize with medical treatment with or without percutaneous drainage; followed by elective PRA without protective stoma if required and/or suitable.
- Above scenario, but non-responder to initial management: two-stage procedure (emergency HP with or without a mucous fistula, followed by elective reversal if suitable) or PRA with or without a de functioning stoma.
- Selected cases Hinchey II-III – LPL.
- Hinchey III not suitable for LPL – PRA or HP.
- Hinchey IV – HP.

On this issue the results of two ongoing studies are waited: one RCT study, LapLand and one multicenter retrospective study on patients submitted to laparoscopic lavage, the LLOStudy [207, 208].

After preliminary promising results [209], future ongoing experiences might confirm the feasibility and demonstrate the safety of laparoscopy and primary anastomosis even in cases of selected, hemodynamically stable, patients with Hinchey IV perforated diverticulitis and feacal peritonitis, if performed by experienced colorectal surgeons [210].

Conclusion

The management of patients with colon perforation from diverticulitis is still evolving. During the late 19th century initial lavage with or without simple suture and drainage was the suggested treatment. The three-stage Mayo Clinic or the two-stage Mickulicz procedures gradually replaced this. Fears of inadequate control of the source of sepsis prompted the implementation of the resection of the affected segment of colon with formation of a colostomy (HP) in the 1970's. The future development of the treatment strategies was driven by the recognition of the high morbidity and mortality associated with HP and the low Hartmann's reversal rates. This led to the wider use of resection with PRA during the 1990's.

The technique of lavage and drainage regained its popularity during the 1960's. It has relatively recently become possible to perform this procedure laparoscopically which takes advantage of the benefits of minimally invasive surgery with faster recovery and shorter hospital stay. Using this strategy allows resection surgery to be postponed or avoided altogether in many patients; moreover, an higher rates of PRA can be achieved avoiding the need for a stoma. The three recent RCTs of LPL reported inconsistent outcomes. These findings warrant further research and debate.

Acknowledgements

We thank Alessandro Quintili for developing the search strategies and for the support in the research of full text.

Funding

None.

Authors' contributions

RC, SA, SDS, GAB were responsible for the study concept and design. RC and SA have written the manuscript, RC and SA carried out the literature search. All authors critically reviewed the manuscript for important intellectual content. AF and GAB were the study supervisors. All authors read and approved the final version of the manuscript.

Competing interests

The authors declare that they have no competing interests.

Strengths and limitations of this study

To our knowledge, this is the first systematic and historical review on the surgical treatment of peritonitis from colonic diverticulitis' perforation.

This systematic review is based on the best evidence published in surgical journals from 1900 to the present day.

The arguments are reported in chronological order, stating how the operations (technique and peri-operative care) were influenced over time.

Limitations of this review include the low level of evidence and the small sample sizes of the included studies.

Most of the studies were performed in Western countries, potentially reducing the external validity and the generalizability of the findings.

Author details
[1]Department of General Surgery, University of Perugia, Terni Hospital, Terni, Italy. [2]Department of General Surgery, Cumberland Infirmary, Carlisle, UK. [3]General (Colorectal) Emergency and Trauma Surgery Service, Maggiore Hospital Regional Emergency Surgery and Trauma Center – Bologna Local Health District, Bologna, Italy. [4]Military Medical Academy, Sofia, Bulgaria. [5]Department of Surgery, Terni Hospital, Terni, Italy. [6]Department of Surgery, University of Ferrara, Ferrara, Italy. [7]Department of Surgery, Macerata Hospital, Macerata, Italy. [8]Department of Emergency Surgery, Parma Hospital, Parma, Italy. [9]Department of Surgery, Forlì Hospital, Forlì, Italy. [10]Department of Gastrointestinal and General Surgery, Medical University of Wrocław, Wrocław, Poland. [11]Section for Surgical Research, Department of Surgery, Medical University of Graz, Graz, Austria. [12]First Department of Surgery, Hippokration University Hospital, University of Athens, Athens, Greece. [13]Department of Surgery, E.O. OspedaliGalliera, Genova, Italy.

References

1. Jacobs DO. Diverticulitis. N Engl J Med. 2007;357(20):2057–66. doi:10.1056/NEJMcp073228.
2. Stollman N, Raskin J. Diverticular disease of the colon. Lancet. 2004;21(363):631–9. doi:10.1016/S0140-6736(04)15597-9.
3. Tursi A. New medical strategies for the management of acute diverticulitis. Expert Rev GastroenterolHepatol. 2015;9(10):1293–304. doi:10.1586/17474124.2015.1075881.
4. Bullard Dunn KM, Rothenberger DA Diverticular disease. In: BrunicardiF, Andersen D (Eds). Schwartz's Principles of Surgery, 10th edition. 2014;1201–3.
5. Hinchey EJ, Schaal PG, Richards GK. Treatment of perforated diverticular disease of the colon. AdvSurg. 1978;12:85–109.
6. Kaiser AM, Jiang JK, Lake JP, Ault G, Artinyan A, Gonzalez-Ruiz C, Essani R, Beart RW. The management of complicated diverticulitis and the role of computed tomography. Am J Gastroenterol. 2005;100(4):910–7. doi:10.1111/j.1572-0241.2005.41154.x.
7. Sher ME, Agachan F, Bortul M, Nogueras JJ, Weiss EG, Wexner SD. Laparoscopic surgery for diverticulitis. SurgEndosc. 1997;11:264–7. doi:10.1007/s004649900340.
8. Kohler L, Sauerland S, Neugebauer E. Diagnosis and treatment of diverticular disease: results of a consensus development conference. The Scientific Committee of the European Association for Endoscopic Surgery. SurgEndosc. 1999;13(4):430–6. doi:10.1007/s004649901007.
9. Vermeulen J, Gosselink MP, Hop WC, Lange JF, Coene PP, Harst E, Weidema WF, Mannaerts GH. Hospital mortality after emergency surgery for perforated diverticulitis. Ned TijdschrGeneesk. 2009;153:1209–14.
10. Horiuchi A, Watanabe Y, Doi T, Sato K, Yukumi S, Yoshida M, Yamamoto Y, Sugishita H, Kawachi K. Evaluation of prognostic factors and scoring system in colonic perforation. World J Gastroenterol. 2007;13(23):3228–31. doi:10.3748/wjg.v13.i23.3228.
11. Vincent J, De Mendoca A, Cantraine F, et al. Use of SOFA score to assess the incidence of organ dysfunction/failure in intensive care units: results of a multicenter, prospective study. Workung group on "sepsis-related problems" of the European Society of Intensive Care Medicine. Crit Care Med. 1998;26(11):1793–800.
12. Jones A, Trzeciak S, Kline J. The Sequential Organ Failure Assessment score for predicting outcome in patients with severe sepsis and evidence of hypoperfusion at the time of emergency department presentation. Crit Care Med. 2009;37(5):1649–54.
13. Mikulicz J. WeitereErfahrungenuber die operative Behanlung der Perforations peritonitis. Arch KlinChir (Berl). 1889;39:756–84.
14. Krukowski ZH, Matheson NA. Emergency surgery for diverticular disease complicated by generalized and faecal peritonitis: a review. Br J Surg. 1984;71:921–7. doi:10.1002/bjs.1800711202.
15. Vermeulen J, Lange JF. Treatment of Perforated Diverticulitis with Generalized Peritonitis: Past, Present, and Future. World J Surg. 2010;34(3):587–93. doi:10.1007/s00268-009-0372-0.
16. Level of evidence proposed from Centre for Evidence-Based Medicine of Oxford. http://www.essentialevidenceplus.com/product/ebmloe.cfm?show= oxford.
17. Liberati A, Altman DG, Tetzlaff J, Mulrow C, Gøtzsche PC, Ioannidis JP, Clarke M, Devereaux PJ, Kleijnen J, Moher D. The PRISMA statement for reporting systematic reviews and meta-analyses of studies that evaluate health care interventions: explanation and elaboration. Ann Intern Med. 2009;151(4):W65–94.
18. Moher D, Liberati A, Tetzlaff J, Altman DG. Preferred reporting items for systematic reviews and meta-analyses: the PRISMA statement. Ann Int Med. 2009;151:264–9. doi:10.7326/0003-4819-151-4-200908180-00135.
19. Lockhart-Mummery P. Disease of the colon and their surgical treatment. Bristol: John Wright and Sons LTD; 1910. p. 181–2.
20. Judd ES, Pollock LW. Diverticulitis of colon. Ann Surg. 1924;80(3):425–38. doi:10.1097/00000658-192409000-00014.
21. Rankin FW, Brown PW. Diverticulitis of the colon. SurgGynecol&Obstet. 1930;30:836–47.
22. Wheeler WI. Perforative diverticulitis of the colon: some problems during the treatment of a fatal case. Br Med J. 1930;4(1):5–6. doi:10.1136/bmj.1.3600.5.
23. Lockhart-Mummery JP. Diseases of the Rectum and colon and their surgical treatment. 2nd ed. London: Baillière, Tindall&Cox; 1934.
24. Eggers C. Diverticulitis and sigmoiditis. Ann Surg. 1931;94(4):648–69. doi:10.1097/00000658-193110000-00020.
25. Conway FM, Hitzrot JM. Diverticulitis of the colon: a report of 36 cases from the New York Hospital. Ann Surg. 1931;94(4):614–39.
26. Hunt VC. Diverticulosis and diverticulitis of the colon. Cal West Med. 1934;40(2):98–102.
27. Smithwick RH. Experiences with the surgical management of diverticulitis of the sigmoid. Ann Surg. 1942;115(6):969–85. doi:10.1097/00000658-194206000-00010.
28. Pemberton JD, Black BM, Maino CR. Progress in the surgical management of diverticulitis of the sigmoid colon. SurgGynecolObstet. 1947;85(4):523–34.
29. Boyden AM. The surgical treatment of diverticulitis of the colon. Ann Surg. 1950;132(1):94–109.
30. Eggers C. Acute diverticulitis and sigmoiditis. Ann Surg. 1941;113(1):15–29. doi:10.1097/00000658-194101000-00003.
31. Arnheim EE. Diverticulitis of the colon with special reference to the surgical complications. Ann Surg. 1940;112(3):352–69. doi:10.1097/00000658-194009000-00004.
32. Gregg RO. The place of emergency resection in the management of obstructing and perforating lesions of the colon. Surgery. 1955;37(5):754–61.
33. Ryan P. Emergency resection and anastomosis for perforated sigmoid diverticulitis. Br J Surg. 1958;45(194):611–6. doi:10.1002/bjs.18004519409.
34. Belding HH. Acute perforated diverticulitis of the sigmoid colon with generalized peritonitis. AMA Arch Surg. 1957;74(4):511–5. doi:10.1001/archsurg.1957.01280100029004.
35. MacLaren IF. Perforated diverticulitis: a survey of 75 cases. J R CollSurgEdinb. 1957;3(2):129–44.
36. Hughes ES, Shaw HM. Acute diverticulitis of the colon with peritonitis. Med J Aust. 1952;1(8):259–60.
37. Lloyd-Davies OV. Diverticulitis. Proc R Soc Med. 1953;46(6):407–16.
38. Welch CE, Allen AW, Donaldson GA. An appraisal of resection of the colon for diverticulitis of the sigmoid. Ann Surg. 1953;138(3):332–43. doi:10.1097/00000658-195313830-00005.
39. Lewis JE, Hurwitz A. Surgical treatment of sigmoid diverticulitis. Surgery. 1953;33(4):481–94.
40. Edwards HC. Intestinal diverticulosis and diverticulitis. Ann R CollSurgEngl. 1954;14(6):371–88.
41. Scarborough RA. Diverticulitis of the colon; surgical treatment. Calif Med. 1954;80(6):445–8.
42. Welch CE. The problem of diverticulitis; surgical management. Calif Med. 1955;83(6):405–9.
43. Ransom HK. Treatment of diverticulitis of the colon: Choice of operation. Am J Surg. 1956;92(5):672–7.
44. Bacon HE, Valiente MA. Surgical management of diverticulitis. Am J Surg. 1956;91(2):178–83. doi:10.1016/S0002-9610(56)80137-2.
45. McGregor RA, Bacon HE. Diverticular disease of the colon. Dis Colon Rectum. 1958;1(3):197–204. doi:10.1007/BF02616832.
46. O'Brien SE, Mustard KI. Surgical management of diverticulitis of the sigmoid colon. Can Med Assoc J. 1959;80(4):257–61.
47. Brown DB, Toomey WF. Diverticular disease of the colon. A review of 258 cases. Br J Surg. 1960;47(205):485–93. doi:10.1002/bjs.18004720506.
48. Greig GW. The Surgical treatment of diverticulitis of the colon. A review of 38 cases. Ulster Med J. 1960;29(2):127–32.
49. Staunton MD. Treatment of Perforated Diverticulitis Coli. Br Med J. 1962;1(5282):916–8. doi:10.1136/bmj.1.5282.916.
50. Smiley DF. Perforated sigmoid diverticulitis with spreading peritonitis. Am J Surg. 1966;111(3):431–4. doi:10.1016/S0002-9610(66)80022-3.
51. Boyden AM. Two-stage Resection of the Sigmoid. Ann Surg. 1961;154 Suppl 6:210–4.

52. Donald DC. Current Trends in the surgical treatment of diverticulitis of the colon: Review of Thirty-Seven Cases. Ann Surg. 1961;153(3):373–7. doi:10.1097/00000658-196103000-00006.
53. Beard RG, Gazet JC. Perforated diverticulitis (of the colon) with generalized peritonitis. Guys Hosp Rep. 1961;110:263–72.
54. Estrada RL, Hoehn RJ, Robertson HR. Diverticulitis of the distal colon; twenty-five years' experience. Postgrad Med. 1962;31:30–6.
55. Hughes ES, Cuthbertson AM, Carden AB. The surgical management of acute diverticulitis. Med J Aust. 1963;50(1):780–2.
56. Linder JM, Hoffman S. Exteriorization in the surgical management of acute free perforations in diverticulitis of the sigmoid colon. SurgGynecolObstet. 1962;114:755–7.
57. Hartley RC. Dangerson of diverticulis Coli. An estimation of the place of resection in avoidance of complications. Br J Surg. 1964;51:45–9.
58. Large JM. Tretment of perforated diverticulitis. Lancet. 1964;22(1):413–4.
59. Madden JL. Primary resection and anastomosis in the treatment of perforated lesions of the colon. Am Surg. 1965;31(12):781–6.
60. Cochrane HL. Diverticula of colon. Postgrad Med J. 1965;41(481):697–8. doi:10.1136/pgmj.41.481.697.
61. Dawson JL, Hanon I, Roxburgh RA. Diverticulitis coli Complicated by diffuse peritonitis. Br J Surg. 1965;52:354–7. doi:10.1002/bjs.1800520509.
62. Bacon HE, Pezzutti JE. Adequate Resection for diverticulitis of the colon. Arch Surg. 1966;92(1):58–9. doi:10.1001/arcsurg.1966.01320190060013.
63. Bolt DE, Hughes LE. Diverticulitis: a follow up of 100 cases. Br Med J. 1966;1:1205–9. doi:10.1136/bmj.1.5497.1205.
64. Byrne RV. Primary resection of the colon for perforated diverticulum. Am J Surg. 1966;112(2):273–8. doi:10.1016/0002-9610(66)90019-5.
65. Watkins GL, Oliver GA. Management of perforative sigmoid diverticulitis with diffusing peritonitis. Arch Surg. 1966;92(6):928–33. doi:10.10001/archsurg.1966.01320240116024.
66. Moseley RV, Ross FP. Sigmoid diverticulitis: evaluation of current practice in a community hospital. Ann Surg. 1966;164(2):275–83. doi:10.1097/00000658-196608000-00014.
67. Giffin JM, Butcher HR, Ackerman LV. Surgical management of colonic diverticulitis. Arch Surg. 1967;94(5):619–26. doi:10.1001/archsurg.1967.01330110035005.
68. Levy SB, Fitts WT, Lench JB. Surgical treatment of diverticular disease of the colon: evaluation of an eleven-year period. Ann Surg. 1967;166(6):947–54. doi:10.1097/00000658-196712000-00010.
69. Localio SA, Stahl WM. Diverticular disease of the alimentary tract. I The colon CurrProbl Surg. 1967;4(12):1–78. doi:10.1016/S0011-3840(67)80010-8.
70. Colcock BP. Surgical treatment of diverticulitis. Twenty years' experience. Am J Surg. 1968;115(2):264–70. doi:10.1016/0002-9610(68)90037-8.
71. Roxburgh RA, Dawson JL, Yeo R. Emergency resection in treatment of diverticular disease complicated by peritonitis. Br Med J. 1968;5616:465–6. doi:10.1136/bmj.3.5616.465.
72. Rodkey GV, Welch CE. Surgical management of colonic diverticulitis with free perforation or abscess formation. Am J Surg. 1969;117(2):265–9. doi:10.1016/0002-9610(69)90313-4.
73. Moore HD. Emergency treatment of diverticulitis of the Sigmoid Flexure. Disease of the colon Rectum. 1969;12(1):22–5. doi:10.1007/BF02617191.
74. Dandekar NV, McCann WJ. Primary resection and anastomosis in the management of perforation of diverticulitis of the sigmoid flexure and diffuse peritonitis. Dis Colon Rectum. 1969;12(3):172–5. doi:10.1007/BF02617805.
75. Fenger C, Nyholm K, Amdrup E. Diverticulitis of the colon. Acta ChirScand Suppl. 1969;396:114–20.
76. Reiss R. Free perforation in sigmoid diverticulitis: two-stage therapy. Dis Colon Rectum. 1969;12(6):453–6. doi:10.1007/BF02617733.
77. Tagart RE. Diverticular disease of the colon. Clinical aspects. Br J Surg. 1969;56(6):417–23. doi:10.1002/bjs.1800560605.
78. Botsford TW, Zollinger RM. Diverticulitis of the colon. SurgGynecolObstet. 1969;128(6):1209–14.
79. Mitty WF, Befeler D, Grossi C, Rousselot LM. Surgical management of complications of diverticulitis in patients over seventy years of age. Am J Surg. 1969;117(2):270–7. doi:10.1016/0002-9610(69)90314-6.
80. Killingkack MJ. Acute diverticulitis: progress report, Australasian survey (1967–1969). Dis Colon Rectum. 1970;13(6):444–7. PMID:5501400.
81. Garnjobst W, Hardwick C. Further criteria for anastomosis in diverticulitis of the sigmoid colon. American J of Surg. 1970;120(2):264–9. doi:10.1016/S0002-9610(70)80122-2.
82. Relly MC. Colonic diverticula. Surgical management. Br Med J. 1970;3(5722):570–3. doi:10.1136/bmj.3.5722.570.
83. Ponka JL. Emergency surgical operations for diverticular diseases. Dis Colon Rectum. 1970;13(3):235–42. doi:10.1007/BF02617215.
84. Barabas AP. Peritonitis due to diverticular disease of the colon: reiew of 44 cases. Proc R Soc Med. 1971;64(3):253–4.
85. Botsford TW, Zollinger RM, Hicks R. Mortality of the surgical treatment of diverticulitis. Am J Surg. 1971;121(6):702–5. doi:10.1016/0002-9610(71)90050-X.
86. Byrne JJ, Garick EI. Surgical treatment of diverticulitis. Am J Surg. 1971;121(4):379–84. doi:10.1016/0002-9610(71)90226-1.
87. Miller DW, Wichern WA. Perforated sigmoid diverticulitis. Appraisal of primary versus delayed resection. Am J Surg. 1971;121(5):536–40.
88. Watkins GL, Oliver GA. Surgical treatment of acute perforative sigmoid diverticulitis. Surgery. 1971;69(2):215–9.
89. Whelan CS, Furcinitti JF, Lavarreda C. Surgical management of perforated lesions of the colon with diffusing peritonitis. Am J Surg. 1971;121(4):374–8. doi:10.1016/0002-9610(71)90225-X.
90. Endrey-Walder P, Judd ES. Acute perforating diverticulitis. Emergency surgical treatment. Minn Med. 1973;56(1):27–30.
91. Labow SB, Salvati EP, Rubin RJ. The Hartman procedure in the treatment of diverticular disease. Dis Colon Rectum. 1973;16(5):392–4.
92. Graves HA, Franklin RM, Robbins LB, Sawyers JL. Surgical management of perforated diverticulitis of the colon. Am Surg. 1973;39(3):142–7.
93. Laimon H. Hartmann resection for acute diverticulitis. Rev Surg. 1974;31(1):1–6.
94. Targart RE General. Peritonitis and haemorrhage complicating colonic diverticular disease. Ann R Surg Engl. 1974;55(4):175–83.
95. Rodkey GV, Welch CE. Colonic diverticular disease with surgical treatment. A study of 338 cases. SurgClin North Am. 1974;54(3):655–74.
96. Ryan P. Emergency resection and anastomosis for perforated sigmoid diverticulitis. Aust N Z J Surg. 1974;44(1):16–20. doi:10.1111/j.1445-2197.1974.tb06511.x.
97. Tolins SH. Surgical treatment of diverticulitis. Experience at a large Municipal Hospital. JAMA. 1975;232(8):830–2. doi:10.1001/jama.232.8.830.
98. Nilsson LO. Surgical treatment of perforations of the sigmoid colon. Acta ChirScand. 1976;142(6):467–9.
99. Berardi RS, Siroospour D. Diverticular disorders of the colon: results of treatment in 128 patients. IntSurg. 1976;61(9):490–3.
100. Saegesser M. ChirurgischeOperationslehre. Bern: Max Ort, Verlag, Jahr; 1975.
101. Classen JN, Bonardi R, O'Mara CS, Finney DC, Sterioff S. Surgical treatment of acute diverticulitis by staged procedures. Ann Surg. 1976;184(5):582–6. doi:10.1097/00000658-197611000-00008.
102. Himal HS, Ashby DB, Duignan JP, Richardson DM, Miller JL, MacLean LD. Management of perforating diverticulitis of the colon. SurgGynecolObstet. 1977;144(2):225–6.
103. Eng K, Ranson JH, Localio SA. Resection of the perforated segment. A significant advance in treatment of diverticulitis with free perforation or abscess. Am J Surg. 1977;133(1):67–72.
104. Nahrwold DL, Demuth WE. Diverticulitis with perforation into the peritoneal cavity. Ann Surg. 1977;185(1):80–3. doi:10.1097/00000658-197701000-00013.
105. Sweatman Jr CA, Aldrete JS. The surgical management of diverticular disease of the colon complicated by perforation. SurgGynecolObstet. 1977;144(1):47–50.
106. Malafosse M, Gallot D, Loygue J. General peritonitis complicating diverticular sigmoiditis. Med Chir Dig. 1978;7(5):397–400.
107. Morgenstern L, Weiner R, Michel SL. 'Malignant' diverticulitis: a clinical entity. Arch Surg. 1979;114(10):1112–6. doi:10.1001/archsurg.1979.01370340018002.
108. Howe HJ, Casali RE, Westbrook KC, Thompson BW, Read RC. Acute perforations of the sigmoid colon secondary to diverticulitis. Am J Surg. 1979;137(2):184–7. doi:10.1016/0002-9610(79)90141-7.
109. Nunes GC, Robnett AH, Kremer RM, Ahlquist Jr RE. The Hartmann procedure for complications of diverticulitis. Arch Surg. 1979;114(4):425–9. doi:10.1001/archsurg.1979.01370280079011.
110. Haglund U, Hellberg R, Johnsén C, Hultén L. Complicated diverticular disease of the sigmoid colon. An analysis of short and long term outcome in 392 patients. Ann ChirGynaecol. 1979;68(2):41–6.
111. Thow GB. Emergency left colon resection with primary anastomosis. Dis Colon Rectum. 1980;23(1):17–24. doi:10.1007/BF02587195.
112. Theile D. The management of perforated diverticulitis with diffuse peritonitis. Aust N Z J Surg. 1980;50(1):47–9. doi:10.1111/j.1445-2197.1980.tb04490.x.
113. Greif JM, Fried G, McSherry CK. Surgical treatment of perforated diverticulitis of the sigmoid colon. Dis Colon Rectum. 1980;23(7):483–7. doi:10.1007/BF02987083.

114. Mikulicz J. ChirurgischeErfahrungen fiber das Darmcarcinom. Arch f klin Chir. 1903;69:28–47.
115. Mayo WJ, Wilson LB, Griffin HZ. Acquired diverticulitis of the large intestine. SurgGynec&Obst. 1907;5:8–15.
116. Hartmann H. Nouveau procédéd'ablation des cancers de la partieterminale du colon pelvien. CongresFrancais de Chirurgia. 1923;30:2241.
117. Painter NS. Diverticular disease of the colon. London: Norgine LTD; 1977.
118. Arnheim EE. Diverticulitis of the colon with special reference to the surgical complication. Ann Surg. 1940;112(3):352–69. doi:10.1097/00000658-194009000-00004.
119. Opelka F. In: Beck DE, editor. Diverticular disease. St Louis: QMP Inc; 1997. p. 217–33.
120. Crile Jr G. Dangers of conservative surgery in abdominal emergencies. Surgery. 1954;35(1):122–3.
121. Marshall JC. Principles of source control in the management of sepsis. Crit Care Clin. 2009;25(4):753–68.
122. Painter NS. Diverticular disease of the colon. London: Heinemann; 1975.
123. Parks TG. Natural history of diverticular disease of the colon. Clin Gastroenterology. 1975;4(1):53–69.
124. Maingot R. Abdominal operations. New York: Appleton; 1955.
125. Krukowski ZH, Matheson NA. Emergency surgery for diverticular disease complicated by generalized and fecal peritonitis: a review. Br J Surg. 1984; 71:921–7.
126. Kronborg O. Treatment of perforated sigmoid diverticulitis: a prospective randomized trial. Br J Surg. 1993;80:505–7. doi:10.1002/bjs.1800800434.
127. Zeitoin G, Laurent A, Rouffet F, Hay J, Fingerhut A, Paquet J, Peillon C, Research TF. Multicentre, randomized clinical trial of primary versus secondary sigmoid resection in generalized peritonitis complicating sigmoid diverticulitis. Br J Surg. 2000;87:1366–74. doi:10.1046/j.1365-2168.2000.01552.x.
128. Nagorney DM, Adson MA, Pemberton JH. Sigmoid diverticulitis with perforation and generalized peritonitis. Dis Colon Rectum. 1985;28(2):71–5. doi:10.1007/BF02552645.
129. Finlay IG, Carter DC. A comparison of emergency resection and staged management in perforated diverticular disease. Dis Colon Rectum. 1987; 30(12):929–33. doi:10.1007/BF02554278.
130. Cirocchi R, Trastulli S, Desiderio J, Listorti C, Boselli C, Parisi A, Noya G, Liu L. Treatment of Hinchey stage III–IV diverticulitis: a systematic review and meta-analysis International. Int J Colorectal Dis. 2013;28(4):447–57. doi:10.1007/S00384-012-1622-4.
131. Wong WD, Wexner SD, Lowry A, Vernava A, Burnstein M, Denstman F, Fazio V, Kerner B, Moore R, Oliver G, Peters W, Ross T, Senatore P, Simmang C. Practice parameters for the treatment of sigmoid diverticulitis–supporting documentation. The Standards Task Force. Dis Colon Rectum. 2000;43(3): 290–7. doi:10.1007/BF02258291.
132. Salem L, Flum DR. Primary anastomosis or Hartmann's procedure for patients with diverticular peritonitis? A systematic review. Dis Colon Rectum. 2004;47(11):1953–64. doi:10.1007/s10350-004-0701-1.
133. Constantinides VA, Tekkis PP, Athanasiou T, Aziz O, Purkayastha S, Remzi FH, Fazio VW, Aydin N, Darzi A, Senapati A. Primary resection with anastomosis vs. Hartmann's procedure in nonelective surgery for acute colonic diverticulitis: a systematic review. Dis Colon Rectum. 2006;49(7):966–81. doi: 10.1007/s10350-006-0547-9.
134. Abbas S. Resection and primary anastomosis in acute complicated diverticulitis, a systematic review of the literature. Int J Colorectal Dis. 2007;22(4):351–7. doi:10.1007/s00384-005-0059-4.
135. Lorusso D, Gilberti A, et al. Non-Elective Surgery for Acute Complicated Diverticulitis. Primary Resection-Anastomosis or Hartmann's Procedure? A Systematic Review and Meta-Analysis. Journal of Surgery. 2016;12(2):43–9. doi:10.7438/1584-9341-12-2-1.
136. Raffety J, Shellito P, Hyman NH, Buie WD. Practice parameters for sigmoid diverticulitis. Dis Colon Rectum. 2006;49(7):939–44.
137. Binda GA, Karas JR, Serventi A, Sokmen S, Amato A, Hydo L, Bergamaschi R. Primary anastomosis vs nonrestorative resection for perforated diverticulitis with peritonitis: a prematurely terminated randomized controlled trial. ColorectalDis. 2012;14(11):1403–10. doi:10.1111/j.1463-1318.2012.03117.x.
138. Oberkofler CE, Rickenbacher A, Raptis DA, Lehmann K, Villiger P, Buchli C, Grieder F, Gelpke H, Decurtins M, Tempia-Caliera AA, DemartinesN HD, Clavien PA, Breitenstein S. A multicenter randomized clinical trial of primary anastomosis or Hartmann's procedure for perforated leftcolonic diverticulitis with purulent or fecal peritonitis. Ann Surg. 2012;256(5): 819–26. doi:10.1097/SLA.0b013e31827324ba. discussion 826–7.
139. Panis Y. A multicenter randomized clinical trial of primary anastomosis or Hartmann's procedure for perforated left colonic diverticulitis with purulent or fecal peritonitis. Ann Surg. 2012;256:826.
140. Hold M, Denck H, Bull P. Surgical management of perforating diverticular disease in Austria. Int J Colorectal Dis. 1990;5(4):195–9. doi:10.1007/BF00303274.
141. Gooszen AW, Gooszen HG, Veerman W, Van Dongen VM, Hermans J, KlienKranenbarg E, Tollenaar RA. Operative treatment of acute complications of diverticular disease: primary or secondary anastomosis after sigmoid resection. Eur J Surg. 2001;167(1):35–9.
142. Schilling MK, Maurer CA, Kollmar O, Büchler MW. Primary vs. secondary anastomosis after sigmoid colon resection for perforated diverticulitis (Hinchey Stage III and IV): a prospective outcome and cost analysis. Dis Colon Rectum. 2001;44(5):699–703. doi:10.1007/BF02234569. discussion 703–5.
143. Regenet N, Pessaux P, Hennekinne S, Lermite E, Tuech JJ, Brehant O, Arnaud JP. Primary anastomosis after intraoperative colonic lavage vs. Hartmann's procedure in generalized peritonitis complicating diverticular disease of the colon. Int J Colorectal Dis. 2003;18(6):503–7. doi:10.1007/s00384-003-0512-1.
144. Richter S, Lindemann W, Kollmar O, Pistorius GA, Maurer CA, Schilling MK. One-stage sigmoid colon resection for perforated sigmoid diverticulitis (Hinchey stages III and IV). World J Surg. 2006;30(6):1027–32. doi:10.1007/s00268-005-0439-5.
145. Trenti L, Biondo S, Golda T, Monica M, Kreisler E, Fraccalvieri D, Frago R, Jaurrieta E. Generalized peritonitis due to perforated diverticulitis: Hartmann's procedure or primary anastomosis? Int J Colorectal Dis. 2011; 26(3):377–84. doi:10.1007/s00384-010-1071-x.
146. Alanis A, Papanicolaou GK, Tadros RR, Fielding LP. Primary resection and anastomosis for treatment of acute diverticulitis. Dis Colon Rectum. 1989; 32(11):933–9.
147. Alizai PH, Schulze-Hagen M, Klink CD, Ulmer F, Roeth AA, et al. Primary anastomosis with a defunctioning stoma versus Hartmann's procedure for perforated diverticulitis–a comparison of stoma reversal rates. Int J Colorectal Dis. 2013;28:1681–8.
148. Blair NP, Germann E. Surgical management of acute sigmoid diverticulitis. Am J Surg. 2002;183:525–8.
149. Berry AR, Turner WH, Mortensen NJ, Kettlewell MG. Emergency surgery for complicated diverticular disease. A 5-year experience. Dis Colon Rectum. 1989;32:849–54.
150. Gawlick U, Nirula R. Resection and primary anastomosis with proximal diversion instead of Hartmann's: evolving the management of diverticulitis using NSQIP data. J Trauma Acute Care. 2012;72:807–14.
151. Herzog T, Janot M, Belyaev O, Sülberg D, Chromik AM, et al. Complicated sigmoid diverticulitis–Hartmann's procedure or primary anastomosis? Acta Chir Belg. 2011;111:378–83.
152. Kourtesis GJ, Williams RA, Wilson SE. Surgical options in acute diverticulitis: value of sigmoid resection in dealing with the septic focus. Aust N Z J Surg. 1988;58:955–9.
153. Mäkelä JT, Kiviniemi H, Laitinen S. Prognostic factors of perforated sigmoid diverticulitis in the elderly. Digest Surg. 2005;22:100–6.
154. Mueller MH, Karpitschka M, Renz B, Kleespies A, Kasparek MS, et al. Co-morbidity and postsurgical outcome in patients with perforated sigmoid diverticulitis. Int J Colorectal Dis. 2011;26:227–34.
155. Pasternak I, Dietrich M, Woodman R, Metzger U, Wattchow DA, et al. Use of severity classification systems in the surgical decision-making process in emergency laparotomy for perforated diverticulitis. Int J Colorectal Dis. 2010;25:463–70.
156. Saccomani GE, Santi F, Gramegna A. Primary resection with and without anastomosis for perforation of acute diverticulitis. Acta Chir Belg. 1993;93:169–72.
157. Smirniotis V, Tsoutsos D, Fotopoulos A, Pissiotis AC. Perforated diverticulitis: a surgical dilemma. Int Surg. 1992;77:44–7.
158. Stumpf MJ, Vinces FY, Edwards J. Is primary anastomosis safe in the surgical management of complications of acute diverticulitis? Am Surg. 2007;73: 787790.
159. Tabbara M, Velmahos GC, Butt MU, Chang Y, Spaniolas K, et al. Missed opportunities for primary repair in complicated acute diverticulitis. Surgery. 2010;148:919–24.
160. Zingg U, Pasternak I, Dietrich M, Seifert B, Oertli D, et al. Primary anastomosis vs Hartmann's procedure in patients undergoing emergency left colectomy for perforated diverticulitis. Colorectal Dis. 2010;12:54–60.
161. Tudor RG, Farmakis N, Keighley M. National audit of complicated diverticular disease: analysis of index cases. Br J Surg. 1994;81:730–2.

162. Vermeulen J, Akkersdijk GP, Gosselink MP, Hop WC, Mannaerts GH, et al. Outcome after emergency surgery for acute perforated diverticulitis in 200 cases. Digest Surg. 2007;24:361–6.
163. O'Sullivan GC, Murphy D, O'Brien MG, Ireland A. Laparoscopic management of generalized peritonitis due to perforated colonic diverticula. Am J Surg. 1996;171:432–34.
164. Myers E, Hurley M, O'Sullivan GC, Kavanagh D, Wilson I, Winter DC. Laparoscopic peritoneal lavage for generalized peritonitis due to perforated diverticulitis. Br J Surg. 2008;95:97–101.
165. Toorenvliet BR, Swank H, Schoones JW, Hamming JF, Bemelman WA. Laparoscopic peritoneal lavage for perforated colonic diverticulitis: a systematic review. Colorectal Dis. 2010;12(9):862–7. doi:10.1111/j.1463–1318.2009.02052.x.
166. Vennix S, Musters GD, Mulder IM, Swank HA, Consten EC, Belgers EH, Van Gelovan AA, Gerhards MF, Goveart MJ, Van Grevenstein WM, Hoofwijk AG, Kruyt PM, Nienhuijs SW, Boemeester MA, Vermeulen J, Van Dieren S, Lange JF, Bemelman WA. Ladies trial collaborators. Laparoscopic peritoneal lavage or sigmoidectomy for perforated diverticulitis with purulent peritonitis: a multicentre, parallel-group, randomised, open-label trial. Lancet. 2015;386: 1269–77. doi:10.1016/S0140-6736(15)61168-0.
167. Angenete E, Thornell A, Burcharth J, Pommergaard HC, Skullman S, Bisgaard T, Jess P, Lackberg Z, Matthiessen P, Heath J, Roesenberg J, Haglind E. Laparoscopic lavage is feasible and safe for the treatment of perforated diverticulitis with purulent peritonitis: the first results from the randomized controlled trial DILALA. Ann Surg. 2016;263:117–22. doi:10.1097/SLA.0000000000001061.
168. Schultz JK, Yaqub S, Wallon C, Blecic L, Forsmo HM, Folkesson J, Buchwald P, Körner H, Dahl FA, Oresland T, SCANDIV Study Group. G. Laparoscopic lavage vs primary resection for Acute perforated diverticulitis: The SCANDIV Randomized Clinica Trial. JAMA. 2015;314(13):1364–75. doi:10.1001/jama.2015.12076.
169. Mandrioli M, Tugnoli G, Di Saverio S. Laparoscopic lavage vs Primary Resection for Perforated Diverticulitis. JAMA. 2016;315(10):1053. doi:10.1001/jama.2015.17864.
170. Slim K. Role of peritoneal lavage for sigmoid perforation peritonitis surgery: What do the meta-analyses tell us? Journal of Visceral Surgery (2016). (in press)
171. Ceresoli M, Coccolini F, Montori G, Catena F, Sartelli M, Ansaloni L. Laparoscopic lavage versus resection in perforated diverticulitis with purulent peritonitis: a meta-analysis of randomized controlled trials. World J Emerg Surg. 2016;30(1):42.
172. Angenete E, Bock D, Rosenberg J, Haglind E. Laparoscopic lavage is superior to colon resection for perforated purulent diverticulitis-a meta-analysis. Int J Colorectal Dis. 2016. (in press)
173. Marshall JR, Buchwald PL, Gandhi J, Schultz JK, Hider PN, Frizelle FA, et al. Laparoscopic Lavage in the Management of Hinchey Grade III Diverticulitis: A Systematic Review. Ann Surg. 2016.
174. Cirocchi R, Weber DG, Di Saverio S, et al. Laparoscopic lavage versus surgical resection for acute diverticulitis with generalised peritonitis: a systematic review and meta-analysis. Techniques in Coloproctology. 2016; 21:93–110
175. Karulf RE. Diverticular disease. Clin Colon Rectal Surg. 2004;17(3):145. doi:10.1055/s-2004-832694.
176. Andreozzi P, Zito FP, Sarnelli G, et al. Management of diverticulitis and prevention of recurrence. EMJ Gastroenterol. 2015;4(1):95–100.
177. Binda GA, Prandi M. Storia naturale della diverticolite del colon. UCP News. 1999;3(S1):14–6.
178. Everhart JE, Ruhl CE. Burden of digestive diseases in the United States Part III: Liver, biliary tract, and pancreas. Gastroenterology. 2009;136(4):1134–44. doi:10.1053/j.gastro.2009.02.038.
179. Khalil H, Yoo J. Colorectal Emergencies: perforated diverticulitis (operative and nonoperative management. J GastrointestSurg. 2014;18(4):865–8. doi:10.1007/s11605-013-2352-9.
180. Papagrigoriadis S, Debrah S, Koreli A, Husain A. A Impact of diverticular disease on hospital costs and activity. Colorectal Dis. 2004;6(2):81–4. doi:10.1111/j.1463-1318.2004.00532.x.
181. Etzioni DA, Mack TM, Beart RW, Kaiser AM. Diverticulitis in the United States: 1998–2005: changing patterns of disease and treatment. Ann Surg. 2009; 249(2):210–7. doi:10.1097/SLA.0b013e3181952888.
182. Solomkin JS, Mazuski JE, Bradley JS, Rodvold KA, Goldstein EJ, Baron EJ, et al. Diagnosis and management of complicated intra-abdominal infection in adults and children: guidelines by the Surgical Infection Society and the Infectious Diseases Society of America. Surg Infect (Larchmt). 2010;11:79–109.
183. Mazuski JE, Sawyer RG, Nathens AB, DiPiro JT, Schein M, Kudsk KA, et al. The Surgical Infection Society guidelines on antimicrobial therapy for intra-abdominal infections: an executive summary. Surg Infect (Larchmt). 2002;3:161–73.
184. Sartelli M, Viale P, Catena F, Ansaloni L, Moore E, Malangoni M, et al. WSES guidelines for management of intra-abdominal infections. World J Emerg Surg. 2013;8:3.
185. Chow AW, Evans GA, Nathens AB, Ball CG, Hansen G, Harding GK, et al. Canadian practice guidelines for surgical intra-abdominal infections. Can J Infect Dis Med Microbiol. 2010;21:11–37.
186. Montravers P, Dupont H, Leone M, Constantin JM, Mertes PM, Société française d'anesthésie et de réanimation (Sfar), et al. Guidelines for management of intra-abdominal infections. Anaesth Crit Care Pain Med. 2015;34:117–30.
187. Sartelli M, Weber DG, Ruppé E, Bassetti M, Wright BJ, Ansaloni L, et al. Antimicrobials: a global alliance for optimizing their rational use in intra-abdominal infections (AGORA). World J Emerg Surg. 2016;15:11–33.
188. Berne J, Velmahos G, Chan L, Asensio JA, Demetriades D. The high morbidity of colostomy closure after trauma: further support for the primary repair of colon injuries. Surgery. 1998;123:157–64. doi:10.1016/S0039-6060(98)70253-3.
189. Antolovic D, Reissfelder C, Özkan T, Galindo L, Büchler MW, Koch M, Weitz J. Restoration of intestinal continuity after Hartmann's procedure– not a benign operation. Are there predictors for morbidity? Langenbeck's Arch Surg. 2011;396(7):989–96. doi:10.1007/s00423-011-0763-1.
190. Roque-Castellano C, Marchena-Gomez J, Hemmersbach-Miller M, Acosta-Merida A, Rodriguez-Mendez A, Fariña-Castro R, Hernandez-Romero J. Analysis of the factors related to the decision of restoring intestinal continuity after Hartmann's procedure. Int J Colorectal Dis. 2007;22(9):1091–6. doi:10.1007/s00384-007-0272-4.
191. Keck JO, Collopy BT, Ryan PJ, Fink R, Mackay JR, Woods RJ. Reversal of Hartmann's procedure: effect of timing and technique on ease and safety. Dis Colon Rectum. 1994;37(3):243–8.
192. Cirocchi R, Trastulli S, Vettoretto N, Milani D, Cavaliere D, Renzi C, Adamenko O, Desiderio J, Burattini MF, Parisi A, Arezzo A, Fingerhut A. Laparoscopic peritoneal lavage: a definitive treatment for diverticular peritonitis or a "bridge" to elective laparoscopic sigmoidectomy? a systematic review. Medicine (Baltimore). 2015; 94(1):e334.
193. Afshar S, Kurer MA. Laparoscopic peritoneal lavage for perforated diverticulitis: are we any further forward? Colorectal Dis. 2016. doi:10.1111/codi.13404.
194. Leff EI, Groff W, Rubin RJ, Eisenstat TE, Salvati EP. Use of ureteral catheters in colonic and rectal surgery. Dis Colon Rectum. 1982;25(5):457–60.
195. Sheikh FA, Khubchandani IT. Prophylactic ureteric catheters in colon surgery- How safe are they? Report of three cases. Dis Colon Rectum. 1990;33:508–10.
196. Kyzer S, Gordon PH. The prophylactic use of ureteral catheters during colorectal operations. Am Surg. 1994;60:212–9.
197. Bothwell WN, Bleicher RJ, Dent TL. Prophylactic ureteral catheterization in colon surgery. A 5-year review. Dis Colon Rectum. 1994;37:330–4.
198. Palaniappa NC, Telem DA, Ranasinghe NE, Divino CM. Incidence of iatrogenic ureteral injury after laparoscopic colectomy. Arch Surg. 2012;147:267–71.
199. Zafar SN, Ahaghotu CA, Libuit L, Ortega G, Coleman PW, et al. Ureteral injury after laparoscopic versus open colectomy. JSLS. 2014;18:3.
200. Chahin F, Dwivedi AJ, Paramesh A, Chau W, Agrawal S, et al. The implications of lighted ureteral stenting in laparoscopic colectomy. JSLS. 2002;6:49–52.
201. Abcarian H, Pearl RK. A safe technique for resection of perforated sigmoid diverticulitis. Dis Colon Rectum. 1990;33:905–6.
202. Schein M, Paladugn R. Diverticulitis. In: Holzheimer RG, Mannick JA (Eds). Surgical Treatment: Evidence-Based and Problem-Oriented. Munich: Zuckschwerdt; 2001. https://www.ncbi.nlm.nih.gov/books/NBK6986/. Accessed 14 Dec 2016.
203. Brandt D, Gervaz P, Durmishi Y, Platon A, Morel P, Poletti PA. Percutaneous CTscan-guided drainage vs. antibiotherapy alone for Hinchey II diverticulitis: acase-control study. Dis Colon Rectum. 2006;49:1533–8.
204. Kumar RR, Kim JT, Haukoos JS, Macias LH, Dixon MR, Stamos MJ, Konyalian VR. Factors affecting the successful management of intra-abdominal abscesses with antibiotics and the need for percutaneous drainage. Dis Colon Rectum. 2006;49:183–9.
205. Siewert B, Tye G, Kruskal J, Sosna J, Opelka F, Raptopoulos V, et al. Impact of CT-guided drainage in the treatment of diverticular abscesses: size matters. AJR Am J Roentgenol. 2006;186:680–6.

206. Lamb MN, Kaiser AM. Elective resection versus observation after nonoperative management of complicated diverticulitis with abscess: a systematic review and meta-analysis. Dis Colon Rectum. 2014;57:1430–40.
207. LapLAND laparoscopic lavage for acute nonfaeculent diverticulitis. 2009. Available at: https://clinicaltrials.gov/ct2/show/NCT01019239. Accessed 28 Dec 2006.
208. Laparoscopic-lavage Observational Study (LLOS). Available at: https://clinicaltrials.gov/ct2/show/NCT02662088?term=NCT02662088&rank=1. Accessed 28 Dec 2006.
209. Vennix S, Lips DJ, Di Saverio S, van Wagensveld BA, Brokelman WJ, Gerhards MF, van Geloven AA, van Dieren S, Lange JF, Bemelman WA. Acute laparoscopic and open sigmoidectomy for perforated diverticulitis: a propensity score-matched cohort. Surg Endosc. 2016;30(9):3889–96. doi:10.1007/s00464-015-4694-8.
210. Di Saverio S, Vennix S, Birindelli A, Weber D, Lombardi R, Mandrioli M, Tarasconi A, Bemelman WA. Pushing the envelope: laparoscopy and primary anastomosis are technically feasible in stable patients with Hinchey IV perforated acute diverticulitis and gross faeculent peritonitis. Surg Endosc. 2016;30(12):5656–64.

22

The open abdomen, indications, management and definitive closure

Federico Coccolini[1*], Walter Biffl[2], Fausto Catena[3], Marco Ceresoli[1], Osvaldo Chiara[4], Stefania Cimbanassi[4], Luca Fattori[5], Ari Leppaniemi[6], Roberto Manfredi[1], Giulia Montori[1], Giovanni Pesenti[5], Michael Sugrue[7,8] and Luca Ansaloni[1]

Abstract

The indications for Open Abdomen (OA) are generally all those situations in which is ongoing the development an intra-abdominal hypertension condition (IAH), in order to prevent the development of abdominal compartmental syndrome (ACS). In fact all those involved in care of a critically ill patient should in the first instance think how to prevent IAH and ACS. In case of ACS goal directed therapy to achieve early opening and early closure is the key: paradigm of closure shifts to combination of therapies including negative pressure wound therapy and dynamic closure, in order to reduce complications and avoid incisional hernia.

There have been huge studies and progress in survival of critically ill trauma and septic surgical patients: this in part has been through the great work of pioneers, scientific societies and their guidelines; however future studies and continued innovation are needed to better understand optimal treatment strategies and to define more clearly the indications, because OA by itself is still a morbid procedure.

Keywords: Open abdomen, Peritonitis, Pancreatitis, Trauma, Management, Closure

Introduction

The first to describe the use of the open abdomen (OA) technique, in a generalized peritonitis was probably Andrew J. McCosh in 1897 [1]. However this clinical approach to a critically ill patient at that time was unusual and while again referred to by Ogilvie in the mid 1940's [2] and only recently became popular in patients undergoing damage control surgery (DCS). The indications for Open Abdomen are generally trauma, abdominal sepsis, severe acute pancreatitis and in general situations in which is ongoing the development an intra-abdominal hypertension condition (IAH), in order to prevent the development of abdominal compartmental syndrome (ACS). The concept of abdominal damage control surgery has two basic components; controlling bleeding and contamination in the abdominal cavity, and leaving the abdomen open, to decompress or facilitate return at planned re-laparotomy. Maintaining the abdomen domain requires a temporary abdominal closure (TAC). Unlike in trauma patients with massive bleeding, the main aims of the OA approach both in severe secondary peritonitis and severe acute pancreatitis (SAP) are sepsis control and expedite subsequent surgical interventions.

Mortality rates are high, usually over >30 % [3] depending on the patient cohort. The challenging situation to manage requires a multidisciplinary approach by the surgeon and the ICU team in a specific staged process (Fig. 1).

Pathophysiology of abdominal compartment syndrome

Definitions

While recognized for over a century ACS was returned to clinical care in the 1980's, when Kron and colleagues [4] described the course of its development following repair of a ruptured abdominal aortic aneurysm. The term was coined by Fietsam in 1989 in patients undergoing abdominal aortic surgery. Since that time, much progress has been made in its management, including the detection, treatment, and prevention [5].

The World Society of the Abdominal Compartment Syndrome convened in 2004 to create a consensus statement on the definition, diagnosis, and treatment of ACS

* Correspondence: federico.coccolini@gmail.com
[1]General Surgery Department, Papa Giovanni XXIII Hospital, Piazza OMS 1, 24127 Bergamo, Italy
Full list of author information is available at the end of the article

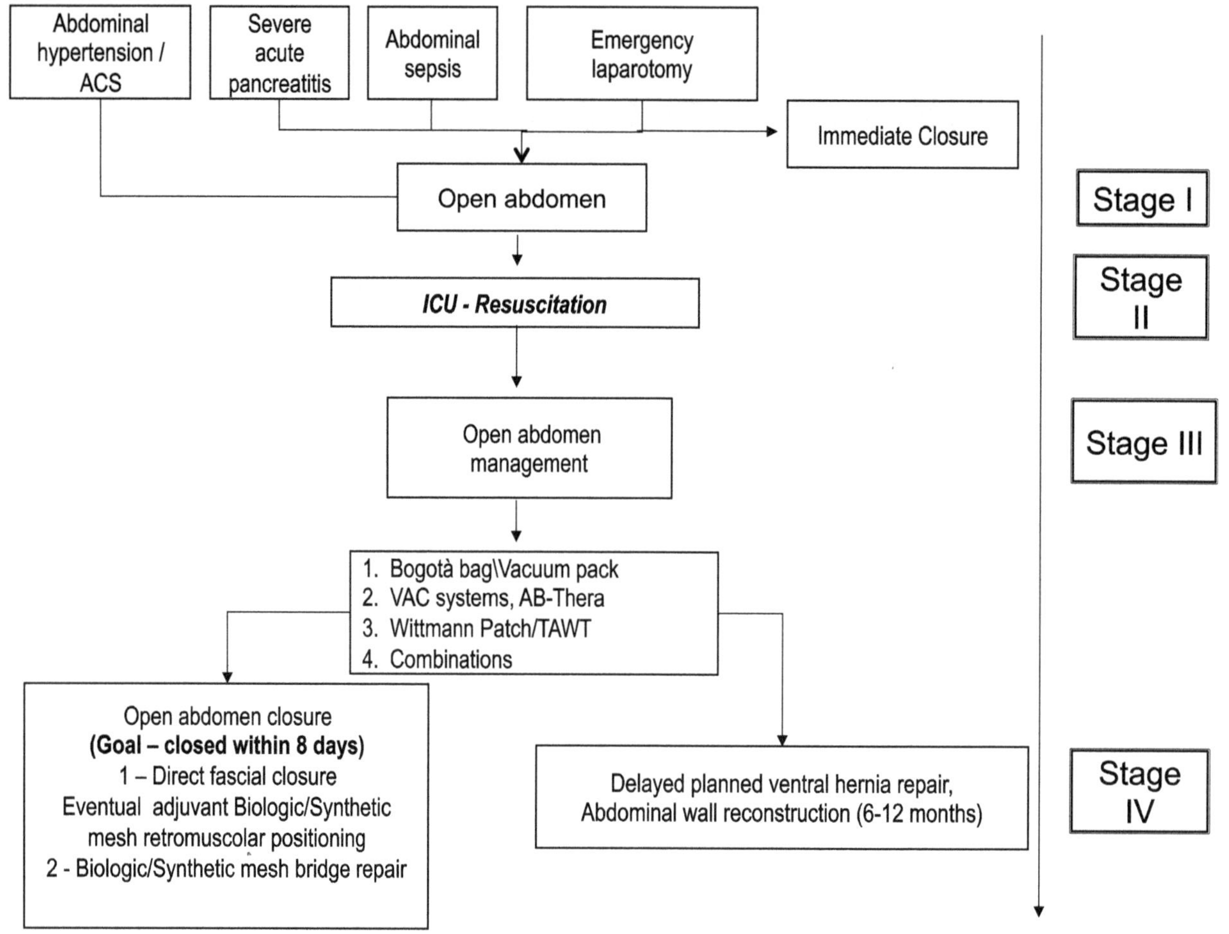

Fig. 1 Schematic flow-chart for the treatment of the open abdomen

[6]. Table 1 contains a partial list of the definitions. The abdomen and pelvis, while anatomically distinct, represent a single space and thus should be considered as one in discussion of intra-abdominal pressure (IAP) and ACS. The abdominopelvic cavity is a closed space, and the elasticity of its walls and the character of its contents determine the IAP. The IAP is fairly uniform throughout and therefore measurement anywhere within the cavity reflects the entire cavity. The IAP varies with diaphragmatic excursion: it increases with diaphragmatic contraction (inspiration) and decreases with expiration. The abdominal perfusion pressure (APP), analogous to the cerebral perfusion pressure, has been proposed as a more accurate predictor of visceral perfusion and consequently a target for intervention. A target APP of ≥60 mmHg is associated with improved survival in the setting of IAH and ACS [6, 7].

Normal IAP is actually below 0 mmHg. In the setting of conditions such as morbid obesity, pregnancy, liver disease with ascites, IAP may be chronically elevated to 10–15 mmHg without evidence of altered physiology [6]. During illness or following surgery, IAP is higher, on

Table 1 Consensus definitions related to intra-abdominal hypertension and abdominal compartment syndrome

IAP	The steady-state pressure concealed within the abdominal cavity. Normal = 5–7 mmHg in critically ill adults
APP	MAP – IAP
IAH	Sustained or repeated pathological elevation of IAP ≥12 mmHg
ACS	Sustained IAP >20 mmHg (with or without APP <60 mmHg) that is associated with a new organ dysfunction or failure
Primary ACS	ACS associated with injury or disease in abdomino-pelvic cavity
Secondary ACS	ACS in absence of conditions originating in the abdomino-pelvic cavity

IAP intra-abdominal pressure, *APP* abdominal perfusion pressure, *MAP* mean arterial pressure, *IAH* intra-abdominal hypertension, *ACS* abdominal compartment syndrome. Adapted from Malbrain et al. [6]

the order of 5–7 mmHg, due to factors such as tissue edema or ileus. The point at which IAP becomes IAH has been a matter of debate; the consensus definition settled on 12 mmHg as this is the lowest point at which pathologic effects are noted [6]. A grading system was proposed by the Denver General Hospital group in 1996, in the interest of guiding interventions [8]. The WSACS consensus definition varies slightly and is as follows: Grade I (12–15 mmHg); Grade II (16–20 mmHg); Grade III (21–25 mmHg); Grade IV (>25 mmHg) (Table 1) [6].

ACS develops as a result of alterations in perfusion related to IAH. Early literature on the syndrome variably defined the ACS; generally speaking, it was felt that ACS represented a pathologic elevation of IAP that was associated with organ dysfunction. The consensus definition selected a sustained IAP >20 mmHg, recognizing that lower levels of IAH may be associated with organ dysfunction. The final common pathway of organ dysfunction is hypoperfusion. The effects and manifestations of IAH on various organ systems are listed in Table 2 [9].

ACS is classified as primary if it is the result of a pathophysiologic process within the abdominopelvic cavity. It may be a result of bleeding, acute accumulation of ascites fluid, rapidly growing tumor or other mass, retroperitoneal edema, packing of visceral injuries, etc. Secondary ACS refers to development of ACS in the absence of a primary abdominopelvic process. In early descriptions, the secondary ACS was identified in patients who had massive resuscitation from hemorrhage or sepsis [10]. Ischemia/reperfusion injury may leads to massive accumulation of ascites, and bowel and retroperitoneal edema from accumulation of extracellular/extravascular fluid [11]. Increasingly it is recognized that secondary ACS is partly iatrogenic secondary to excessive fluid resuscitation.

Diagnosis and treatment

The role of elevated IAP is fundamental in understanding the evolution from IAH to ACS. Basing on the different patients and the setting into which they are admitted the measurement of IAP can be less or more helpful but in any case it remains a cornerstone. Recently Starkopf et al. found that the risk of IAH in mechanically ventilated patients is very low especially if they have a positive end expiratory pressure (PEEP) < 10 cm H2O, PaO2/FiO2 > 300 and BMI < 30 kg/m2 and without pancreatitis, hepatic failure/cirrhosis with ascites, gastrointestinal bleeding or laparotomy and the use of vasopressor/inotropes at admission [12]. In all those patients with the aforementioned characteristics the measurement of IAP might be considered.

According to the World Society of the Abdominal Compartment Syndrome 2013 consensus guidelines, IAP should be measured when there are at least 2 known risk factor for IAH/ACS in critically ill or injured patients [13]. Serial measurements should be performed during the patient's critical illness, preferably every 4–6 h. To measure the IAP the bladder pressure is considered the gold standard and should be taken at end-expiration with the patient supine and the transducer zeroed at the midaxillary line after an instillation of saline into the bladder. Another option available, if the bladder pressure is contraindicated (due to a constitutive augmented bladder pressure, e.g. in pelvic hematoma), is the measurement with the stomach technique [14]. Moreover exist the possibility to measure the intra-abdominal pressure via rectal, vaginal, inferior vena cava and direct intra-peritoneal measurement.

In treating patients with IAH, key principles include: optimization of systemic perfusion and organ function, institution of specific medical procedures to reduce IAP, and prompt surgical decompressive laparotomy for refractory IAH. Great emphasis has been placed on prevention, with early, prompt haemostatic control, aggressive balancing of resuscitation to include abundant coagulation factors. Tailoring the response for individual patients is essential to ensure that optimal outcomes are achieved. Further measures to alleviate IAH include sedation, analgesia, and neuromuscular blockade can be used to decrease IAP. Is it has been shown that persistent IAH of >18 mmHg is an independent cause of renal failure in general surgical patients admitted to ICU [15].

When employing early goal-directed fluid resuscitation is crucial to remember that correction of hypovolemia must be balanced carefully to avoid an iatrogenic secondary abdominal compartment syndrome. The keys in the end are prompt return to status quo, hemorrhage control,

Table 2 The effects of IAH on various organ systems, and clinical manifestations of ACS

System	Effect	Manifestation
Renal	Renal vein compression, cortical arteriolar compression	Oliguria, rising creatinine
Pulmonary	Upward pressure on diaphragm, decreased compliance and functional residual capacity, increased air way resistance	Hypoxia, hypercarbia, elevated airway pressure, decreased tidal volume
Cardiovascular	Decreased venous return, increased afterload	Decreased cardiac output
Cerebral	Increased intrathoracic pressure with decreased cerebral venous outflow	Elevated Intra Cranial Pressure
Splanchnic	Decreased perfusion of liver and intestine	Metabolic acidosis, bowel ischemia

eradication of sepsis, removal of fluid either by percutaneous catheter drainage and finally decompression.

Open abdomen in trauma

The management of complex problems in major trauma patients using OA and TAC techniques has gained popularity and become a valuable tool for the emergency surgeon. Notwithstanding the evolution of supportive care and the development of new and sophisticated commercial devices for TAC have significantly simplified clinical management, OA is still associated with serious complications such as nutritional problems with fluid and protein loss, loss of abdominal domain secondary to fascial retraction, frozen abdomen and entero-atmospheric fistulas (EAF). For these reasons, OA should be reserved for selected cases only and with the aim of obtaining early abdominal closure, possibly with primary fascial repair [16]. In trauma patients frequent indications for OA after injury are the prevention or treatment of ACS, the need for a "second look" operation in abdominal injuries, post-injury septic abdomen and injury with partial or entire loss of the abdominal wall.

Prevention and treatment of IAH/ACS

The prevalence of ACS in trauma patients has fallen in centers with advanced medical care, some reporting falls from 30 to almost 0 % [5]. Where trauma and emergency surgery systems are not so advanced IAH and ACS can be expected to occur in up to 40 % of ICU admission respectively. Risk factors for IAH/ACS in trauma patients are: (i) increased intra-retroperitoneal contents consequent to hemorrhage from organ or pelvic injury, or emergency surgery with packing procedures, (ii) increased intraluminal contents occurring in post-injury bowel paresis, (iii) decreased abdominal wall compliance when abdominal injury occurs in patients with high body mass index or for an associated third degree burn of the abdominal wall and (iv) increased visceral edema following massive fluid/blood resuscitation. Untreated post-injury ACS is an independent predictor of organ failure [17] that is often difficult to reverse, and should be prevented using different strategies. delayed decompression may not reverse the sequalae of IAH and ACS [18]. At the end of a damage control operation, it would be ideal to measure IAP to decide for fascial closure: however this is technically difficult unless a continuous IAP technique is used [5]. Some authors prefer to left open the abdomen for 24–48 h if the value is greater than 12 mmHg Moreover, in trauma patients with elevated IAP (with or without previous surgery) every medical strategy to reduce IAP should be applied: ng tube, colonic decompression, prokinetic medications, supine position, negative fluid balance starting from post-injury day one, percutaneous drainage of fluid collections and sedation and muscle relaxation.

Need for a "second look" operation

A second look procedure is planned when the initial operation has been stopped in a damage control setting for physiologic exhaustion of the patient, bleeding from remote areas not amenable to surgical correction, vascular injuries of visceral vessels with risk of bowel ischemia, resected and closed bowel with subsequent need for anastomosis or stoma, complex liver injury treated with packing, and the need for transfer to a higher level facility. All these cases require TAC that allows for a simple re-operation for definitive abdominal care.

Post-injury septic abdomen

Septic abdomen may develop following hollow viscus injuries for penetrating or blunt trauma, particularly in cases of delayed diagnosis or leakage after primary repair of colonic wounds. Unusual conditions are septic evolutions of complex duodeno-pancreatic injuries. Recent clinical series suggest that OA associated with negative pressure therapy (NPT) improves observed survival compared with P-POSSUM expected survival in severe peritonitis [19]. In a porcine model of peritoneal fecal contamination, NPT reduced systemic inflammation thereby improving organ function [20].

Loss of abdominal wall

This is an unusual condition following penetrating injuries caused by high velocity military weapons or blast injuries. It is sometimes a consequence of extensive surgical debridement after soft tissue infection by necrotizing germs that have spread to the abdominal wall. The abdomen is of necessity open and requires TAC until it is possible to reconstruct the wall.

Open abdomen in abdominal sepsis and pancreatitis

The main aims of the open abdomen approach in severe secondary peritonitis and severe acute pancreatitis (SAP) are to facilitate the clearance of the infectious material, expedite subsequent surgical interventions and prevent the development of abdominal compartment syndrome (ACS).

Abdominal sepsis

In severe secondary peritonitis, a staged approach may be required for three different reasons, although they are often used in combinations.

Firstly, the inability to control the source of contamination in a single operation: Instead of the traditional model of one definitive operation and possible reoperation only performed as needed (relaparotomy on-demand strategy), there are two other options to manage a severely contaminated peritoneal cavity. One, termed planned relaparotomy refers to a technique where the need for a second operation is recognized and decided at the initial operation. Another option, the open abdomen technique, is leaving the abdomen open and treating the infected peritoneal cavity like an "open abscess" with frequent irrigations and TAC techniques [21].

Secondly, if the surgeon feels the patient wont tolerate a definitive repair and/or abdominal wall closure, the operation is deliberately abbreviated due to the severe physiological derangement and suboptimal local conditions for healing, and restoration of intestinal continuity is deferred to the second operation (deferred anastomosis technique) This is particularly important in hypotensive patients who are already received ionotropes [22].

Thirdly, the presence of extensive visceral edema may increase the risk of ACS development, if primary fascial closure is attempted [23]. To prevent ACS, the abdominal incision is left open and the viscera are covered with one of the TAC methods. ACS can develop from a number of complications related to intra-abdominal sepsis including but not limited to large volume fluid resuscitation resulting in visceral edema and intra-abdominal free fluid collection, retroperitoneal, intra-abdominal and abdominal wall bleeding and ileus, pseudo-obstruction and mechanical obstruction of the bowel.

Severe acute pancreatitis

Since the late 1970s a treatment option for SAP was an open management with frequent dressing changes in order to facilitate the clearance of infection and an adequate drainage analogously to the open management of an incised abscess.

Patients underwent surgical interventions to achieve control of the infection source, the infected peripancreatic necrosis. If the source control at the initial operation was incomplete and if repeated measures to achieve it were needed, the abdomen was left open between procedures. Gradually the cavity decreased in size and often healed by secondary intention after formation of granulation tissue. Even in the case of an enteric fistula secondary to the open abdomen treatment, expectant management often resulted in acceptable results, although the open management was associated with poorer results than the closed drainage methods [24–27].

It was suggested that a significant proportion of patients with SAP dying of early multiple organ dysfunction syndrome in effect died of unrecognized and untreated ACS caused by massive fluid resuscitation, capillary leak and visceral edema [28, 29].

Although percutaneous drainage of pancreatic ascites can, in some cases, decrease IAP at least temporarily, surgical decompression is the most reliable method to relieve IAH and restore vital organ functions, especially in the pulmonary, cardiovascular and renal systems.

There are three options for surgical decompression in patients with no recent abdominal incision (that often is the case in SAP). A long vertical midline incision is most commonly used and it has been showed to decrease IAP effectively: it is rapid and easy to perform, but it is associated with a risk of intestinal fistulas and in many cases failure to close the fascia requiring complex reconstructive surgery at a later stage [30]. Transverse laparostomy is a promising alternative and isolated reports have shown its effectiveness in reducing IAP [31]. Although it takes slightly longer to perform than midline laparostomy, same principles of managing the open abdomen can be applied without additional equipment.

A third alternative used in SAP is the subcutaneous linea alba fasciotomy, where the fascia is incised through three small skin incisions leaving the rest of the skin and the peritoneum intact [32]. Although it eliminates the OA, it might not be always effective enough [33]. In addition, the subcutaneous fasciotomy always results in a ventral hernia requiring repair later on.

Infected pancreatic necrosis is an established indication for surgical necrosectomy, ideally postponed until 4 weeks after the onset of symptoms and performed most commonly through a midline incision [34]. Because ACS usually commences during the first few days of the disease and the (usually) sterile necrosis is unripe, there are no indications to explore the pancreas or the peripancreatic spaces further. In addition to causing significant bleeding, it could also introduce an infection to the peri-pancreatic space [28]. Although both midline and transverse incisions could later be utilized for necrosectomy, transverse subcostal incision could be justified for decompression when concomitant necrosectomy is planned or anticipated in patients with late onset ACS.

Management of OA and its definitive closure

The management of patients with OA is a particularly challenging issue that requires compulsorily a multidisciplinary approach with a strength interaction among the surgeon and the intensive care unit (ICU) team in order to offer the best treatment to these critical patients.

ICU management

A management plan to reduce risk of ACS developing, both primary and secondary, should ideally begin before the patient gets to the emergency room e from there get to the operatory room where the surgeon decide to leave open the abdomen.

In the ICU a patient with OA requires a specific management. Coagulopathy should be treated with balanced transfusion [35] with a restrictive fluid management strategy in order to prevent acute lung injury (ALI) and acute respiratory distress syndrome (ARDS) [36–39]; in trauma the application of a Exsanguination Protocol with massive transfusion showed a decreased mortality with lower incidence of severe sepsis/septic shock and multi organ failure (MOF) and lower ventilator associated pneumonitis (VAP), ventilatory failure, and ACS [35, 40].

pH should be maintained > 7.2 and checked with a frequent measurement of arterial lactate level. The heat loss in a patient with OA is a problem that should be constantly kept in mind. Hypothermia should be treated reaching an ideal temperature > 37 °C with passive rewarming, air warmers and Bair Hugger Therapy [38].

These patients should receive a tailored ventilatory support with a low tidal volume in order to prevent ALI and ARDS that can be exacerbated by VAP and transfusion-related ALI [41]. Infectious complications, not only in the abdomen, are associated with failed abdominal closure [42, 43]: an adequate antibiotic therapy should be directed toward the underlying disease that culminated in the OA with an empirical anti-enterococcal coverage in patients with prior antibiotic exposure [44]. Another important issue in the ICU is the pain control with a consequent reduction in agitation, stress and fear. Adequate sedation levels should be maintained and strictly monitored in order to reduce the recall of unpleasant experiences and the awareness.

Fluid balance and nutrition

Other fundamental issues in critically ill patient with OA are fluid and electrolytes balance and nutrition support. Patients with OA have an increased insensible fluid loss. In addition, these wounds are open into the peritoneal cavity, adding significantly to the amount of fluid loss across the wound surface. Hydration and volume status should be meticulously monitored, ideally the patients weight should be documented daily. The negative pressure wound therapy contributes to a decrease in fluid losses across the open wound surfaces by significantly reducing evaporation [45] and draining into a dedicated canister as V.A.C pack or Ab-thera (KCI, San Antonio, TX), facilitates fluid collection and allows a more accurate estimation of fluid losses from the wound and peritoneal cavity. The measured fluid losses can then be more precisely replaced, and hypovolemia can be minimized or potentially avoided.

Generally a critically ill patient is in a hypercatabolic state that's associated with muscle proteolysis, acute protein malnutrition, impairment in immune function, and subclinical development of MOF. Moreover OA is a significative source of nitrogen loss in the critically ill patient with an estimate loss of 2 g of nitrogen per liter of abdominal fluid output [46] requiring an adjusted integration. A patient with OA represents one of the sickest, most inflamed, and subsequently most hypermetabolic among surgical patients. A particular attention must be given to this critical aspect: once the resuscitation is near complete and the GI tract allows it enteral nutrition should be initiated as soon as possible, with a clear benefit for the patient in a lower time to fascia closure and a lower pneumonia and fistula rate [47–49].

Temporary abdominal closure techniques

Several different TAC techniques to left open the abdomen exist. The ideal one should be easy to apply and remove, should allow rapid access to a surgical second-look, should drain secretions, should ease primary closure and should has morbidity and mortality acceptable, should allow easy nursing, and last but not least should be readily available and cheap. During years, different methods for TAC have been proposed. From late '70s and during '80s, abdominal dressings for OA were quite simple, and the attention during treatment was focused only on protection and control of the bowel outside the abdomen. Through years, the attention of surgeons moved from protection of the ileus to preservation of the peritoneal space and prevention of lateral retraction of the fascia, which are the most important obstacles against the reconstruction of the abdominal wall at the end of the treatment.

One of the simplest and most inexpensive way to cover the viscera is approximating only the skin with a simple running suture or using towel clips. Another easy method is the plastic silo, also known as Bogotà bag, with a non-adherent plastic sheet, usually from sterile 3 lt. urology irrigation bag, sutured between the fascial edges or the skin.

In the 1993 Wittmann described a new technique (Witmann patch, Star Surgical, Burlington, Vt) consisting in two opposite Velcro sheets sutured to the fascia and connected on the middle allowing an easy and fast access to the abdominal cavity, with a simple traction, and a stepwise reapproximation preventing the fascia retraction [50].

Barker and colleagues in 1995 described another technique, the vacuum pack, where a perforated plastic sheet covers the viscera, sterile surgical towels are placed in the wound, a surgical drain connected with a continue negative pressure is placed on the towels and all is covered by an airtight seal; the dressing should be changed every 2–3 days in operative room but also in the ICU. The negative pressure allows a collection of excess fluid and keeps constant tension on the fascia with a limited cost (50$) [51] with a reported primary fascia closure rate of 68,1 % with a total complication rate of 15 %. [52]. The vacuum pack was then developed with the use of a polyurethane sponge and an adjustable pump to set the negative pressure (KCI V.A.C. Pack, San Antonio, TX) with some advantages as reduced need for frequent dressing changes, increased vascularity of the wound, decreased bacterial counts and extended opportunity for definitive fascial closure (Fig. 2).

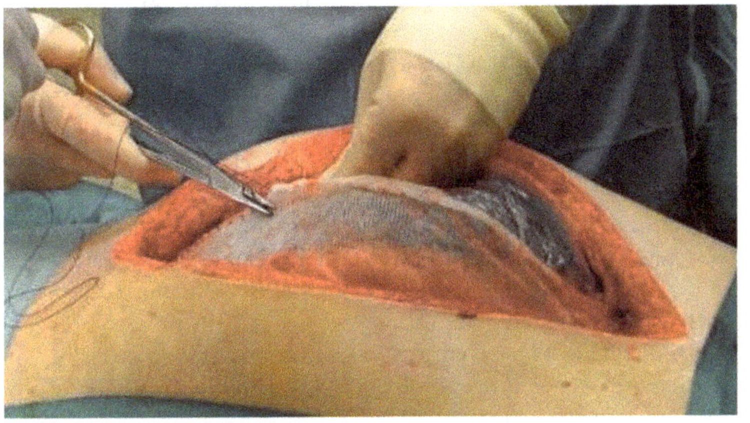

Fig. 2 Synthetic mesh sutured to the fascial edges to maintain the traction and prevent the fascial retraction with a plastic sheet posed under in direct contact with the intrabdominal content to protect the bowel

Another implementation of the system was introduced by the AB-Thera (KCI, San Antonio, TX) with the use of spider-like sponge that allow a better fluid drainage and a better wound contraction and with a reported primary fascia closure rate of 89 % [53, 54]. When OA is prolonged for more than two days, the AB-Thera system obtains better results [55]. In a prospective observational open-label study involving 20 trauma centers across the USA, was demonstrated that AB-Thera was associated with higher primary fascial closure rate and lower 30 day all-cause mortality, possibly because of the improved peritoneal cytokine removal with this system [55].

A recent modification of the Wittmann patch was described by Dennis et al. in the 2013: the burr like sheet are sutured not directly on the medial fascia but to the underside of the abdominal wall, lateral to the rectus sheath, using external blosters; on the wound is applied a vacuum pack dressing. With this technique they showed a primary fascia closure in 100 % of the patients [56].

Burlew et al. described similar results using the VAC system (KCI, San Antonio, TX) with a polydioxanone (PDS) suture keeping the fascia in a moderate tension and a sequential closure of the abdomen during the following change of dressing, every 2 days [57].

Acosta described a combined technique using VAC system (KCI, San Antonio, TX) with a polypropylene mesh applied on the fascia edge to keep it in traction and reported a fascia closure rate of 76.6 % [58] (Fig. 3).

Another combined technique consist in the use of the ABRA system (Canica Design Inc, Almonte, Ontario, Canada), which consist in a dynamic fascial tension device with elastomers anchored to the abdominal wall with plastic "button anchors" with the VAC system (KCI, San Antonio, TX) with interesting results and a reported fascial apposition rate of 83 % [59, 60].

Which is the best and the correct management of a patient with OA nowadays is still unclear: the technique is relatively new and in the literature the data and the casuistic reported are too various and too heterogeneous to assess. With these criticisms the techniques seamed to be associated with the best rate of primary closure and minor complication rate are the Negative Pressure Wound therapy and the Wittmann patch but grounded data are needed [61, 62].

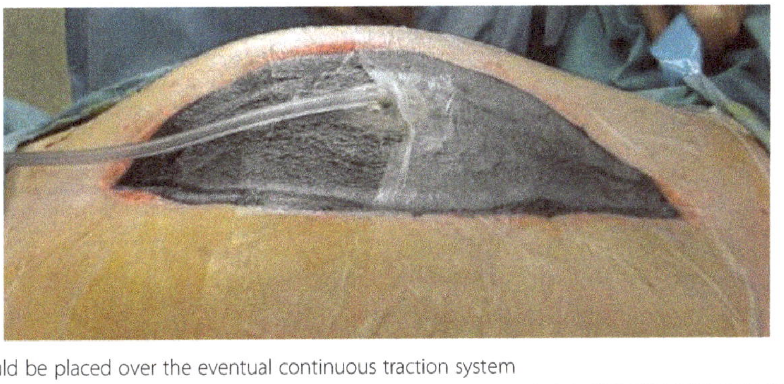

Fig. 3 Aspiration system could be placed over the eventual continuous traction system

Definitive closure

In the management of OA with TAC the primary goal is to close the wound within 8 days: indeed Miller reported in a large case series, a progressive complication rate increase after the 8th day of OA and increased morbidity and mortality were also reported if the fascia was closed under undue tension [63]. If the primary closure is still impossible to reach the surgeon has different chance. Before the introduction of the temporary closure technique the wounds were closed with, component separation, with granulation tissue with split-thickness skin grafting or with the use of synthetic mesh: in the first case it's been created a planned ventral hernia that requires a later surgical correction; in the second case the use of a synthetic mesh required a sufficient skin to cover it and exposed the patient to the risk of fistula, adhesion formation and the risk of infection, especially in contaminated fields [64]. A very interesting alternative is the use of Biological Prosthesis (BP) [65, 66]: BP are collagen mesh derived from allogenic or xenogenic sources and they work as a scaffold where the host tissue can growth, covering the wall defect activating a remodelling process in which the host remodels the prosthesis with new healthy tissue. The use of BP gives some advantages: the lowest adhesiogenic potential among the prosthetic material [67], allows blood, growth and pro/anti-inflammatory factors and drugs to reach the surgical field during the healing process enhancing the effect against contamination or infections. They could be divided in cross-linked and non-cross-linked [68, 69]. The crosslinked biological meshes are treated, after the decellularization, in order to obtain crosslinks between and inside the collagen chains: the presence of these bridges prolongs the lengthening of resorption of the mesh ensuring better tensile strength; however, this process slows the fibroblast invasion and angiogenesis, making more difficult the integration with the host tissue and increasing the foreign body response by the prosthesis. The non-crosslinked meshes have a better profile of tissue integration and local inflammatory response, but are subject to a faster resorption process [70]. The Italian Biological Prosthesis Work Group (IBPWG) proposed a decisional model to choose which BP use, cross-linked or not-cross-linked, creating a score on the basis of the presence of infection and the dimension of wall defect. [71] in order to facilitate the decisional process and to obtain the better outcome for the patients.

Conclusions

All those involved in care of a critically ill patient should in the first instance think how to prevent IAH and ACS. In case of ACS goal directed therapy to achieve early opening and early closure is the key: paradigm of closure shifts to combination of therapies including NPWT and dynamic closure, in order to reduce complications and avoid incisional hernia.

There have been huge studies and progress in survival of critically ill trauma and septic surgical patients: this in part has been through the great work of pioneer and scientific societies, as the WSACS and their guidelines; however future studies and continued innovation are needed to better understand optimal treatment strategies and to define more clearly the indications, because OA by itself is still a morbid procedure.

Consensus statement

Written informed consent was obtained from the patient for the publication of the images.

Competing interests

All authors declare to have no conflict of interest.

Author's contributions

FCo, FCa, LA designed research; FCo, WB, FCa, MC, OC, SC, LF, AL, RM, GM, GP, MS analyzed data; FCo, WB, OC, SC, LF, AL, GP wrote the paper. All authors read and approved the final manuscript.

Author details

[1]General Surgery Department, Papa Giovanni XXIII Hospital, Piazza OMS 1, 24127 Bergamo, Italy. [2]Denver Health Medical Center, Denver, CO, USA. [3]General surgery Department, Ospedale Maggiore, Parma, Italy. [4]Niguarda Trauma Center, Ospedale Niguarda Ca'Granda, Milan, Italy. [5]Unità Operativa di Chirurgia d'Urgenza, Azienda Ospedaliera "San Gerardo", Monza, Italy. [6]Department of Abdominal Surgery, University of Helsinki, Helsinki, Finland. [7]Letterkenny Hospital and the Donegal Clinical Research Academy, Donegal, Ireland. [8]University College Hospital, Galway, Ireland.

References

1. McCosh II AJ. The treatment of general septic peritonitis. Ann Surg. 1897;25:687–97.
2. Ogilvie WH. The late complications of abdominal war wounds. Lancet. 1940;2:253–6.
3. Perez D, Wildi S, Demartines N, Bramkamp M, Koehler C, Clavien PA. Prospective evaluation of vacuum-assisted closure in abdominal compartment syndrome and severe abdominal sepsis. J Am Coll Surg. 2007;205(4):586–92.
4. Kron IL, Harman PK, Nolan SP. The measurement of intra-abdominal pressure as a criterion for abdominal re-exploration. Ann Surg. 1984;199:28–30.
5. Balogh ZJ, Lumsdaine W, Moore E, Moore FA. Postinjury abdominal compartment syndrome: from recognition to prevention. The Lancet. 2014;384(9952):1466–75.
6. Malbrain ML, Cheatham ML, Kirkpatrick A, Sugrue M, Parr M, De Waele J, et al. Results from the international consensus of experts on intra-abdominal hypertension and abdominal compartment syndrome. I. Definitions. Intensive Care Med. 2006;32:1722–32.
7. Cheatham ML, White MW, Sagraves SG, Johnson JL, Block EF. Abdominal perfusion pressure: A superior parameter in the assessment of intra-abdominal hypertension. J Trauma. 2000;49:621–6.
8. Burch JM, Moore EE, Moore FA, Franciose R. The abdominal compartment syndrome. Surg Clin North Am. 1996;76:833–42.
9. Carr JA. Abdominal compartment syndrome: A decade of progress. J Am CollSurg. 2013;216:135–46.
10. Burrows R, Edington J, Robbs JV. A wolf in wolf's clothing—the abdominal compartment syndrome. S Afr Med J. 1995;85(1):46–8.
11. Biffl WL, Moore EE, Burch JM, Offner PJ, Franciose RJ, Johnson JL. Secondary abdominal compartment syndrome is a highy lethal event. Am J Surg. 2001;182:645–8.

12. Starkopf J, Tamme K, Blaser AR. Should we measure intra-abdominal pressure in every intensive care patient? Ann Intensive Care. 2012;2 Suppl 1:S9. doi:10.1186/2110-5820-2-S1-S9.
13. Kirkpatrick AW, Roberts DJ, De Waele J, Jaeschke R, Malbrain MLNG, De Keulenaer B, et al. Intra-abdominal hypertension and the abdominal compartment syndrome: updated consensus definitions and clinical practice guidelines from the World Society of the Abdominal Compartment Syndrome. Intensive Care Med. 2013;39:1190–206.
14. Malbrain MLNG. Different techniques to measure intra-abdominal pressure (IAP): time for a critical re-appraisal. In: Applied Physiology in Intensive Care Medicine. Berlin Heidelberg: Springer; 2009. p. 143–57.
15. Sugrue M, Jones F, Deane SA, Bishop G, Bauman A, Hillman K. Intra-abdominal hypertension is an independent cause of post-operative renal impairment. Arch Surg. 1999;134:1082–805.
16. Cothren Burlew C. The open abdomen: practical implications for the practicing surgeon. Am J Surg. 2012;204:826–35.
17. Balogh ZJ, van Wessem K, Yoshino O, Moore FA. Post injury abdominal compartment syndrome: are we winning the battle? World J Surg. 2009;33:1134–41.
18. Sugrue M, Jones F, Janjua KJ, Deane SA, Bristow P, Hillman K. Temporary abdominal closure: a prospective evaluation of its effects on renal and respiratory physiology. J Trauma. 1998;45:914–21.
19. Horwood J, Akbar F, Maw A. Initial experience of laparostomy with immediate vacuum therapy in patients with severe peritonitis. Ann R Coll Surg Eng. 2009;91:681–7.
20. Kubiak BD, Albert SP, Gatto LA, Snyder KP, Maier KG, Vieau CJ, et al. Peritoneal negative pressure therapy prevents multiple organ injury in a chronic porcine sepsis and ischemia/reperfusion model. Shock. 2010;34:525–34.
21. Schein M. Surgical management of intra-abdominal infection: is there any evidence? Langenbeck's Arch Surg. 2002;387:1–7.
22. Ordonez CA, Sanchez AI, Pineda JA, Badiel M, Mesa R, Cardona U, et al. Deferred primary anastomosis versus diversion in patients with severe secondary peritonitis managed with staged laparotomies. World J Surg. 2010;34:169–76.
23. Plantefeve G, Hellmann R, Pajot O, Thirion M, Bleichner G, Mentec H. Abdominal compartment syndrome and intra-abdominal sepsis: two of the same kind? Acta Clin Belg. 2007;62 Suppl 1:162–7.
24. Bradley III EL. Management of infected pancreatic necrosis by open drainage. Ann Surg. 1987;206:542–8.
25. Fugger R, Schultz F, Rogy M, Herbst F, Mirza D, Fritsch A. Open approach in pancreatic and infected pancreatic necrosis: laparostomies and preplanned revisions. World J Surg. 1991;15:516–21.
26. Fugger R, Götzinger P, Sautner T, Mittlböck M, Rogy M, Adamer K, et al. Necrosectomy and laparostomy – a combined therapeutic concept in acute necrotizing pancreatitis. Eur J Surg. 1995;161:103–7.
27. Bosscha K, Hulstaert PF, Hennipman A, Visser MR, Gooszen HG, van Vroonhoven TJMV, et al. Fulminant acute pancreatitis and infected necrosis: results of open management of the abdomen and "planned" reoperations. J Am Coll Surg. 1998;187:255–62.
28. De Waele J, Hoste E, Blot S, Decruyenaere J, Colardyn F. Intraabdominal hypertension in patients with severe acute pancreatitis. Crit Care. 2005;9:R452–7.
29. Keskinen P, Leppäniemi A, Pettilä V, Piilonen A, Kemppainen E, Hynninen M. Intra-abdominal pressure in severe acute pancreatitis. World J Emerg Surg. 2007;2:2.
30. De Waele JJ, Hoste EAJ, Malbrain MLNG. Decompressive laparotomy for abdominal compartment syndrome – a critical analysis. Crit Care. 2006;10:R51.
31. Leppäniemi A, Mentula P, Hienonen P, Kemppainen E. Transverse laparostomy is feasible and effective in the treatment of abdominal compartment syndrome in severe acute pancreatitis. In press.
32. Leppäniemi AK, Hienonen PA, Siren JE, Kuitunen AH, Lindström OK, Kemppainen EA. Treatment of abdominal compartment syndrome with subcutaneous anterior abdominal fasciotomy in severe acute pancreatitis. World J Surg. 2006;30:1922–4.
33. Leppäniemi A, Hienonen P, Mentula P, Kemppainen E. Subcutaneous linea alba fasciotomy, does it really work? Am Surg. 2011;77:99–102.
34. Werner J, Hartwig W, Hackert T, Buchler MW. Surgery in the treatment of acute pancreatitis – open pancreatic necrosectomy. Scand J Surg. 2005;94:1130–4.
35. Gunter Jr OL, Au BK, Isbell JM, Mowery NT, Young PP, Cotton BA. Optimazing outcomes in damage control resuscitation: identifying blood product ratiosassociated with Improved survival. J Trauma. 2008;65(3):527–34.
36. Borgman MA, Spinella PC, Perkins JG, Grathwohl KW, Repine T, Beekley AC, et al. The ratio of blood products transfused affects mortality in patients receiving massive transfusions at a combat support hospital. J Trauma. 2007;63(4):805–13.
37. Kauvar DS, Lefering R, Wade CE. Impact of hemorrhage on trauma outcome: an overview of epidemiology, clinical presentations, and therapeutic considerations. J Trauma. 2006;60(6 Suppl):S3–11.
38. Dutton WD, Diaz Jr JJ, Miller RS. Critical care issues in managing complex open abdominal wound. J Intensive Care Med. 2012;27(3):161–71.
39. Stewart RM, Park PK, Hunt JP, McIntyre Jr RC, McCarthy J, Zarzabal LA, et al. Less is more: improved outcomes in surgical patients with conservative fluid administration and central venous catheter monitoring. J Am Coll Surg. 2009;208(5):725–35. discussion 735–7.
40. Cotton BA, Au BK, Nunez TC, Gunter OL, Robertson AM, Young PP. Predefined massive transfusion protocols are associated with a reduction in organ failure and postinjury complications. J Trauma. 2009;66(1):41–8.
41. Rosenberg AL, Dechert RE, Park PK, Bartlett RH, NIH NHLBI ARDS Network. Review of a large clinical series: association of cumulative fluid balance on outcome in acute lung injury: a retrospective review of the ARDSnet tidal volume study cohort. J Intensive Care Med. 2009;24(1):35–46.
42. Teixeira PG, Salim A, Inaba K, Brown C, Browder T, Margulies D, et al. A prospective look at the current state of open abdomens. Am Surg. 2008;74(10):891–7.
43. Vogel TR, Diaz JJ, Miller RS, May AK, Guillamondegui OD, Guy JS, et al. The open abdomen in trauma: do infectious complications affect primary abdominal closure? Surg Infect (Larchmt). 2006;7(5):433–41.
44. Harbarth S, Uckay I. Are there patients with peritonitis who require empiric therapy for enterococcus? Eur J Clin Microbiol Infect Dis. 2004;23(2):73–7.
45. Caro A, Olona C, Jimenez A, Vadillo J, Feliu F, Vicente V. Treatment of the open abdomen with topical negative pressure therapy: a retrospective study of 46 cases. Int Wound J. 2011;8:274–9.
46. Cheatham ML, Safcsak K, Brzezinski SJ, Lube MW. Nitrogen balance, protein loss, and the open abdomen. Crit Care Med. 2007;35(1):127–31.
47. Collier B, Guillamondegui O, Cotton B, Donahue R, Conrad A, Groh K, et al. Feeding the open abdomen. J Parenter Enter Nutr. 2007;31(5):410–5.
48. Dissanaike S, Pham T, Shalhub S, Warner K, Hennessy L, Moore EE, et al. Effect of immediate enteral feeding on trauma patients with an open abdomen: protection from nosocomial infections. J Am Coll Surg. 2008;207(5):690–7.
49. Cothren CC, Moore EE, Ciesla DJ, Johnson JL, Moore JB, Haenel JB, et al. Postinjury abdominal compartment syndrome does not preclude early enteral feeding after definitive closure. Am J Surg. 2004;188(6):653–8.
50. Wittmann DH, Aprahamian C, Bergstein JM, Edmiston CE, Frantzides CT, Quebbeman EJ, et al. A burr-like device to facilitate temporary abdominal closure in planned multiple laparotomies. Eur J Surg. 1993;159(2):75–9.
51. Brock WB, Barker DE. Burns RPTemporary closure of open abdominal wounds: the vacuum pack. Am Surg. 1995;61(1):30–5.
52. Barker DE, Green JM, Maxwell RA, Smith PW, Mejia VA, Dart BW, et al. Experience with vacuum-pack temporary abdominal wound closure in 258 trauma and general and vascular surgical patients. J Am Coll Surg. 2007;204(5):784–92.
53. Lindstedt S, Malmsjö M, Hlebowicz J, Ingemansson R. Comparative study of the microvascular blood flow in the intestinal wall, wound contraction and fluid evacuation during negative pressure wound therapy in laparostomy using the V.A.C. abdominal dressing and the ABTheraopen abdomen negative pressure therapy system. Int Wound J. 2013. doi:10.1111/iwj.12056. [Epub ahead of print].
54. Frazee RC, Abernathy SW, Jupiter DC, Hendricks JC, Davis M, Regner JL, et al. Are commercial negative pressure systems worth the cost in open abdomen management? J Am Coll Surg. 2013;216(4):730–3.
55. Cheatham ML, Demetrides D, Fabian TC, Kaplan MJ, Miles WS, Schreiber MA, et al. Prospective study examining clinical outcomes associated with negative pressure wound therapy system and Barker's vacuum packing technique. World J Surg. 2013;37:2018–30.
56. Dennis A, Vizinas TA, Joseph K, Kingsley S, Bokhari F, Starr F, et al. Not so fast to skin graft: transabdominal wall traction closes most "domain loss" abdomens in the acute setting. J Trauma Acute Care Surg. 2013;74(6):1486–92.
57. Burlew CC, Moore EE, Biffl WL, Bensard DD, Johnson JL, Barnett CC. One hundred percent fascial approximation can be achieved in the postinjury open abdomen with a sequential closure protocol. J Trauma Acute Care Surg. 2012;72(1):235–41.

58. Petersson U, Acosta S, Björck M. Vacuum-assisted wound closure and mesh-mediated fascial traction–a novel technique for late closure of the open abdomen. World J Surg. 2007;31(11):2133–7.
59. Salman AE, Yetişir F, Aksoy M, Tokaç M, Yildirim MB, Kiliç M. Use of dynamic wound closure system in conjunction with vacuum-assisted closure therapy in delayed closure of open abdomen. Hernia. 2014;18(1):99–104.
60. Haddock C, Konkin DE, Blair NP. Management of the open abdomen with the Abdominal Reapproximation Anchor dynamic fascial closure system. Am J Surg. 2013;205(5):528–33.
61. Boele van Hensbroek P, Wind J, Dijkgraaf MG, Busch OR, Goslings JC. Temporary closure of the open abdomen: a systematic review on delayed primary fascial closure in patients with an open abdomen. World J Surg. 2009;33(2):199–207.
62. Roberts DJ, Zygun DA, Grendar J, Ball CG, Robertson HL, Ouellet JF, et al. Negative-pressure wound therapy for critically ill adults with open abdominal wounds: a systematic review. J Trauma Acute Care Surg. 2012;73(3):629–39.
63. Miller RS, Morris Jr JA, Diaz Jr JJ, Herring MB, May AK. Complications after 344 damage-control open celiotomies. J Trauma. 2005;59(6):1365–71.
64. Dinsmore RC, Calton Jr WC, Harvey SB, Blaney MW. Prevention of adhesions to polypropylene mesh in a traumatized bowel model. J Am Coll Surg. 2000;191(2):131–6.
65. Rosen MJ, Krpata DM, Ermlich B, Blatnik JA. A 5-year clinical experience with single-staged repairs of infected and contaminated abdominal wall defects utilizing biologic mesh. Ann Surg. 2013;257(6):991–6.
66. Campanelli G, Catena F, Ansaloni L. World Journal of Emergency Surgery. World J Emerg Surg. 2008;3:33.
67. Catena F, Ansaloni L, D'Alessandro L, Pinna A. Adverse effects of porcine small intestine submucosa (SIS) implants in experimental ventral hernia repair. Surg Endosc. 2006;21(4):690.
68. Deeken CR, Melman L, Jenkins ED, Greco SC, Frisella MM, Matthews BD. Histologic and biomechanical evaluation of crosslinked and non-crosslinked biologic meshes in a porcine model of ventral incisional hernia repair. J Am Coll Surg. 2011;212(5):880–8.
69. Melman L, Jenkins ED, Hamilton NA, Bender LC, Brodt MD, Deeken CR, et al. Early biocompatibility of crosslinked and non-crosslinked biologic meshes in a porcine model of ventral hernia repair. Hernia. 2011;15(2):157–64.
70. Orenstein SB, Qiao Y, Klueh U, Kreutzer DL, Novitsky YW. Activation of human mononuclear cells by porcine biologic meshes in vitro. Hernia. 2010;14(4):401–7.
71. Coccolini F, Agresta F, Bassi A, Catena F, Crovella F, Ferrara R, et al. Italian Biological Prosthesis Work-Group (IBPWG): proposal for a decisional model in using biological prosthesis. World J Emerg Surg. 2012;7(1):34.

The current management of acute uncomplicated appendicitis: should there be a change in paradigm?

Samuel Ho Ting Poon[1], Jennifer Wah Yan Lee[1], Ka Man NG[1], Gloria Wing Yan Chiu[1], Brian Yung Kong Wong[1], Chi Chung Foo[2*] and Wai Lun Law[2]

Abstract

Introduction: Appendectomy has long been the mainstay of intervention for acute appendicitis, aiming at preventing perforation, peritonitis, abscess formation and recurrence. With better understanding of the disease process, non-operative management (NOM) with antibiotics alone has been proved a feasible treatment for uncomplicated appendicitis. This article aimed at systematically reviewing the available literatures and discussing the question whether NOM should replace appendectomy as the standard first-line treatment for uncomplicated appendicitis.

Method: A search of the Embase, Pubmed and Cochrane Library was performed using the keywords 'acute appendicitis' and 'antibiotic therapy'. Meta-analysis with inverse variance model for continuous variable and Mantel Haenzel Model for dichotomous variable was performed to evaluate the one year treatment efficacy, morbidities rate, sick leave duration and length of hospital stay associated with emergency appendectomy and NOM.

Results: Six randomized control trials were identified out of 1943 publications. NOM had a significant lower treatment efficacy rate at one year, 0.10 (95% CI 0.03–0.36, $p < 0.01$), when compared to appendectomy. The morbidities rate was comparable between the two interventions. The length of hospital stay was longer, with a mean difference of 1.08 days (95% CI 0.09–2.07, $p = 0.03$), and the sick leave duration was shorter, a mean difference of 3.37 days (95% CI -5.90 to −0. 85 days, $p < 0.01$) for NOM.

Conclusion: The paradigm remains unchanged, that appendectomy is the gold standard of treatment for uncomplicated appendicitis, given its higher efficacy rate when compared to NOM.

Keywords: Appendicitis, Antibiotic therapy, Appendectomy, Non operative management

Background

Acute appendicitis is one of the commonly encountered acute surgical conditions. Worldwide incidences range from 7.5 to 22.71 per 10,000 and the lifetime risk is around 16.3% [1, 2]. Untreated appendicitis can progress into gangrene or perforation with resultant peritonitis or abscess formation. Since the very first successful appendectomy performed by Claudius Amyand in 1735 [3], it has long been the gold standard of treatment for acute appendicitis. This surgical dogma was first challenged by Fitz in 1886, who suggested that patients with appendicitis may resolve without surgical intervention as evidence of previous appendicitis were found in many autopsy specimens [4]. Coldrey first reported successful treatment of 471 patients with acute appendicitis using antibiotics alone in 1956 [5]. Since then, a number of studies investigated the role of using antibiotics alone, non-operative management (NOM), in the management

* Correspondence: ccfoo@hku.hk
[2]Department of Surgery, The University of Hong Kong, Queen Mary Hospital, 102 Pokfulam Road, Hong Kong, China
Full list of author information is available at the end of the article

of acute uncomplicated appendicitis with promising results [6–8]. Appendectomy, albeit a routine surgical procedure with low mortality [9], has a complication rate of 5 to 28% [10]. Given the evidence that supports NOM, should the paradigm of treatment for uncomplicated appendicitis changed from operative to non-operative? This review focused on the current available evidence in the literature comparing NOM and appendectomy for the treatment of acute uncomplicated appendicitis in adults in order to answer this question.

Methodology

All studies that evaluated the effectiveness of NOM over appendectomy in managing uncomplicated acute appendicitis were retrieved from Medline (PubMed), Embase (1980-) and Cochrane Library electronic databases. The search was carried out on 15th June, 2017. The MeSH term "acute appendicitis" & "antibiotic therapy" were used as search terms. Only two terms were used with the intention to include more literatures for preliminary screening. "antibiotic therapy" was chosen since operative management had been considered as the gold standard for treating appendicitis and trials working on performance of NOM should have compared NOM with the gold standard. It is reasonable to assume using "antibiotic therapy" as search term can identify all trials that compared NOM with appendectomy.

Search mode was set as best matched and "full text" for Pubmed searching. The search terms were used as subject heading for searching in Cochrane and Embase (1980-). Editorials, case reports, expert opinions, letters to the editor, reviews without original data, conference abstract and studies solely on pediatric population were excluded. The screening and selection criteria of studies were summarized in Table 1.

Table 1 A summary of the screening and selection criteria of studies

Inclusion Criteria	1. Uncomplicated Acute Appendicitis - Excluded perforation - Excluded intra-abdominal abscess 2. Mainly focus on adult population 3. Full article published in English 4. Randomized control trials & prospective comparative studies
Exclusion	1. Studies that solely involved the pediatric population (Subjects' age < 18) 2. Studies that only compared elective surgery and conservative management
Search engine	1. PubMed 2. Embase (1980-) 3. Cochrane Library
Keywords	1. Acute appendicitis 2. Antibiotic therapy

Inclusion criteria

Studies that meet the following criteria were included: 1) Uncomplicated acute appendicitis (Excluding perforation & intra-abdominal abscess); 2) Mainly focused on the adult population; 3) Full article published in English; 4) Randomized control trials (RCT) & observational comparative studies.

Exclusion criteria

Studies were excluded if they have the following: 1) Studies that solely involved the pediatric population (Subjects' age < 18); 2) Studies that only compared elective surgery with conservative management.

Data searches and quality assessments

Embase (1980-), Cochrane Library and Pubmed database were searched by Poon & Wong. The search process was conducted independently and the findings were filled in a preset Excel document. Authors subsequently combined the search result and duplications were removed. Literatures were independently assessed by the authors and then subsequently reviewed together. Consensus was achieved on the inclusion of articles. Quality assessments was performed by Poon and reviewed by Wong.

The primary outcomes that were measured included the success rate, morbidities rate, length of hospital stay and loss of work associated with the two treatment modalities.

Statistical analysis

Cochrane Review Manager (RevMan) Version 5.3.5 (Copenhagen: The Nordic Cochrane Centre, The Cochrane Collaboration, 2014) was used for evaluating the studies' results and constructing the forest plots & funnel plots. Odds ratio (OR) of successfully treated cases in patients with NOM when compared to the appendectomy group had been employed to evaluate the outcomes of the two interventions. 95% confidence intervals (95% CI) were decided to evaluate the statistical significance of the OR. An OR of greater than one dictates a superior outcome for the NOM group, and the value of OR was considered statistically significant at the $p = 0.05$ level. Heterogeneity was accounted by the I-square test. Fixed effect model of Mantel Haenzel method was used for analyzing dichotomous data. The analysis of continuous data employed random effect model of inverse variance with regard to the great heterogeneity.

Results

Search result

In total, 1943 records were identified from the databases (Fig. 1). 1545 were identified from Pubmed, while 369

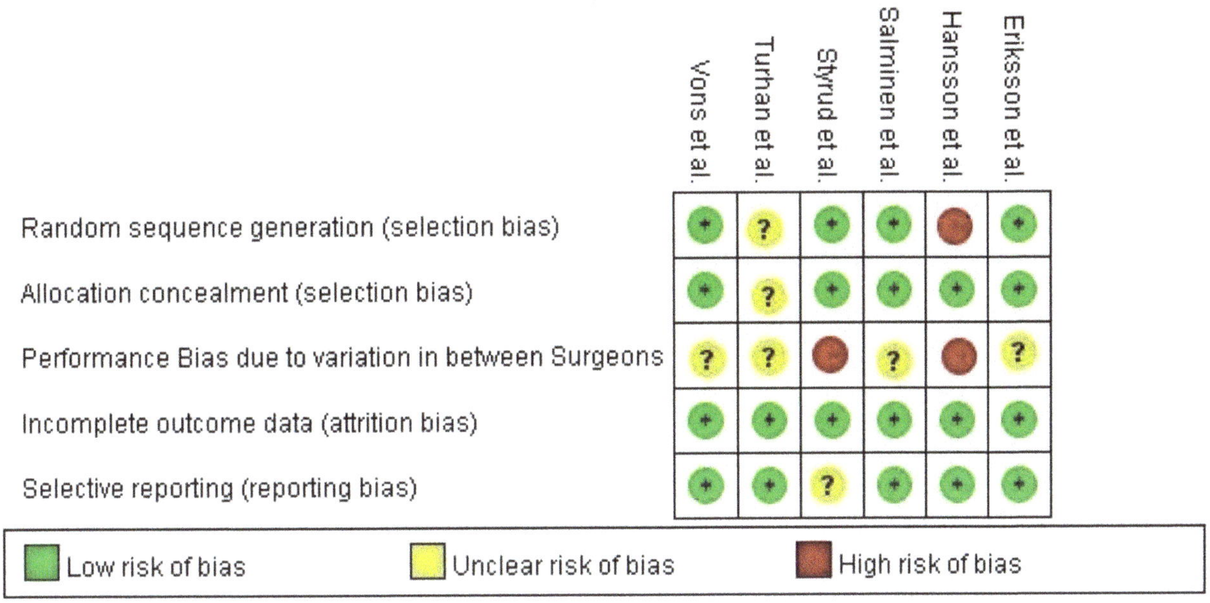

Fig. 1 Bias assessment of the included RCTs

were identified from Embase. The remaining was identified from Cochrane Library of Systematic Review. After excluding the reviews without original data, letters to editor, case reports, conference abstracts and non-comparative studies, 388 items were left from the three databases. 106 articles were found after screening of titles and abstracts of the 388 items. An addition of six articles were excluded due to duplication. 16 studies were identified for qualitative synthesis. Out of those 16 studies, seven RCTs fulfilling the preset criteria were identified. One RCT was excluded as the article was subsequently retracted due to plagiarism [11]. The included studies were summarized in Table 2.

Critical appraisal of the studies

Figure 2 summarized the bias assessment of the included studies. Eriksson et al. [6] was the first randomized trial that compared the outcome of NOM with appendectomy. The study was limited by small sample size, with only 40 patients recruited. The diagnoses were based on clinical signs and ultrasonographic findings and none had a computer tomography (CT) scan prior to surgery. Diagnostic inaccuracy is one of the main pitfalls of many studies published in the literature as some of the recruited patients were indeed suffering from complicated appendicitis. There is a chance of underestimating the efficacy of NOM in uncomplicated appendicitis and partly explains the high recurrence rate of 35% after 7 months of follow-up in the NOM group.

Styrud et al. conducted the first large scale randomized trial and it was the follow-up RCT of Eriksson's pilot study [12]. It reported a failure rate of NOM up to 12% at 24 h after the initiation of treatment. Among those patients, 47% of them were subsequently found to have perforated appendicitis. In this study, the randomization process and demographics of the excluded patients were clearly stated. However only male subjects and patients younger than 50 were included in view of ethical concerns from the local ethics committee. This limited its ability to address the role of NOM in elderly patients. The diagnosis of uncomplicated acute appendicitis was made on clinical grounds alone, without the use of imaging studies. There was a relatively high post-operative complication rate in the appendectomy group, 14%, mainly due to wound infection. It was difficult to generalize its results in the era of minimally invasive surgery as the author indiscriminately included both laparoscopic and open approaches.

Hansson et al. published their study in 2009 [13]. The diagnosis of uncomplicated appendicitis was based on clinical grounds with or without the use of imaging studies. This study adopted an unclassical method of subject randomization; using the date of birth of patients, with uneven date being the NOM group. This resulted in a huge difference in the number of subjects among the two groups and resulted in high selection bias. Furthermore, the study had a high crossover rate from the NOM arm to the appendectomy arm. Nearly half of the patients (96 out of 202) assigned to NOM were crossed over to surgery because of either surgeons' preference or patients' request. Besides, only less than half of the patients in the NOM group were followed up one year later. The rate of recurrence in patients treated with NOM was therefore likely underestimated. The study

Table 2 A summary of the studies comparing non-operative management and appendectomy

Study, Study Design	Year of publication	Medical Treatment	Surgical Treatment	No. of Patients	Outcome	Remarks
Eriksson et al. [6] Pilot RCT	1995	IV cefotaxime 2 g BID and tinidazole 800 mg daily for 2 days, followed by oral ofloxacin 200 mg BID and tinidazole 500 mg BID for 8 days	Open appendectomy	S:20 + M:20 = T:40	NOM was superior to Appendectomy in pain control NOM had a recurrence rate of 35% in 17 months NOM could effectively manage AUA	CT not applied for diagnosis of appendicitis
Styrud et al. [12] RCT	2006	IV cefotaxime for 2 days and tinidazole 800 mg daily, followed by ofloxacin 200 mg	Open or laparoscopic approach on surgeon preference	S:124 + M:128 = T: 252	Appendectomy had a higher complication rate NOM could successfully manage AUA	Female patients excluded
Hansson et alia [13] RCT	2009	IV cefotaxime 1 g BID and metronidazole 1·5 g q24hr for 1 day, followed by oral ciprofloxacin 500 mg BID and metronidazole 400 mg TID for 10 days	Open or laparoscopic approach as surgeons' usual practice	S:167 + M:202 = T:369	NOM was safe in AUA NOM had a recurrence rate of 13.9% in 1 year Appendectomy was 3 folds higher in major complication rate Minor complication rate was similar	This study has a high cross over rate from NOM to appendectomy.
Malik et al. [11] RCT	2009	IV ciprofloxacin 500 mg BID and metronidazole 500 mg TID for 2 days, followed by oral ciprofloxacin 500 mg BID and tinidazole 600 mg BID for 7 days	Approach not specified	S:40 + M:40 = T:80	NOM was superior to Appendectomy in pain control NOM was superior in lowering white cell count and temperature in early course NOM had more recurrence	This article was retracted due to plagiarism.
Turhan et al. [14] RCT	2009	IV ampicillin 1 g QID, gentamicin 160 mg daily and metronidazole 500 mg TID for 3 days, followed by oral antibiotics for 10 days	Open or laparoscopic appendectomy	S:183 + M:107 = T: 290	Appendectomy was superior to NOM in length of hospital stay NOM cost less than Appendectomy No difference in morbidity	
Vons et al. [15] RCT	2011	Amoxicillin and clavulanic Acid of 3 g or 4 g according to weight, with route and duration according to clinical symptoms	Open or laparoscopic approach on surgeon preference	S:123 + M:120 = T: 243	Appendectomy was superior to NOM	
Salminen et al. [19] RCT	2015	IV ertapenem 1 g daily for 3 days, followed by oral levofloxacin 500 mg daily and metronidazole 500 mg TID for 7 days	Open appendectomy	S:273 + M:257 = T: 530	Appendectomy had a higher overall complication rate than NOM NOM had longer hospital stay NOM failed to demonstrate non-inferiority No significant difference in treatment efficacy	

S = Number of surgically managed patients; M = Number of medically managed patients T = Total number of patients involved in the study
NOM = Non-operative management; AUA = Acute uncomplicated appendicitis
Superior refers to statistically significant in clinical outcome by parameter used by the authors of the respective studies

suggested that NOM was a safe alternative to appendectomy. However, the aforementioned factors made the trial less reliable.

Turhan et al. published their result in 2009 [14]. This study specified itself as a randomized control trial. Nevertheless, the randomization process was not clearly

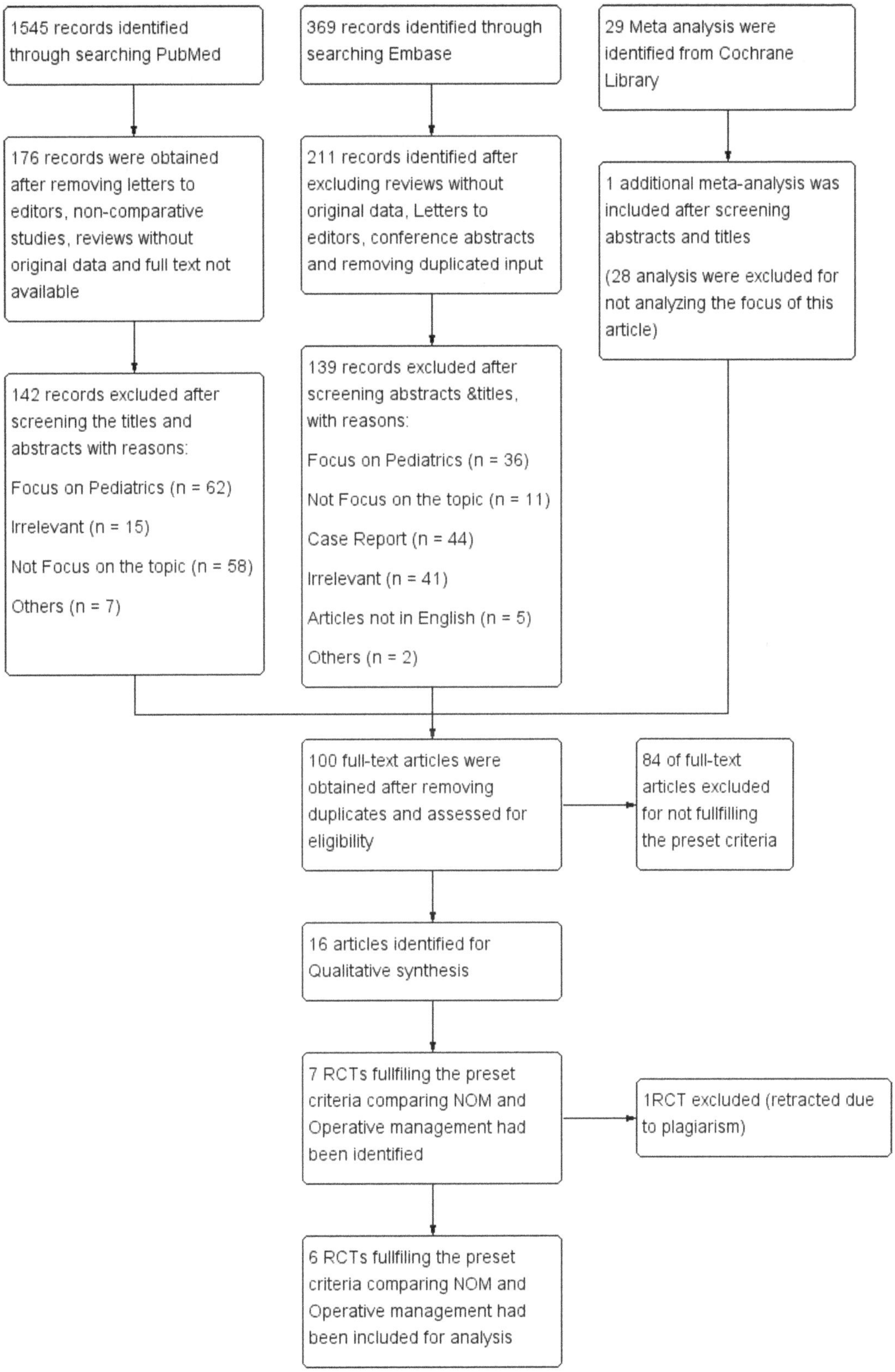

Fig. 2 PRISMA flow diagram

stated. This might result in potential bias. The diagnosis of uncomplicated acute appendicitis was confirmed by either ultrasonography or computed tomography.

The study published by Vons et al. involved patients from six hospitals [15]. Vons et al. used clearly defined diagnostic criteria with the aid of high quality CT scan to confirm the diagnoses in the study. Despite this, there was still an incidence of 18% for perforated appendicitis on upfront surgery. Randomization method and the results of the trials were well documented. The study also evaluated the risk factors associated with the absence of improvement of appendicitis in the NOM group. Despite no multivariate regression performed, fever at initial presentation, high presenting serum C-reactive protein level and intraluminal fecolith, were likely predictors for poor response to NOM. The antibiotics of choice in the NOM group in this study was amoxicillin and clavulanic acid, with an initial failure rate of 11.7%, which was relatively high compared to other studies. This might be explained by the fact that, *Escherichia coli*, being the most common bacterial isolates from patients with acute appendicitis, have a high percentage of resistance to amoxicillin and clavulanic acid [16, 17]. This regime is currently not recommended for the treatment of acute appendicitis [18].

The study performed by Salminen et al. is the largest available RCT focusing on this topic to date [19]. It included 530 patients recruited in Finland. The study documented well the reason for excluding patients from the trial. Other components including the process of randomization, standardization between different hospitals and diagnostic criteria were clearly stated. These found the reliability of the results of this trial. Ertapenem was the antibiotics of choice in this study. It was preferred due to its efficacy as a single agent for abdominal infections [19]. The initial failure rate was 5.7%. Despite the fact that it demonstrated a significant shorter hospital study for the operated group, the postoperative sick leave period was significantly longer in the appendectomy group. The study failed to demonstrate non-inferiority for NOM over appendectomy in terms of treatment efficacy. Nevertheless, the setting of a 24% non-inferiority margin was challenged [20].

Treatment success rate

Treatment success was defined as resolution of appendicitis without the development of complications or recurrence necessitating interventions. The majority of the comparative studies favored appendectomy in this regard. Hasson et al. demonstrated a 48% one-year success rate for NOM, compared to 89.2% for appendectomy [13]. Salminen et al. reported a higher success rate of 70.4% for NOM [19]. Similar result was published by Vons et al., where the successful rate of NOM was 67.5% [15]. The same study also demonstrated that the presence of fecolith on CT scan, was associated with higher chance of failure for NOM (50% vs 14%). Overall, the recurrence rate ranged from 13.9 to 35% in the first year [6, 12, 13, 15, 19].

Pooled analysis of one year treatment efficacy was performed by the random effect model of Mantel Haenzel method with respect to the high heterogeneity (Fig. 3.3). The sample sizes of patients were included in the above analysis. It demonstrated a significant advantage in surgically managed patients when compared to those with NOM. The odds ratio for successful treatment in the NOM group at one year was only 0.10 (95% CI 0.03–0.36, $p < 0.01$), when compared with the surgically managed group. Sensitivity test, which remained in favor of surgical management, was performed by alternatively removing the largest and smallest study. Both tests resulted in significant advantages for the operated group.

Morbidities

Except the one from Eriksson et al..., all studies provided the incidence of overall complications following each intervention. The results from Turhan et al. & Vons et al's studies supported appendectomy while the remaining three studies favored NOM. Analysis was performed with Mantel Haenszel random effect model. The overall complication rate after excluding recurrence was compared. The analysis demonstrated a comparable result between appendectomy and NOM with a risk ratio of 0.60 (95%CI: 0.23–1.59, $p = 0.31$), favoring NOM. The majority of these complications were related to infections. A high heterogeneity was noted with regard to the results. It might be accounted by the difference in antibiotic regimes and the surgical approaches used. Sensitivity tests were performed by excluding the largest and smallest studies alternatively. The complication rate remained comparable between the two interventions. Separate analysis for major and minor complications was not performed as only Hasson et al. clearly listed the nature of complications.

Length of hospital stay

Pooled analysis of the length of stay for the initial admission demonstrated a significant longer hospital stay in the NOM group. A total of 1720 patients were included in the analysis. Random effect model was employed with regard to the high heterogeneity in the studies included. The standardized mean difference in hospital stay after pooled analysis was 1.08 (95% CI 0.09–2.07, $p = 0.03$). Sensitivity test was performed by removing the largest and smallest study respectively. A significant advantage was still noted after removing the smallest scaled study by Eriksson et al. [6]. The significance disappeared after removing the study by Salminen et al. [19].

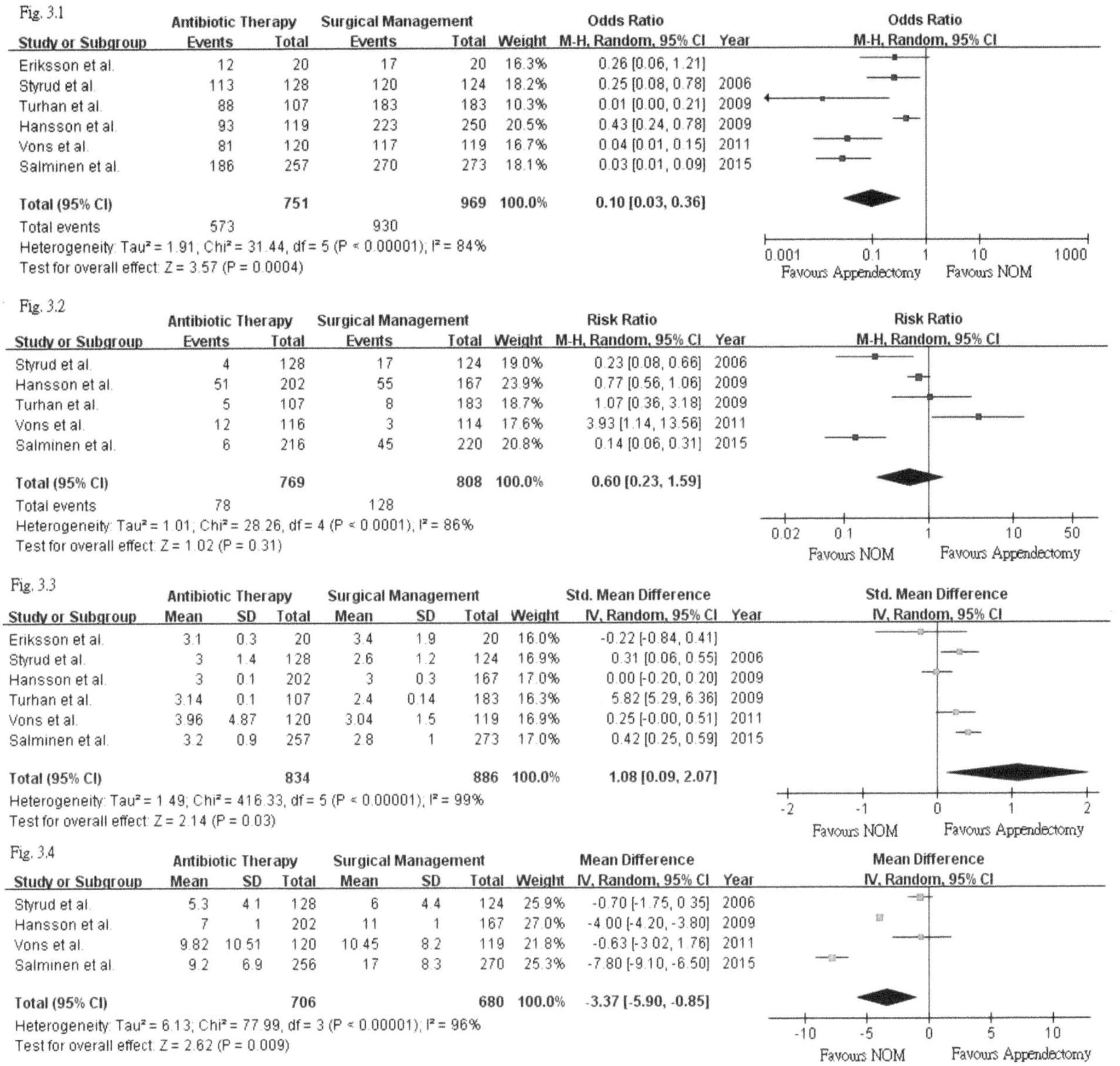

Fig 3.1 Forest plot for analysis of 1 year treatment efficacy,
Fig 3.2 Forest plot for analysis of overall treatment morbidities
Fig 3.3 Forest plot for analysis of total hospital stay in the first admission
Fig 3.4 Forest plot for analysis of total sick leave duration following first discharge

Fig. 3 Forest plots of meta-analysis results

Loss of work

The duration of sick leave was significantly shorter in the NOM group, with a mean difference of 7.8 days (95% CI 6.5 to 9.1) in Salminen's study [19]. This is in line with the pooled analysis of four RCTs in this review. The analysis of the total sick leave duration after the first admission included a sample size of 1380. Random effect model was employed with regard to the high heterogeneity in the studies included. Significance was detected between the two intervention groups with a trend favoring NOM. The mean difference noted from the analysis was 3.37 days less for the NOM group with 95% CI of −5.90 to −0.85 day, p value <0.01 was noted. Sensitivity test was not performed as only 4 studies were included for analysis.

Discussion

This review demonstrated a higher efficacy for appendectomy and was consistent with earlier meta-analysis [21, 22]. In the meta-analysis by Sallinen et al., including five RCTs, one on pediatric patients, 8.5% of the patients treated with NOM required appendectomy within the first month [23]. Wilms et al. published a meta-analysis involving five RCTs and 901 patients [24]. Although 73.4% of the patients treated with NOM had resolution of acute appendicitis without major complications and recurrence in the following year, as compared to 97.4% in the appendectomy group, the author could not demonstrate non-inferiority of NOM and concluded that more than one out of five patients treated with NOM would develop either complications or recurrence requiring surgery in the following year. A consensus statement was issued by the expert panel at the 3rd World Congress of the World Society of Emergency Surgery held in Jerusalem, Israel in 2015, which stated that NOM could be successful in selected patients with uncomplicated appendicitis who wish to avoid surgery and accept a higher risk, up to 38%, of recurrence [25].

The complications rate of appendectomy was generally higher than NOM in the literature. In Mason's meta-analysis [26], NOM was shown to be protective for major and minor complications with an odds ratio of 0.54 (95% CI 0.37 to 0.78). This is contrary to results from some non-randomized studies. Data from a national database involving the treatment of 436,400 cases of acute appendicitis over a 8-year period showed a significantly higher rate of in-hospital complications (27.8% vs. 7%, $p < 0.001$) and longer hospital stay (3 vs. 2 days, p < 0.001) in the NOM group [27]. It is unfortunate that all RCTs comparing NOM and surgery, except one [15], had a high rate of open appendectomy, ranging from 82 to 100% [6, 12, 14, 19]. Further, the choice of operative approach was not standardized and was often up to surgeons' discretion. It is difficult to generalize these results in terms of morbidities from the available RCTs as the majority of patients, up to over 90%, with acute appendicitis were operated with the laparoscopic approach nowadays [28]. Previous RCTs and systematic reviews have shown that laparoscopic approach was associated with fewer wound complications, less postoperative pain and shorter hospital stay [29] but with a higher incidence of intra-abdominal collection [30].

The results of the earlier RCTs did not show a difference between NOM and surgery in terms of hospital stay [6, 12, 13]. The two latest RCTs published in 2011 and 2015 showed shorter hospital stay in the appendectomy group [15, 19]. A meta-analysis showed shorter hospital stay in the appendectomy group, with a mean difference of 0.41 days (95% CI 0.26 to 0.57) [23]. This is in line with the result of this review, which the surgically treated patients had a shorter hospital stay than those with NOM. Nevertheless, two other meta-analysis failed to demonstrate a significant difference in hospital stay when only adult RCTs were included [21, 22]. As mentioned above, the percentage of patients operated with the laparoscopic approach in the RCTs was far less than expected. Shorted hospital stay and faster return to work would be expected in laparoscopic appendectomy. On the other hand, the use of oral antibiotics in NOM, as demonstrated in the Non Operative Treatment for Acute Appendicitis (NOTA) study conducted in Italy, would largely reduce the length of hospital stay [31]. It is difficult to draw a conclusion whether NOM has an advantage over appendectomy based on the current evidence.

In terms of long term efficacy, results beyond one year from the published RCTs were not available in the literature. A retrospective study on 3236 patients treated with NOM revealed a long-term recurrence rate of 4.4% at a mean follow up of 7 ± 3.9 years [32]. Another study on 118 patients treated with NOM showed a 10.2% recurrence at a median follow-up of 23 months [33]. The NOTA study suggested a long term efficacy of 83% up to two years with NOM [34].

Given the aforementioned one-year recurrence rate of 13.9 to 35%, the majority of the patients primarily treated with NOM would remain symptoms-free. Routine interval appendectomy after resolution of symptoms was therefore not necessary. On the other hand, the morbidities rate of interval appendectomy was low. In the study by Salminen, none of the patients suffered from intra-abdominal abscess after interval appendectomy [19]. The surgical complication rate of elective interval appendectomy was lower than primary appendectomy by 13.4%.

Apart from a higher treatment efficacy rate, appendectomy offers definitive histology and provides a chance to diagnose rare appendiceal and extra-appendiceal pathologies. Connor reported the presence of appendiceal tumors in 0.9% of 7970 appendectomy specimens [35]. Another study reported a 2.7% and 1.1% incidence of appendiceal diverticulitis and appendiceal tumors, which included carcinoid tumors, adenocarcinoma, mucinous cystadenoma etc. [36].

Conclusion

NOM is definitely a feasible and effective alternative for uncomplicated appendicitis. The majority of patients primarily treated with NOM would be spared from post-operative pain, surgical risks and wound complications. The paradigm remains unchanged, however, that appendectomy should be the gold standard of treatment given its higher treatment success rate and shorter hospital stay. Current evidence in the literature mainly focused on comparing NOM with open appendectomy. With widespread adoption of the laparoscopic approach, high quality evidence is still needed in the comparison of primary laparoscopic appendectomy and NOM. Studies evaluating factors that could affect the rate of success in NOM is needed for clinical reference and to tailor treatment on an individual basis. Until then, patients should be well informed of the available treatment options, their pros and cons, so as to make informed decision and benefit from the optimal treatment.

Acknowledgements
None.

Funding
There is no funding support in conducting this study.

Authors' contributions
Drs. SHTP and BYKW were responsible for the acquisition, analysis and interpretation of data, drafting of manuscript and final approval of the manuscript. Drs. JWYL, KMN and GWYC were responsible for the acquisition of data, preparation and final approval of the manuscript. Dr. CCF was responsible for the design of the study, analysis and interpretation of data, preparation and final approval of the manuscript. LWL was responsible for the analysis and interpretation of data and final approval of the manuscript.

Competing interests
The authors declare that they have no competing interests.

Author details
[1]The Li Ka Shing Faculty of Medicine, The University of Hong Kong, Hong Kong, China. [2]Department of Surgery, The University of Hong Kong, Queen Mary Hospital, 102 Pokfulam Road, Hong Kong, China.

References

1. Lee JH, Park YS, Choi JS. The epidemiology of appendicitis and appendectomy in South Korea: national registry data. J Epidemiol. 2010; 20:97–105.
2. Al-Omran M, Mamdani M, McLeod RS. Epidemiologic features of acute appendicitis in Ontario, Canada. Can J Surg. 2003;46:263–8.
3. Meljnikov I, Radojcic B, Grebeldinger S, Radojcic N. History of surgical treatment of appendicitis. Med Pregl. 2009;62:489–92.
4. FITZ R. On perforating inflammation of the vermiform appendix with special reference to its early diagnosis and treatment. N Engl J Med. 1935;213:245–8.
5. Coldrey E. Treatment of acute appendicitis. Br Med J. 1956;2:1458–61.
6. Eriksson S, Granstrom L. Randomized controlled trial of appendicectomy versus antibiotic therapy for acute appendicitis. Br J Surg. 1995;82:166–9.
7. Gurin NN, Slobodchuk IS, Gavrilov IF. The efficacy of the conservative treatment of patients with acute appendicitis on board ships at sea. Vestn Khir Im I I Grek. 1992;148:144–50.
8. Winn RD, Laura S, Douglas C, Davidson P, Gani JS. Protocol-based approach to suspected appendicitis, incorporating the Alvarado score and outpatient antibiotics. ANZ J Surg. 2004;74:324–9.
9. Guller U, Hervey S, Purves H, Muhlbaier LH, Peterson ED, Eubanks S, Pietrobon R. Laparoscopic versus open appendectomy: outcomes comparison based on a large administrative database. Ann Surg. 2004; 239:43–52.
10. Masoomi H, Nguyen NT, Dolich MO, Mills S, Carmichael JC, Stamos MJ. Laparoscopic appendectomy trends and outcomes in the United States: data from the Nationwide inpatient sample (NIS), 2004-2011. Am Surg. 2014; 80:1074–7.
11. Malik AA, Bari SU. Conservative management of acute appendicitis. J Gastrointest Surg. 2009;13:966–70.
12. Styrud J, Eriksson S, Nilsson I, Ahlberg G, Haapaniemi S, Neovius G, Rex L, Badume I, Granstrom L. Appendectomy versus antibiotic treatment in acute appendicitis. A prospective multicenter randomized controlled trial. World J Surg. 2006;30:1033–7.
13. Hansson J, Korner U, Khorram-Manesh A, Solberg A, Lundholm K. Randomized clinical trial of antibiotic therapy versus appendicectomy as primary treatment of acute appendicitis in unselected patients. Br J Surg. 2009;96:473–81.
14. Turhan AN, Kapan S, Kutukcu E, Yigitbas H, Hatipoglu S, Aygun E. Comparison of operative and non operative management of acute appendicitis. Ulus Travma Acil Cerrahi Derg. 2009;15:459–62.
15. Vons C, Barry C, Maitre S, Pautrat K, Leconte M, Costaglioli B, Karoui M, Alves A, Dousset B, Valleur P, et al. Amoxicillin plus clavulanic acid versus appendicectomy for treatment of acute uncomplicated appendicitis: an open-label, non-inferiority, randomised controlled trial. Lancet. 2011;377:1573–9.
16. Andersen BR, Kallehave FL, Andersen HK. Antibiotics versus placebo for prevention of postoperative infection after appendicectomy. Cochrane Database Syst Rev. 2005;(3):CD001439.
17. Oteo J, Campos J, Lazaro E, Cuevas O, Garcia-Cobos S, Perez-Vazquez M, de Abajo FJ. Increased amoxicillin-clavulanic acid resistance in Escherichia Coli blood isolates, Spain. Emerg Infect Dis. 2008;14:1259–62.
18. Solomkin JS, Mazuski JE, Bradley JS, Rodvold KA, Goldstein EJ, Baron EJ, O'Neill PJ, Chow AW, Dellinger EP, Eachempati SR, et al. Diagnosis and management of complicated intra-abdominal infection in adults and children: guidelines by the surgical infection society and the Infectious Diseases Society of America. Surg Infect. 2010;11:79–109.
19. Salminen P, Paajanen H, Rautio T, Nordstrom P, Aarnio M, Rantanen T, Tuominen R, Hurme S, Virtanen J, Mecklin JP, et al. Antibiotic therapy vs appendectomy for treatment of uncomplicated acute appendicitis: the APPAC randomized clinical trial. JAMA. 2015;313:2340–8.
20. Di Saverio S, Sartelli M, Catena F, Birindelli A, Tugnoli G. Renewed interest in acute appendicitis: are antibiotics non-inferior to surgery or possibly clinically superior? What is long-term follow-up and natural evolution of appendicitis treated conservatively with "antibiotics first"? Surg Infect. 2016;17:376–7.
21. Podda M, Cillara N, Saverio SD, et al. Antibiotics-first strategy for uncomplicated acute appendicitis in adults is associated with increased rates of peritonitis at surgery. A systematic review with meta-analysis of randomized controlled trials comparing appendectomy and non-operative management with antibiotics. Surgeon. 2017;15(5):303-14.
22. Rollins KEVK, Neal KR, Lobo DN. Antibiotics versus appendicectomy for the treatment of uncomplicated acute appendicitis: an updated meta-analysis of randomised controlled trials. World J Surg. 2016;40:2305–18.
23. Sallinen V, Akl EA, You JJ, Agarwal A, Shoucair S, Vandvik PO, Agoritsas T, Heels-Ansdell D, Guyatt GH, Tikkinen KA. Meta-analysis of antibiotics versus appendicectomy for non-perforated acute appendicitis. Br J Surg. 2016; 103(6):656-67.
24. Wilms IM, de Hoog DE, de Visser DC, Janzing HM. Appendectomy versus antibiotic treatment for acute appendicitis. Cochrane Database Syst Rev. 2011;(11):CD008359.
25. Di Saverio S, Birindelli A, Kelly MD, Catena F, Weber DG, Sartelli M, Sugrue M, De Moya M, Gomes CA, Bhangu A, et al. WSES Jerusalem guidelines for diagnosis and treatment of acute appendicitis. World J Emerg Surg. 2016;11:34.
26. Mason RJ, Moazzez A, Sohn H, Katkhouda N. Meta-analysis of randomized trials comparing antibiotic therapy with appendectomy for acute uncomplicated (no abscess or phlegmon) appendicitis. Surg Infect. 2012;13:74–84.
27. Khalil M, Rhee P, Jokar TO, Kulvatunyou N, O'Keeffe T, Tang A, Hassan A, Gries L, Latifi R, Joseph B. Antibiotics for appendicitis! Not so fast. J Trauma Acute Care Surg. 2016;80:923–32.
28. Co-ordinating Committee in Surgery CETMD, Quality & Safety Division. Surgical outcomes monitoring & improvement program (SOMIP) report. Hong Kong: Hospital Authority; 2016.
29. Ohtani H, Tamamori Y, Arimoto Y, Nishiguchi Y, Maeda K, Hirakawa K. Meta-analysis of the results of randomized controlled trials that compared laparoscopic and open surgery for acute appendicitis. J Gastrointest Surg. 2012;16:1929–39.
30. Sauerland S, Jaschinski T, Neugebauer EA. Laparoscopic versus open surgery for suspected appendicitis. Cochrane Database Syst Rev. 2010; (10):CD001546.

31. Di Saverio S, Sibilio A, Giorgini E, Biscardi A, Villani S, Coccolini F, Smerieri N, Pisano M, Ansaloni L, Sartelli M, et al. The NOTA study (non operative treatment for acute appendicitis): prospective study on the efficacy and safety of antibiotics (amoxicillin and clavulanic acid) for treating patients with right lower quadrant abdominal pain and long-term follow-up of conservatively treated suspected appendicitis. Ann Surg. 2014;260:109–17.
32. McCutcheon BA, Chang DC, Marcus LP, Inui T, Noorbakhsh A, Schallhorn C, Parina R, Salazar FR, Talamini MA. Long-term outcomes of patients with nonsurgically managed uncomplicated appendicitis. J Am Coll Surg. 2014; 218:905–13.
33. Kirkil C, Yigit MV, Aygen E. Long-term results of nonoperative treatment for uncomplicated acute appendicitis. Turk J Gastroenterol. 2014;25:393–7.
34. Saverio SD, Sibilio A, Giorgini E, et al. The NOTA study (non operative treatment for acute appendicitis). Ann Surg. 2014;260:109–17.
35. Connor SJ, Hanna GB, Frizelle FA. Appendiceal tumors: retrospective clinicopathologic analysis of appendiceal tumors from 7,970 appendectomies. Dis Colon Rectum. 1998;41:75–80.
36. Ma KW, Chia NH, Yeung HW, Cheung MT. If not appendicitis, then what else can it be? A retrospective review of 1492 appendectomies. Hong Kong Med J. 2010;16:12–7.

24

On table POCUS assessment for the IVC following abdominal packing

Fikri M. Abu-Zidan

Abstract

Background: Some surgeons may lack proper experience in abdominal packing. Overpacking may directly compress the inferior vena cava (IVC). This reduces the venous return and possibly causes hypotension. Here, a new on table Point-of-Care Ultrasound application that has been recently used to assess the effect of abdominal packing on the IVC diameter is described. Following abdominal packing, a small print convex array probe with low frequency (2–5 MHz) is used to visualize the IVC. Using the B mode, the IVC can be directly evaluated through a hepatic window between the ribs. The ultrasound beam should be vertical to the IVC longitudinal section at its midpoint. The abdominal towels will be in front of the IVC. This will enable us to judge whether there was overpacking on the IVC.

Results: Our method demonstrates that overpacking does not compress the IVC in a patient whose blood pressure has improved. The IVC diameter progressively increases on table and in the ICU with active resuscitation implying that bleeding stopped and the resuscitation was successful. Furthermore, presence of intra-peritoneal fluid can be excluded.

Conclusions: This new application of ultrasound evaluation of IVC patency after abdominal packing is simple, practical, easily reproducible, and can guide a less experienced surgeon in determining if overpacking of the abdomen is the cause of hypotension. Ultrasound findings should be correlated with the clinical picture to be useful.

Keywords: Abdomen, Point-of-care ultrasound, IVC, Packing

Abbreviations: IVC, Inferior vena cava; POCUS, Point-of-care ultrasound; ICU, Intensive care unit; DCS, Damage control surgery

Background

Abdominal packing is a useful simple technique which is used in damage control surgery (DCS) to stop severe bleeding in multiply injured patients who are acidotic, hypothermic and coagulopathic [1]. This stabilises the patient and gives time to restore the physiological derangement through damage control resuscitation [2]. Finally, the patient can be timely reoperated upon to restore the functional anatomy [3]. In addition, surgeon-performed Point-of-Care Ultrasound (POCUS) has become an important critical decision making tool in managing critically-ill patients [4, 5]. Both DCS and POCUS have been used successfully in the military and prehopsital settings [3, 6].

Some surgeons may lack proper experience in abdominal packing and possibly overpack the abdomen. Overpacking has side effects. The packs and its associated increased intra-abdominal pressure may directly compress the inferior vena cava (IVC). This reduces the venous return and may cause hypotension. Furthermore, transportation time can be long before arriving to a proper hospital. It is therefore reasonable to aim at proper intra-abdominal packing that stops bleeding but without obliterating the IVC. Sonographic measurement of the IVC diameter has been recently advocated in the evaluation of patients in hemorrhagic or septic shock [7, 8]. POCUS machines are now usually available in surgical theatres because they are used routinely in inserting sonographic guided central lines. It would be then attractive to evaluate the IVC patency by POCUS following abdominal packing for DCS. The author of the present paper has recently reviewed the literature on the use of ultrasound measurement of IVC diameter in resuscitation [7]. The relative change of IVC diameter in trauma patients could differentiate

Correspondence: fabuzidan@uaeu.ac.ae
Department of Surgery, College of Medicine and Health Sciences, UAE University, Al-Ain, United Arab Emirates

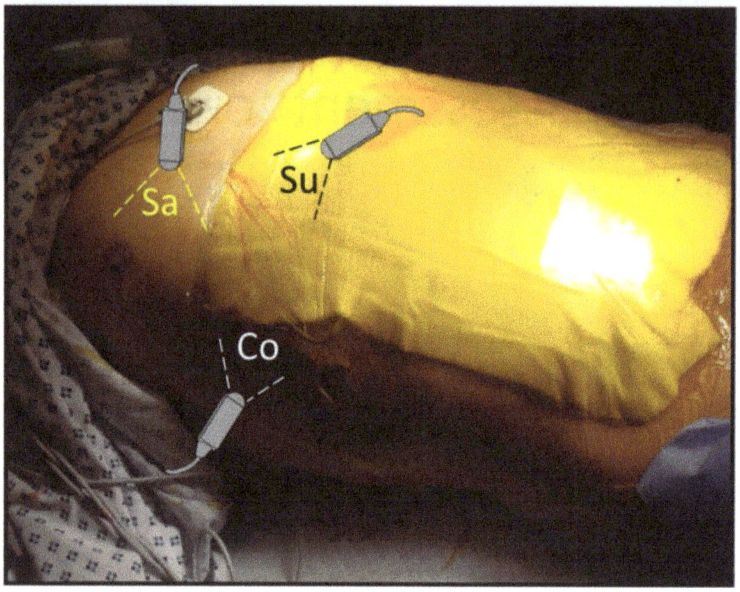

Fig. 1 There are three windows in which we can measure the IVC: The subxiphoid (Su), the direct sagittal (Sa), and the coronal view (Co). The only useful approach after DCS is the direct sagittal approach

between proper resuscitation responders from transient responders who develop recurrent shock [9]. IVC measurement was feasible in 92 % of patients having septic shock [10]. Using ultrasound in evaluating the IVC following abdominal packing was not described before. The present paper describes a recent on table POCUS application that can be used to assess the effect of abdominal packing on the IVC diameter following DCS.

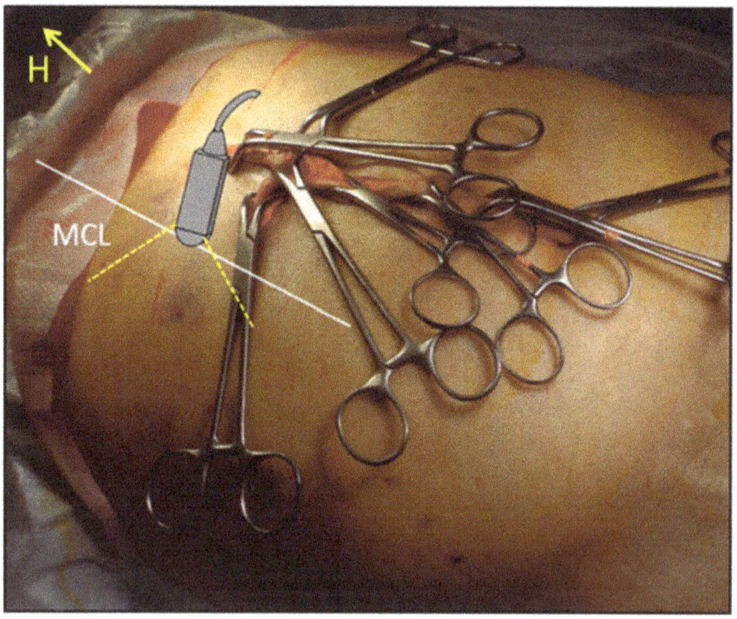

Fig. 2 A diagram demostrating the technique to visualize the IVC by ultrasound in a longitudinal section following damage control surgery with abdominal packing. The skin was closed with towel clips following abdominal packing without closure of the fascia. A small print convex array probe with low frequency (2–5 MHz) should be used. The probe is located at the right mid-clavicular line (MCL) at the lower chest wall vertical to the skin. H = location of the head

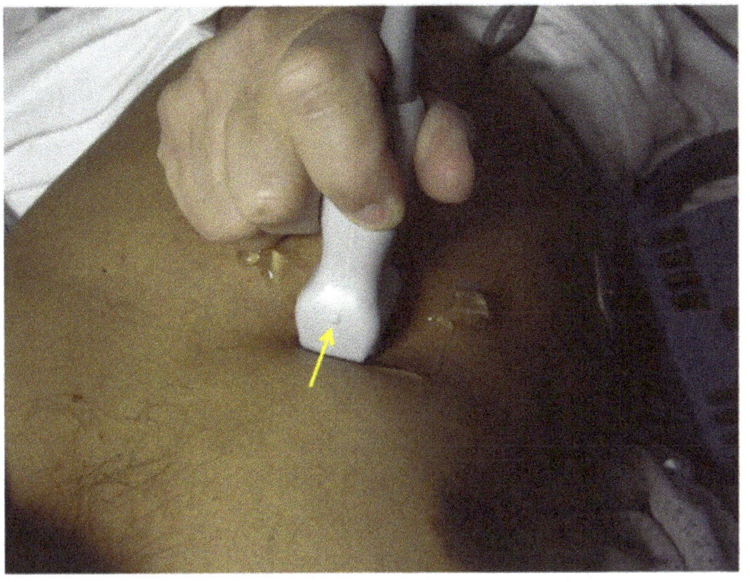

Fig. 3 The marker of the probe should point proximally towards the head of the patient (arrow). It may be required to tilt the probe a little towards the right shoulder to be parallel to the IVC

Methods

A small print convex array probe with low frequency (2–5 MHz) should be used. Ultrasound waves are generated perpendicular to the surface of this probe. This probe has deep sonographic penetration and wide view. It will enable sonographic visualization of the IVC between the ribs and through a hepatic window to directly measure the antero-posterior section of the IVC [11]. There is usually no intra-peritoneal sonographic air barrier hindering the view if this approach was used.

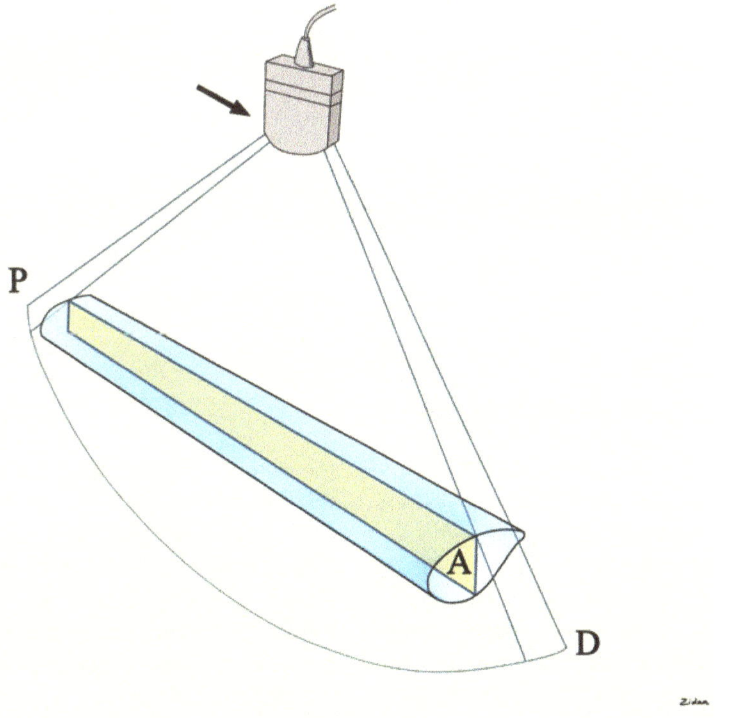

Fig. 4 The ultrasound beam should be vertical to the IVC longitudinal section (A) at its midpoint. P = proximal, D = distal, Black arrow = marker of the probe

The probe should be covered by sterile gel and plastic sleeve. Sufficient sterile gel should be used to have proper contact with the skin so that the air does not disturb the view. There are three windows in which we can visualize the IVC by ultrasound: the subxiphoid, the direct sagittal and the coronal view (Fig. 1). The marker of the probe should point proximally towards the head. This will be on the right side of the ultrasound screen. The probe is located at the right mid-clavicular line, at the lower chest wall, and vertical to the skin (Fig. 2). It is then *shifted* in both lateral directions to locate the IVC. Gentle slow lateral *fanning* movements may be needed to locate the IVC. It may be required to *tilt* the probe a little towards the right shoulder to be parallel to the IVC (Fig. 3). The commonly used subxiphoid view cannot be used following damage control laparotomy for different reasons. *First,* the midline laparotomy and its dressing will be in the way. *Second,* the presence of distended stomach and free intra-peritoneal air will hinder the view, and *third,* the abdomen may be left open. The coronal section will cut the IVC transversely and will not measure the antero-posterior diameter of the IVC.

Using the B mode, the IVC can be evaluated in its longitudinal diameter. The ultrasound beam should be vertical to the IVC longitudinal section at its midpoint (Figs. 4 and 5). The IVC will be black in color on the B mode ultrasound image. The abdominal towels will appear as whitish linear layers without shadowing (behaving like a fibrous tissue) anterior to the IVC. This will show whether the IVC is compressed or not (Fig. 6).

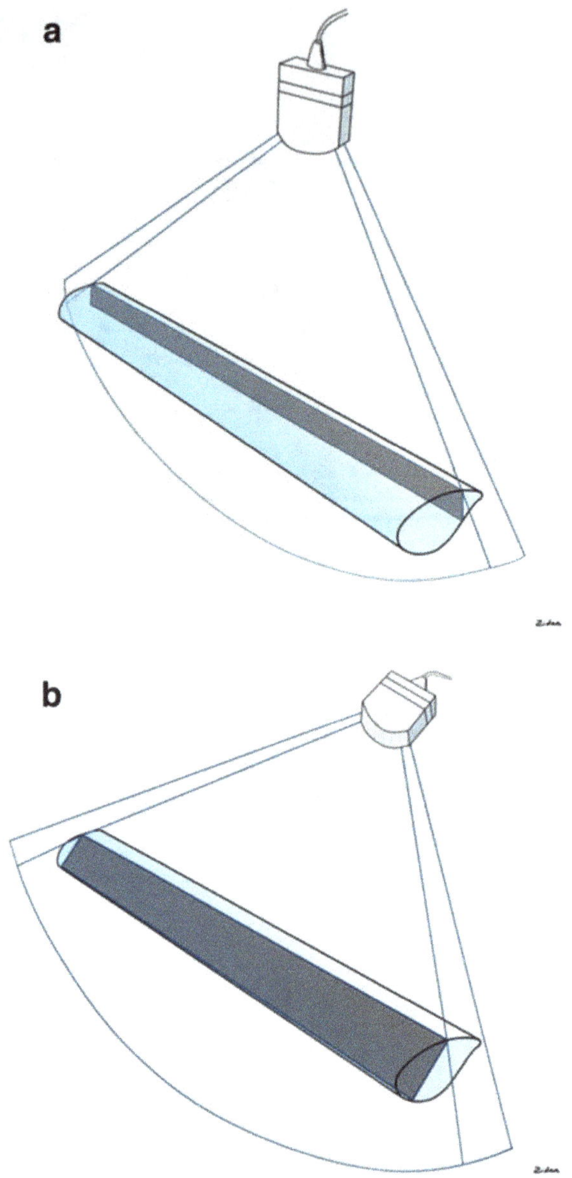

Fig. 5 The two common pitfalls in visualizing the IVC by ultrasound are cutting it at the periphery **a** giving a false impression that it is small **a** or cutting it obliquely giving a false impression that it is large **b**

Results

Our method serves to assess excessive pressure on the IVC in abdominal packing (Fig. 6). The IVC diameter progressively increases on table and in the ICU with active resuscitation implying that bleeding stopped and the resuscitation was successful (Fig. 7). Furthermore, presence of intra-peritoneal fluid can be detected.

Discussion

The value of POCUS in the management of patients in hemorrhagic or septic shock using specific protocols is well-established [5, 8]. Our group routinely follows the Rapid Ultrasound in Shock (RUSH) protocol which examines the pump (heart), tubes (great vessels) and reservoir (free intra-peritoneal or intra-thoracic fluid) [5]. Performing an on table RUSH protocol directly following DCS is very attractive. Using the same approach, it would be logical to evaluate the IVC patency by POCUS following abdominal packing. POCUS is quick, done bedside and does not interfere with reuscitation. It may yield very useful information during the continuation of damage control resuscitation on the operating table after the damage control laparotomy and before transferring the patient to the ICU.

The skin was closed with towel clips following abdominal packing without closure of the fascia in the patient shown in Fig. 2 because we were anticipating to close the fascia within 48 hours without the development of postoperative abdominal hypertension. There are different methods for temporary abdominal closure that has been recently detailed in a position paper published by the World Society of Emergency Surgery [12]. Advantages and disadvantages of each of these techniques were

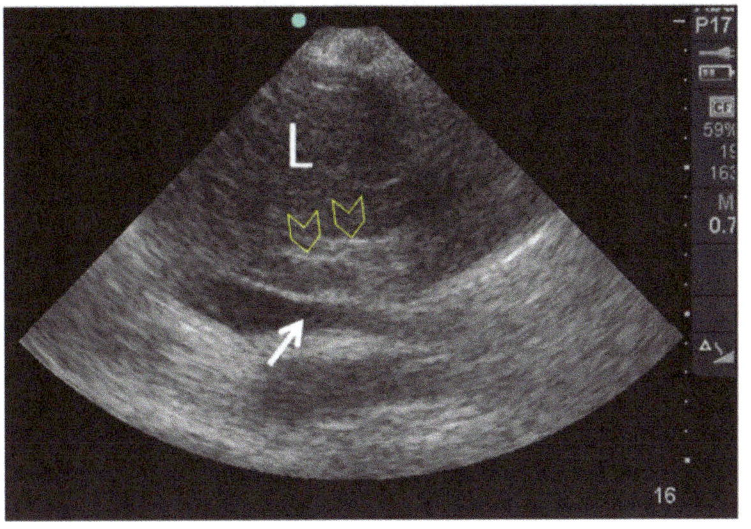

Fig. 6 Using the hepatic window, a two dimensional B mode image shows that the IVC was patent (white arrow). The abdominal towels appear as whitish linear layers without shadowing (yellow arrow heads) anterior to the IVC. L = liver

described in detail in that paper which is beyond the scope of the present communication. These techniques included the plastic silo, negative pressure therapy (NPT), and the combined NPT with fascial approximation. The most extensively used method is NPT while the most promising one is the combined NPT with fascial approximation. Using our described ultrasound approach, POCUS can be applied with all these different techniques of closing the abdomen because a transthoracic hepatic ultrasound window is away from the wound.

Sonographic appearance of intra-peritoneal free air has been described in detail [13]. They result from reflections of the ultrasound waves at the interface between the soft tissue and air. This is accompanied by a reverberation artefact. This artefact typically appears as increased echogenicity of a peritoneal stripe accompanied by posterior reverberation parallel echogenic lines having equal distances that will hide the organs. This image can be changed by changing the patient's position. The echogenic appearance of the intra-abdominal towels (as shown in Fig. 6) is different. The echogenic lines are not parallel, not of the same length, not at equal distances, and finally they do not hide the liver. Although these ultrasound fine details can be observed by an experienced

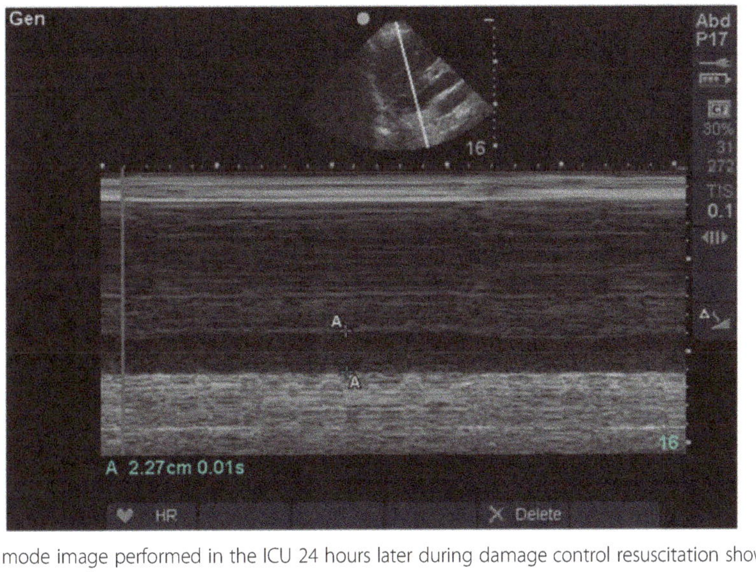

Fig. 7 A two dimensional B mode image performed in the ICU 24 hours later during damage control resuscitation shows that the IVC diameter (A-A) increased to 2.27 cm. The patient had a blood pressure of 130/80 mmHg and had adequate urine output. Hypothermia, acidosis, and coagulopathy were corrected at this stage

sonographer, they are not needed for evaluating the IVC diameter which can be done by a less experienced sonographer.

Weekes et al. [14] prospectively studied trauma patients and found that gross appearance of the IVC size agreed with the actual measured IVC diameter during resuscitation. A meta-analysis, which included a total of 86 hypovolemic patients and 189 controls, found that IVC diameter was significantly less in hypovolemic patients compared with controls [15]. A recent prospective randomized controlled trial in injured patients having hypotension or tachycardia treated in a Level I trauma center [16] found that focused ultrasound studies of the heart and IVC significantly reduced the IV fluid requirements and the time to surgery. We have recently reported that increased intra-abdominal pressure in abdominal compartment syndrome causes direct pressure on the IVC which reduces the antero-posterior IVC diameter [17].

Our method is logically more useful when the blood pressure of the patient improves. Its value may be questionnable when the patient significantly continues to bleed because the sonographic IVC diameter will be small. Nevertheless, we have to clarify that active intra-abdominal arterial bleeding does not respond to packing and should be actually dealt with surgically. However, on table POCUS is useful in detecting an on going intraperitoneal bleeding. In a patient with improving blood pressure, the IVC diameter will increase indicating that IVC was not overpacked, bleeding stopped, and the resuscitation was successful.

Conclusions

This new application of ultrasound evaluation of IVC patency after abdominal packing is simple, practical, easily reproducible, and can guide a less experienced surgeon in determining if overpacking of the abdomen is the cause of hypotension. Ultrasound findings should be correlated with the clinical picture to be useful.

Acknowledgements
The author thanks Mr Cyrus Tariq Gill, RCS, RDCS (ADULT ECHO), Adult Echocardiographer, Department of Medicine, College of Medicine and Health Sciences, UAE University, Al-Ain, United Arab Emirates, for fruitfull discussions during writing this manuscript.

Funding
None.

Authors' contribution
The author performed the Point-of-Care Ultrasound studies and surgery, read the literature, wrote first version of the paper, edited it, and approved its final version.

Competing interest
The author declares no conflict of interest.

References

1. Bashir MM, Abu-Zidan FM. Damage control surgery for abdominal trauma. Eur J Surg. 2003;168 Suppl 588:8–13.
2. Kaafarani HM, Velmahos GC. Damage control resuscitation in trauma. Scand J Surg. 2014;103:81–8.
3. Blackbourne LH. Combat damage control surgery. Crit Care Med. 2008;36(7 Suppl):S304–10.
4. Abu-Zidan FM. Point-of-care ultrasound in critically ill patients: Where do we stand? J Emerg Trauma Shock. 2012;5:70–1.
5. Perera P, Mailhot T, Riley D, Mandavia D. The RUSH exam: rapid ultrasound in SHock in the evaluation of the critically ill. Emerg Med Clin North Am. 2010;28:29–56.
6. Dittrich K, Abu-Zidan FM. Role of ultrasound in mass-casualty situations. Int J Disaster Med. 2004;2:18–23.
7. Abu-Zidan FM. Optimizing the value of measuring inferior vena cava diameter in shocked patients. World J Crit Care Med. 2016;5:7–11.
8. Seif D, Mailhot T, Perera P, Mandavia D. Caval sonography in shock: a noninvasive method for evaluating intravascular volume in critically ill patients. J Ultrasound Med. 2012;31:1885–90.
9. Yanagawa Y, Sakamoto T, Okada Y. Hypovolemic shock evaluated by sonographic measurement of the inferior vena cava during resuscitation in trauma patients. J Trauma. 2007;63:1245–8.
10. Coen D, Cortellaro F, Pasini S, Tombini V, Vaccaro A, Montalbetti L, Cazzaniga M, Boghi D. Towards a less invasive approach to the early goal-directed treatment of septic shock in the ED. Am J Emerg Med. 2014;32:563–8.
11. Abu-Zidan FM, Hefny AF, Corr P. Clinical ultrasound physics. J Emerg Trauma Shock. 2011;4:501–3.
12. Sartelli M, Abu-Zidan FM, Ansaloni L, et al. The role of the open abdomen procedure in managing severe abdominal sepsis: WSES position paper. World J Emerg Surg. 2015;10:35.
13. Hefny AF, Abu-Zidan FM. Sonographic diagnosis of intraperitoneal free air. J Emerg Trauma Shock. 2011;4:511–3.
14. Weekes AJ, Tassone HM, Babcock A, Quirke DP, Norton HJ, Jayarama K, Tayal VS. Comparison of serial qualitative and quantitative assessments of caval index and left ventricular systolic function during early fluid resuscitation of hypotensive emergency department patients. Acad Emerg Med. 2011;18:912–21.
15. Dipti A, Soucy Z, Surana A, Chandra S. Role of inferior vena cava diameter in assessment of volume status: a meta-analysis. Am J Emerg Med. 2012;30:1414–1419.e1.
16. Ferrada P, Evans D, Wolfe L, Anand RJ, Vanguri P, Mayglothling J, Whelan J, Malhotra A, Goldberg S, Duane T, Aboutanos M, Ivatury RR. Findings of a randomized controlled trial using limited transthoracic echocardiogram (LTTE) as a hemodynamic monitoring tool in the trauma bay. J Trauma Acute Care Surg. 2014;76:31–7.
17. Abu-Zidan FM, Idris K. Sonographic measurement of the IVC diameter as an indicator for fluid resuscitation: beware of the intra-abdominal pressure. World J Surg. 2015;39:2608–9.
18. Abu-Zidan FM, Idris K, Khalifa M. Strangulated epigastric hernia in a 90-year-old man: Point-of-Care Ultrasound (POCUS) as a saving kit: case report. Int J Surg Case Rep. 2016;22:19–22.

Development of a reconditioning program for elderly abdominal surgery patients: the Elder-friendly Approaches to the Surgical Environment–BEdside reconditioning for Functional ImprovemenTs (EASE-BE FIT)

Alyssa McComb[1], Lindsey M. Warkentin[2], Margaret L. McNeely[1] and Rachel G. Khadaroo[2,3*]

Abstract

Background: Elderly individuals who are hospitalized due to emergency abdominal surgery spend over 80% of their recovery time in bed, resulting in early and rapid muscle loss. As these elderly individuals have a lower physiological reserve, the impact of muscle wasting on function may be profound. The objectives of this study are to (1) create an independently led post-surgical reconditioning program and (2) pilot its implementation, while assessing the feasibility and safety of the program.

Methods: The BE FIT program was generated with hospital rehabilitation staff to target lower limb strength, balance, and endurance. This pilot study was assessed using a sequential before and after trial, with a cohort of patients aged ≥ 65 years enrolled in the Elder-friendly Approaches to the Surgical Environment (EASE) study. Change in 30-s sit-to-stand performance between postoperative day 2 and discharge was compared between Usual Care pre- and post-BE FIT participants.

Results: A total of 66 patients participated in the sub-study, 33 Usual Care and 33 BE FIT. Mean (SD) age was 76.2 (8.78); 44 (67%) were female, with 11 (17%) reporting mild/moderate frailty on the CHSA Clinical Frailty Scale. BE FIT participants had a median of three rehab days and self-reported completing an average of 83% of the exercises. The adjusted between group difference showed that the BE FIT patients were able to complete more stands than the Usual Care (1.9 stands (0.94), $p = 0.05$). There were no reported adverse events.

Conclusion: The reconditioning program was shown to be safe and feasible within the hospital setting for the elderly emergency abdominal surgery patients. More rigorous assessment is needed to confirm this effectiveness and to better assess patient adherence to self-directed exercise.

Keywords: Reconditioning, Rehabilitation, Elderly, Abdominal, Surgery, Emergency, Physiotherapy, Bed rest

* Correspondence: khadaroor@gmail.com
[2]Department of Surgery, University of Alberta, Edmonton, Alberta, Canada
[3]Department of Critical Care Medicine, University of Alberta, Edmonton, Alberta, Canada
Full list of author information is available at the end of the article

Background

With our rapidly aging population and advancements to allow surgery as a viable option for those with increased age, a greater number of surgical procedures are now performed on seniors (≥ 65 years) in Canada and the USA [1–3]. Unfortunately, the increased prevalence of pre-existing vulnerabilities and the precipitating insults associated with surgery (polypharmacy, catheters, and bed rest) result in higher rates of adverse events in the elderly population compared to their younger counterparts [4, 5]. Occurrence of these adverse events often leads to longer hospital stays, more intensive care, greater resource expenditure, and an increased risk of mortality [4–9].

The traditional approach to postoperative surgical care has largely centralized around activity restrictions to optimize wound healing. However, prolonged bed rest is not a viable option for the frail elderly as evidence strongly supports its detrimental effects on muscle mass that can compromise independence [10]. Currently, there is no consensus on the necessary level or type of activities that should be restricted following surgery and current physical therapy practices focus on mobilization and discharge practices, as opposed to enhancing muscular strength [10].

The American College of Surgeons National Surgical Quality Improvement Program (ACS-NSQIP) Best Practices Guideline suggests early mobilization with a focus on positioning assistance, balance, and gait training [11]. Newer enhanced recovery after surgery care pathways encourage early mobilization with the suggestions that patients dangle their legs on the day of surgery, then ambulate every 4 to 6 h each day while they are awake until discharge beginning on postoperative day 1 [12]; however, even in well-established enhanced recovery programs, mobilization adherence is low [13], with seniors having lower adherence than non-senior adults [14]. Adult patients often do not sit upright until postoperative day 1 and take an average of 5.3 days to independently mobilize [15]; previous research by Browning et al. [15] reported total median uptime was 3.0 (IQR 8.2) min for the first postoperative day, increasing to only 4.4 (IQR 65.6) min on the fourth postoperative day.

For these reasons, new rehabilitation strategies are needed to improve functional outcomes in older adults following abdominal surgery, especially for those done urgently when pre-admission optimization is not feasible [16]. The objective of this pilot was to develop and test an exercise program that considered patient healing and safety, promoted self-management, and was resource neutral in terms of the workload impact on hospital staff.

Methods

Development of the BE FIT rehabilitation program

Prior to program development, the author AM, a kinesiologist, shadowed in-hospital physical and occupational therapists who were responsible for the standard physical therapy of the population group of interest. The purpose of this was to familiarize the author with current hospital rehabilitation practices, safe movement with recent incision sites, common areas of physical weakness for elderly inpatients, and the accessibility of the hospital ward. The program was based around the progressive use of multi-disciplinary teams within Alberta's Health Care system. The goal of the program was to provide a uniform transitional program that all members of the health-care team would be knowledgeable about and comfortable using. The program was designed with input from exercise physiologists, physical therapists, occupational therapists, and surgeons.

An initial list of exercises was selected by authors AM and MM, based on expert opinion and the American College of Sports Medicine's recommendations for elderly individuals [17], with the guiding intention that the exercises were simple enough that a lay person could teach, be taught, or perform the exercises with minimal guidance. These exercises targeted lower limb strength, balance, and endurance and would be expected to support participants in independent living and ambulation once discharged. The exercises chosen were reviewed by all authors, as well as the in-hospital physical and occupational therapists, and consensus was reached for all exercises included in the final program, after several rounds of edits and discussion. Three exercise levels, of increasing difficulty, of the program were generated, and visual instructional materials and patient logbooks were created (Table 1). The program materials were trialed with non-study participant elderly surgical inpatients prior to implementation for user feedback and refinement.

Pilot feasibility and safety assessment: study design

Testing of the BEdside reconditioning for Functional ImprovemenTs (BE FIT) program was done using a prospective, sequential before-and-after sub-study of the Elder-friendly Approaches to the Surgical Environment (EASE) study [18]. The main EASE study's aim is to

Table 1 BE FIT reconditioning program exercises

CHSA Clinical Frailty Scale [19]	BE FIT exercises
Very fit/well	Standing-based program • Sit-to-stand • Calf raises • Hip marching
Managing well/vulnerable	Chair-based program • Bed rolls • Sit-to-stand (with assist) • Leg extensions
Mild/moderately frail	Bed-based program • Quad extensions • Butt squeezes • Triceps extensions

Participants were instructed to complete each exercise 10 times, thrice daily assess the impact of an elder-friendly surgical unit through capacity alignment, an interdisciplinary care team, an evidence-informed care pathway, the BE FIT reconditioning program, and transition optimization. The full protocol of the EASE study is published, and the Human Research Ethics Boards of the University of Alberta granted ethics approval (Pro00047180) [18].

Participants for EASE-BE FIT sub-study were consecutively enrolled elderly patients (≥ 65 years old) who had been referred directly to Acute Care Surgery services for emergency abdominal surgery at the University of Alberta Hospital in Edmonton, Canada, from May 2015 to May 2016. Patients were excluded if they (1) received elective or palliative surgery, (2) were admitted due to trauma, (3) were dependent in three or more activities of daily living or were non-ambulatory prior to admission, and (4) could not read/speak or comprehend English. The research coordinator approached the eligible patients prior to their surgery, and willing participants were consented.

Participants included prior to the implementation of the BE FIT program received only usual care, which may have included physical therapy if it was requested by the clinical team (Usual Care cohort). The physiotherapist would assess the frequency and timing of the clinical physiotherapy involvement, independent of the study. Participants included after the BE FIT program implementation received usual care plus the BE FIT reconditioning program beginning on postoperative day 2 (BE FIT cohort). The appropriate level of the program was determined using the participant's frailty within 2 weeks prior to admission, assessed using CHSA Clinical Frailty Scale [19], along with informal interview of the participant on postoperative day 2. The exercises were demonstrated to the participant, and the first set of exercises was supervised to ensure they were being performed safely. The participants were instructed to perform the exercises three times per day until discharged, and the visual diagram of the exercises was provided to remind the participant of proper technique. The logbook was provided to encourage compliance, and the participants were told to notify the clinical or study team if they needed re-teaching of the exercises or modifications; however, as the program was intended to be self-directed, the study team did not initiate follow-up with the participant nor monitor adherence to the exercises.

Data collection

Chart review was completed to determine age, sex, race, marital status, living situation prior to admission, type of surgery, postoperative physical and occupational therapy intervention, any occurrence of in-hospital falls, discharge status, and length of stay.

Participants completed a 30-s sit-to-stand (STS) test on postoperative day 2 (prior to receiving the BE FIT program for the BE FIT cohort) and again on the day of discharge. The STS test is a measurement used to assess functional lower extremity strength in older adults [20]. Briefly, a participant rises to a full stand from being seated in a chair, without the use of their arms, and then returns back to the initial seated position. The number of full repetitions that are completed in 30 s is recorded. As all participants had recent abdominal incisions, participants were permitted to use their arms to assist them into a standing position if they felt necessary. More repetitions are indicative of better functional performance.

Six weeks after discharge, for those participants who returned for their scheduled follow-up with their surgeon, a Timed Up and Go (TUG) test was completed [21]. The TUG test is a commonly used screening tool for falls risk. The participant is timed while they rise from a chair, walk 3 m at a comfortable and safe pace, turn and walk back to the chair, and sit down again. Faster time indicates a better functional performance.

Sample size

Sample size was calculated based on the few normative values currently published in scientific literature, along with the established minimal clinically important difference scores (2.6 stands in the STS [22] and 3.5 s in the TUG [23]). For a statistical significance of $p = 0.05$ and a power value of 0.90, the necessary value for the STS tests was based on the mean and standard deviation values normalized by Jones et al. [24] on community-dwelling older adults, suggesting a minimum sample of 11. For the TUG, using mean and standard deviation scores normalized by Steffen et al. [25], a sample size of 22 is suggested. We therefore attempted to enroll a minimum of 60 participants (30 in each group) to increase power and attempt to have equivalent distribution of baseline characteristics between groups.

Analyses

Change in functional status

Participants were included in the analysis regardless of their length of stay or adherence to the program. Descriptive statistics were calculated and compared between Usual Care and BE FIT groups using the t test/Mann-Whitney test for continuous variables and chi-squared/Fisher exact test for categorical. Change in STS was calculated by subtracting postoperative day 2 STS from the discharge STS within participants. Change in STS and post-discharge TUG test results were compared between Usual Care and BE FIT groups first by using a two-sample t test, then in multivariable linear regression models in order to adjust for sex, CHSA Clinical Frailty Scale, and surgery type.

Adherence and informal feedback

Adherence was calculated by averaging number of times they self-reported completing the reconditioning program a day (maximum 3) by the number of possible rehab days (discharge date minus postoperative day 2 date). Informal feedback and participant comments about the program were captured on the logbook and notes written by the research coordinator during final testing at discharge.

Results

Participant characteristics

A total of 66 participants were enrolled in the study with 33 participants in each group. The Usual Care group had more intestinal revision or resection surgeries ($p = 0.001$), had fewer cholecystectomies ($p = 0.04$), were more often mild or moderately frail ($p = 0.02$), and received more physical or occupational therapy intervention ($p = 0.009$) compared to the BE FIT group (see Table 2). Four participants in the BE FIT group did not perform the reconditioning program, as they were discharged on postoperative day 2; for those who completed the program ($n = 29$), median number of possible rehab days was 3 (IQR 1–6) and mean (SD) adherence was reported as 2.56 (0.65), suggesting that participants completed 83% of their exercises. The logbook was completed by 18 (55%) of BE FIT participants. Two falls occurred during the duration of the study (one Usual Care, one BE FIT), but neither was associated with performance of the functional testing or completion of the BE FIT program.

Table 2 Participant characteristics

Characteristics	Usual Care $n = 33$	BE FIT $n = 33$	*P* value
Age (years)*	77.3 (9.56)	75.1 (7.92)	0.31
Female	22 (67)	22 (67)	1.0
White	31 (94)	29 (88)	0.22
Married	19 (58)	17 (52)	0.621
CHSA Clinical Frailty Scale			0.07
Very fit/well	9 (27)	12 (36)	
Managing well/vulnerable	15 (45)	19 (58)	
Mild/moderately frail	9 (27)	2 (6)	
Procedure			0.02
Appendectomy	1 (3)	2 (6)	
Cholecystectomy	4 (12)	11 (33)	
Hernia repair	3 (9)	5 (15)	
Intestine resection/revision	25 (76)	12 (36)	
Other	0 (0)	3 (9)	
PT/OT visit	16 (48)	6 (33)	0.009
Falls	1 (3)	1 (3)	1.0
Length of stay (days)†	9 (7–13)	6 (3–11)	0.02

Reported as *n* (%) unless indicated otherwise
*Mean (SD)
†Median (IQR)

Participant feedback on program

Several BE FIT participants responded with comments such as "More exercises," "Enjoyed the program, wish I could take it home," and "Please provide this to other hospitals" in the logbook and commented that it was helpful to be given direction on moving after surgery, as they felt unsure if it was allowed. However, four (12%) of participants felt that postoperative day 2 was too soon to complete exercises after surgery (either due to pain or beliefs that bed rest would be most beneficial to them) and either delayed beginning the program or chose not to complete the exercises during their hospital stay. No concerns were brought forth by the clinical team regarding the program.

Sit to stand

Overall, 10 (15%) of participants completed the STS reps without using their arms, 37 (56%) completed their STS reps with the assistance of using their arms, and 19 (29%) used a combination of without-arm and with-arm reps. Combining all reps, regardless of arm use, the BE FIT group completed 5.0 (3.9) more stands at discharge compared to postoperative day 2, while the Usual Care group completed 2.7 (3.0) (between group difference 2.3 (0.45) stands, $p = 0.01$). After adjusting for sex, Clinical Frailty Scale, and surgery type, the difference of difference was 1.9 (0.94) ($p = 0.05$) (see Fig. 1).

Timed Up and Go

Loss to follow-up at 6 weeks post-discharged occurred for 19 (56%) participants in the Usual Care group and

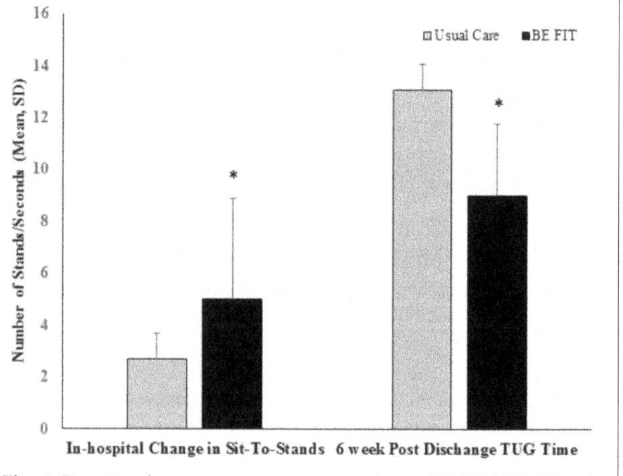

Fig. 1 Functional status outcomes pre- and post-BE FIT. TUG, Timed Up and Go. *$p < 0.05$ compared to Usual Care, after adjusting for sex, CHSA Clinical Frailty Scale, and surgery type

10 (30%) participants in the BE FIT group. BE FIT participants completed the TUG in 9.0 (2.8) s, while the Usual Care completed it in 13.1 (5.2) s (difference between groups, 4.0 (1.3), $p = 0.004$). After adjusting for sex, Clinical Frailty Scale, and surgery type, the difference between groups remained significant (mean difference 4.1 (1.4), $p = 0.006$) (see Fig. 1).

Discussion

This is one of the first pilot studies to develop a structured postoperative reconditioning program for elderly emergency surgery patients. Using an integrated knowledge translation approach to generating the BE FIT program contributed to the successful implementation for the program. The reconditioning program was feasible and safe within our hospital setting. There were no reported associated adverse events, and the self-directed nature of the program and use of a progress monitoring via logbook allowed us to remain resource neutral. Both the change in STS between postoperative day 2 and discharge and the TUG at 6 weeks post-discharged showed greater improvement in the BE FIT group, compared to Usual Care, even after adjusting for sex, clinical frailty, and surgery type. Leaving the hospital in a better functional state places BE FIT participants to a reduced risk of injury and falls and loss of physical independence [6].

As there are few studies of this nature available in the literature, similar results are limited; however, improvement in STS scores due to early exercise interventions has been found in patients undergoing elective hip and knee arthroplasty [26], elderly acute general medical patients [27, 28], sedentary community-dwelling older adults [29], and nursing home residents [30].

Most participants were eager and willing to perform the exercises as often as they felt they could; however, a small portion of participants felt that they should not be performing exercises so soon after surgery and therefore did not complete the program. Self-reported adherence was adequate, though overall use of the logbook was variable. While this was not formally assessed, we expect barriers to logbook use likely include time constraints, misunderstanding around logbook use, or sensory impairments (example, eye glasses for reading unavailable at bedside). Unfortunately, participants who did not perform the program also did not complete the logbook, creating reporting bias and limiting our knowledge of the barriers to exercise in this group. Participants' informal feedback regarding exercise after surgery prompts us to believe that the lack of education and sharing information around postoperative mobility exists at the level of not only heath care providers but patients and their families as well. Education opportunities for health-care staff may increase uptake of postoperative mobility programs and should be assessed and incorporated into further research.

Unfortunately, the concurrent EASE interventions, small sample size, and unclear adherence due to poor completion rates of logbooks limit our interpretation of this sub-study. For these reasons, a dedicated study is required to determine the optimal program and resources necessary to improve patient outcomes. Our future work will be to perform a pragmatic randomized controlled trial examining our exercise intervention, tailored to frailty.

Conclusions

As this sub-study included a small cohort and occurred in the setting of the concurrent implementation of other elder-friendly initiatives, our ability to interpret our finding and report unequivocal success is limited. However, our pilot reconditioning program results show promise in helping offset declines in physical function in elderly patients following emergency abdominal surgery and warrants further, more rigorous investigation to assess patient uptake and adherence, safety, and effectiveness.

Abbreviations

BE FIT: BEdside reconditioning for Functional ImprovemenTs; EASE: Elder-Friendly Approaches to the Surgical Environment; STS: Sit-to-stand; TUG: Timed Up and Go

Acknowledgements

Financial support was provided by Alberta Innovates Health Solutions—Partnership for Research and Innovation in the Health and Alberta Health Services Surgery Strategic Clinical Network. We also would like to thank the University of Alberta Hospital's Surgery physiotherapist and occupational therapists for their assistance in developing this program and dedication to caring for patients.

Authors' contributions

AM was active in writing the majority of the manuscript. LW provided the majority of the data analysis and was active in writing the document. MM and RK both edited the manuscript. All authors read and approved the final manuscript.

Competing interests

The authors declare that they have no competing interests.

Author details

[1]Faculty of Rehabilitation Medicine, University of Alberta, 1-38 Corbett Hall, 8205-114 St NW Edmonton, Edmonton, Alberta T6G 2G4, Canada. [2]Department of Surgery, University of Alberta, Edmonton, Alberta, Canada. [3]Department of Critical Care Medicine, University of Alberta, Edmonton, Alberta, Canada.

References

1. PomPei P. Geriatric review syllabus—a core curriculum in geriatric medicine. New York: American Geriatrics Society; 2006.
2. Robinson TN, et al. Accumulated frailty characteristics predict postoperative discharge institutionalization in the geriatric patient. J Am Coll Surg. 2011; 213:37–42.

3. Kwok AC, et al. The intensity and variation of surgical care at the end of life: a retrospective cohort study. Lancet. 2011;378(9800):1408–13.
4. Gillick MR, Serrell NA, Gillick LS. Adverse consequences of hospitalization in the elderly. Soc Sci Med. 1982;16:1033–8.
5. Creditor MC. Hazards of hospitalization of the elderly. Ann Intern Med. 1993; 118:219–23.
6. Inouye SK, et al. A controlled trial of a nursing-centered intervention in hospitalized elderly medical patients: the Yale Geriatric Care Program. J Am Geriatr Soc. 1993;41:1353–60.
7. Turrentine FE, et al. Surgical risk factors, morbidity, and mortality in elderly patients. J Am Coll Surg. 2006;203(6):865–77.
8. Lidsky ME, et al. Advanced age is an independent predictor for increased morbidity and mortality after emergent surgery for diverticulitis. Surgery. 2012;152(3):465–72.
9. Joseph B, et al. Superiority of frailty over age in predicting outcomes among geriatric trauma patients: a prospective analysis. JAMA Surg. 2014; 149(8):766–72.
10. Nygaard IE, Hamad NM, Shaw JM. Activity restrictions after gynecologic surgery: is there evidence? Int Urogynecol J. 2013;24(5):719–24.
11. Mohanty S, et al. Optimal perioperative management of the geriatric patient: a best practices guideline from the American College of Surgeons NSQIP and the American Geriatrics Society. J Am Coll Surg. 2016;222(5):930–47.
12. Pearsall E, McCluskey S, Aarts MA, McLeod R. Enhanced Recovery After Surgery: ERAS for All. 2017. Retreived from http://bestpracticeinsurgery.ca/wpcontent/uploads/2017/11/ERAS_BPS_FINAL_Nov2017.pdf.
13. Gustafsson UO, et al. Adherence to the enhanced recovery after surgery protocol and outcomes after colorectal cancer surgery. Arch Surg. 2011; 146(5):571–7.
14. Kisialeuski M, et al. Enhanced recovery after colorectal surgery in elderly patients. Videosurgery Miniinvasive Tech. 2015;10(1):30–6.
15. Browning L, Denehy L, Scholes RL. The quantity of early upright mobilisation performed following upper abdominal surgery is low: an observational study. Aust J Physiother. 2007;53(1):47–52.
16. Etzioni DA, et al. The aging population and its impact on the surgery workforce. Ann Surg. 2003;238:170–7.
17. Symons TB, Swank AM. Exercise testing and training strategies for healthy and frail elderly. ACSMs Health Fit J. 2015;19(2):32–5.
18. Khadaroo RG, et al. Optimizing senior's surgical care—Elder-friendly Approaches to the Surgical Environment (EASE) study: rationale and objectives. BMC Health Serv Res. 2015;15(1):338.
19. Rockwood K, et al. A global clinical measure of fitness and frailty in elderly people. CMAJ. 2005;173:489–95.
20. Rehab measures: 30 second sit to stand test. January 31, 2014 [cited 2015 June 10, 2015]; Available from: http://www.rehabmeasures.org/Lists/RehabMeasures/DispForm.aspx?ID=1122.
21. Barry E, et al. Is the Timed Up and Go test a useful predictor of risk of falls in community dwelling older adults: a systematic review and meta- analysis. BMC Geriatr. 2014;14 https://doi.org/10.1186/1471-2318-14-14.
22. Wright AA, et al. A comparison of 3 methodological approaches to defining major clinically important improvement of 4 performance measures in patients with hip osteoarthritis. J Orthop Sports Phys Ther. 2011;41(5):319–27.
23. Huang SL, et al. Minimal detectable change of the timed "up & go" test and the dynamic gait index in people with Parkinson disease. Phys Ther. 2011; 91(1):114–21.
24. Jones CJ, Rikli RE, Beam WC. A 30-s chair-stand test as a measure of lower body strength in community-residing older adults. Res Q Exerc Sport. 1999; 70(2):113–9.
25. Steffen TM, Hacker TA, Mollinger L. Age- and gender-related test performance in community-dwelling elderly people: Six-Minute Walk Test, Berg Balance Scale, Timed Up & Go Test, and gait speeds. Phys Ther. 2002;82(2):128–37.
26. Munin MC, et al. Early inpatient rehabilitation after elective hip and knee arthroplasty. JAMA. 1998;279(11):847–52.
27. Jones CT, et al. A randomised controlled trial of an exercise intervention to reduce functional decline and health service utilisation in the hospitalised elderly. Australas J Ageing. 2006;25(3):126–33.
28. Sullivan DH, et al. Progressive resistance muscle strength training of hospitalized frail elderly. Am J Phys Med Rehabil. 2001;80(7):503–9.
29. Roma MF, et al. Effects of resistance training and aerobic exercise in elderly people concerning physical fitness and ability: a prospective clinical trial. Einstein (Sao Paulo). 2013;11(2):153–7.
30. Slaughter SE, Estabrooks CA. Optimizing the mobility of residents with dementia: a pilot study promoting healthcare aide uptake of a simple mobility innovation in diverse nursing home settings. BMC Geriatr. 2013;13(1):110.

26

The impact of early surgical intervention in free intestinal perforation

Andreas Hecker[1*†], E. Schneck[2†], R. Röhrig[2], F. Roller[3], B. Hecker[2], J. Holler[1], C. Koch[2], M. Hecker[4], M. Reichert[1], C. Lichtenstern[2], G. A. Krombach[3], W. Padberg[1] and M. A. Weigand[2]

Abstract

Purposes: An abdominal inflammatory focus is the second most often source of sepsis with a high risk of death in surgical intensive care units. By establishing evidence-based bundled strategies the surviving sepsis campaign provided an optimized rapid and continuous treatment of these emergency patients. Hereby the hospital mortality decreased from 35 to 30 %. Sepsis treatment is based on three major therapeutic elements: surgical treatment (source control), antiinfective treatment, and supportive care. The international guidelines of the surviving sepsis campaign were updated recently and recommend rapid diagnosis of the infection and source control within the first 12 h after the diagnosis (grade 1c). Interestingly this recommendation is mainly based on studies on soft tissue infections.

Methods: In this retrospective analysis 76 septic patients with an intraabdominal inflammatory focus were included. All patients underwent surgery at different time-points after diagnosis.

Results: With 80 % patients of the early intervention group had an improved overall survival (vs. 73 % in the late intervention group).

Conclusions: Literature on the time dependency of early source control is rare and in part contradicting. Results of this pilot study reveal that immediate surgical intervention might be of advantage for septic emergency patients. Further multi-center approaches will be necessary to evaluate, whether the TTI has any impact on the outcome of septic patients with intestinal perforation.

Keywords: Time-to-intervention, Free intestinal perforation, Sepsis

Introduction

Despite modern diagnostic and therapeutic developments the in-hospital mortality of septic patients still remains inacceptably high. With 60 % mortality rates in cases of severe sepsis and septic shock a continuous optimization of treatment and rapid diagnosis is necessary and life-saving.

In up to 25 % of all septic patients an intraabdominal inflammation can be detected [1]. Results of the PROWESS study reveal, that in 66,5 % of the surgical patients the peritoneal cavity was affected by an inflammatory focus [2]. On a surgical intensive care unit the secondary peritonitis due to an intestinal perforation or an anastomotic leakage with extraintestinal air in the radiographic imaging is the main cause for an intraabdominal sepsis and sepsis-associated death. In a post mortem analysis of 235 patients, who died on surgical intensive care units, a persistent, continuous septic intraabdominal focus was found in 32,5 % of cases [1]. Compared to patients from medical intensive care units septic patients from surgical intensive care units have a 7 day longer length of hospital stay and higher cost rates [3].

While an intestinal perforation on its own leads to a mortality of about 14 %, a septic clinical progress is associated with an increase in mortality to 30 %. Among

* Correspondence: andreas.hecker@chiru.med.uni-giessen.de
†Equal contributors
1Department of General and Thoracic Surgery, University Hospital Giessen, Rudolf-Buchheim-Street 7, 35392 Giessen, Germany
Full list of author information is available at the end of the article

the patients suffering from secondary peritonitis the postoperative, secondary peritonitis bears the highest risk of a lethal outcome (1-year mortality >70 %) [4].

In February 2013 the new Surviving Sepsis Guideline was published, which underlines the multimodal, rapid treatment for the septic patient with an intraabdominal focus [5]. According to the recent guideline the sepsis therapy can be subdivided into four different subtypes: surgical source control, the antiinfectious therapy, the supportive intensive care medicine and adjunctive therapeutic approaches.

Surgical approaches for the treatment of intraabdominal infections are mainly based on principle and tradition. Over the last decade evidence-based medicine has emerged to assure best clinical practice, based on a review of literature, quality of research and therapeutic impact. Only few surgical strategies have been evaluated by randomized, prospective and controlled trials. Intraoperative circumstances are often unique and require a flexible, somtimes even unstandardized reaction by the surgeon.

Surgical source control is the only causal treatment option for patients suffering from peritonitis and intraabdominal sepsis. If source control is not possible during the initial emergency operation, mortality increases from 13 to 27 % [6].

In 2004 Barie et al. showed that an inadequate surgical removal of the intraabdominal inflammatory focus leads to a mortality of more than 90 % [7]!

The recent Surviving Sepsis Guideline from 2013 recommends an early source control within 12 h after diagnosis (evidence grade 1C) [5]:

> *"A specific anatomical diagnosis of infection requiring consideration for emergent source control be sought and diagnosed or excluded as rapidly as possible, and intervention be undertaken for source control within the first 12 hr after the diagnosis is made, if feasible."*

While a time-dependency in the early phase of hospital admission has been shown for an antimicrobial treatment at least in some studies, it remains nebulous, if a time-dependency of surgical source control and the outcome of the septic patient could be detected. These effects have never been analyzed before for the surgical patient with intestinal perforation. Interestingly, the guideline recommendation is based on literature mainly dealing with necrotisizing soft tissue infections [8–10]. Furthermore, the necrosectomy of peripancreatic necrosis is citated as one rationale for a conservative, delayed surgical intervention [11, 12]. To our surprise there is hardly any literature, analyzing the influence of the time to intervention on the outcome of critically ill septic patients with an intestinal perforation. For that reason we performed this time-to-intervention pilot study to investigate, if surgical source control in the very early phase of early-goal directed sepsis therapy is of benefit for our surgical intensive care patients.

Materials and methods

This study was approved by the local ethical committee and was designed as a retrospective cohort analysis of clinical data from 76 septic patients (45 males and 31 females) with a mean age of 59.64 years (range 21–88 years) suffering from intestinal perforation. Observational period was between August 2008 and February 2012. Subjects were included, if intestinal perforation was detected by radiographic imaging (computertomography scan or x-ray of the abdomen) and confirmed during surgery. Intestinal perforation was diagnosed in cases of free intraabdominal air and/or extravasation of contrast medium into the peritoneal cavity. Patients were included, if they showed either free intestinal perforation or an anastomotic leakage. They were excluded, if the intraoperative and radiologic findings were discordant, of if there was a contained perforation. In addition, patients must have met the sepsis criteria of the ACCP/SCCM consensus conference on sepsis [13] [Fig. 1].

Patients were excluded from the study if the radiological diagnosis of an intestinal perforation was discordant to the intraoperative finding. Further exclusion criteria were postoperative perforations due to anastomotic leakage, age < 18 years and perforations, which were treated interventionally (e.g. CT-guided drainage, Endo-VAC-Systems). Patients with an open abdomen were furthermore excluded from the study.

"Time-to-intervention" is defined as the time span between the diagnosis by radiographic imaging (CT scan/x-ray) and the start of surgical intervention ("cut of the scin"). Due to the time to intervention the study group was subdivided into three groups: under 3 h, 3 to 9 h and longer than 9 h. These time intervals were chosen in order to represent usual hospital procedures. In daily routine a time to intervention of less than 3 h reflects the situation, when the surgeon is waiting for the next operation room available (high urgency). Patients who were operated between 3 and 9 h represent urgent cases, which were operated within one hospital working shift. More than 9 h of time to intervention represent a situation of a delayed diagnosis and/or treatment of the intestinal perforation.

Clinical data were collected by the regular hospital documentation software (IMESO KisData and ICUData version 7.7.0.1590, KAOS desktop version 3.0.0.1, MEDOS Nexus .med RIS Client version 9.3.2276). Parameters of interest were length of hospital stay, ventilatory time, pre- and postoperative blood parameters, amount of cristalloids and catecholamine consumption. Furthermore, the

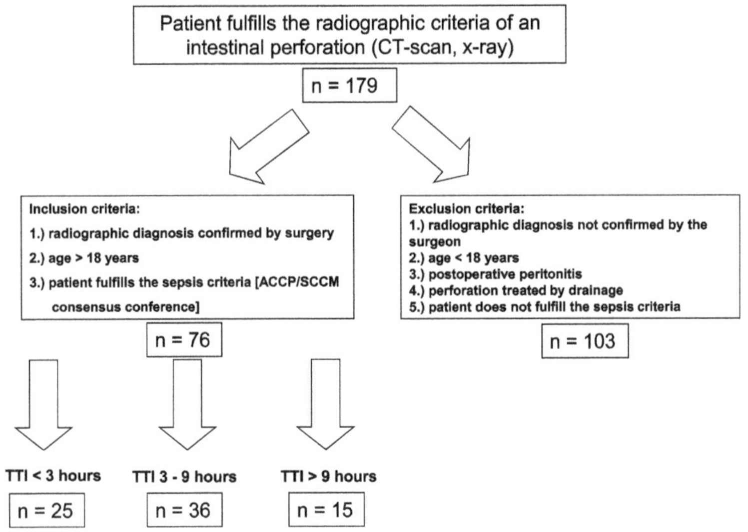

Fig. 1 Study protocoll of this retrospective analysis of patients with an intestinal perforation at our university hospital: Of 179 patients with the diagnosis of a perforation in the GI-tract 79 met the inclusion criteria of this pilot study. These patients were attributed to the three study arms according to their time-to-intervention

application of blood transfusions was analyzed. Different protein serum levels (lactate, pH, base excess, blood glucose, creatinine, urea, c-reactive protein, procalcitonin), hemoglobin and the amount of leukocytes were measured on admission in the emergency room and immediately after surgical source control. Both the in-hospital mortality and the overall motality were calculated. Additionally radiologic methods and surgical specifications (cause and location of perforation, surgical technique) were collected. The amount and type of infusion and transfusion were determined for the first 24 h after surgery. ICU prognostic scores (SAPS II, SOFA, APACHE II) were also calculated for the first postoperative 24 h according to the established protocols published before [14–16].

Baseline characteristics were expressed as mean ± standard deviation in normal and as median ± interquantile range in not normally distributed data. A p-value of $p < 0.05$ was considered as significant. Descriptive analysis was performed with contingency tables, while Chi-Squared-Test was used to describe the distribution of discrete parameters in proportion to the time to intervention. Mann–Whitney-U-Test was used to test metric values. All statistical analyses were performed with Microsoft® Excel® and IBM®SPSS®Statistics (version 21.0.0.0).

Results

From 179 patients with radiographic signs of an intestinal perforation 76 septic patients fulfilled the inclusion criteria. 31 female and 45 male septic patients with an intestinal perforation entered this retrospective monocenter study. Figure 2 shows the location of the intraabdominal inflammatory. With 36 cases most patients were operated between 180 and 540 min after diagnosis (study group II). In 25 patients surgery was performed in less than 180 min (study group I). In study group III (TTI > 540 min) 15 cases were included.

In the majority of cases (97 %) the diagnosis was based on an emergency computertomography scan. In two cases free intraabdominal air in the conventional x-ray of the abdomen led to the indication for surgical intervention.

Sixty patients developed respiratory failure requiring mechanical ventilation in the postoperative course. The duration of the operation did not differ between the three groups. In addition, the absolute time of mechanical ventilation and the amount of catecholamines applied did not depend on the time between diagnosis and surgical intervention (Fig. 3). Revisions had to be performed in 38 % of the cases (study group 1 44 % vs. study group 2 39 % vs. study group 3 27 %). In case of perforation of the small intestine segmental resection with a side-to-side anastomosis were performed. Perforations of the sigmoid colon were resected. Due to the impression of the emergency surgeon a Hartmann operation was done. Alternatively the colorectum was reconstructed by a descendorectostomy. In some cases (deep distal anastomosis) a diverting protective ileostomy was implemented.

Perforations of the ascending colon were reconstructed by a ileotransversostomy. In cases of anastomotic leakage either discontinuous or continuous reconstructions were performed due to the surgeon's impression.

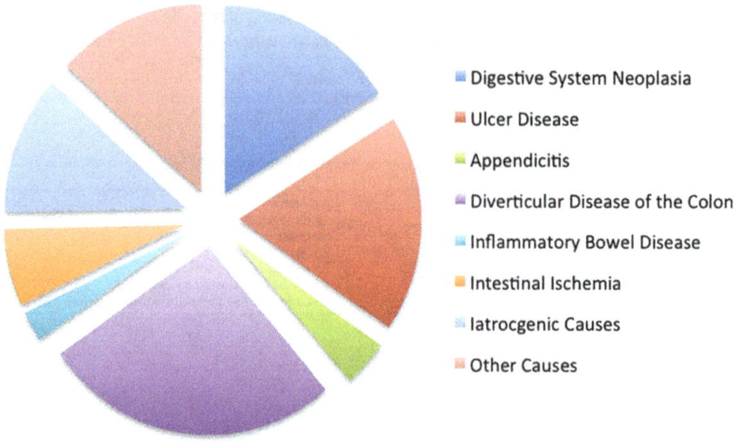

Fig. 2 The different reasons for the perforation reflects the typical pattern of a European university hospital

Concerning the 30-day in hospital mortality (non-significant) differences between the three study groups were detected: While patients of study group I had a 80 % survival, patients with a time-to-intervention of more than three hours (study group II and III) showed a survival of 73 % each. The overall survival was 80 % for the early intervention group, compared to 75 % (study group II) and 73 % (study group) respectively.

Tables 1, 2 and 3 provide the descriptive parameters, retrospectively analyzed in this study.

The time-courses of the serum CRP, urea, creatinine and lactate are presented in Fig. 4. Significant differences between the three study groups could not be detected.

Discussion

Despite the risks of a specific surgical intervention (fistulas, SIRS, bleeding) it is common surgical practice, that emergency patients with intestinal perforation are initially stabilized and transferred to the operation room.

In our pilot study 76 septic patients were analyzed concerning the time-dependency between surgical intervention and patient's mortality and morbidity. It thus provides insights into the surgical management in the very early phase after hospital admission:

More than 80 % of the patients with an intestinal perforation underwent surgical source control within the first 9 h after hospital admission. About one third of the patients was operated within 3 h. In the great majority of cases we met the 12-h intervall of surgical source

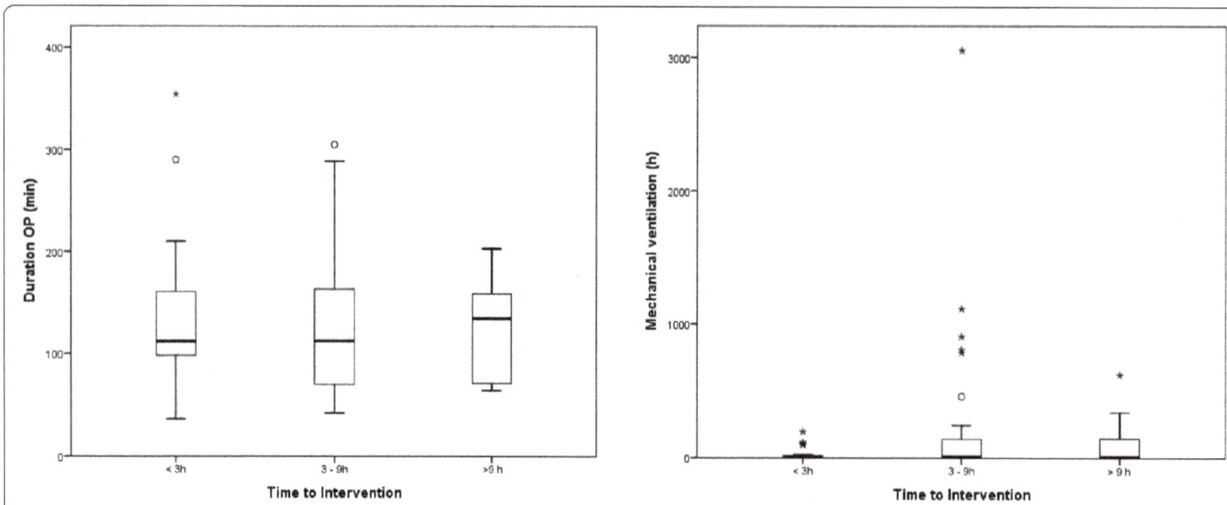

Fig. 3 All study groups were equal concerning the duration of surgical source control. The time-to-intervention had no significant impact on the time of mechanical ventilation or the amount of catecholamins adiministered after surgery. o and * represent single spike values

Table 1 Characteristics of the three study groups

		<3 h				3–9 h				>9 h				
	N	*n*	Mean	SD	Median [IQR]	*n*	Mean	SD	Median [IQR]	*n*	Mean	SD	Median [IQR]	*p*-Value
Age	76	25	59,64	18,775	63 [50, 74]	36	64,36	14,934	65 [56.25;76.5]	15	68,8	14,586	69 [61;80]	0,205
Length of hospital stay	76	25	20,64	14,731	22 [10, 28]	36	28,75	32,056	17,5 [11;29]	15	20,27	14,235	16 [11;27]	0,921
Duration of surgery (minutes)	76	25	135,2	73,005	112 [97, 165.5]	36	126,58	68,393	112,5 [70;170.25]	15	127,07	47,596	135 [70; 160]	0,744
Ventilatory time (hours)	76	25	29,524	51,3765	6,2 [0.5, 19.2]	36	228,253		9,9 [5.175; 148.75]	15	105,94	186,3957	7,7 [3.9;276]	0,141
Katecholamins (within 24 h)	76	25	7102,32	15541,449	450 [0, 9330]	36	31294,5	80932,459	1911 [0; 9700]	15	4570,8	8733,606	0 [0; 2340]	0,604
Bikarbonate	76	25	84	123,929	0 [0, 155]	36	65,56	91,634	50 [0; 100]	15	40	54,116	0 [0;100]	0,656
Kristalloids	76	25	2876	1416,945	2600 [1600, 4125]	36	2564,17	1364,581	2525 [1562.5; 31^37.5]	15	1990	978,373	1800 [1500; 2100]	0,184
Kolloids	76	25	854	1951,384	500 [0, 1000]	36	326,39	421,813	0 [0; 500]	15	400	430,946	500 [0; 500]	0,13
Substitution of erythrocyte concentrates	76	25	276	465,725	0 [0, 1020]	36	283,33	411,617	0 [0; 990]	15	260	0	437,199 [0; 1200]	0,839
Thrombocyte concentrates	76	25	20	70,711	0	36	20,83	71,088	0	15	33,33	129,099	0	1
Fresh frozen plasma	76	25	100	322,749	0	36	187,5	432,497	0	15	133,33	296,808	0	0,322
Glucose substitution within24h	76	25	15,2	76	0	36	15,2	76	0	15	40	129,835	0	0,987
Bicarbonate substitution within 24 h	76	25	70	119,024	0 [0, 100]	36	48,53	101,865	0	15	53,33	104,312	0 [0; 50]	0,335
Kistralloid substitution within 24 h	76	25	2990,8	2348,709	2800 [1720, 3700]	36	3198,61	1712,078	2800 [2000; 4500]	15	2536,67	1155,649	2250 [1700; 3000]	0,79
Kolloid substitution within 24 h	76	25	380	505,8	0 [0, 500]	36	328,57	404,076	0 [0; 500]	15	833,33	1531,417	0 [0; 1000]	0,869
Erythrocyte concentrates within 24 h	76	25	108	285,657	0	36	233,33	424,937	0 [0; 300]	15	260	337,639	0 [0; 600]	0,056
Thrombocyte concentrates within 24 h	76	25	12	60	0	36	12	60	0	15	8,33	50	0	0,604
FFP within 24 h	76	25	48	132,665	0	36	177,78	390,685	0 [0; 350]	15	26,67	103,28	0	0,283
SAPS_II score after source control	76	25	42,36	15,508	43 [29.5, 50.5]	36	44,28	15,161	46 [31.25; 55.75]	15	41,53	13,674	38 [34; 46]	0,894
APACHE II score after soruce control	76	25	21,08	8,026	21 [14, 26]	36	21,86	6,69	21,5 [17.25; 26.5]	15	19,87	5,718	20 [16; 25]	0,79
SOFA score after source control	76	25	6,32	4,059	6 [3, 9.5]	36	7,28	3,377	7 [5; 10]	15	6,27	3,127	6 [4; 9]	0,479
Gastric reflux within 24 h (ml)	76	25	166	225,074	30 [0, 300]	36	266,94	436,347	100 [0; 400]	15	163,33	227,272	80 [0; 250]	0,57

***FFP* fresh frozen plasma, *SAPS* Simplified Acute Physiology Score, *APACHE* Acute Physiology and Chronic Health Evaluation II-score, *SOFA* Sequential Organ Failure Assessment score**

Table 2 Descriptive analysis of different parameters of the three study groups

		<3 h				3–9 h				>9 h				
	N	*n*	Mean	SD	Median [IQR]	*n*	Mean	SD	Median [IQR]	*n*	Mean	SD	Median [IQR]	*p*-Value
Before surgery														
Serum lactate	46	9	2,45	1,66193	1,9 [1.2, 3.2]	28	2,6404	2,67295	1,8 [1.175; 2.875]	9	1,9733	0,99991	1,7 [1.235; 2.645]	0,661
pH	49	17	7,34	0,05374	7,33 [7.3, 7.375]	23	7,3422	0,10904	7,38 [7.24; 7.41]	9	7,4144	0,04613	7,43 [7.4; 7.445]	0,074
BE	49	17	−3,3824	2,56131	−3,8 [−5.35, −0.9]	23	−4,8	6,70271	−3,8 [−8.5; 0.4]	9	−1,0778	6,41693	−2,2 [−5.4; 1.4]	0,95
Glucose	55	11	152,684	70,4683	138 [101, 166]	33	150,494	73,9948	136 [100; 165]	11	163,909	68,9775	148 [107; 176]	0,869
Hemoglobin	75	24	12,417	3,0039	12,6 [9.7, 14.65]	36	13,681	13,8924	11 [9.475; 13.575]	15	10,593	1,9036	9,9 [9.1; 11.8]	0,11
Creatinine	76	25	1,352	1,138	1 [0.8, 1.25]	36	7,136	34,2748	1 [0.8; 2.05]	15	1,347	0,9782	1 [0.8; 1.5]	0,781
Urea	76	25	59,68	54,4225	41 [25, 83]	36	64,764	62,7524	42,5 [32.25; 73.75]	15	76,133	41,8857	63 [43; 108]	0,175
Leukocytes	76	25	12,276	7,2799	12,3 [7.25, 17.2]	36	12,328	8,8553	9,25 [7.975; 15.775]	15	11,373	7,0199	9,3 [6.1; 12.9]	0,808
CRP	75	25	141,6148	157,91994	74,3 [9.05, 253]	36	168,0072	131,14877	149,175 [42.32; 250.28]	14	181,7514	137,22675	155,7 [56.28; 320.4]	0,176
PCT	12	3	13,267	14,584	10,6 [0.2, 0	7	8,714	12,3999	0,8 [0.4; 15]	2	12,95	15,3442	12,95 [2.1; 0]	1
After Surgery														
Serum lactate	66	15	2,9718	2,19183	2,25 [1.35, 4]	36	1,9333	1,41219	1,4 [1.1; 2.775]	15	2,3867	1,92423	1,8 [1.2; 2.2]	0,06
pH	74	23	7,302	0,082848	7,308 [7.231, 7.37]	36	7,346	0,079749	7,35 [7.31; 7.4]	15	7,33233	0,080053	7,31 [7.265; 7.4]	0,072
BE	74	23	−5,4348	3,49488	−5,1 [−8.4, −3]	36	−3,7389	3,98929	−3,8 [−5.4; −2.2]	15	−3,8467	5,18871	−4,5 [−6.2; −2.3]	0,059
Glucose	75	24	126,288	42,1621	122 [1104, 145.75]	36	130,717	51,9907	134,5 [107.25; 144.75]	15	172,467	54,1702	175 [138; 221]	0,118
Hemoglobin	75	24	16,438	22,6004	11,9 [10.25, 13.68]	36	17,181	28,0558	10,65 [9.425; 13.08]	15	10,367	2,4555	10,4 [9.6; 11.6]	0,065
Creatinine	75	24	1,304	1,1035	1 [0.9, 1.12]	36	1,45	0,7865	1,2 [0.825; 1.7]	15	1,267	0,8156	0,9 [0.8; 1.6]	0,319
Urea	75	24	54,67	47,416	39,5 [26.25, 49.5]	36	71,08	56,263	59 [36; 78]	15	74,13	43,083	67 [47; 83]	0,025
Leukocytes	75	24	10,129	5,9572	9,4 [4.95, 13.4	36	10,597	6,5088	8,45 [6.43; 13.2]	15	12,02	7,4694	12,9 [4.6; 16.9]	0,759
CRP	75	24	137,0608	110,5366	140,93 [31.2, 229.4]	36	168,595	107,2545	156,555 [76.8; 228.5]	15	182,9213	104,25169	184,2 [115; 256]	0,175
PCT	13	3	20,933	20,9381	17,7 [1.8, 0]	9	20,933	20,9381	17,7 [5.35; 29.6]	1	26,356	34,8009	14,4 [9.75; 30.5]	1

***BE* base excess, *CRP* C-reactive protein, *PCT* procalcitonin**

Table 3 General description of the three study groups conerning OP technique, antibiotics and others

	Total		Up to 3 h.		3 to 9 h.		More than 9 h.	
Gender	n	%	n	%	n	%	n	%
Female	31	41 %	8	32 %	13	36 %	10	67 %
Male	45	59 %	17	68 %	23	64 %	5	33 %
Total	76	100 %	25	100 %	36	100 %	15	100 %
Ventilation	N	%	n	%	n	%	n	%
Not ventilated	16	21 %	5	20 %	8	22 %	3	20 %
Ventilated	60	79 %	20	80 %	28	78 %	12	80 %
Total	76	100 %	25	100 %	36	100 %	15	100 %
OP-method	N	%	n	%	n	%	n	%
Laparascopic	2	3 %	2	8 %	0	0 %	0	0 %
Open	74	97 %	24	92 %	35	97 %	15	100 %
Converted	2	3 %	0	0 %	1	3 %	0	0 %
Total	76	100 %	26	100 %	36	100 %	15	100 %
Antibiotics	N	%	n	%	n	%	n	%
No antibiotics	2	3 %	0	0 %	0	0 %	2	13 %
Antibiotics	74	97 %	25	100 %	36	100 %	13	87 %
Total	76	100 %	25	100 %	36	100 %	15	100 %
Revision	N	%	n	%	n	%	n	%
No revision	47	62 %	14	56 %	22	61 %	11	73 %
Revision	29	38 %	11	44 %	14	39 %	4	27 %
Total	76	100 %	25	100 %	36	100 %	15	100 %
Ischemia	N	%	n	%	n	%	n	%
No ischemia	67	88 %	22	88 %	31	86 %	14	93 %
Ischemia	9	12 %	3	12 %	5	14 %	1	7 %
Total	76	100 %	25	100 %	36	100 %	15	100 %

control strongly recommended by the Surviving Sepsis Campaign [5]. The overall survival was 80 % for study group I and decreased to 75 % (study group II) and 73 % (study group III) respectively.

In a multivariate analysis of septic patients with necrotizing soft tissue infections Boyer et al. was able to show that a delayed surgical intervention > 14 h after diagnosis was a negative prognostic predictor, associated with a 34-fold increase in hospital mortality [9]. Hospital mortality was 40.6 %. Forty-one percent of the patients were septic on admission.

Delayed operation is recognized as a contributor to adverse outcome in many fields of emergency surgery. A prospective trial from Kollef could determine the delay in diagnostics followed by surgical intervention as one independent negative predictor for the survival of intensive care patients [17]. Reasons for delayed surgical intervention were analyzed in a retrospective study by North et al. and by the Danish National Indicator Project in 2009: out-hospital perforation, masked clinical signs of peritonitis, late surgical attendance and a missing pulseoxymetry on admission were independent prognostic factors for a bad outcome.

In a study from the field of pediatric surgery all children, who survived a necrotizing fasciitis had undergone surgical source control within three hours after admission [8]. These data are supported by a retrospective cohort study by Gajic et al., who could identify delays in surgical evaluation and therapy as critical contributors to mortality on medical intensive care units: A delay of more than 48 h led to a dramatic decline in patients' survival (41 % vs. 73 % in the early intervention group) [18].

Despite some evidence for a conservative treatment of perforated peptic ulcera [19] surgery is still the gold standard for gastric perforation [20]. For patients with perforations of the upper GI tract Buck et al. could detect a strong dependency of the delay of surgical treatment after hospital admission on the 30 day survival rates [21]. Over the first 24 h after admission each hour

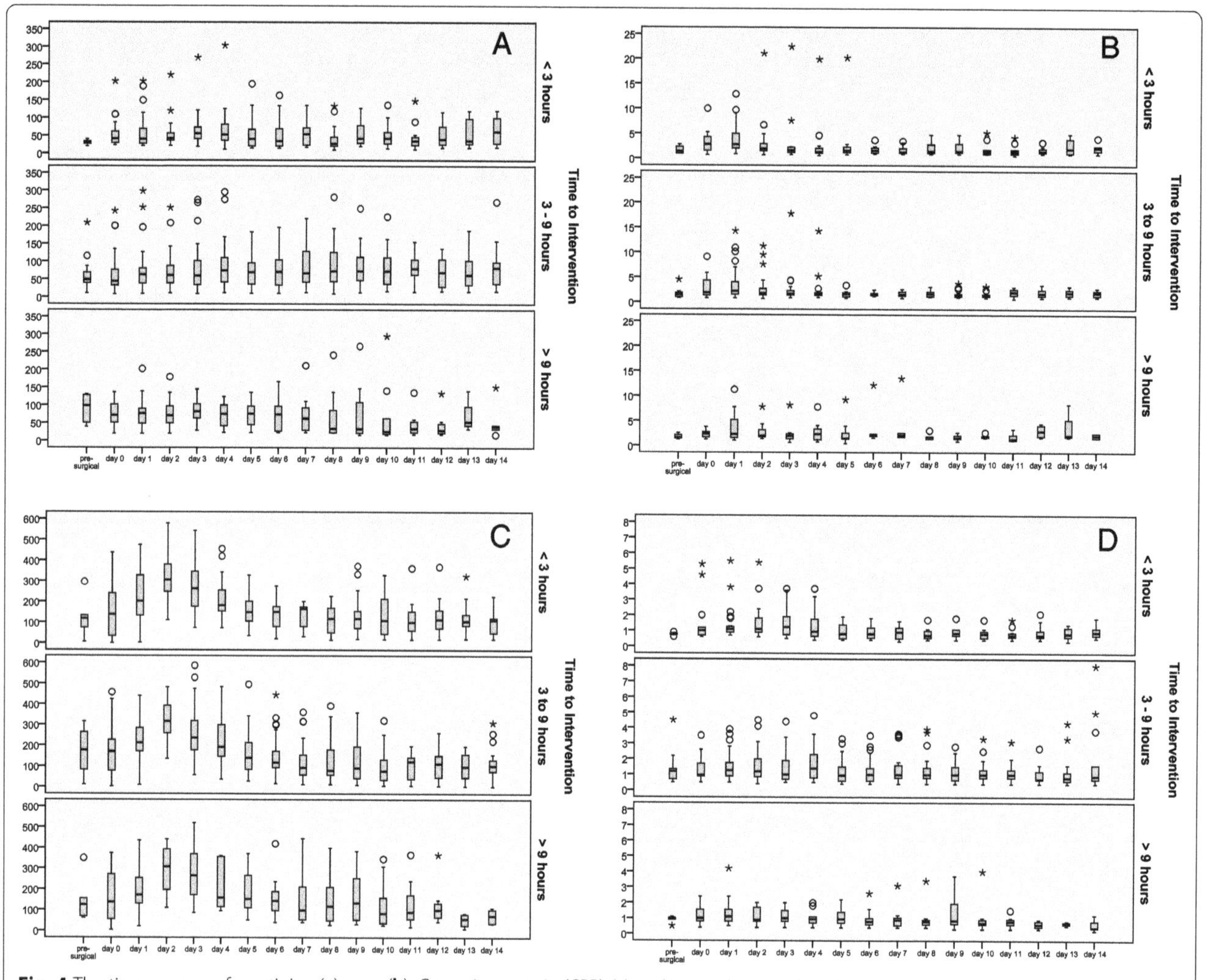

Fig. 4 The time-courses of creatinine (**a**), urea (**b**), C-reactive protein (CRP) (**c**) and serum lactate (**d**) before surgical source control and in the postoperative phase. o and * represent single spike values

of surgical delay was associated with a 2 % decrease in patient survival [21]. The amount of septic patients in the study group remains unclear. About 16 % were hypotensive on admission.

This strong time-dependency conflicts the recommendation of the new guidelines of the Surviving Sepsis Campaign, which advises a time-to-intervention of 12 h from diagnosis to source control. These very early hours after hospital admission are still nebulous concerning the influence of the velocity of diagnostics and surgical source control on patients'survival.

Due to the very limited number of septic patients included in this pilot study we potentially failed to find a significant influence of the TTI on the mortality. Nevertheless with prolonged TTI mortality rates showed an increasing tendency to higher levels. While 30-day mortality was 20 % in Study group I, it was 27 % in group III. Hospital mortality confirmed this tendency (study group I 20 % vs. Study group II 33 % vs. Study group III 33 %).

In contrast to Wachta et al., who investigated 14 % mortality for patients with peritonitis after intestinal perforation, our study revealed a higher overall mortality (31 %). This can be explained by the inclusion of only septic patients with increased APACHE II scores > 20 (vs. APACHE II 14.3). Besides the lack of prospective randomized studies a comparison of studies on surgical source control ist nearly impossible. This is due to incoherence in the group of patients with intestinal perforation: While patients with perforations requiring intensive care have a very poor prognosis, patients with iatrogenic perforation show an improved survival [18, 22]. Perforations due to an ischemia of the bowel have a very bad prognosis. With a 1 year-mortality of more than 70 % patients with secondary peritonitis due to postoperative complications have the worst outcome [4]. Generally peritonitis is a negative predictor for patients' outcome after intestinal perforation. In our study an early surgical intervention tends to result in lower rates of peritonitis (group I 88 % vs. Group II 92 % vs. Group III 100 %). This goes in line with the differences in mortality we could determine.

To minimize the incoherence of the study group the patients with complications after surgery like anastomotic leakage or ischemia were excluded from the study cohort. Nevertheless this important group of patients for the surgeons everyday-life should be analyzed in future studies.

This incoherence in the group of septic patients in general also reflects the contradictory results on the impact of a rapid or delayed initiation of antimicrobial therapy on the mortality of septic patients: The prospective, objective multicenter study from Ferrer et al. revealed, that only an early broad-spectrum antibiotic treatment within one hour is life-saving for the septic patient [23]. However, source control was not tested in this study. These data underline the results of Kumar et al., who determined the impact of delays in initiation of an effective antibiotic treatment on the mortality of septic shock patients. Each hour of delay in the adminitration of antimicrobials was associated with a decreased survival of 5–10 % [24]. Despite its wide adoption, whether this practice is of benefit for all septic patients is still controversial. Hranjec et al. analyzed 1483 patients concerning an aggressive (early start of antimcirobial treatment) vs. conservative (start of antibiotics as soon as the infection objectively was confirmed) treatment modality. Interestingly, the benefitial effects of an early administration of antibiotics were not detectable in the hemodynamic stable surgical patient [25]. Detailed analysis of the study protocols reveals that the beneficial effects of a rapid initiation of antimicrobial pharmacotherapy especially can be found for the subgroup of patients with a septic shock, a group, which also received antibiotics in the Hranjec study immediately.

From these data one could deduce that not the standardized, strictly time-dependent, but the personalized antimicrobial therapy could be trend-setting.

The originality of our study is supported by several differences to trials published previously: First only those patients were included, who met the sepsis criteria of the ACCP/SCCM consensus conference on sepsis. Second, all patients had an intestinal perforation. The locations of the perforations and its reasons reflect the spectrum of a typical European university hospital. Third, all study groups showed no differences concerning their catecholamine consumption or APACHE II scores. Thus the groups are comparable concerning the severity of sepsis.

This small unicenter study is a pilot-study to turn the focus on citically ill, septic surgical patients, which – so far – are not reflected by the recent sepsis guidelines.

Due to the retrospective study design the analysis of the patients suffering from severe abdominal sepsis bears the risk of an important bias: It is probable, that those patients, who were staged as very critical in the emergency room were transferred into the operation room more rapidly than those, who presented as relatively stable concering their clinical situation. We tried to minimalize this bias by analysing the consumption of catecholamines, the analysis of preoperative labarotory parameters and clinical scores (e.g. APACHE II). Our study was designed and performed in only one surgical center and thus only a very limited number of septic patients were included. Results can only show tendencies, which underlines, that multicenter approaches are necessary to analyze this group of critically ill surgical patients in the very early phase of emergency and intensive care treatment.

Conclusions

Despite its relevance literature on the time dependency of early surgical intervention in intestinal perforation is rare and contradictory. In this pilot study there is a tendency that immediate surgical intervention might be of advantage for septic emergency patients. Further multicenter approaches will be necessary to evaluate, whether the TTI has any impact on the outcome of septic patients with intestinal perforation.

Abbreviations

APACHE: acute physiology and chronic health evaluation; SAPS: simplified acute physiology score II; SOFA: sepsis-related organ failure assessment; TTI: time to intervention.

Competing interests

Andreas Hecker and other co-authors have no conflict of interest.

Authors' contributions

AH, ES, RR and RF designed the study and wrote the manuscript. BH, JH, CK and MR were involved in statistical analysis of the data. MR and CL participated in the coordination and helped to draft the manuscript. GAK, WP and MAW were involved in the final corrections. All authors read and approved the final manuscript.

Author details

[1]Department of General and Thoracic Surgery, University Hospital Giessen, Rudolf-Buchheim-Street 7, 35392 Giessen, Germany. [2]Department of Anesthesiology, Surgical Intensive Care Medicine and Pain Therapy, University Hospital Giessen, Rudolf-Buchheim-Street 7, 35392 Giessen, Germany. [3]Department of Radiology, University Hospital Giessen, Rudolf-Buchheim-Street 7, 35392 Giessen, Germany. [4]Department of Internal Medicine, University Hospital Giessen, Rudolf-Buchheim-Street 7, 35392 Giessen, Germany.

References

1. Torgersen C, Moser P, Luckner G, Mayr V, Jochberger S, Hasibeder WR, et al. Macroscopic postmortem findings in 235 surgical intensive care patients with sepsis. Anesth Analg. 2009;108(6):1841–7.
2. Bernard GR, Vincent JL, Laterre PF, LaRosa SP, Dhainaut JF, Lopez-Rodriguez A, et al. Efficacy and safety of recombinant human activated protein C for severe sepsis. N Engl J Med. 2001;344(10):699–709.
3. Angus DC, Wax RS. Epidemiology of sepsis: an update. Crit Care Med. 2001;29(7 Suppl):S109–116.

4. Hartl W, Kuppinger D, Vilsmaier M. Secondary peritonitis. Zentralbl Chir. 2011:136(1):11–7.
5. Dellinger RP, Levy MM, Rhodes A, Annane D, Gerlach H, Opal SM, et al. Surviving sepsis campaign: international guidelines for management of severe sepsis and septic shock. Crit Care Med. 2012;41(2):580–637.
6. Seiler CA, Brugger L, Forssmann U, Baer HU, Buchler MW. Conservative surgical treatment of diffuse peritonitis. Surgery. 2000;127(2):178–84.
7. Barie PS, Williams MD, McCollam JS, Bates BM, Qualy RL, Lowry SF, et al. Benefit/risk profile of drotrecogin alfa (activated) in surgical patients with severe sepsis. Am J Surg. 2004;188(3):212–20.
8. Moss RL, Musemeche CA, Kosloske AM. Necrotizing fasciitis in children: prompt recognition and aggressive therapy improve survival. J Pediatr Surg. 1996;31(8):1142–6.
9. Boyer A, Vargas F, Coste F, Saubusse E, Castaing Y, Gbikpi-Benissan G, et al. Influence of surgical treatment timing on mortality from necrotizing soft tissue infections requiring intensive care management. Intensive Care Med. 2009;35(5):847–53.
10. Bufalari A, Giustozzi G, Moggi L. Postoperative intraabdominal abscesses: percutaneous versus surgical treatment. Acta Chir Belg. 1996;96(5):197–200.
11. Mier J, Leon EL, Castillo A, Robledo F, Blanco R. Early versus late necrosectomy in severe necrotizing pancreatitis. Am J Surg. 1997;173(2):71–5.
12. van Santvoort HC, Besselink MG, Bakker OJ, Hofker HS, Boermeester MA, Dejong CH, et al. A step-up approach or open necrosectomy for necrotizing pancreatitis. N Engl J Med. 2010:362(16):1491–502.
13. Levy MM, Fink MP, Marshall JC, Abraham E, Angus D, Cook D, et al. 2001 SCCM/ESICM/ACCP/ATS/SIS international sepsis definitions conference. Intensive Care Med. 2003;29(4):530–8.
14. Vincent JL, Moreno R, Takala J, Willatts S, De Mendonca A, Bruining H, et al. The SOFA (Sepsis-related Organ Failure Assessment) score to describe organ dysfunction/failure. On behalf of the Working Group on Sepsis-Related Problems of the European Society of Intensive Care Medicine. Intensive Care Med. 1996;22(7):707–10.
15. Knaus WA, Draper EA, Wagner DP, Zimmerman JE. APACHE II: a severity of disease classification system. Crit Care Med. 1985;13(10):818–29.
16. Le Gall JR, Lemeshow S, Saulnier F. A new Simplified Acute Physiology Score (SAPS II) based on a European/North American multicenter study. JAMA. 1993;270(24):2957–63.
17. Kollef MH, Allen BT. Determinants of outcome for patients in the medical intensive care unit requiring abdominal surgery: a prospective, single-center study. Chest. 1994;106(6):1822–8.
18. Gajic O, Urrutia LE, Sewani H, Schroeder DR, Cullinane DC, Peters SG. Acute abdomen in the medical intensive care unit. Crit Care Med. 2002;30(6):1187–90.
19. Crofts TJ, Park KG, Steele RJ, Chung SS, Li AK. A randomized trial of nonoperative treatment for perforated peptic ulcer. N Engl J Med. 1989;320(15):970–3.
20. Sartelli M, Viale P, Catena F, Ansaloni L, Moore E, Malangoni M, et al. WSES guidelines for management of intra-abdominal infections. World J Emerg Surg. 2013;8(1):3.
21. Buck DL, Vester-Andersen M, Moller MH. Surgical delay is a critical determinant of survival in perforated peptic ulcer. Br J Surg. 2013:100(8):1045–9.
22. Gedebou TM, Wong RA, Rappaport WD, Jaffe P, Kahsai D, Hunter GC. Clinical presentation and management of iatrogenic colon perforations. Am J Surg. 1996;172(5):454–7. discussion 457–458.
23. Ferrer R, Artigas A, Suarez D, Palencia E, Levy MM, Arenzana A, et al. Effectiveness of treatments for severe sepsis: a prospective, multicenter, observational study. Am J Respir Crit Care Med. 2009;180(9):861–6.
24. Kumar A, Roberts D, Wood KE, Light B, Parrillo JE, Sharma S, et al. Duration of hypotension before initiation of effective antimicrobial therapy is the critical determinant of survival in human septic shock. Crit Care Med. 2006;34(6):1589–96.
25. Hranjec T, Rosenberger LH, Swenson B, Metzger R, Flohr TR, Politano AD, et al. Aggressive versus conservative initiation of antimicrobial treatment in critically ill surgical patients with suspected intensive-care-unit-acquired infection: a quasi-experimental, before and after observational cohort study. Lancet Infect Dis. 2012:12(10):774–80.

Important CT findings for prediction of severe appendicitis: involvement of retroperitoneal space

Kumiko Kitaoka*†, Kazuhiro Saito† and Koichi Tokuuye†

Abstract

Background: Determination of the severity of appendicitis and differentiation between complicated and uncomplicated appendicitis are clinically important. Severe appendicitis frequently affects extraperitoneal spaces. We have investigated CT findings of retroperitoneal space (RPS) in patients with appendicitis to create a model for identification of complicated appendicitis.

Method: CT images of 223 patients with pathologically proven appendicitis were reviewed. The total number of the segments in RPS where inflammatory changes were located (RPS count) was obtained as well as appendiceal diameter, appendicolithiasis, WBC count, and CRP level. Data were analyzed to identify factors indicating complicated appendicitis. Univariate analysis was conducted to identify statistically significant variables. A multivariable logistic regression analysis was performed in order to find independent predictors of complicated appendicitis.

Results: Patients with complicated appendicitis were more likely to have higher RPS count ($P < 0.001$), appendicolithiasis ($P = 0.002$), higher CRP level ($P < 0.001$), and greater appendix diameter ($P < 0.001$) than patients with uncomplicated appendicitis. Statistical analysis showed RPS count was the most helpful predictor of complicated appendicitis.

Conclusion: Radiologists and surgeons should be aware of the importance of CT findings in RPS when treating patients with appendicitis. Complicated appendicitis can be predicted by RPS count, diameter of the appendix, appendicolithiasis, and CRP level.

Keywords: Appendicitis, Complicated, Retroperitoneal space, Extraperitoneal space, CT

Introduction

Appendicitis, a very common surgical condition, has been traditionally considered as a surgical emergency and a clinical challenge [1]. With the advent of computed tomography (CT), the diagnostic accuracy of appendicitis has dramatically improved. So far, CT findings, such as enlargement of the appendix, appendicolithiasis, and phlegmon, have been reported to successfully identify cases of acute appendicitis and these findings are relatively easy to identify [2-4]. Other researchers have reported that laboratory markers are useful in making diagnosis [5]. Recently, one systematic review and meta-analysis reported imperfect accuracy of procalcitonin, C-reactive protein (CRP) and white blood cell count (WBC) in uncomplicated or complicated appendicitis [6].

In patients with complicated appendicitis, a significant increase in mortality rate has been reported [7,8]. Accordingly, accurate determination of the severity of appendicitis, and differentiation between complicated and uncomplicated appendicitis is clinically warranted. CT could help surgeons recognize the location of appendix, confirm the diagnosis and other intra-abdominal conditions requiring other procedures, such as perforation, abscess, and peritonitis [9]. Some previous studies have investigated the implication of various CT findings in the context of severity of appendicitis [10-17]. Clinical application of such findings, however, may not be easy, because they can be subtle, and subjective.

The appendix is usually located in the anterolateral portion of pelvic cavity, and inflammation of the appendix

* Correspondence: kumiko_kitaoka@yahoo.co.jp
†Equal contributors
Department of Radiology Tokyo Medical University Hospital, 6-7-1 Nishishinjuku, Shinjuku-ku, Tokyo 160-0023, Japan

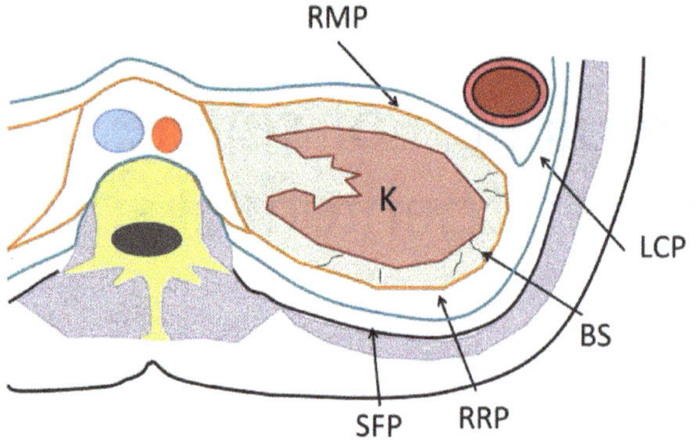

Figure 1 Transverse diagram showing segments in RPS. Retromesenteric plane (RMP), lateral conal plane (LCP), retrorenal plane (RRP), subfascial plane (SFP), combined fascial plane (CFP), and bridging septa (BS) constitute retroperitoneal space (RPS) around the kidney (K). RMP is an interfascial space bounded by the anterior pararenal space and the perirenal space. RRP is located between the perirenal space and the posterior pararenal space. RMP and RRP extend caudally to form CFP below the kidney. RMP and RRP continue anterolaterally to LCP. BP is a lamellar structure having connection with the anterior and posterior renal fasciae. SFP is a potential space between the pararenal space and the transversalis fascia.

can trigger inflammatory process in pelvic extraperitoneal space (PEPS). Recent studies have discovered more precise anatomical relationship between retroperitoneal space (RPS) and PEPS [18-20].

Methods

Approval was obtained by the institutional review board of our university before initiation of this study. All

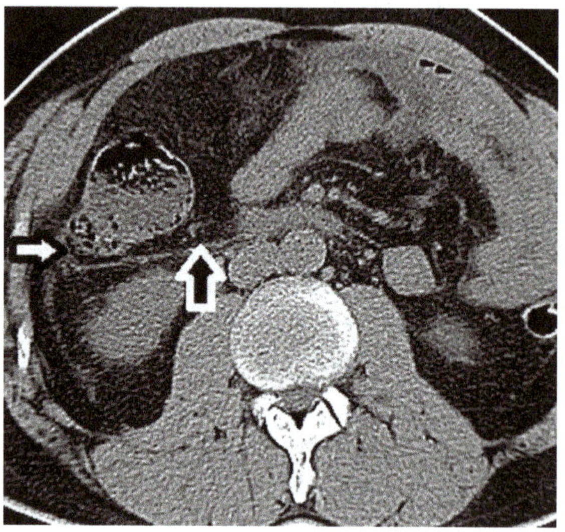

Figure 2 Transverse CT image of 46-year-old man with complicated appendicitis. Retrorenal plane, retromesenteric plane (black arrow), lateral conal plane (white arrow), subfascial plane, and bridging septa are involved.

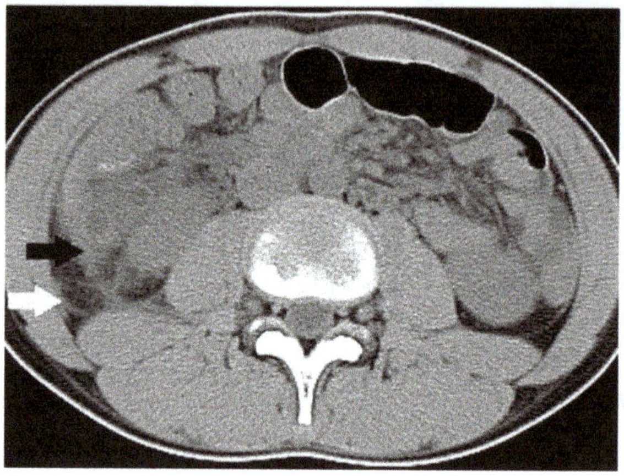

Figure 3 Transverse CT image of 13-year-old boy with complicated appendicitis. The picture shows enlarged appendix with fluid collection in retrorenal plane, subfascial plane (white arrow), lateral conal plane (black arrow), and bridging septa.

consecutive patients who underwent an appendectomy for suspected acute appendicitis at our university hospital between January 1, 2007 and December 31, 2012 were eligible. All eligible patients were chosen by searching a pathology database with an appropriate code for appendix or appendectomy. The eligibility criteria were a histology report showing acute appendicitis (n = 231). Patients were excluded when pathologists made a diagnosis of chronic appendicitis (n = 7), or when there was no preoperative, non-focused, abdominopelvic CT examination available in our picture archiving and communication system (PACS) at the time of the study that had been obtained before a surgery (n = 1). Written informed consent was obtained from the patient on admission for the publication of clinical report and any accompanying images performed during their medical treatment.

We reviewed the patients' medical, surgical, and pathology records. All multidetector non-contrast or contrast CT images were obtained to visualize structures in ileocecal area. All patients were scanned using a 16 or 64 multi-detector helical scanner, (Bright Speed Elite; Right Speed VCT General Electric Health Care). The abdomen was scanned helically (pitch of 1.375:1, rotation time 0.4 sec, 120kVp, auto mAs) with a 5-mm collimation.

The images were retrospectively reviewed at a PACS workstation and interpreted by consensus of two radiologists (K.S. 23 years of experience, specialized in abdominal radiology; K.K. 3 years of experience) who were blinded to the patients' surgical or pathological results.

We selected six sections within RPS without discriminating the right from the left. These sections included (a) lateral conal plane (LCP), (b) retromesenteric plane (RMP), (c) retrorenal plane (RRP), (d) bridging septa (BS), (e) subfascial plane (SFP), and (f) combined fascial plane (CFP) [21] (Figures 1, 2 and 3). These segments

Table 1 Distribution of observed radiological changes in RPS segments

		LCP	RRP	RMP	BS	SFP	CFP
Complicated appendicitis (true positive)	≧16y	49	38	33	12	12	82
	<16y	4	5	3	1	5	17
Uncomplicated appendicitis(false positive)	≧16y	7	7	5	2	1	46
	<16y	6	3	3	0	0	15
PPV	≧16y	0.88	0.84	0.87	0.86	0.92	0.64
	<16y	0.40	0.63	0.50	1.0	1.0	0.53
NPV	≧16y	0.53	0.47	0.46	0.40	0.41	0.48
	<16y	0.60	0.63	0.61	0.61	0.65	0.72

Significantly more segments were involved (i.e. radiographical changes were observed) in complicated appendicitis group. CFP, which is closest to the pelvic extraperitoneal space, was predominantly involved. Positive predictive value (PPV) of complicated appendicitis was highest for SFP in older patient group while PPV was highest for SFP and BS in younger patient group.

were evaluated for signs of inflammation, such as thickening of the fascial plane (Figures 2 and 3). We regarded recognizable thickening of fascial planes of any degree as pathological as well as fluid accumulation. RPS segments where signs of inflammation could be located and the total number of involved RPS segments (RPS count) were recorded for each patient. In addition, maximal diameter of the appendix on an axial image was measured, and presence or absence of appendicolithiasis was determined. Patients were divided into two groups a complicated appendicitis group and an uncomplicated appendicitis group. The complicated appendicitis group consisted of patients whose surgical reports either described the presence of a perforated appendix, abscess formation, or purulent peritoneal fluid, or whose histology reports indicated a perforated appendix, abscess formation, peritonitis, or gangrenous appendicitis.

We analyzed data using the Statistical Package for the Social Sciences (SPSS) ver. 16.0 (SPSS Inc., Chicago, IL). Univariate analysis was performed by comparing characteristics between complicated and uncomplicated appendicitis. Analysis was also repeated for two subgroups, the younger patients (age <16 years, n = 68) and the older patients (age ≧16 years, n = 155).

A multivariable logistic regression analysis was performed in order to find factors for indicating complicated appendicitis.

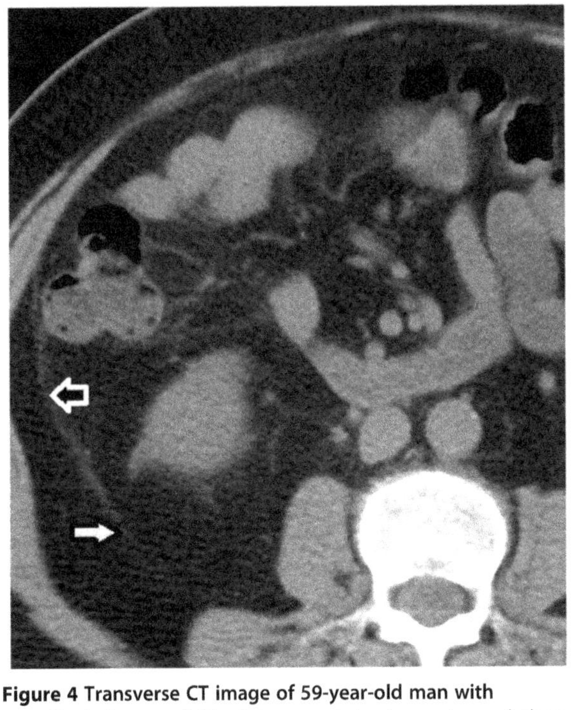

Figure 4 Transverse CT image of 59-year-old man with complicated appendicitis. Retromesenteric plane, retrorenal plane (white arrows), and lateral conal plane (black arrow) were involved.

Results

A total number of 223 patients with pathologically proven appendicitis, 78 female, 145 male, were included. The

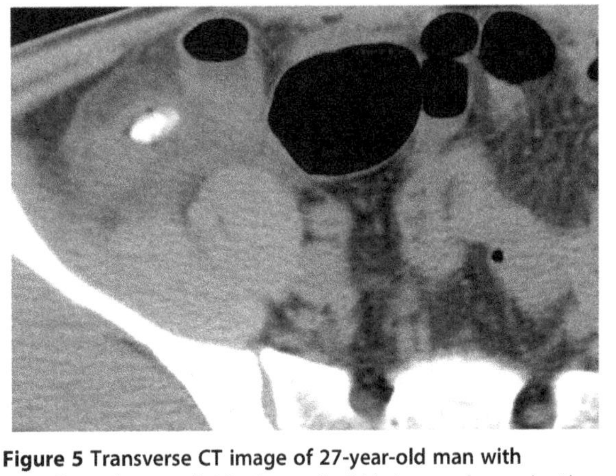

Figure 5 Transverse CT image of 27-year-old man with complicated appendicitis. Appendicolithiasis was observed with involvement of combined fascial plane.

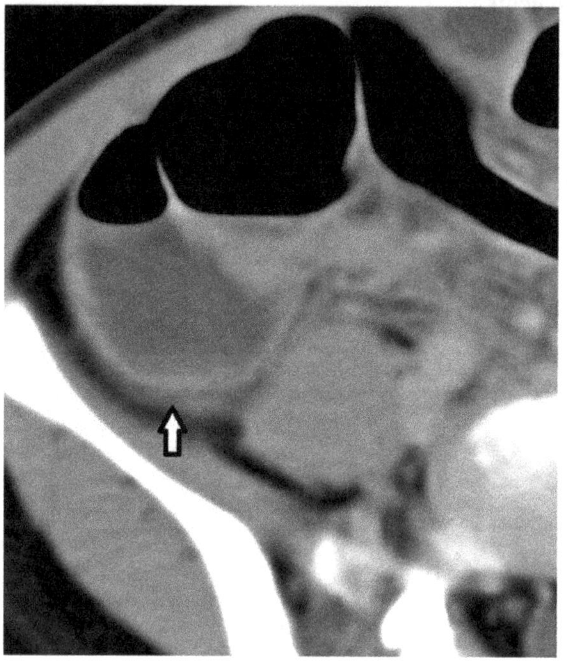

Figure 6 Transverse CT image of 6-year-old patient with complicated appendicitis and ileus. Identification of RPS and other extraperitoneal spaces was difficult due to the patient's younger age and ileus. Combined fascial plane (white arrow) involvement was observed.

mean age of the patients was 31.4 years old (4–94 year old). 123 patients had complicated appendicitis (55.2%).

Observed distribution of changes in each segment of RPS for the complicated/uncomplicated appendicitis group was summarized (Table 1). Significantly more RPS segments were involved in the complicated appendicitis group compared with the uncomplicated appendicitis group (Figures 2, 3, 4 and 5). Involvement of RPS segments was

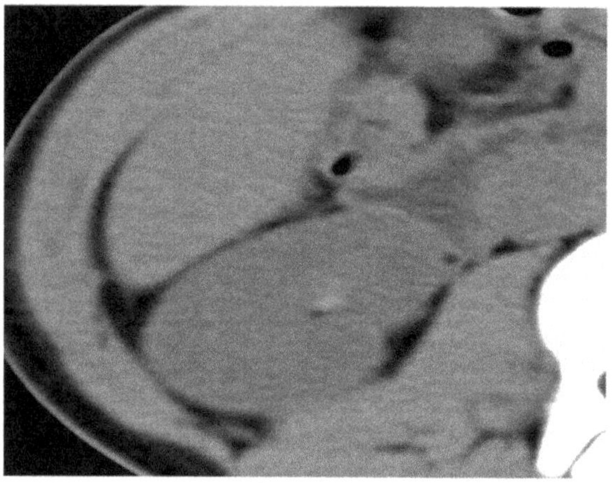

Figure 7 Transverse CT image of 12-year-old patient with phlegmonous appendicitis. No change can be observed in RPS.

Table 2 Results of univariate analysis of variables between groups

	Complicated (n = 123)	Uncomplicated (n = 100)	P value
Appendix diameter*† (mm)	13.4 (10.4-16.0)	10.6 (8.6-13.1)	<0.001
RPS count*†	2 (1-3)	1(0-1)	<0.001
WBC count† (×10^9 cells/L)	13.7 (11.3-17.0)	13.7 (11.1-16.5)	>0.05
CRP level*† (nmol/L)	45.7 (11.4-131.4)	12.4 (4.8-36.2)	<0.001
Age*†(years old)	34(18-51)	23 (11-34.8)	<0.001
Appendicolithiasis*‡			0.002
Gender‡			>0.05

*P value <0.05 was considered significant.
†Medians are shown with 25th percentile and 75th percentile between brackets.
‡Data were analyzed using Fishers' exact test.

more identifiable in the older patient (age ≧16 years) group than in the younger patient group (age <16 years) because segments of RPS are sometimes difficult to be observed (Figures 6 and 7).

Positive predictive value (PPV) was relatively high (0.64-0.92) for segments of RPS among older patients. The most frequently involved segment was CFP, which had Negative predictive value (NPV) of 0.72 among younger patients. The least frequently involved segment, SFP had PPV of 0.92 among older patients (Table 1).

Univariate analysis revealed that patients with complicated appendicitis were more likely to have higher RPS count ($P < 0.001$), higher CRP level ($P < 0.001$), greater appendix diameter ($P < 0.001$), and appendicolitiasis ($P = 0.002$) (Table 2). No statistically significant differences were noted between both groups with respect to gender and WBC count.

In the older patient group, patients with complicated appendicitis were more likely to have higher RPS count ($P < 0.001$), higher CRP level ($P < 0.001$), greater appendix diameter ($P = 0.002$), appendicolitiasis ($P = 0.04$), and advanced age ($P = 0.01$). In the younger patient group, patients with complicated appendicitis were more likely to be female ($P = 0.02$), more likely to have appendicolitiasis ($P = 0.01$), greater appendix diameter ($P = 0.02$), and higher CRP level ($P = 0.03$).

Variables of age, RPS count, diameter of appendix, appendicolithiasis, and CRP level were entered into the initial logistic regression model.

The final model included RPS count, diameter of appendix, appendicolithiasis, and CRP level, and was characterized by a Nagelkerke R-square value of 0.31 and a Hosmer and Lemeshow level of fit with a $\chi 2$ value of 7.9 and a P value of 0.45.

The regression coefficients for the final regression models are shown in Table 3. Obtained ROC curve showed the largest area under the curve (AUROC) for

Table 3 Logistic regression model for probability of complicated appendicitis

	P value	Regression coefficient	Odds ratio
RPS count	0.004	0.419	1.52
Appendix diameter	0.06	0.088	1.09
Appendicolithiasis	0.09	0.863	0.42
CRP level	0.08	0.076	1.709

RPS (AUROC = 0.70), followed by CRP level (AUROC = 0.69) (Figure 8). The optimal cutoff value of RPS count for complicated appendicitis was calculated around 1 to 2 (sensitivity = 0.521, specificity 0.786 at RPS = 1.5).

Analysis was repeated for the older patient group and RPS count was found to be a better indicator of complicated appendicitis than other variables. The final model included only RPS count, appendicolithiasis, and CRP level. AUROC was largest for RPS (AUROC = 0.71).

Discussion

This study showed a complicated appendicitis can be predicted by a combination of clinical variables, the number of involved segments of RPS, the maximal diameter of the appendix on CT examination, existence of appendicolithiasis, and the CRP levels. Based on our data, CT analysis has strong predictive power for the severity of appendicitis [21]. This finding is similar to the pancreatitis severity scoring system [22], which determines the severity of pancreatitis based on the extent of inflammation on CT. The appendix, being located in the proximity of PEPS, can cause inflammation-related CT changes in RPS as well by way of CFP.

Compared with laboratory markers, CT findings of appendicitis have been found helpful because of their specificity. Noncontrast CT scan in adults had reasonably high sensitivity and specificity for clinical decision making. Previous radiologists who studied severity of appendicitis limited the scope of observation to findings observed in the vicinity of the appendix, such as involvement of periappendiceal fat and appendicolithiasis [9-17]. Although these results are important, these findings are not always reproducible. For example, contrast medium is contraindicated in some patients while many of these findings are sometimes difficult to be identified without contrast enhancement. Furthermore, not every clinician is familiarized with subtle CT changes. Contrary to these limitations, the key elements of CT findings that we presented in this article can be interpreted more objectively and in a semiquantitative manner in almost every patient once clinicians know where to look at.

The present study included 123 cases of complicated appendicitis in 223 cases of pathologically proven appendicitis (55.2%). The ratio of complicated appendicitis is relatively high compared with other previous reports (20-40%) [9,16,17]. There was no appendicitis-associated death observed among the study subjects.

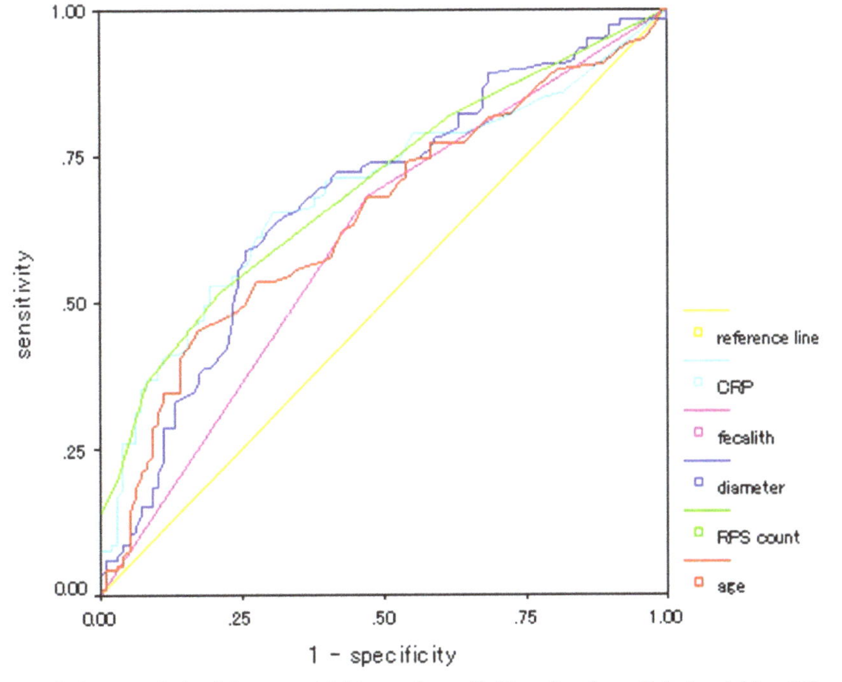

Figure 8 Receiver characteristic curve derived from sensitivities and specificities of various clinical variables. RPS count is plotted in light green line with the following variables: CRP level (light blue), appendicolithiasis (pink), appendiceal diameter (dark blue), and age (red). Yellow line is a reference line. RPS count had the largest area under the curve of 0.70.

Potential limitations of this study include difficulty of identifying anatomical structures in pediatric patients. We acknowledge that this method may be more useful in patients who are at the age of 16 or higher. CT exposes patients to a risk of ionizing radiation. Therefore, CT is less indicated in the young and female patients due to its high level of irradiation and may be more helpful in the elderly age group, but there is still a 10-20% negative appendectomy rate despite the use of CT [23-25]. However, most importantly we can utilize this diagnostic method without specialized training or it can be employed irrespective of use of contrast medium once its practical utility is properly understood.

Conclusion

In conclusions, radiographical findings of RPS segments are important for the diagnosis of appendicitis and the prediction of severity of acute appendicitis because numerosity of the involved RPS segments (for example ≥2) is indicative of severe appendicitis. Complicated appendicitis can be predicted by RPS count, diameter of the appendix, appendicolithiasis, and CRP level. The possibility of false positivity remains, but RPS count would be more useful than other CT findings because administration of contrast medium is not required and it can be utilized in almost every clinical setting. Radiologists and clinicians should continue appropriate measures to minimize irradiation for susceptible patients.

Competing interest

The authors declare that they have no competing interests. No external financial support was provided.

Authors' contribution

Study concept and design: KK and KS. Acquisition of data: KK. Analysis and interpretation of data: KK, KS, and KT, Drafting of the manuscript: KK. Critical revision of the manuscript for important intellectual content: KS and KT. All authors take responsibility for the integrity of the data and the accuracy of the data analysis. All authors read and approved the final manuscript.

References

1. Agresta F, Ansaloni L, Catena F, Verza LA, Prando D: **Acute appendicitis: position paper, WSES, 2013.** *World J Emerg Surg* 2014, **9**(1):26.
2. Ives EP, Sung S, McCue P, Durrani H, Halpern EJ: **Independent predictors of acute appendicitis on CT with pathologic correlation.** *Acad Radiol* 2008, **15**(8):996–1003.
3. Lane MJ, Liu DM, Huynh MD, Jeffrey RB Jr, Mindelzun RE, Katz DS: **Suspected acute appendicitis: nonenhanced helical CT in 300 consecutive patients.** *Radiology* 1999, **213**(2):341–346.
4. Raman SS, Lu DS, Kadell BM, Vodopich DJ, Sayre J, Cryer H: **Accuracy of nonfocused helical CT for the diagnosis of acute appendicitis: a 5-year review.** *Am J Roentgenol* 2002, **178**(6):1319–1325.
5. Xharra S, Gashi-Luci L, Xharra K, Veselaj F, Bicaj B, Sada F, Krasniqi A: **Correlation of serum C-reactive protein, white blood count and neutrophil percentage with histopathology findings in acute appendicitis.** *World J Emerg Surg* 2012, **7**(1):27.
6. Yu CW, Juan LI, Wu MH, Shen CJ, Wu JY, Lee CC: **Systematic review and meta-analysis of the diagnostic accuracy of procalcitonin, C-reactive protein and white blood cell count for suspected acute appendicitis.** *Br J Surg* 2013, **100**(3):322–329.
7. Aprahamian CJ, Barnhart DC, Bledsoe SE, Vaid Y, Harmon CM: **Failure in the nonoperative management of pediatric ruptured appendicitis: Predictors and consequences.** *J Pediatr Surg* 2007, **42**(6):934–938. discussion 938.
8. Velanovich V, Satava R: **Balancing the normal appendectomy rate with the perforated appendicitis rate: Implications for quality assurance.** *Am Surg* 1992, **58**(4):264–269.
9. Hansen AJ, Young SW, De Petris G, Tessier DJ, Hernandez JL, Johnson DJ: **Histologic severity of appendicitis can be predicted by computed tomography.** *Arch Surg* 2004, **139**(12):1304–1308.
10. Oliak D, Sinow R, French S, Udani VM, Stamos MJ: **Computed tomography scanning for the diagnosis of perforated appendicitis.** *Am Surg* 1999, **65**(10):959–964.
11. Foley TA, Earnest F, Nathan MA, Hough DM, Schiller HJ, Hoskin TL: **Differentiation of nonperforated from perforated appendicitis: accuracy of CT diagnosis and relationship of CT findings to length of hospital stay.** *Radiology* 2005, **235**(1):89–96.
12. Bixby SD, Lucey BC, Soto JA, Theysohn JM, Ozonoff A, Varghese JC: **Perforated versus nonperforated acute appendicitis: accuracy of multidetector CT detection.** *Radiology* 2006, **241**(3):780–786.
13. Pinto Leite N, Pereira JM, Cunha R, Pinto P, Sirlin C: **CT evaluation of appendicitis and its complications: imaging techniques and key diagnostic findings.** *Am J Roentgenol* 2005, **185**(2):406–417.
14. Tsuboi M, Takase K, Kaneda I, Ishibashi T, Yamada T, Kitami M, Higano S, Takahashi S: **Perforated and Nonperforated Appendicitis: Defect in enhancing appendiceal wall – depiction with Multi-Detector Row CT.** *Radiology* 2008, **246**(1):142–147.
15. Mori Y, Yamasaki M, Furukawa A, Takahashi M, Murata K: **Enhanced CT in the diagnosis of acute appendicitis to evaluate the severity of disease: comparison of CT findings and histological diagnosis.** *Radiat Med* 2001, **19**(4):197–202.
16. Tsukada K, Miyazaki T, Katoh H, Masuda N, Ojima H, Fukuchi M, Manda R, Fukai Y, Nakajima M, Ishizaki M, Motegi M, Ohsawa H, Mogi A, Okamura A, Tsunoda Y, Sohda M, Ohno T, Moteki T, Sekine T, Kuwano H: **CT is useful for identifying patients with complicated appendicitis.** *Dig Liver Dis* 2004, **36**(3):195–198.
17. Miki T, Ogata S, Uto M, Nakazono T, Urata M, Ishibe R, Shinyama S, Nakajo M: **Enhanced Multidetector-row Computed Tomography (MDCT) in the diagnosis of acute appendicitis and its severity.** *Radiat Med* 2005, **23**(4):242–255.
18. Korobkin M, Silverman PM, Quint LE, Francis IR: **CT of the extraperitoneal space: normal anatomy and fluid collections.** *Am J Roentgenol* 1992, **159**(5):933–942.
19. Beaulieu CF, Mindelzun RE, Dolph J, Jeffrey RB Jr: **The infraconal compartment: a multidirectional pathway for spread of disease between the extraperitoneal abdomen and pelvis.** *J Comput Assist Tomogr* 1997, **21**(2):223–228.
20. Lee SL, Ku YM, Rha SE: **Comprehensive reviews of the interfascial plane of the retroperitoneum: normal anatomy and pathologic entities.** *Emerg Radiol* 2010, **17**(1):3–11.
21. Sartelli M, Viale P, Catena F, Ansaloni L, Moore E, Malangoni M, Moore FA, Velmahos G, Coimbra R, Ivatury R, Peitzman A, Koike K, Leppaniemi A, Biffl W, Burlew CC, Balogh ZJ, Boffard K, Bendinelli C, Gupta S, Kluger Y, Agresta F, Di Saverio S, Wani I, Escalona A, Ordonez C, Fraga GP, Junior GA, Bala M, Cui Y, Marwah S, *et al*: **WSES guidelines for management of intra-abdominal infections.** *World J Emerg Surg* 2013, **8**(1):3.
22. Ishikawa K, Idoguchi K, Tanaka H, Tohma Y, Ukai I, Watanabe H, Matsuoka T, Yokota J, Sugimoto T: **Classification of acute pancreatitis based on retroperitoneal extension: application of the concept of interfascial planes.** *Eur J Radiol* 2006, **60**(3):445–452.
23. Chandrasekaran TV, Johnson N: **Acute appendicitis. Intestinal Surgery II.** *Surgery* 2014, **32**(8):413–417.
24. Wray CJ, Kao LS, Millas SG, Tsao K, Ko TC: **Acute Appendicitis: controversies in diagnosis and management.** *Curr Probl Surg* 2013, **50**(2):54–86.
25. Omari AH, Khammash MR, Qasaimeh GR, Shammari AK, Yaseen MK, Hammori SK: **Acute appendicitis in the elderly: risk factors for perforation.** *World J Emerg Surg* 2014, **9**(1):6.

28

Stump appendicitis: a retrospective review of 3130 consecutive appendectomy cases

Enis Dikicier[1*], Fatih Altintoprak[1], Kayhan Ozdemir[2], Kemal Gundogdu[2], Mustafa Yener Uzunoglu[2], Guner Cakmak[2], Feyyaz Onuray[2] and Recai Capoglu[2]

Abstract

Background: Stump appendicitis is inflammation of remnant appendix tissue due to incomplete removal of the appendix. Due to appendectomy history, stump appendicitis diagnosis is usually delay and that can cause increase morbidity.

Methods: Medical records of patients who had surgery for acute appendicitis at a single center from 2008 to 2017 were retrospectively reviewed. During the evaluation of medical records, patients that had a previous operation for acute appendicitis or had "stump appendicitis" as an exploratory finding in operation notes were included.

Results: Appendectomy was performed in 3130 patients (2630 open surgeries and 380 laparoscopic surgeries). Stump appendicitis was diagnosed in five patients (0.15%). The appendectomies had been performed 4, 5, 7, 7, and 11 years previously. Mean time taken for surgery was 36 h after symptoms began. Open surgery was performed in three patients, laparoscopic procedures in others.

Conclusion: Awareness of stump appendicitis before radiological examinations may facilitate accurate diagnosis and decrease the duration of the decision-making process, leading to decreased morbidity.

Keywords: Appendicitis, Stump appendicitis, Remnant appendicitis

Background

Appendectomy is currently the most common surgical operation worldwide [1]. Stump appendicitis is a rare condition beside the other common post-operative complications of appendectomy which are wound infection, bleeding, and intestinal obstruction.

Stump appendicitis is inflammation of remnant appendix tissue due to incomplete removal of the appendix [2]. This condition, which can be considered as recurring of acute appendicitis, may occur due to some technical and anatomical factors. Clinical findings are similar with acute appendicitis, as abdominal pain located on the right inferior quadrant is the most common sign [3]. This condition is not usually considered as preliminary diagnosis by clinicians at first referral due to previous appendectomy history. A delayed diagnosis may lead to delays in treatment and subsequently to an increase in morbidity.

In this retrospective study, four stump appendicitis cases out of 3130 consecutive appendectomies were evaluated and the medical histories of the subjects were reviewed.

Methods

The charts of patients who had surgery for acute appendicitis at the General Surgery Clinics of Sakarya University Faculty of Medicine from 2008 to 2017 were retrospectively reviewed. During the evaluation of medical records, patients that had a previous operation for acute appendicitis or had "stump appendicitis" as an exploratory finding in operation notes were included. For these patients, we reviewed demographic data, time after the initial operation, symptoms at the time of referral, laboratory and radiological findings, and operation findings. Previous operation and pathology reports were reviewed, and previous appendectomy was confirmed.

* Correspondence: enisdikicier@gmail.com
[1]Department of General Surgery, Istinye University Faculty of Medicine, Istanbul, Turkey
Full list of author information is available at the end of the article

Results

Appendectomy was performed in 3130 patients with a diagnosis of acute appendicitis between January 2008 and November 2017 (2630 open surgeries and 380 laparoscopic surgeries). Perforated appendicitis in 621 (19.8%) patients, acute appendicitis in 2024 (64.6%) patients, and normal appendix (negative appendectomy) in 476 (%15.2) patients were found.

Stump appendicitis was diagnosed in five patients (0. 15%). Three patients (60%) were male and two (40%) were female. The mean age was 32 (range 19–45). The appendectomies were performed 4, 5, 7, and 7 and 11 years previously using a conventional McBurney incision (open surgery). In the previous operation notes, the cases were recorded as perforated appendicitis in four patients (80%) and acute appendicitis in one patient (20%). In one of the patients who had been operated and confirmed due to perforated acute appendicitis, the localization of the appendix was recorded as retrocecal. The localization of the appendices of the other three patients was not recorded. The length of the appendices also was not recorded; the mean length of these appendices was 5.9 cm (4.9–7.2 cm) according to histopathologic reports.

The histopathological examination results were benign, and only inflammatory changes were observed in all patients.

One patient (20%) was referred to our clinic directly, and the remaining four patients (80%) were referred from other centers after an average of 2 days (range 1–3 days) of medical follow-up. During patient assessment at our clinic, three patients (60%) had classical physical examination findings consistent with acute appendicitis (tenderness and rebound in right lower abdominal quadrant) and the remaining two patients (40%) had acute abdomen (general tenderness, abdominal guarding, and rebound tenderness) and fever. An increase in the white blood cell (WBC) count was a common laboratory finding. The average WBC count was 14,300/mm^3 (range 12,800–18,700/mm^3).

Conventional radiographic imaging results were normal in all patients. Abdominal ultrasonography (USG) exams revealed acute appendicitis in two patients (40%). In the remaining three patients (60%), USG revealed inflammatory changes around the pericecal region. In these patients, the appendix was not observed; therefore, abdominal computerized tomography (CT) was performed, which revealed inflammation around the pericecal region, localized abscess formation, and thickening of the remnant appendix wall (Figs. 1 and 2).

On average, patients had surgery 36 h (range 24–72) after symptoms began. During surgery, one patient (20%) was under spinal anesthesia, and the remaining four patients (80%) were under general anesthesia. In three patients (60%), the surgeries were held as open operations

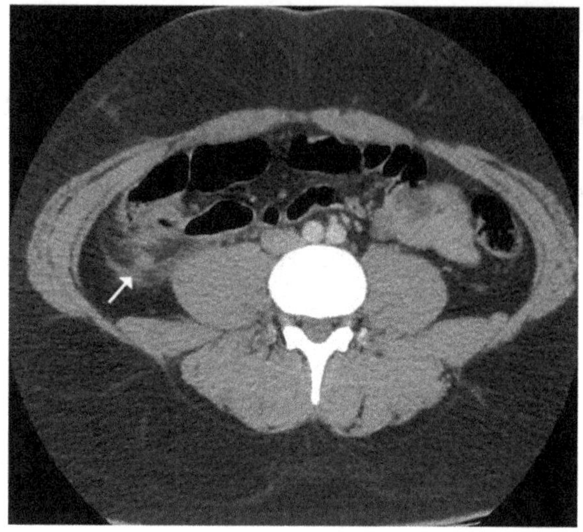

Fig. 1 Abdominal CT scan. In the right lower quadrant, inflammation in the pericecal region and tip of the remnant appendix tissue (arrow) is observed

using a McBurney incision line. In the other two patients (40%), diagnostic laparoscopy was performed. In the two diagnostic laparoscopy patients, one procedure (50%) was converted to open surgery due to dense attachments at the appendectomy lodge. In the other patient, operation was completed as laparoscopic. Perforation did not occur in any of the patients. Localized abscess formation was observed in three patients, and only inflammatory changes were observed in the other two patients.

In three patients (60%), the location of the remnant appendix was subserous, and in two patients (40%), there was still a residual remnant appendix tissue (Fig. 3) although the location was not subserous. No remnant meso-appendix was detected within remnant appendix tissues. Remnant tissue was isolated through the entrance part on the cecum and ligated with 2/0 absorbable suture on that localization. The mean length of the remnant

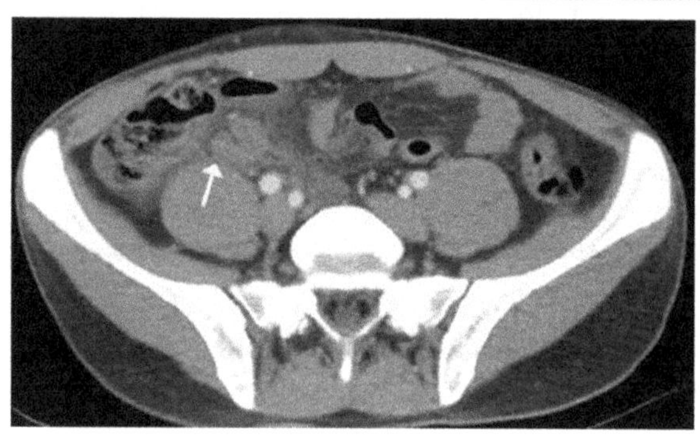

Fig. 2 Abdominal CT scan. In the right lower quadrant, remnant appendix tissue in the pericecal region and fecalitis within the appendix tissue are observed

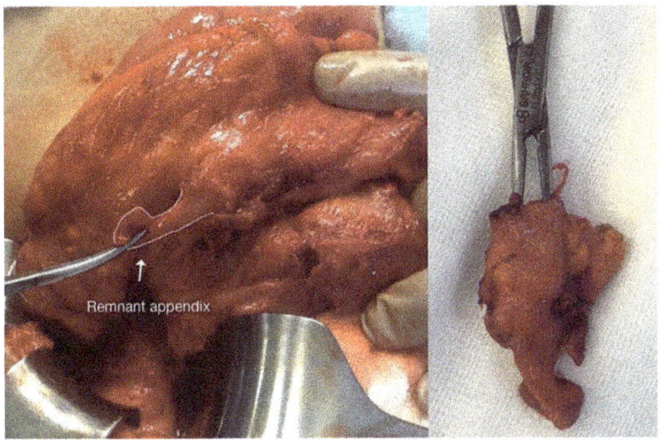

Fig. 3 Intraoperative view of stump appendicitis due to remnant appendix tissue

appendix was 2.7 cm (range 1.8–4.2). In all patients, the remnant appendix tissue was easily excised; the appendix radix was tied with a double tie using 2/0 Vicryl and was not inverted into the cecum. The post-op period was normal, and patients were discharged from the hospital within 2 days on average (range 1–4). Histopathological exams revealed acute stump appendicitis in all cases.

Discussion

Appendectomy is currently the most common surgical operation worldwide [2]. After appendectomy, various morbidities including wound infection may be encountered. Remnant appendix tissue inflammation after appendectomy is called stump appendicitis, a very rare condition. The lifelong probability of developing acute appendicitis is estimated at 7%, but the probability of developing stump appendicitis is much lower (1/50,000) [3]. In our study, this rate was very low (0.15%).

As expected, the symptoms and signs of stump appendicitis are the same as for classical acute appendicitis [4]. As such, clinicians usually do not suspect or, worse, disregard a probable diagnosis of stump appendicitis in patients with a history of appendectomy who present with clinical signs of acute appendicitis. This may lead to a delay in diagnosis, which may lead to future complications. Kumar et al. [5] reported suppurative appendicitis during laparoscopic exploration in a patient with a previous history of appendectomy and abdominal pain at the time of referral. Manoglu et al. [6] described a patient with cecal necrosis secondary to stump appendicitis who was referred to the hospital two times with complaints of abdominal pain. In our study, the average time to surgery was 2 days after referral of the patient. This is consistent with previous findings that stump appendicitis is difficult to diagnose. In three of our cases (60%), abscesses were detected during surgery; however, more complicated conditions were not encountered.

In a literature review conducted by Kanona et al. [7], the time it took for stump appendicitis to develop in patients with inadequate appendectomy ranged from 9 weeks to 50 years. In addition, Onder et al. [8] conducted two case studies and found that a history of appendectomy dated back to 4 months in one patient and 4 years in the other patient. In our study, the shortest time from first appendectomy to the development of stump appendicitis was 4 years; however, a much shorter time period is possible.

Establishing a diagnosis of stump appendicitis is difficult, and delayed diagnosis is established only after a certain period of clinical follow-up [5]. Even in the patient whose first referral was to our clinic, the patient underwent surgery 24 h after referral because, although a radiological exam done in the initial referral suggested stump appendicitis, a second radiological exam and second opinion were deemed necessary to confirm the diagnosis. This observation suggests that a delay in surgical decision in cases of stump appendicitis is due not only to the difficulty of establishing a diagnosis during the first referral, but also to the desire of the surgeons to feel confident about the diagnosis.

Clinical signs and laboratory findings of stump appendicitis are similar to those of primary acute appendicitis; therefore, radiological methods are more useful for differential diagnosis. In USG, remnant appendix tissue can be detected as a tube extending from the right iliac fossa or retrocecal region to the cecum [9, 10]. In abdominal CT, inflammation in the pericecal region, abscesses, thickening of the cecum and terminal ileum, and free-floating fluid at the pericecal and paracolic region are the likely findings [11–13]. In some cases, the appendix stump may be inflamed and edematous, and in other cases, fecalitis may occur [14]. In all of our cases, preoperative radiological exam findings revealed remnant appendix tissue and inflammation.

According to the literature, remnant appendix tissue > 5 mm in length is a risk factor for fecalitis and stump appendicitis [15]. The length of the remnant appendix ranges from 0.5 to 6.5 cm in patients who have undergone surgery with a diagnosis of stump appendicitis [8, 12]. In our study, the mean length of the remnant appendix was 2.3 cm. In addition to the lack of experience of the surgeon, reasons for longer remnant tissue include a subserous or retrocecal position of appendix tissue and inadequate dissection during laparoscopic appendectomy [16, 17]. A retrocecal position of remnant appendix tissue was found in three out of four patients in our study. This suggests the anatomic location of the appendix is a significant factor in the development of stump appendicitis.

There are some comments in the literature that appendectomy is performed by incomplete exposure of the radix of the appendix, so excess residual part is left and stump appendicitis takes place after laparoscopic appendectomy

[1]. However, most of the stump appendicitis in the literature are reported after open appendectomies. [3]. The important thing is performing the appendectomy after complete exposure of the meso-appendix, taenia coli of the cecum, and appendico-cecal junction and ligation of recurrent or accessory branch of the appendiceal artery (artery of Seshachalam), independent from the choice of method: laparoscopic or open [18, 19].

Histopathologic examination revealed no remnant meso-appendeceal tissue. Perforation was present in the four of the stump appendicitis cases. The inflammation may be a risk factor for stump appendicitis. We suggest that intensive inflammation during appendectomy may prevent to recognize the subserosal localization of appendix or makes it difficult to isolate the appendix through the cecal entrance area; each of the situations may increase the risk of stump appendicitis. The rate of stump appendicitis after perforating appendicitis in our study (4/621, 0.64%) is similar with the rates reported in the literature. Remnant tissue was sub-serosal in the three of these four cases. These findings support our suggestion.

There is no standardized surgical approach for probable stump appendicitis, but it has been reported that laparoscopy is superior to open surgery because it provides a better viewing angle, which leads to a better differential diagnosis [20].

Conclusion

Delays in the diagnosis of stump appendicitis continue to be an issue. Awareness of stump appendicitis before radiological examinations may facilitate accurate diagnosis and decrease the duration of the decision-making process, leading to decreased morbidity.

Key message

Appendectomy history does not exclude re-acute appendicitis (stump appendicitis) possibility.

Stump appendicitis possibility should be kept in mind in patients who have acute appendicitis signs even if there is appendectomy history.

Authors' contributions

KÖ, MYU, and KG collected the data analyzed. GÇ, FO, and RÇ made the statistical analysis. ED and FA made the study design and completed the writing process. All authors read and approved the final manuscript.

Competing interests

The authors declare that they have no competing interests.

Author details

[1]Department of General Surgery, Istinye University Faculty of Medicine, Istanbul, Turkey. [2]Department of General Surgery, Sakarya University Research and Educational Hospital, Sakarya, Turkey.

References

1. Subramanian A, Liang MK. A 60-year literature review of stump appendicitis: the need for a critical view. Am J Surg. 2012 Apr;203(4):503–7. https://doi.org/10.1016/j.amjsurg.2011.04.009.
2. Anderson KD, Parry RL. Appendicitis. In: O'Neill JA, Rowe MI, Grosfeld JL, Fonkalsurd EW, Coran AG, editors. Pediatric surgery. 5th ed. London: Mosby; 1998. p. 1369–79.
3. Liang MK, Lo HG, Marks JL. Stump appendicitis: a comprehensive review of literature. Am Surg. 2006;72:162–6.
4. Truty MJ, Stulak JM, Utter PA, Solberg JJ, Degnim AC. Appendicitis after appendectomy. Arch Surg. 2008;143:413–5.
5. Kumar A, Sharma A, Khullar R, Soni V, Baijal M, Chowbey PK. Stump appendicitis: a rare clinical entity. J Minim Access Surg. 2013;9(4):173–6.
6. Manoglu B, Niflioglu GG, Uysal E. A rare case: appendectomy after connected stump appendicitis perforation of the cecum. J Clin Anal Med. 2015;6(4):539–41.
7. Kanona H, Samaraee AA, Nice C, Bhattacharya V. Stump appendicitis: a review. Int J Surg. 2012;10(9):425–8.
8. Onder A, Kapan M, Boyuk A, Tekbas G, Gumus M. Stump appendicitis after appendectomy. Kolon Rektum Hast Derg. 2010;20(4):188–91.
9. O'Leary DP, Myers E, Coyle J, Wilson I. Case report of recurrent acute appendicitis in a residual tip. Cases J. 2010;3:14.
10. Baldisserotto M, Cavazzola S, Cavazzola LT, Lopes MHI, Mottin CC. Acute edematous stump appendicitis diagnosed preoperatively on sonography. AJR Am J Roentgenol. 2000;175:503–4.
11. Shin LK, Halpern D, Weston SR, Meiner EM, Katz DS. Prospective CT diagnosis of stump appendicitis. AJR Am J Roentgenol. 2005;184:62–4.
12. Erzurum VZ, Kasirajan K, Hashmi M. Stump appendicitis: a case report. J Laparoendosc Adv Surg Tech A. 1997;7(6):389–91.
13. Rao PM, Sagarin MJ, McCabe CJ. Stump appendicitis diagnosed preoperatively by computed tomography. Am J Emerg Med. 1998;16(3):309–11.
14. Al-Dabbagh AK, Thomas NB, Haboubi N. Stump appendicitis. A diagnostic dilemma. Tech Coloproctol. 2009;13:73–4.
15. Durgun AV, Baca B, Ersoy Y, Kapan M. Stump appendicitis and generalized peritonitis due to incomplete appendectomy. Tech Coloproctol. 2003;7:102–4.
16. Uludag M, Isgor A, Basak M. Stump appendicitis is a rare delayed complication of appendectomy: a case report. World J Gastroenterol. 2006;12:5401–3.
17. Devereaux DA, MC Dermott JP, Caushaj PF. Recurrent appendicitis following laparoscopic appendicectomy. Dis Colon rectum. 1994;37:719–20.
18. Leff DR, Sait MR, Hanief M, Salakianathan S, Darzi AW, Vashisht R. Inflammation of the residual appendix stump: a systematic review. Color Dis. 2012;14(3):282–93. https://doi.org/10.1111/j.1463-1318.2010.02487.x.
19. Constantin V, Popa F, Carap A, Socea B. Stump appendicitis- an overlooked clinical entity. Chirurgia (Bucur). 2014;109(1):128–31.
20. Roberts K, Starker L, Duffa A, Bell R, Bohkari J. Stump appendicitis: a surgeon's dilemma. JSLS. 2011;15(3):373–8.

Permissions

All chapters in this book were first published in WJES, by BioMed Central; hereby published with permission under the Creative Commons Attribution License or equivalent. Every chapter published in this book has been scrutinized by our experts. Their significance has been extensively debated. The topics covered herein carry significant findings which will fuel the growth of the discipline. They may even be implemented as practical applications or may be referred to as a beginning point for another development.

The contributors of this book come from diverse backgrounds, making this book a truly international effort. This book will bring forth new frontiers with its revolutionizing research information and detailed analysis of the nascent developments around the world.

We would like to thank all the contributing authors for lending their expertise to make the book truly unique. They have played a crucial role in the development of this book. Without their invaluable contributions this book wouldn't have been possible. They have made vital efforts to compile up to date information on the varied aspects of this subject to make this book a valuable addition to the collection of many professionals and students.

This book was conceptualized with the vision of imparting up-to-date information and advanced data in this field. To ensure the same, a matchless editorial board was set up. Every individual on the board went through rigorous rounds of assessment to prove their worth. After which they invested a large part of their time researching and compiling the most relevant data for our readers.

The editorial board has been involved in producing this book since its inception. They have spent rigorous hours researching and exploring the diverse topics which have resulted in the successful publishing of this book. They have passed on their knowledge of decades through this book. To expedite this challenging task, the publisher supported the team at every step. A small team of assistant editors was also appointed to further simplify the editing procedure and attain best results for the readers.

Apart from the editorial board, the designing team has also invested a significant amount of their time in understanding the subject and creating the most relevant covers. They scrutinized every image to scout for the most suitable representation of the subject and create an appropriate cover for the book.

The publishing team has been an ardent support to the editorial, designing and production team. Their endless efforts to recruit the best for this project, has resulted in the accomplishment of this book. They are a veteran in the field of academics and their pool of knowledge is as vast as their experience in printing. Their expertise and guidance has proved useful at every step. Their uncompromising quality standards have made this book an exceptional effort. Their encouragement from time to time has been an inspiration for everyone.

The publisher and the editorial board hope that this book will prove to be a valuable piece of knowledge for researchers, students, practitioners and scholars across the globe.

List of Contributors

Massimo Sartelli
Department of Surgery, Macerata Hospital, Italy

Pierluigi Viale and Fabio Tumietto
Clinic of Infectious Diseases, Department of Internal Medicine Geriatrics and Nephrologic Diseases, St Orsola-Malpighi University Hospital, Bologna, Italy

Kaoru Koike
Department of Primary Care & Emergency Medicine, Kyoto University Graduate School of Medicine, Japan

Federico Pea
Institute of Clinical Pharmacology and Toxicology, Azienda O spedaliera Universitaria Santa Maria Misericordia, Department of Experimental and Clinical Pathology and Medicine, University of Udine, Italy

Harry van Goor
Department of Surgery, Radboud University Nijmegen Medical Centre, The Netherlands

Gianluca Guercioni
Department of Surgery, "Mazzoni" Hospital, Ascoli Piceno Italy

Angelo Nespoli
Department of Surgical Sciences San Gerardo Hospital, Monza, University of Milano-Bicocca, Italy

Cristian Tranà
Department of Surgery, University of Ancona, Italy

Fausto Catena and Antonio Daniele Pinna
Department of General and Transplant surgery, St Orsola-Malpighi University Hospital, Bologna, Italy

Luca Ansaloni
Department of Surgery, "Ospedali Riuniti" Hospital, Bergamo, Italy

Ari Leppaniemi
Department of Surgery, Helsinki University Central Hospital, Finland

Walter Biffl and Ernest E Moore
Department of Surgery, Denver Health Medical Center, USA

Frederick A Moore
Department of Surgery, University of Texas Health Science Center, Houston, USA

Renato Poggetti
Emergency Surgery Department, University of São Paulo, Brazil

Rao R Ivatury
Surgery, Virginia Commonwealth University Health System, Richmond, VA, USA

Frederick A Moore
Acute Care Surgery, University of Florida, Gainesville, FL, USA

Walter Biffl
Surgery, Denver Health Medical Center, University of Colorado School of Medicine, 777 Bannock St., MC 0206, Denver, CO 80204, USA

Ari Leppeniemi
Surgery, Meilahti Hospital, Haartmaninkatu 4, Helsinki, Finland

Luca Ansaloni
Surgery I, Papa Giovanni XXIII Hospital, Piazza OMS 1, 24127 Bergamo, Italy

Fausto Catena
Department of Emergency Surgery, Parma University Hospital, Parma, Italy

Andrew Peitzman
Department of CSurgery, University of Pittsburgh, Pittsburgh, USA

Ernest E Moore
University of Colorado Denver, Denver, CO 80206, USA

Zainna C Meyer, Jennifer MJ Schreinemakers and Lijckle van der Laan
Department of Surgery, Amphia Hospital, Breda, the Netherlands

Massimo Sartelli
Department of Surgery, Macerata Hospital, Macerata, Italy

Fausto Catena
Emergency Surgery, Maggiore Parma Hospital, Parma, Italy

Luca Ansaloni
Department of General Surgery, Ospedali Riuniti, Bergamo, Italy

Ernest Moore
Department of Surgery, Denver Health Medical Center, Denver, CO, USA

Rafael Díaz-Nieto
Department of General and Digestive Surgery, Virgen de la Victoria, University Hospital, Malaga, Spain

Damien Massalou
Department of General Surgery and Surgical Oncology, Université de Nice Sophia-Antipolis, Universitary Hospital of Nice, Nice, France

Matej Skrovina
Department of Surgery, Hospital and Oncological Centre, Novy Jicin, Czech Republic

Ihor Gerych
Department of General Surgery, Lviv Emergency Hospital, Lviv, Ukraine

Ahmed O Hamedelneel
Department of Surgery, Our Lady of Lourdes Hospital, Drogheda, Ireland

Noel Naidoo
Department of Surgery, Port Shepstone Hospital, Port Shepstone, South Africa

Abdul Rashid Kayode Adesunkanmi
Department of Surgery, College of Health Sciences, Obafemi Awolowo University Hospital, Ile-Ife, Nigeria

Yoshiro Kobe
Department of Emergency and Critical Care Medicine, Chiba University Hospital, Chiba, Japan

Karim Ibn majdoub Hassani, Said Ait laalim, El Bachir Benjelloun, Imane Toughrai and Khalid Mazaz
Department of Surgery, School of Medicine and Pharmacy of Fez, Sidi Mohammed Ben Abdellah University, BP: 1893; Km2.200, Route de Sidi Hrazem, Fez 30000, Morocco

Chee Siong Wong and Syed Altaf Naqvi
Department of Surgery, Mid Western Regional Hospital, Dooradoyle, Co. Limerick, Ireland

James Frydman, Hany Bahouth and Yoram Kluger
Department of General Surgery, Rambam Health Care Campus, 31096 Haifa, Israel

Maxim Leiderman and Amos Ofer
Depatment of Radiology, Rambam Health Care Campus, 31096 Haifa, Israel

Paola Di Carlo, Giuliana Guadagnino and Daniela Cabibi
Department of Sciences for Health Promotion and Mother-Child Care "G. D'Alessandro", University of Palermo, Via del Vespro 127, I- 90127 Palermo, Italy

Gaetano Di Vita
Department of Surgery and Oncology Sciences, General Surgery Unit, University of Study of Palermo, Italy, Via del Vespro 127, I- 90127 Palermo, Italy

Gianfranco Cocorullo
Department of General Surgery, Urgency and Organ Transplantation, University of Palermo, Via del Vespro 127, I- 90127 Palermo, Italy

Roberta Villa, Stefano Costa, Sibilla Focchi, Carlo Corbellini, Massimo Vigorelli and Ettore Contessini Avesani
Department of General and Emergency Surgery, Fondazione IRCCS Ca' Granda Ospedale Maggiore Policlinico, Milan, Italy
Faculty of Medicine, Università degli Studi di Milano, Milano, Italy

Peter Vasas, Tom Wiggins, Asif Chaudry, Catherine Bryant and Frances S Hughes
Academic Surgical Department, Barts and the London NHS Trust, Whitechapel, London (E1 1BB), United Kingdom

Okiemute F Emanuwa, Abraham A Ayantunde and Tony W Davies
Department of Surgery, Queen Mary's Hospital, Frognal Avenue, Sidcup, DA14 6LT, London, UK

Slobodan Krstic, Ana Sijacki, Vladimir Djukic, Zlatibor Loncar and Aleksandar Karamarkovic
University of Belgrade, Belgrade, Serbia Clinic for Emergency Surgery, Emergency center, Clinical centre of Serbia, Belgrade, Serbia

Tamara Alempijevic
Clinic for Gastroenterology, Clinical Center of Serbia, Belgrade, Serbia

Aleksandar Resanovic
Surgery Department, Medical Center "Bezanijska kosa", Belgrade, Serbia

Somsubhra Datta Roy, Dawood Khan and Krishna K De
Department of surgery, Medical College Hospital, 88, College Street, Kolkata 73, India

Utpal De
Dankuni Housing Complex, L-4/9, Ph 3, Dankuni, Hooghly 713211, India

Phillipo L Chalya, Joseph B Mabula, Geofrey Giiti and Japhet M Gilyoma
Department of Surgery, Catholic University of Health and Allied Sciences-Bugando, Mwanza, Tanzania

Mheta Koy, Johannes B Kataraihya and Hyasinta Jaka
Department of Internal Medicine, Catholic University of Health and Allied Sciences-Bugando, Mwanza, Tanzania

Stephen E Mshana and Mariam Mirambo
Department of Microbiology and Immunology, Catholic University of Health and Allied Sciences-Bugando, Mwanza, Tanzania

Mabula D Mchembe
Department of Surgery, Muhimbili University of Health and Allied Sciences, Dar Es Salaam, Tanzania

Aldo M Marini and Paolo De Rai
General and Emergency Surgery Unit, Fondazione IRCCS Cà Granda Ospedale Maggiore Policlinico di Milano, via F. Sforza 35-20100, Milano, Italy

Arianna Zefelippo, Paola M Bertazzoni and Ettore Contessini-Avesani
General Surgery Post-graduation School, University of Milan, via F. Sforza 35-20100, Milano, Italy

Gökhan Ertuğrul, Murat Coşkun, Mahsuni Sevinç and Behzat Yelimlieş
Department of General Surgery, Düzce Atatürk State Hospital, Muncurlu, Düzce, Turkey

Fisun Ertuğrul
Department of Anesthesiology and Reanimation, Düzce Atatürk State Hospital, Muncurlu, Düzce, Turkey

Toygar Toydemir
Department of General Surgery, İstanbul Surgery Hospital, Nişantaşı, İstanbul, Turkey

Peter Ambe
Helios Klinikum Wuppertal, Department of Surgery II, Witten/Herdecke University, Heusner Strasse 40, 42283 Wuppertal, Germany

Sebastian A Weber
Department of Internal Medicine, St. Elisabeth Hospital Hohenlind, 50377 Köln, Germany

Hildegard Christ
Department of medical statistics and epidemiology, University of Cologne, Cologne, Germany

Dirk Wassenberg
Department of General, visceral and thoracic surgery, St. Remigius Hospital Opladen, An St. Remigius 26, 51379 Leverkusen, Germany

Federico Coccolini, Giulia Montori and Marco Ceresoli
General, Emergency and Trauma Surgery dept., Papa Giovanni XXIII Hospital Piazza OMS, 24127 Bergamo, Italy

Fausto Catena
Emergency and Trauma Surgery, Parma Maggiore hospital, Parma, Italy

Ernest E. Moore
Denver Health, Denver, CO 80204, USA.

Rao Ivatury
Trauma Surgery, Virginia Commonwealth University, Richmond, VA 23284 USA

Vladimir Khokha
General Surgery, Mozir Hospital, Mozir City, Belarus

Manu Malbrain
ICU and High Care Burn Unit, Ziekenhius Netwerk Antwerpen, Antwerpen, Belgium

Vanni Agnoletti
ICU Department, Bufalini Hospital, Cesena, Italy

Ignacio Martin-Loeches
Critical Care Centre, Corporasiò Sanitaria Park Tauli, Sabdel, Spain

Tino M. Valetti
ICU Department, Papa Giovanni XXIII Hospital, Bergamo, Italy

Thomas Scalea
Trauma Surgery department, University of Maryland School of Medicine, Baltimore, MD 21201, USA

Osvaldo Chiara
Emergency and Trauma Surgery department, Niguarda Hospital, Milan, Italy

Jeffry L. Kashuk
General Surgery department, Assuta Medical Centers, Tel Aviv, Israel

Camila Menezes Souza Pessoa, Flavia Nunes Dias Campos
Intensive Care Unit, Hospital Israelita Albert Einstein, São Paulo, Brazil

Leonardo Lima Rocha and Milton Steinman
Telemedicine Service, Hospital Israelita Albert Einstein, Av. Albert Einstein, 2 andar, bloco D, São Paulo CEP: 05651-901, Brazil

Felipe Martin Bianco Rossi, Carlos Eduardo Fonseca Pires and Milton Steinman
Surgery Department, Hospital Israelita Albert Einstein, São Paulo, Brazil

Massimo Sartelli
Department of Surgery, Macerata Hospital, Macerata, Italy

Fikri M. Abu-Zidan
Department of Surgery, College of Medicine and Health Sciences, UAE University, Al-Ain, United Arab Emirates

Fausto Catena
Department of Emergency Surgery, Maggiore Hospital, Parma, Italy

Ewen A. Griffiths
General and Upper GI Surgery, Queen Elizabeth Hospital, Birmingham, UK

Martin Hutan
82nd Surgical Department of Medical Faculty Comenius University, University Hospital Bratislava, Bratislava, Slovakia

Orestis Ioannidis
2nd Surgical Department, General Hospital of Kavala, Kavala, Greece

Arda Isik
Department of Surgery, Mengucek Gazi Training Research Hospital, Erzincan, Turkey

Yoshimitsu Izawa
Department of Emergency and Critical Care Medicine, Jichi Medical University, Shimotsuke, Japan

Tonguç Utku Yilmaz
Department of Surgery, Kocaeli University Training and Research Hospital, Kocaeli, Turkey

Kuo-Ching Yuan
Trauma and Emergency Surgery Department, Chang Gung Memorial Hospital, Taoyuan City, Taiwan

Sanoop Koshy Zachariah
Department of Surgery, MOSC Medical College Kolenchery, Cochin, India

Maurice Zida
General and Digestive Surgery Department, Teaching Hospital Yalgado Ouedraogo, Ouagadougou, Burkina Faso

Roberto Cirocchi
Department of General Surgery, University of Perugia, Terni Hospital, Terni, Italy

Sorena Afshar
Department of General Surgery, Cumberland Infirmary, Carlisle, UK

Salomone Di Saverio and Gregorio Tugnoli
General (Colorectal) Emergency and Trauma Surgery Service, Maggiore Hospital Regional Emergency Surgery and Trauma Center - Bologna Local Health District, Bologna, Italy

Georgi Popivanov
Military Medical Academy, Sofia, Bulgaria

Angelo De Sol
Department of Surgery, Terni Hospital, Terni, Italy

Francesca Gubbiotti
Department of Surgery, University of Ferrara, Ferrara, Italy

Massimo Sartelli
Department of Surgery, Macerata Hospital, Macerata, Italy

Fausto Catena
Department of Emergency Surgery, Parma Hospital, Parma, Italy

David Cavaliere
Department of Surgery, Forlì Hospital, Forlì, Italy

Renata Taboła
Department of Gastrointestinal and General Surgery, Medical University of Wrocław, Wrocław, Poland

Abe Fingerhut
Section for Surgical Research, Department of Surgery, Medical University of Graz, Graz, Austria First Department of Surgery, Hippokration University Hospital, University of Athens, Athens, Greece

Gian Andrea Binda
Department of Surgery, E.O. OspedaliGalliera, Genova, Italy

Federico Coccolini, Marco Ceresoli, Roberto Manfredi, Giulia and Luca Ansaloni
General Surgery Department, Papa Giovanni XXIII Hospital, Piazza OMS 1, 24127 Bergamo, Italy

Walter Biffl
Denver Health Medical Center, Denver, CO, USA

Fausto Catena
General surgery Department, Ospedale Maggiore, Parma, Italy

Osvaldo Chiara and Stefania Cimbanassi
Niguarda Trauma Center, Ospedale Niguarda Ca'Granda, Milan, Italy

Luca Fattori and Giovanni Pesenti
Unità Operativa di Chirurgia d'Urgenza, Azienda Ospedaliera "San Gerardo", Monza, Italy

Ari Leppaniemi
Department of Abdominal Surgery, University of Helsinki, Helsinki, Finland

Montori Michael Sugrue
Letterkenny Hospital and the Donegal Clinical Research Academy, Donegal, Ireland. 8University College Hospital, Galway, Ireland

Samuel Ho Ting Poon, Jennifer Wah Yan Lee, Ka Man NG, Gloria Wing Yan Chiu and Brian Yung Kong Wong
The Li Ka Shing Faculty of Medicine, The University of Hong Kong, Hong Kong, China

Chi Chung Foo and Wai Lun Law
Department of Surgery, The University of Hong Kong, Queen Mary Hospital, 102 Pokfulam Road, Hong Kong, China

Fikri M. Abu-Zidan
Department of Surgery, College of Medicine and Health Sciences, UAE University, Al-Ain, United Arab Emirates

Alyssa McComb and Margaret L. McNeely
Faculty of Rehabilitation Medicine, University of Alberta, 1-38 Corbett Hall, 8205-114 St NW Edmonton, Edmonton, Alberta T6G 2G4, Canada

Lindsey M. Warkentin and Rachel G. Khadaroo
Department of Surgery, University of Alberta, Edmonton, Alberta, Canada

Rachel G. Khadaroo
Department of Critical Care Medicine, University of Alberta, Edmonton, Alberta, Canada

Andreas Hecker, M. Reichert and W. Padberg
Department of General and Thoracic Surgery, University Hospital Giessen, Rudolf-Buchheim-Street 7, 35392 Giessen, Germany

E. Schneck, R. Röhrig, B. Hecker, J. Holler, C. Koch, C. Lichtenstern and M. A. Weigand
Department of Anesthesiology, Surgical Intensive Care Medicine and Pain Therapy, University Hospital Giessen, Rudolf-Buchheim-Street 7, 35392 Giessen, Germany

G. A. Krombach and F. Roller
Department of Radiology, University Hospital Giessen, Rudolf-Buchheim-Street 7, 35392 Giessen, Germany

M. Hecker
Department of Internal Medicine, University Hospital Giessen, Rudolf-Buchheim-Street 7, 35392 Giessen, Germany

Kumiko Kitaoka, Kazuhiro Saito and Koichi Tokuuye
Department of Radiology Tokyo Medical University Hospital, 6-7-1 Nishishinjuku, Shinjuku-ku, Tokyo 160-0023, Japan

Enis Dikicier and Fatih Altintoprak
Department of General Surgery, Istinye University Faculty of Medicine, Istanbul, Turkey

Kayhan Ozdemir, Kemal Gundogdu, Mustafa Yener Uzunoglu, Guner Cakmak, Feyyaz Onuray and Recai Capoglu
Department of General Surgery, Sakarya University Research and Educational Hospital, Sakarya, Turkey

Index